MICROBIOLOGICALLY SAFE FOODS

MICROBIOLOGICALLY SAFE FOODS

NORMA HEREDIA
Facultad de Ciencias Biológicas
Universidad Autónoma de Nuevo León
Monterrey, N. L. México

IRENE WESLEY
National Animal Diseases Center
U.S. Department of Agriculture
Ames, Iowa

SANTOS GARCÍA
Facultad de Ciencias Biológicas
Universidad Autónoma de Nuevo León
Monterrey, N. L. México

WILEY
A JOHN WILEY & SONS, INC., PUBLICATION

Published by John Wiley & Sons, Inc., Hoboken, New Jersey.
Published simultaneously in Canada.

Library of Congress Cataloging-in-Publication Data:

Microbiologically safe foods / edited by Norma Heredia, Irene Wesley, and Santos García.
p. ; cm.
Includes bibliographical references and index.
ISBN 978-0-470-05333-1 (cloth)
1. Food–Preservation. 2. Food–Microbiology. 3. Food–Safety measures. I. Heredia, Norma. II. Wesley, Irene. III. García, Santos, 1961–
[DNLM: 1. Food Handling–standards. 2. Food Contamination–prevention & control. 3. Food Microbiology–standards. 4. Food, Genetically Modified. 5. Safety. WA 695 M626 2009]
TP371.2M53 2009
664′.028–dc22

2008045639

Printed in the United States of America

10 9 8 7 6 5 4 3 2 1

To our families

CONTENTS

CONTRIBUTORS

JUDD AIKEN, Center for Prions and Protein Folding Diseases, 204 Environmental Engineering Bldg., University of Alberta, Edmonton, Alberta T6G 2M8, Canada

ROBIN C. ANDERSON, U.S. Department of Agriculture, Agricultural Research Service, Southern Plains Agricultural Research Center, College Station, TX 77845

FELIPE ASCENCIO-VALLE, Centro de Investigaciones Biológicas del Noroeste, S.C. La Paz, BCS 23090 México

PETER K. BEN EMBAREK, Department of Food Safety, Zoonoses and Foodborne Diseases, World Health Organization, 20 Avenue Appia, CH-1211 Geneva 27, Switzerland

DEANN L. BENESH, 3M Company, 3M Center, St. Paul, MN 55144-1000

LARRY R. BEUCHAT, Center for Food Safety, Department of Food Science and Technology, University of Georgia, 1109 Experiment Street, Melton Building, Griffin, GA 30223-1797

ANDREIA BIANCHINI, Department of Food Science and Technology, University of Nebraska – Lincoln, Lincoln, NE 68583-0919

GLEYN E. BLEDSOE, Food Science and Human Nutrition, Washington State University, P.O. Box 646376, Pullman, WA 99164-6376

ROBERT L. BUCHANAN, FDA/CFSAN HFS-006, 5100 Paint Branch Parkway, College Park, MD 20740-3835

MARTIN W. BUCKNAVAGE, Department of Food Science, Penn State University, 438 Food Science Building, University Park, PA 16802

Lloyd B. Bullerman, Department of Food Science and Technology, University of Nebraska – Lincoln, Lincoln, NE 68583-0919

Genisis Iris Dancer, Research Development and Engineering, Ecolabs, 8300 Capital Dr., Greensboro, NC 27409

Jean-Yves D'Aoust, Division de la Recherche en Microbiologie, Centre de Recherches Sir F.G. Banting, Tunney' Pasture Santé Canada, Repre Postal: 22 04 A2, Ottawa, Ontario K1A 0L2, Canada

James S. Dickson, Iowa State University, 215F Meat Laboratory, Ames, IA 50011-3150

Peter Feng, U.S. Food and Drug Administration, DMS, HFS-516, 5100 Paint Branch Parkway, College Park, MD 20740-3835

Lucio Galaviz-Silva, Facultad de Ciencias Biológicas, UANL, Laboratorio de Parasitología, Ciudad Universitaria, San Nicolás, N.L. 66451 México

Santos Garcia, Facultad de Ciencias Biológicas, UANL, Apartado Postal 124-F, Ciudad Universitaria, San Nicolás, N.L. 66451 México

Gracia Gómez-Anduro, Centro de Investigaciones Biológicas del Noroeste, S.C., La Paz, BCS 23090 México

Mansel W. Griffiths, Canadian Research Institute for Food Safety, University of Guelph, 43 McGilvray Street, Guelph, Ontario N1G 2W1, Canada

Fidel Guevara-Lara, Centro de Ciencias Básicas, Universidad Autónoma de Aguascalientes, Boulevard Universidad 940, Aguascalientes, Ags. 20100 México

Jung (John) H. Han, Department of Food Science, Faculty of Agricultural and Food Sciences, 238 Ellis Building, University of Manitoba, Winnipeg, Manitoba R3T 2N2, Canada

Norma Heredia, Facultad de Ciencias Biológicas, UANL, Apartado Postal 124-F, Ciudad Universitaria, San Nicolás, N.L. 66451 México

Shane M. Horrocks, U.S. Department of Agriculture, Agricultural Research Service, Southern Plains Agricultural Research Center, Food and Feed Safety Research Unit, College Station, TX 77845

Keith A. Ito, Laboratory for Research in Food Preservation, University of California, 6665 Amador Plaza Road, Suite 207, Dublin, CA 94568

Lee-Ann Jaykus, 339-A Schaub Hall, Department of Food, Bioprocessing and Nutrition Sciences, North Carolina State University, Raleigh, NC 27695

Michael G. Johnson, Center for Food Safety–IFSE, Department of Food Science, University of Arkansas, Fayetteville, AR 72704

Dong-Hyun Kang, Department of Food Science and Human Nutrition, Washington State University, P.O. Box 646376, Pullman, WA 99164-6376

KEVIN KEENER, Department of Food Science, Purdue University, 745 Agriculture Mall Drive, West Lafayette, IN 47907-2009

TATIANA KOUTCHMA, Food Process Engineering, Agriculture and Agri-Food Canada/Agriculture et Agroalimentaire Canada, 93 Stone Road West, Guelph, Ontario NIG 5C9, Canada

RONALD G. LABBÉ, Food Science Department, University of Massachusetts, Amherst, MA 01003

JUAN S. LEÓN, Hubert Department of Global Health, Rollins School of Public Health, Emory University, 1518 Clifton Road, NE 7th Floor, Atlanta, GA 30322

BWALYA LUNGU, Center for Food Safety–IFSE, Department of Food Science, University of Arkansas, Fayetteville, AR 72704

DEBBIE MCKENZIE, Center for Prions and Protein Folding Diseases, 204 Environmental Engineering Bldg., University of Alberta, Edmonton, Alberta T6G 2M8, Canada

MARIANNE D. MILIOTIS, FDA/CFSAN HFS-006, 5100 Paint Branch Parkway, College Park, MD 20740-3835

GAY Y. MILLER, College of Veterinary Medicine, University of Illinois at Urbana–Champaign, 2001 South Lincoln, Room 2635, Urbana, IL 61802

CHRISTINE L. MOE, Hubert Department of Global Health, Emory University, 1518 Clifton Road, NE 7th floor, Atlanta, GA 30322

ZINNIA J. MOLINA-GARZA, Facultad de Ciencias Biológicas, UANL, Laboratorio de Parasitología. Ciudad Universitaria, San Nicolás, N.L. 66451 México

CATHERINE NETTLES CUTTER, Department of Food Science, Pennsylvania State University, 202 Food Science Building, University Park, PA 16802

DAVID J. NISBET, U.S. Department of Agriculture, Agricultural Research Service, Southern Plains Agricultural Research Center, Food and Feed Safety Research Unit, College Station, TX 77845

LINDA L. NOLAN, Food Science Department, University of Massachusetts, Amherst, MA 01003

CHRISTY OLIVER, Department of Animal and Range Sciences, North Dakota State University, Fargo, ND 58105

OLGA I. PADILLA-ZAKOUR, Department of Food Science and Technology, New York State Agricultural Experiment Station, 630 West North Street, Geneva, NY 14456

MICKEY E. PARISH, Nutrition and Food Science, 0112 Skinner Building, University of Maryland, College Park, MD 20742-7521

NINA G. PARKINSON, 684 Willow Creek Terrace, Brentwood, CA 94513

BARBARA A. RASCO, Food Science and Human Nutrition, Washington State University, P.O. Box 646376, Pullman, WA 99164-6376

STEVEN C. RICKE, Center for Food Safety–IFSE, Department of Food Science, University of Arkansas, Fayetteville, AR 72704

EDUARDO SÁNCHEZ-GARCIA, Facultad de Ciencias Biológicas, UANL, Apartado Postal 124-F, Ciudad Universitaria, San Nicolás, N.L. 66451 México

JAMES MARK SIMMERMAN, Influenza Surveillance and Control, World Health Organization, 63 Tran Hung Dao Street, Hoan Kiem District, Ha Noi, Viet Nam

JOHN N. SOFOS, Center for Meat Safety and Quality, Food Safety Cluster of Infectious Diseases Supercluster, Department of Animal Sciences, Colorado State University, 1171 Campus Delivery, Fort Collins, CO 80523-1171

LUISA Y. SOLÍS-SOTO, Facultad de Ciencias Biológicas, UANL, Apartado Postal 124-F, Ciudad Universitaria, San Nicolás, N.L. 66451 México

MARK L. TAMPLIN, Australian Food Safety Centre of Excellence, Sandy Bay, Tasmania 7005, Australia

IRENE V. WESLEY, National Animal Diseases Center, USDA, 2300 Dayton Road, Ames, IA 50010

FOREWORD

Food safety has become a worldwide concern that affects international trade and relations due to its impact on human health and economics, especially in recent years when the number and complexity of food safety issues has increased substantially. This is evidenced by the large number of new, emerging, reemerging, or evolving pathogenic microorganisms (e.g., *Escherichia coli* O157:H7 and other Shiga toxin–producing *E. coli* serotypes, *Salmonella* serotypes Enteritidis and Typhimurium DT 104, *Campylobacter jejuni/coli*, *Yersinia enterocolitica*, *Listeria monocytogenes*, and *Enterobacter sakazakii*, parasitic agents such a *Cryptosporidium* and *Cyclospora*, Noroviruses) which have become food safety concerns after the 1970s, 1980s, and even 1990s. Another alarming development is the increasing number of types of foods being involved in outbreaks, including products not usually associated with confirmed foodborne illness episodes in the past (e.g., fruit juices, lettuce, spinach, other produce, mayonnaise, various berries, sautéed onions, clam chowder, ice cream). Simultaneously, controlling bacterial pathogens, which are the most important food safety concern relative to number of deaths and economic losses, has become more complicated as accumulating evidence indicates development of resistance to antibiotics and potential adaptation and cross-resistance or cross-protection to traditional food preservation barriers, such as acidity, thermal processing, cold temperature storage, dry or low-water-activity environments, and chemical additives. In addition, evidence indicates the existence of pathogenic strains with enhanced ability for survival in their hosts, lower infectious doses, and increased virulence.

Modern food safety issues and concerns appear to multiply and become more significant when considered in association with societal changes and our transformation as consumers. Our societies have become more urbanized, populations continue to increase dramatically, human life expectancy increases, and as lifestyles are changing, consumer food preferences and expectations related to food characteristics are different than they were just a few decades ago. As aging populations increase, they include more immunosuppressed and chronically ill persons who are more sensitive to foodborne illnesses and their consequences. Modern advances in medical treatments improve human survival rates from various illnesses but are also associated with increasing numbers of people with reduced immunity to infection. As a consequence, it is logical that food safety risks become even greater and more acute for consumers who are more sensitive to microbial infection. Thus, ongoing microbial evolution, coupled with societal changes including consumer food preferences, lack of adequate food-handling education, increases in at-risk human populations, complex food distribution patterns, increased international trade, and better methods of testing for microbial detection, bring microbial food safety to the forefront of our societal concerns. These developments have certainly increased interest in food safety among scientists, regulatory officials, industry, and public health agencies at the national and international level, especially as they become of more interest to news-reporting media and public-interest groups. This increased publicity leads to public awareness, concern, and more interest in food safety issues worldwide. The result is increased pressure on the private and public sectors to accelerate efforts that may lead to enhanced microbial food safety.

Initiatives undertaken by regulatory and public health agencies, industry, and research organizations in recent years have targeted microbial food safety as a worldwide public health issue. Important developments include establishment of new regulations, based on the concept and principles of hazard analysis of critical control points (HACCP) for the inspection of meat, poultry, seafood, and fruit juice–processing operations in the United States, as well as similar efforts undertaken by countries in various parts of the world. Furthermore, efforts are undertaken to improve international collaboration, coordination, and harmonization of food safety assurance programs. Parallel efforts and accomplishments include scientific research and development for better control of pathogens in order to reduce risks. The knowledge base generated by research is necessary for regulatory decision making, development of industry approaches for solutions to food safety problems, worker training, and public education in food safety. These scientific efforts have contributed not only significant new knowledge in pathogen ecology, detection, and control, but have also generated new approaches for development of novel control strategies based on microbial predictive modeling and risk assessments. These new avenues of thinking and addressing food safety issues should facilitate adoption of evolving concepts such as food safety objectives and associated process and product criteria needed for assurance of desired levels of food protection.

In light of these concerns and related developments, a book providing comprehensive coverage to all microbial food safety issues is very timely and needed. *Microbiologically Safe Foods* is a comprehensive book of worldwide interest written by an impressive group of international experts. It addresses all aspects of microbial food safety that are of interest to scientists, regulators, public health officials, and industry worldwide. The strength of this book is its comprehensive nature and the excellent expertise of the authors. It is a book that I have always considered as needed because it deals with all aspects of microbial food safety: bacterial, fungal, parasitic, and viral, including various emerging concerns. It is comprehensive because it covers all known foodborne pathogens, including those that usually receive little or no coverage in most available books on food microbiology because they may not be of major concern in certain developed countries. The other unique feature that makes this book extremely valuable is that in addition to covering a long list of pathogens and other modern food safety issues, it includes specific chapters on food safety problems associated with all types of food commodities or groups of food products. Additional topics of current interest covered by the book include microbiological risk assessment, various programs for pathogen control, HACCP, novel pathogen control technologies, traditional and modern microbial detection approaches, laboratory accreditation, bioterrorism, genetically modified organisms, and predictive microbiology. Overall, this book should be extremely valuable to all those interested in food safety, as a single comprehensive source covering modern microbial food safety concerns of international interest.

Colorado State University
Fort Collins, Colorado

JOHN N. SOFOS

PREFACE

The seed for this book was planted, germinated, and nurtured in Monterrey, Mexico, during the International Conference of Food Safety hosted in this city. The goal was to compile a "mini" encyclopedia of microbial food safety to span the proverbial farm-to-fork continuum. With the advent of NAFTA and the global commerce of food, it was only natural that the book would acquire an international flavor. This publication surveys foodborne pathogens and food safety issues, including those that usually receive little or no coverage in most books because they may be of local concern. However, with the global exchange of commodities, these are now of interest worldwide.

The book addresses the contamination of foods in the production chain and presents approaches and state-of-the-art technologies to harvest microbiologically safe foods for our global dinner table. Each chapter summarizes and updates scientific advances of importance to professionals involved in all aspects of food science, especially pre- and post-harvest food safety, processing, quality control, and regulatory matters.

Production processes of a variety of foods, including dairy, eggs, beef, and poultry, and the recognition of fruits and vegetables as major vehicles of the transmission of human foodborne diseases are surveyed. The growing market in processed foods, as well as interventions, including innovative food packaging and high technologies to inhibit spoilage organisms and prolong shelf life, is addressed. Recent foodborne outbreaks and recalls involving a particular product and incriminated microbial hazards are summarized.

Other current issues that broaden readership are the role of genetically modified organisms in food safety, predictive microbiology, emerging foodborne pathogens, and good manufacturing practices. The emergence of bioterrorism is tracked. Novel approaches to pre-harvest food safety, such as the potential of competitive exclusion cultures in livestock and poultry, are examined. The impact of HACCP strategies on enhancing the microbial quality of foods is chronicled. The critical issue of microbiological laboratory accreditation to assure compliance with performance standards is described. The applications of molecular biology, encompassing rapid methods to detect, characterize, and enumerate pathogens, abound throughout.

Authors were selected on the basis of their scientific stature, their presentations at international conferences, and the recommendations of commodity groups. Some were active participants in the Monterrey conferences, shared our dream of compiling this book, and urged us on to publication. The coeditors added, revised topics, and updated chapters in response to the prevailing trends in the food safety community. Hence, we included a chapter on avian influenza because of its potential implications for food safety. It was during the final editing of the 31 chapters that we realized the enormity (and significance!) of the undertaking.

Although the task of selecting topics and authors was daunting, we are indebted to the participants of the international conferences held in Mexico, whose interest was a catalyst in the final selection of authors and chapter topics. We thank Wiley for their encouragement along the way and for realizing the publication of this book.

We encourage the reader to suggest topics and offer improvements for future editions of this international collaboration.

Monterrey, Mexico NORMA HEREDIA
Ames, Iowa IRENE WESLEY
SANTOS GARCÍA

PART I

MICROBIAL FOOD HAZARDS

CHAPTER 1

PUBLIC HEALTH IMPACT OF FOODBORNE ILLNESS: IMPETUS FOR THE INTERNATIONAL FOOD SAFETY EFFORT

IRENE V. WESLEY

1.1 INTRODUCTION

Microbial food safety has emerged as a global concern because of its effect on consumer health and the financial losses in the food industry due to product recalls and trade barriers. In the United States the economic impact of foodborne illness, although secondary to the loss of lives, is driven by medical care, legal fees, public health investigation, lost wages, loss of market share, and loss of consumer confidence and is estimated at \$20 to \$43 billion each year (USDHHS, continuously updated). In this chapter we survey the impact of foodborne pathogens—viral, bacterial, fungal, and protozoan—at the global dinner table and provide a brief overview of foodborne morbidity and mortality with examples based primarily on data for the United States. This will set the table for more in-depth descriptions in the following chapters of the epidemiology, food safety issues in specific commodities, methods for detection, prevention and control strategies, risk assessments, and global impact of each pathogen on the food supply.

1.2 STATISTICAL ESTIMATES

The World Health Organization (WHO) estimates that in 2005, 1.8 million people died from diarrheal disease, with a significant proportion of these cases following the consumption of contaminated food and drinking water (WHO, continuously updated-a). In the United States up to 30% of the population experiences foodborne illnesses,

Microbiologically Safe Foods, Edited by Norma Heredia, Irene Wesley, and Santos García

TABLE 1 Estimated Public Health Impact of Foodborne Illnesses in the United States and the Proportion for Which an Etiology Is Known

	Cases	Hospitalizations	Deaths
Etiology unknown	62 million	265,000	3,200
Etiology known	14 million	60,000	1,800
Total	76 million	325,000	5,000

Source: Mead et al. (1999).

as evidenced by the 76 million cases, 325,000 hospitalizations, and 5000 deaths estimated annually (Table 1).

Nearly 81.6%—62 million cases, 265,000 hospitalizations, and 3200 deaths—have no known cause (Table 1). For the approximately 18% of foodborne illnesses for which an etiology is known (Table 2) viruses such as norovirus, rotavirus, and hepatitis virus cause the overwhelming majority (79.3%) of human morbidity followed by bacteria (13.5%) and protozoans (6.6%) (Mead et al., 1999).

Foodborne illnesses occur as single sporadic cases or as outbreaks involving two or more persons who consumed the same product in the same time interval. Based on data from the Centers for Disease Control and Prevention (CDC), the vehicles of transmission causing 67% of U.S. outbreaks remain unknown. Of the remaining 33% of outbreaks for which an etiology was identified, fruits, vegetables, and salads, including ready-to-eat packaged products (22%), shellfish (22%), and poultry (5%) rank as the top three vehicles of transmission (CDC, continuously updated).

Recently published attribution data and per capita consumption provide insight into the relative importance of specific commodities as vehicles of foodborne pathogens (Table 3). As illustrated in the following chapters, multiple pathogens contaminate a variety of food types. Thus, *Listeria monocytogenes*, which has been described in major epidemics involving dairy products, is associated with cases incriminating contaminated ready-to-eat delicatessen items, seafood, and produce.

TABLE 2 Estimated Morbidity and Mortality of Foodborne Illnesses in the United States

	Cases	Deaths
Norwalk-like viruses	9,200,000	124
Campylobacter	1,963,141	91
Salmonella	1,342,532	556
Toxoplama gondii	112,500	375
Yersinia	86,731	2
E. coli O1578:H7	62,458	52
E. coli STEC	31,229	26
Listeria monocytogenes	2,493	449

Source: Mead et al. (1999).

TABLE 3 Mean Number of Cases of Foodborne Illness Attributed to Specific Foods and Estimated per Capita Consumption

	Total Cases	Percent	Per Capita Consumption[a] (lb)
Produce	3,800,929	29.4	688.6
Seafood	3,200,976	24.8	16.1
Poultry	2,036,156	15.8	73.5
Luncheon meats	921,538	7.1	NA
Breads, bakery items	543,714	4.2	192.3
Dairy	535,566	4.1	38.0
Eggs	446,964	3.5	253.9
Beverages (nondairy)	444,020	3.4	142 gal
Beef	437,051	3.4	62.4
Pork	402,217	3.1	46.4
Game	140,473	1.1	NA

Source: Hoffman et al. (2007), USDA-ERS (2007a).
[a]NA, per capita consumption not available from USDA Economic Research Service.

TABLE 4 U.S. Public Health Service Targeted Reductions in Major Foodborne Pathogens (Cases per 100,000 U.S. Population)

	1987	2000	2010
Campylobacter jejuni	50	25	12.3
Salmonella spp.	18	16	6.8
E. coli O157:H7	8	4	1.0
Listeria monocytogenes	0.7	0.5	0.25

Source: USDHHS (continuously updated).

To improve the overall health of the nation, the U.S. Department of Health and Human Services has set national goals for reducing human illness attributed to each of the major bacterial foodborne pathogens (Table 4). Targeted reductions use the 1987 baseline data for comparison and to project the goals to be achieved in Healthy People 2010 and in Healthy People 2020.

1.3 IMPACT OF REPRESENTATIVE FOODBORNE PATHOGENS

1.3.1 *Campylobacter jejuni*

Campylobacter jejuni is the leading cause of human bacterial foodborne illness worldwide. In 2004, the 25 member states of the European Union (EU) reported 183,961 cases of campylobacteriosis. The overall incidence of 47.6 cases/100,000 population represented a 31% increase from 2003. A trend toward increasing incidence was observed in the 13 of the original 15 member states, with only Spain and Sweden reporting a decline. In the EU, 20 to 50% of all clinical isolates were resistant to fluoroquinolones, tetracyclines, and penicillin. Thus, the use of fluoroquinolones in food animals was banned to prevent the emergence of fluoroquinolone resistance (El Amin, 2006).

In the United States the nearly 2 million human campylobacteriosis cases account for an estimated $1.2 billion in productivity losses annually. Based on attribution data, contaminated poultry (72%), dairy products (7.8%), and red meats, including beef (4.3%) and pork (4.4%), are vehicles of transmission and acknowledged risk factors (Hoffman et al., 2007; Miller and Mandrell, 2005). In the Netherlands, Campylobacter Risk Management and Assessment (CARMA) is a multidisciplinary project to integrate information from risk assessments, epidemiology, and economics. CARMA estimates the cost of campylobacateriosis at 21 million euros annually, with an estimated 20 to 40% of cases attributed to contaminated poultry (Havelaar et al., 2007). The importance of pork in the transmission of *Campylobacter* (as well as of *Salmonella* and *Yersinia*) has been reviewed (Fosse et al., 2008). Other factors, such as water, contact with pets, and worldwide travel, loom as significant.

Campylobacteriosis has been linked with the onset of Guillain–Barré syndrome (GBS) (Buzby et al., 1997). Of an estimated 2628 to 9575 patients diagnosed with GBS in the United States, 526 to 3830 (20 to 40%) are triggered by *Campylobacter* infection in the 1 to 2 weeks prior to the onset of neurological symptoms (Rees et al., 1995). No single factor appears to cause a greater proportion of GBS cases than recent *Campylobacter* infections.

The availability of the total genome map (1.5×10^6 base pairs, ca. 1.5 megabases, Mb) of *C. jejuni* (Parkhill et al., 2000) and other food-associated *Campylobacter* species has expedited molecular-based methods for their detection, epidemiology, and pathogenesis. The impact of modern agricultural production practices on the convergence of *C. jejuni* and *C. coli* into a single species has been described (Sheppard et al., 2008). *Arcobacter butzleri*, a close relative of *Campylobacter*, is an emerging foodborne pathogens whose genetic makeup encodes traits to (2.34 Mb) ensure survival in a potentially hostile environment (Miller et al., 2007) such as a packing plant.

1.3.2 Nontyphoidal *Salmonella*

There are about 2500 serotypes of *Salmonella enterica*. Of these, a small fraction account for the majority of 1,343,000 cases of foodborne illness resulting in about 15,000 hospitalizations and 500 deaths annually in the United States (Mead et al., 1999). CDC has targeted reduction of human salmonellosis from 18 cases per 100,000 population in 1987 to 6.8 cases per 100,000 by the year 2010 (Table 4). In the EU, 192,703 cases of salmonellosis were reported during 2004. The 2004 incidence (42.4 cases/100,000 population) is an increase over 2003 prior to the admission of 10 new member states. Eggs, poultry, and pork are major sources of contamination; surveys show high *Salmonella* contamination in herbs and spices. The implementation of control programs in the original member states has resulted in a decline in salmonellosis (El Amin, 2006).

In the United States, human salmonellosis follows consumption of contaminated poultry (35%), eggs (22%), and produce (12%), as well as beef (23.2%) and pork (5.7%), (Hoffman et al., 2007). The U.S. Department of Agriculture (USDA) Economic Research Service (ERS) estimates the annual losses in illness and productivity at $2.9 billion (USDA-ERS, 2007b).

Hazard analysis of critical control points (HACCP) was initiated in 1996 in USDA-inspected processing plants. In 1998, 10.65% of the overall number of regulatory samples analyzed by the USDA Food Safety and Inspection Service (FSIS) yielded *Salmonella*, compared with 4.29% in 2002 (Rose et al., 2002). The decline in human morbidity during this interval coincided with the reduction of *Salmonella* isolated from meat and poultry and may be attributed to the HACCP plans implemented by the industry (Eblen et al., 2005; USDA-FSIS, 1999). Because reduction of human salmonellosis is lagging behind that of other bacterial foodborne infections, in 2007 the USDA-FSIS further accelerated the targeted reduction of human salmonellosis by 50%.

The availability of the full *Salmonella* genome (4.8 Mb) will yield robust techniques for elucidating its pathogenesis and molecular epidemiology. Advances in rapid detection, serotyping, and virulence characterization will contribute significantly to comprehensive risk assessments and to evaluating the effectiveness of HACCP interventions both on-farm and during processing.

1.3.3 *E. coli* O157:H7

Human infections have been attributed to beef (67%) as well as to fruit juices, sprouts, lettuce, and spinach (18.4%) (Hoffman et al., 2007). Hemolytic uremic syndrome (HUS), a rare sequela of *E. coli* O157:H7 infection, is now listed as a separate entity targeted for reduction in the Healthy People 2010 document. For the year 2000, USDA-ERS calculated the costs of *E. coli* O157:H7 ($659 million) and non-O157:H7 ($329.7 million) (USDA-ERS, 2007b). The genome of enterohemorrhagic *E. coli* is estimated at 5 Mb. The significance of pathogenic *E. coli* is detailed in subsequent chapters.

1.3.4 *Listeria monocytogenes*

Listeria monocytogenes accounts for about 2500 cases, 2289 hospitalizations, and 449 deaths each year in the United States. The mortality rate of *L. monocytogenes* (ca. 28%) remains the highest of all foodborne pathogens (Table 2). The USDA-ERS estimates the cost of acute illness at $2.3 billion annually (USDA-ERS, 2007b). In the EU, 12,678 cases of listeriosis were reported in 2004, an incidence rate of 0.3 case/100,000 population. In countries with several years of data, the incidence of listeriosis increased compared with the preceding five years. In the EU, significant contamination (100 *L. monocytogenes*/gram) was reported in fishery products, meats, cheeses, and ready-to-eat products, thus banning their import into the United States, which maintains a "zero tolerance" policy (El Amin, 2006).

Major human listeriosis epidemics have been linked to consumption of dairy products (Painter and Slutsker, 2007). Product recalls, sporadic cases, and outbreaks have incriminated ready-to-eat delicatessen items. Recent data attribute human listeriosis to consumption of contaminated delicatessen meats (54%), dairy products, including cheeses (24%), and produce (8.7%) (Hoffman et al., 2007). In France, listeriosis outbreaks have been traced to pickled pork tongue and involved 279 human cases (33% pregnancy-related) (Jacquet et al., 1995).

The full genome of *L. monocytogenes* (2.9 Mb) was published in 2001 by Glaser and colleagues (Glaser et al., 2001). This led to the development of microarray technologies to compare virulence attributes of strains and to single nucleotide polymorphism (SNP) analysis to track listeriosis dissemination. In addition, *prfA* virulence gene cluster sequence analysis assigned *L. monocytogenes* isolates to groups or lineages: clinical (lineage 1) and food-processing environments (lineage 3) (Ward et al., 2004). Earlier, molecular methods established that *Listeria* spp. persist in processing environments, including chilling and cutting rooms, knives, conveyer belts, and floor drains (Giovannacci et al., 1999). By pulsed field gel electrophoresis (PFGE), a multistate outbreak of human listeriosis, ascribed to serotype 4 (101 cases, resulting in 22 deaths), was linked to delicatessen meats prepared in a contaminated processing plant (CDC, 1998).

1.3.5 *Yersinia enterocolitica*

Pigs are the major animal reservoir for strains of *Y. enterocolitica* which are pathogenic to humans (Andersen et al. 1991; Bottone, 1997, 1999; Nielsen and Wegener, 1997). *Y. enterocolitica* is isolated from porcine tongue, tonsils, cecum, rectum, feces, and gut-associated lymphoid tissue, as well as from chitterlings and retail-purchased pork.

Attribution data link human yersiniosis to consumption of pork (71%), dairy products (12.2%), and seafoods (4.7%) (Hoffman et al., 2007). The public health risks associated with *Yersinia* on hog carcasses have been detailed (Fosse et al., 2008). Foodborne outbreaks have involved consumption or handling of contaminated raw or undercooked ground pork, pork tongues, and chitterlings (Bottone, 1999). During 1982, 172 cases of *Y. enterocolitica* serotype O:13a,13b were traced to pasteurized milk possibly contaminated with pig manure during transport (Robins-Browne, 2001). In addition to pork consumption, the risk of human yersiniosis in Auckland increased with contact with untreated water and sewage (Satterthwaite et al., 1999).

In the United States, human yersiniosis (96,368 cases, 1228 hospitalizations) is one of the seven major foodborne diseases under surveillance by CDC. According to FoodNet, the yersiniosis case rate (cases per 100,000 population) varies from 0.5 (California) to 3 (Georgia). The hospitalization rate for yersiniosis (32% of cases) is second only to that of listeriosis (94% of cases) (CDC, 2006). In 2004, the 25

TABLE 5 Percent Change of the Seven Bacterial Pathogens Under FoodNet Surveillance

	Cases/100,000	Percent Change	Confidence (%) Interval
Yersinia	0.36	−49	36–59
Shigella	4.67	−43	18–60
Listeria	0.30	−32	16–45
Campylobacter	12.72	−30	25–35
STEC 0157	1.06	−29	12–42
Salmonella	14.55	−9	2–15
Vibrio	0.27	+41	3–92

Source: CDC (2006).

member states of the EU reported 10,000 cases of human yersiniosis. The genome of *Y. enterocolitica* is estimated at 4.6 Mb by the Sanger Institute.

1.3.6 *Vibrio*

Vibrio cholerae is a major public health problem in developing countries. In addition to water, contaminated rice, vegetables, and seafoods have been implicated in cholera outbreaks (WHO, continuously updated-a). *Vibrio vulnificus* and *V. parahaemolyticus* are discussed in later chapters. In the United States, despite the overall reduction in foodborne pathogens since FoodNet was initiated in 1996, only seafood-related *Vibrio parahaemoliticus* cases have increased: by 41% (Table 5).

1.3.7 Parasites

FoodNet initiated national surveillance of parasitic infections in 1997. *Cyclospora cayetanensis* was first recognized as a foodborne pathogen in raspberries imported from Central America in 1996. Human cases are attributed to contaminated produce (96%), with fewer attributed to beverages (1.5%) (Hoffman et al., 2007). *Cryptosporodium parvum*, linked to municipal water supply outbreaks, has been also been traced to produce (59%) and beverages (9%) (Hoffman et al., 2007).

Toxoplasma gondii, which is transmitted between cats and domestic livestock and wildlife, has been associated with human infections traced to pork (41%), beef (23.2%), and produce (7%). Cats excrete the resistant oocysts in their feces. Infection occurs when pigs or other livestock ingest the oocysts, which invade skeletal muscle or other organs (i.e., brain, heart, liver). Humans become infected when eating contaminated meat or by inhaling or ingesting the oocyst released by the feline host. In the EU, 2000 cases of toxoplasmosis were reported in 2004; 225,000 cases were estimated in the United States (Mead et al., 1999). The genome of *T. gondii* is estimated at 30 Mb.

In 2004 the EU reported between 300 and 400 cases of *Trichinella*; 52 cases were estimated in the United States. In the EU, 300 to 400 cases due to *Echinocococcus* were reported in 2004.

1.4 NATIONAL MICROBIAL BASELINE SURVEYS

In 1996–1998, the USDA Food Safety and Inspection Service conducted nationwide microbial baseline surveys of beef, hogs, poultry, and turkey carcasses and their respective ground meat products (see Chapter 8, Table 1). The data show the highest contamination of poultry carcasses with *Campylobacter* (90%), distribution of *Salmonella* across commodities, and *L. monocytogenes* in ground products, which may reflect contamination of the processing environment.

Baseline prevalence estimates will change for each pathogen as bacteriological methods for their isolation and molecular protocols for their detection improve and HACCP strategies in the plant evolve. Data obtained during these nationwide baseline studies are the basis for performance standards which serve as benchmarks for the industry as they optimize their HACCP strategies. Although the current emphasis is pathogen reduction at the processing level, reducing the on-farm prevalence of potential human pathogens will clearly result in an overall decline in human foodborne illness.

1.5 GLOBAL MARKETPLACE

In 2004, international trade in agricultural products (including food) was estimated at $783 billion, with the EU ($374 billion) being the largest importer. The United States imports 13% of its annual food or food ingredients, an estimated 260 lb of its yearly per capita diet, valued at $70 billion, principally from the EU, Canada, and Mexico. Approximately 1% of foods imported into the United States are inspected or tested by the U.S. Food and Drug Administration (FDA). Because of the emergence of China as an exporter of agricultural products, the FDA now has personnel assigned to Beijing.

International standards for food hygiene are coordinated through the multinational *Codex Alimentarius* (FAO/WHO, continuously updated). The *Codex* was founded in 1962 by the Food and Agriculture Committee of the United Nations and the World Health Organization. *Codex* committees set standards to protect the health of the global consumer and to ensure fair trade practices. *Codex* provides guidance to governments on methods to be used between laboratories to determine equivalencies, especially for export and import concerns.

To estimate the human burden of foodborne illnesses worldwide, the World Health Organization (WHO) coordinates efforts to compile laboratory, outbreak, and surveillance data from member nations (Flint et al., 2005; WHO, continuously updated-a). WHO Global Sal-Surv (WHO, continuously updated-b) collects prevalence data for *Salmonella*, *Campylobacter*, *Shigella*, bovine spongiform encephalopathy (BSE), and antimicrobial drug resistance profiles. In 2000, Australia launched OzFood Net to more accurately determine the burden of foodborne illness. This effort estimated that 5.4 million cases of foodborne gastroenteritis occur each year in Australia (AGDHA, 2005). Fourteen pathogens (11 bacterial and 3 viral) were monitored during 2000.

Major causes of gastroenteritis were pathogenic *E. coli* (38%), noroviruses (30%), and *Campylobacter* (14%).

FoodNet continuously monitors seven bacterial foodborne pathogens in 10 U.S. states, representing 44.5 million people or 15% of the population (Table 5) (Jones et al., 2007; Scallan et al., 2007). Six of the seven bacterial pathogens have shown reductions since FoodNet was initiated in 1997. Only seafood-related *Vibrio* cases have increased significantly (CDC, 2006).

Molecular-based approaches have accelerated detection and characterization of foodborne pathogens (Hytia-Trees et al., 2007; Withee and Dearfield, 2007). The availability of published full genome sequences available on the World Wide Web for *V. cholerae* (2.9 Mb), *Cryptosporidium* (9.1 Mb), and the protozoan *Giardia lamblia* (11.19 Mb), as well as of potential foodborne pathogens such as *Mycobacterium avium* subspecies paratuberculosis, will identify novel sequences for their rapid identification and hasten assessment of their human public health significance.

In the future, international multilaboratory and mulitnational collaborations utilizing state-of-the-art molecular protocols will yield reliable estimates of the morbidity and mortality associated with foodborne infections. Prevalence data for rigorous risk assessments will ensure the integrity of the global food supply.

When reviewing the following chapters the reader should be mindful that as-yet-unidentified foodborne pathogens may appear in future editions of this book. In addition, the global marketplace is confounded with production issues including limitations for the on-farm use of antimicrobials, transport of pathogens due to world travel, and animal welfare concerns. All of these affect the microbial food safety of the final product in the global market.

REFERENCES

AGDHA (Australian Government Department of Health and Ageing) (2005): Foodborne illness in Australia: annual incidence circa 2000. http://www.ozfoodnet.org.au/internet/ozfoodnet/publishing.nsf/Content/reports-1/$FILE/foodborne_report.pdf. Accessed June 2008.

Andersen JK, Sorensen R, Glensbjerg M (1991): Aspects of the epidemiology of *Yersinia enterocolitica*: a review. *Int J Food Microbiol.* 13:231–237.

Bottone EJ (1997): *Yersinia enterocolitica*: the charisma continues. *Clin Microbiol Rev.* 10:257–276.

——— (1999): *Yersinia enterocolitica*: overview and epidemiologic correlates. *Microb Infect.* 1:323–333.

Buzby JC, Roberts T, Allos BM (1997): *Estimated Annual Costs of* Campylobacter-*Associated Guillain–Barré Syndrome*. Publication 756. USDA-ERS, Washington, DC.

CDC (Centers for Disease Control and Prevention) (1998): Multistate outbreak of listeriosis—United States. *MMWR Morb Mortal Wkly Rep.* 47:1085–1086.

——— (2006): Preliminary FoodNet data on the incidence of infection with pathogens transmitted commonly through food: 10 states, United States, 2005. *MMWR Morb Mortal Wkly Rep.* 55:392–395.

——— (continuously updated): Outbreak surveillance data. http://www.cdc.gov/foodborneoutbreaks/outbreak_data.htm. Accessed May 2008.

Eblen DR, Levine P, Rose BE, Saini P, Mageau R, Hill WE (2005): Nationwide microbiological baseline data collected by sponge sampling during 1997 and 1998 for cattle, swine, turkeys, and geese. *J Food Prot*. 68:1848–1852.

El Amin A (2006): Foodborne *Campylobacter* infections increase. http://www.food-productiondaily.com/news/ng.asp?n=64828-food-safety-zoonoses-campylobacteria. Accessed June 2008.

FAO/WHO (Food and Agriculture Organization/World Health Organization) (continuously updated): *Codex Alimentarius*. http://www.codexalimentarius.net/web/index_en.jsp. Accessed June 2008.

Flint JA, vam Duynhoven YT, Angulo FJ, et al. (2005): Estimating the burden of acute gastroenteritis, foodborne disease, and pathogens commonly transmitted by food: an international review. *Clin Infect Dis*. 41:698–704.

Fosse J, Seegers H, Magras C (2008): Foodborne zoonoses due to meat: a quantitative approach for a comparative risk assessment applied to pig slaughtering in Europe. *Vet Res*. 39, E-pub ahead of print.

Giovannacci I, Ragimbeau C, Quequiner S, et al. (1999): *Listeria monocytogenes* in pork slaughtering and cutting plants: use of RAPD, PFGE and PCR-REA for tracing and molecular epidemiology. *Int J Food Microbiol*. 53:127–140.

Glaser P, Fangeul L, Buchrieser C, et al. (2001): Comparative genomics of *Listeria* species. *Science*. 294:849–852.

Havelaar AH, Mangen MJ, de Koeijer AA, et al. (2007): Effectiveness and efficiency of controlling *Campylobacter* on broiler chicken meat. *Risk Anal*. 27:831–844.

Hoffman S, Fischbeck P, Krupnick A, McWilliam M (2007): Using expert elicitation to link foodborne illnesses in the United States to foods. *J Food Prot*. 70:1220–1229.

Hytia-Trees EK, Cooper K, Ribot EM, Gerner-Smidt P (2007): Recent developments and future prospects in subtyping of foodborne bacterial pathogens. *Future Microbiol*. 2: 175–185.

Jacquet C, Catimel BR, Brosch R, et al. (1995): Investigations related to the epidemic strain involved in the French listeriosis outbreak in 1992. *Appl Environ Microbiol*. 61:2242–2246.

Jones TF, Scallan E, Angulo FJ (2007): FoodNet: overview of a decade of achievement. *Foodborne Pathol Dis*. 4:60–66.

Mead PS, Slutsker L, Dietz V, et al. (1999): Food-related illness and death in the United States. *Emerg Infect Dis*. 5:607–625.

Miller WG, Mandrell RE (2005): Prevalence of *Campylobacter* in the food and water supply: incidence, outbreaks, isolation, and detection. In: Ketley J, Konkel ME (Eds.). Campylobacter: *Molecular and Cellular Biology*. Horizon Bioscience, Norfolk, UK, pp. 101–163.

Miller WG, Parker CT, Rubenfield M, et al. (2007): The complete genome sequence and analysis of the epsilonproteobacterium *Arcobacater butzleri*. *PLoS One*. 26e1358.

Nielsen B, Wegener HC (1997): Public health and pork and pork products: regional perspectives of Denmark. *Rev Sci Tech Off Int Epizoot*. 16; 513–524.

Painter J, Slutsker L (2007): Listeriosis in humans. In: Marth E, Ryser E (Eds.). *Listeria, Listeriosis and Food Safety*, 3rd ed. CRC Press, Boca Raton, FL, pp. 85–109.

Parkhill J, Wren BW, Mungall K, et al. (2000): The genome sequence of the food-borne pathogen *Campylobacter jejuni* reveals hypervariable sequences. *Nature*. 402:665–668.

Rees JH, Soudain SE, Gregson NA, Hughes RAC (1995): *Campylobacter jejuni* infection and Guillain–Barré syndrome. *N Engl J Med.* 333:1374–1379.

Robins-Browne RM (2001): *Yersinia enterocolitica.* In: Doyle MP, Beuchat LR, Montville TJ (Eds.). *Food Microbiology: Fundamentals and Frontiers*, 2nd ed. ASM Press, Washington, DC, pp. 215–245.

Rose BE, Hill WE, Umholtz R, Ransom GM, James WO (2002): Testing for *Salmonella* in raw meat and poultry products collected at federally inspected establishments in the United States, 1998 through 2000. *J Food Prot.* 65:937–947.

Satterthwaite P, Pritchard K, Floyd D, Law B (1999): A case–control study of *Yersinia enterocolitica* infections in Auckland. *Aust NZ J Public Health.* 23:482–485.

Scallan E (2007): Activities, Achievements and lessons learned during the first 10 years of the Foodborne Dieases Active Surveillance Network: 1996–2005. *Clin Infect Dis.* 44:718–725.

Sheppard SK, McCarthy ND, Falush D, Maiden MVC (2008): Convergence of *Campylobacter* species; implications for bacterial evolution. *Science.* 320:237–239.

USDA-ERS (U.S. Department of Agriculture–Economic Research Service) (2007a): Food availability (per capita) data system. http://www.ers.usda.gov/data/foodconsumption. Accessed May 2008.

——— (2007b): Briefing rooms. http://www.ers.usda.gov/briefing/FoodSafety. Accessed May 2008.

USDA-FSIS (U.S. Department of Agriculture–Food Safety and Inspection Service) (1999): HACCP Implementation: first year *Salmonella* test results. http://www.fsis.usda.gov/OPHS/haccp/salmdata.htm. Accessed June 2008.

USDHHS (U.S. Department of Health and Human Services) (continuously updated): Healthy People 2010. http://www.healthypeople.gov/Data. Accessed February 2008.

Ward TJ, Gorski L, Borucki MK, Mandrell RE, Hutchins J, Pupedis K (2004): Intraspecific phylogeny and lineage group identification based on the *prfA* virulence gene cluster of *Listeria monocytogenes. J Bacteriol.* 186:4994–5002.

WHO (World Health Organization) (continuously updated-a): Media Centre. http://www.who.int/mediacentre/en. Accessed June 2008.

——— (continuously updated-b): Global Salm-Surv (GSS) site. http://www.who.int/salmsurv/en. Accessed June 2008.

Withee J, Dearfield KL (2007): Genomics-based food-borne pathogen testing and diagnostics: possibilities for the US Department of Agriculture's Food Safety and Inspection Service. *Environ Mol Mutagen.* 48:363–378.

CHAPTER 2

FOODBORNE PATHOGENS AND TOXINS: AN OVERVIEW

SANTOS GARCÍA and NORMA HEREDIA

2.1 INTRODUCTION

In this section we describe the main foodborne pathogens and toxins involved in food contamination. It is a prelude to the following chapters, in which foods specifically affected by these pathogens or toxins are discussed. For descriptions of *Enterobacter sakazakii*, prion diseases, and avian influenza viruses, consult Chapters 3, 4, and 5, respectively.

2.2 *AEROMONAS*

2.2.1 The Organism

Aeromonas spp. comprise an emerging waterborne pathogen that is widely distributed in the environment and has gained importance as a human pathogen, causing intestinal and extraintestinal infections. This organism is one of the causative agents of diarrheal infections in children and immunocompromised patients (Daskalov, 2006; Fernández-Escartín and García, 2001).

Aeromonas is now classified within the family Aeromonadaceae, which can be divided into a psychrotrophic group and a mesophilic group. The psychrotrophic group contains the fish pathogen *A. salmonicida*, whereas the *Aeromonas* spp. regarded as potential human pathogens belong to the motile mesophilic group (Fernández-Escartín and García, 2001).

A. hydrophila, *A. caviae,* and *A. veronii* have been suggested as the main causes of *Aeromonas*-mediated human gastroenteritis, although other species have also been linked to cases of human enteric diseases (i.e., *A. trota* and *A. jandaei*). In addition, *A. schubertii* and *A. hydrophila* may also be isolated from human wound infections. In immunocompromised individuals, *A. septicaemia* may prove fatal (Daskalov, 2006).

Microbiologically Safe Foods, Edited by Norma Heredia, Irene Wesley, and Santos García

Aeromonas spp. grow at the temperature range 0 to 42°C; for example, *A. hydrophila* grows optimally around 28°C. However, of concern for microbial food safety, many strains grow at refrigeration temperatures (sometimes as low as 0.1°C). *Aeromonas* spp. have the ability to grow anaerobically and are gram-negative, nonspore-forming, rod-shaped bacteria (Daskalov, 2006; Fernández-Escartín and García, 2001).

Disease-associated strains possess a large number of virulence factors, many of which have been linked to *Aeromonas*-associated pathogenesis. Among them are matrix-binding proteins; elastases; proteases; cytotonic, cytolytic, and cytotoxic toxins; hemolysins; aldolase; chitinase; lipases; and type IV pilus adhesins. These strains also possess the ability to form a capsulelike outer layer (Daskalov, 2006).

2.2.2 The Illness

The major infections caused by *Aeromonas* spp. in humans can be classified in two major groups: septicemia, a general infection caused mainly by *A. veronii* subsp. *sobria* and *A. hydrophila*; and gastroenteritis, which is due primarily to *A. hydrophila* and *A. veronii* (Daskalov, 2006; Fernández-Escartín and García, 2001).

Aeromonas spp. may play a significant role in "summer diarrhea," a worldwide seasonal problem affecting children under 5 years old, the elderly, and travelers particularly. Acute self-limited diarrhea is more frequent in young children, whereas in older patients, chronic enterocolitis may also be observed. Fever, vomiting, and fecal leukocytes or erythrocytes (colitis) may be present in these types of infections. Furthermore, *Aeromonas* spp. have been responsible for extraintestinal infections, including meningitis and pulmonary and wound infections, and have been linked to cases of hemolytic uremic syndrome (Fernández-Escartín and García, 2001).

2.2.3 Contamination of Foods

Mesophilic aeromonads have been found in a wide variety of aquatic environments, including drinking water, sewage, groundwater, and streams and rivers. These pathogens have also been isolated from many foodstuffs, including green vegetables, raw milk, ice cream, beef, lamb, chicken, fish, and seafood (Daskalov, 2006; Fernández-Escartín and García, 2001).

2.2.4 Prevention and Control

Although *Aeromonas* spp. are resistant to food preservation techniques such as cooling, these species are sensitive to temperature (heating), low pH (<4.5), salt ($>5\%$), phosphates, nitrites, and other factors. Therefore, multiple-hurdle technology, which utilizes a combination approach (temperature, pH, NaCl, $NaNO_2$) to control foodborne pathogens, could be appropriate to control *Aeromonas* in foods. Furthermore, plant extracts, smoking, and a modified atmosphere could be used in combination with other methods to control the organism (Daskalov, 2006; Fernández-Escartín and García, 2001).

2.3 *ARCOBACTER*

2.3.1 The Organism

The genus *Arcobacter* has been placed in the family Campylobacteraceae, which includes the genera *Campylobacter*. The family is characterized as fastidious, gram-negative, non-spore-forming, motile, microaerobic, spiral-shaped organisms. *A. butzleri*, *A. cibarius*, *A. cryaerophilus*, *A. halophious*, *A. skirrowii*, *A. nitrofigilis*, and *A. sulfidicus* are components of the genus, and three of these species, *A. butzleri*, *A. cryaerophilus*, and *A. skirrowii*, have been associated with human and animal enteric diseases. *Arcobacter* spp. grow in the presence of atmospheric oxygen (aerotolerant) and at 15 to 30°C (Fera et al., 2004; Lehner et al., 2005).

2.3.2 The Illness

Arcobacter species have frequently been isolated from clinically healthy and ill animals, meats, and humans with enteritis. *A. butzleri* and *A. cryaerophilus* have been associated with enteritis and occasionally, bacteriemia or septicemia in humans. They have also been associated with mastitis, diarrhea, reproductive abnormalities, abortion, septicemia, gastritis, and enteritis of farm animals. *A. butzleri* and *A. cryaerophilus* have been isolated from stool samples of patients with acute diarrhea (Lehner et al., 2005). *Arcobacter* spp. account for up to 4% of *Campylobacter*-like organisms (CLOs) isolated from human stools in Europe (Vandenberg et al., 2004; Prouzet-Mauleon et al., 2006).

2.3.3 Contamination of Foods

It has been suggested that water may play an important role in the transmission of *Arcobacter* spp. to animals and humans, and drinking water has been cited as a major risk factor in acquiring diarrheal illness associated with these bacteria. The organism has been isolated from drinking water reservoirs, water treatment plants, rivers, canal water, sewage, and well water (Fera et al., 2004; Lehner et al., 2005).

Although difficult to isolate from the live bird, poultry carcasses in particular are commonly contaminated with high levels of *Arcobacter* species. In contrast, *Arcobacter* spp. have been isolated from the intestine and feces of healthy dairy cattle, pigs, sheep, and horses as well as from meats originating from these species.

2.3.4 Prevention and Control

Risk factors for human infection include handling of raw meats, especially poultry, and consumption of undercooked contaminated meats and water. Preventive measures include hygiene, HACCP, good manufacturing and handling practices in the processing plant (especially during slaughter), and family education (Lehner et al., 2005).

2.4 *BACILLUS CEREUS*

2.4.1 The Organism

The *Bacillus cereus* group of organisms contains *B. cereus, B. thuringiensis,* and *B. anthracis*. *B. cereus* is ubiquitous in nature and is often associated with two forms of human food poisoning, characterized by either diarrhea and abdominal distress or nausea and vomiting (Dierick et al., 2005; Rasko et al., 2005).

B. cereus is a gram-positive, motile, spore-forming rod. The cells are 1.0 to 1.2 μm in diameter by 3.0 to 5.0 μm in length and grow at a wide range of temperatures. As an important attribute, *B. cereus* can survive and grow at low temperatures. In fact, strains could be divided into those with a high-temperature growth range (10 to 42°C) and those with a low-temperature growth range (4 to 37°C). Strains may also be distinguished by their ability to grow below 7°C (psychrotrophs with an optimal temperature of 25 to 30°C) and those that cannot (mesophiles with optimal temperature around 37°C). The organism has also been reported to survive and grow in the pH range 4.3 to 9.3 (Rasko et al., 2005).

The endospores allow the bacterium to enhance its resistance to wet heat, dry heat, radiation, desiccation, extreme pH, chemicals, enzymes, and high pressure. This resistance could enable the bacterium to survive commercial food pasteurization and cooking at ambient pressure. In addition, sublethal heat treatment of foods containing *B. cereus* spores can actually select for the pathogen among other microorganisms that might be present (Rasko et al., 2005).

2.4.2 The Illness

B. cereus causes diarrheal and emetic types of food poisoning, which originate from different toxins (Rajkovic et al., 2006). Diarrheal symptoms are caused by heat-labile enterotoxins produced during vegetative growth of *B. cereus* in the small intestine. Five of these enterotoxins have been characterized: the three-component hemolysin BL enterotoxin, the three-component and nonhemolytic enterotoxin, and three enterotoxic proteins: enterotoxin T, cytotoxin K, and enterotoxin FM (Rajkovic et al., 2006; Rasko et al., 2005).

The emetic syndrome (intoxication) is caused by cereulide, a pH- and thermostable (1.2 kDa) cyclic peptide toxin. A sufficient amount of toxin to cause illness 0.5 to 6 h after ingestion can be produced by 10^5 CFU/g; however, cereulide production is dependent on the *B. cereus* strain involved (Rajkovic et al., 2006; Rasko et al., 2005). Typically, the diarrheal syndrome is relatively mild and short-lived, although cytotoxin K was implicated in an outbreak in which people died. This syndrome is generally characterized by abdominal cramps with profuse watery diarrhea, rectal tenesmus, and occasionally, nausea, which rarely results in vomiting. It has an incubation period within the range 8 to 16 h, and the symptoms generally disappear in 12 to 24 h (Rasko et al., 2005).

The second type of illness, described as the emetic type of intoxication, caused by *B. cereus* is characterized by an acute attack of vomiting that occurs 1 to 5 h after consumption of contaminated food. Concentrations of cereulide, ranging from 0.01

to 1.280 mg/g, have been reported in foods implicated in emetic-type food poisoning (Rajkovic et al., 2006; Rasko et al., 2005). Fulminant liver failure has also been associated with the emetic toxin. Recently, a fatal case due to liver failure occurred after the consumption of pasta salad, which resulted in vomiting, respiratory distress, severe pulmonary hemorrhage, coma, diffuse bleeding, and severe muscle cramps in the patient (Dierick et al., 2005); *B. cereus* was detected in six food samples and the vomit of the deceased girl. Although the presence of cereulide in the pasta salad was not demonstrated directly, its production at a high level was indirectly proven in cytotoxicity tests of the isolates (Dierick et al., 2005).

2.4.3 Contamination of Foods

The bacterium is ubiquitous in nature and can be isolated from soil, dust, water, and diverse foods. *B. cereus* has been detected in heat-processed or cooked foods such as baking chocolate, baked bread, cooked rice, pasta, meats, milk, and dairy products, and its presence in spices, raw vegetables, salad dressing, and seafood has also been reported. Furthermore, an association between farinaceous foods and cereulide-related foodborne poisonings has been established (Dierick et al., 2005; Rajkovic et al., 2006; Rasko et al., 2005).

2.4.4 Prevention and Control

The widespread occurrence of *B. cereus* and the factors that favor its survival and presence in foods could make this bacterium difficult to control. Cells can attach to stainless steel surfaces and are especially capable of forming biofilms, while spores are even more adherent. Importantly, spores and vegetative cells embedded in biofilms are more protected against inactivation by sanitizers (Rasko et al., 2005). The high resistance to heat (126°C over 90 min), extreme pH (pH 2 to 11), and proteolytic enzymes makes cereulide difficult to eradicate or inactivate in foods; consequently, cereulide preformed in foods is an important risk for the consumer.

Another important risk is that refrigeration cannot prevent outgrowth of psychrotrophic *B. cereus* (Rajkovic et al., 2006; Rasko et al., 2005). Heat, irradiation treatment, low temperatures, low a_w, (water activity), or low pH in foods could destroy or greatly reduce growth or spore germination of enterotoxigenic *Bacillus* spp., thereby preventing toxin formation in foods. Therefore, proper handling, heating, and holding precautions should be employed to reduce the chance of foodborne illness by *B. cereus* (Rasko et al., 2005).

2.5 *BRUCELLA*

2.5.1 The Organism

The brucelleae are gram-negative, 0.5 to 0.7 μm in size, nonmotile, strict aerobes, ovoid rods, or cocco-bacilli. They are obligate parasites of animals and humans, and cause brucellosis (Fernández-Escartin and García, 2001). Brucellosis is a zoonosis of world distribution, and *Brucella* has host specificity among animals: *B. abortus* in cattle, *B. melitensis* in goats and sheep, and *B. suis* in pigs. *B. melitensis* is prevalent in the Mediterranean area and in Mexico (Fernández-Escartin and García, 2001).

2.5.2 The Illness

Infection can result after consumption of contaminated food or direct contact with infected animals (e.g., in the case of farmers, veterinarians, and slaughterhouse workers). Brucellosis, also known as undulant fever or Malta fever, is an insidious illness with varied symptomology in humans. The incubation period ranges from 3 to 21 days and occasionally, up to 7 months. Acute cases show fever, sweating, chills, weakness, chest pain, migraine, arthralgia, anorexia, and weight loss (Fernández-Escartin and García, 2001).

2.5.3 Contamination of Foods

The common sources of infection for humans are unpasteurized milk and cheese and undercooked meat or vegetables that have been in contact with feces or urine from infected animals (Fernández-Escartin and García, 2001; Tantillo et al., 2001).

2.5.4 Prevention and Control

The application of common germicides at the concentrations recommended for plant sanitation reliably inactivates the microorganism. Chlorine- or iodine-based compounds are recommended for disinfection of areas exposed to infected animals. Control of the microorganism is achieved by avoiding food contamination and assuring its destruction, mainly using heat (pasteurization or boiling). Appropriate acidification of cheeses during maturation inhibits *Brucella*. Control of the disease resides essentially in eliminating the source of primary infection, such as ill animals (Fernández-Escartin and García, 2001).

2.6 *CAMPYLOBACTER*

2.6.1 The Organism

Campylobacter spp. were not recognized as human pathogens until the 1970s; however, data suggest that they have probably caused illness in humans for centuries (Butzler, 2004). This organism is recognized as the most common cause of foodborne bacterial gastroenteritis in humans in many countries and possibly worldwide. Its low infective dose in humans and its potentially severe sequelae make this bacterium a significant public health hazard.

The family Campylobacteraceae comprises *Campylobacter, Arcobacter,* and *Bacteroides ureolyticus* and occurs primarily as a commensal in domestic animals (Snelling et al., 2005). *Campylobacter* spp. are S-shaped rods (0.2 to 0.8 μm wide and 0.5 to 5.0 μm long), gram-negative, non-spore-forming, and motile with a characteristic corkscrew-like motion. This species requires complex growth media, as it is not able to oxidize or ferment carbohydrates, has no lipase or lecithinase activity, and is oxidase positive. Campylobacters are unable to grow below 30°C, below pH 4.9, or in a 2% concentration of sodium chloride. Furthermore, these bacteria are very sensitive to desiccation and do not survive well on dry surfaces (Butzler, 2004; Snelling et al., 2005).

Although *C. jejuni*, *C. coli*, *C. upsaliensis*, *C. lari*, *C. concisus*, *C. fetus* subsp. *fetus*, *C. jejuni* subsp. *doylei*, and *C. hyointestinalis* have been shown to cause diarrhea, the vast majority of reported cases of diarrhea are attributed to *C. jejuni* (90 to 95%) and *C. coli* (5 to 10%). *Campylobacter* strains associated with dysentery-like illnesses have been shown to be more invasive and cytotoxic than other *Campylobacter* strains in in vitro assays (Butzler, 2004; Snelling et al., 2005).

Campylobacters are generally microaerophilic and may be cultured in atmospheres with 3 to 15% oxygen supplemented with 2 to10% CO_2. The hippuricase gene is found only in *C. jejuni*, although some *C. jejuni* isolates are hippuricase-negative, making it impossible to differentiate *C. coli* from hippuricase-negative *C. jejuni* using purely biochemical tests (Snelling et al., 2005).

2.6.2 The Illness

Campylobacter spp. have an infective dose of between 500 and 10,000 organisms and an incubation period of 1 to 7 days and cause either asymptomatic infections, watery diarrhea, or dysentery-type illnesses in humans. Although most infections are self-limiting (lasting up to 7 days) and rarely cause death, some are associated with chronic, debilitating sequelae such as arthritis, Reiter syndrome, and Guillain–Barré syndrome (Butzler, 2004; Snelling et al., 2005). Symptoms of the gastrointestinal illness can include diarrhea, fever, and abdominal cramps (sometimes the severe abdominal pain may mimic appendicitis), headache, asthenia, and anorexia. Fresh blood, pus, or mucus may appear in the stools, and vomiting is rare.

Adherence to and invasion of host mucosal surfaces were proposed as crucial steps in the pathogenesis of these gastrointestinal illnesses, in which chemotaxis, motility, adhesins, hemolytic activity, lipooligosaccharide, capsular antigens, and cytolethal-distending toxin could play an important role (Butzler, 2004; Snelling et al., 2005).

Over 90% of human campylobacteriosis cases are sporadic, and most of them occur in the summer. It affects people of all ages but with a distinctive bimodal distribution, affecting particularly children less than 4 years of age and young adults aged 15 to 44 years. A recent study from the United States estimated the number of cases at 2 million with about 100 deaths at an annual economic cost of $1.3 to 6.2 billion (Butzler, 2004; Mead et al., 1999; Snelling et al., 2005).

2.6.3 Contamination of Foods

Epidemiological studies indicate that handling or consumption of chicken or poultry is an important risk factor for sporadic cases of human campylobacteriosis, and many studies have identified common types of *Campylobacter* from poultry and humans; however, several studies have suggested that pork may also be an important source of human infection (Fosse et al., 2008). Additionally, *C. jejuni* has been isolated from a range of food sources, including poultry, red meat, and milk (Miller and Mandrell, 2005). Almost all parts of poultry carcasses, whether fresh, chilled, or frozen, are frequently contaminated with *C. jejuni*. Raw or undercooked beef, hamburgers, sausages, and clams have also been implicated in *Campylobacter* enteritis (Butzler, 2004; Snelling et al., 2005). *C. jejuni* is found in the normal gastrointestinal flora of poultry (and probably all avians), swine, and cattle, and epidemiological evidence suggests that these may be reservoirs for strains infecting humans. The primary reservoir for *C. coli* is pig, whereas *C. coli* constitute only a minimal percentage of the *Campylobacter* isolates from chicken and cattle (Butzler, 2004).

2.6.4 Prevention and Control

Prevention should aim at reducing infection at all stages of poultry production. On farms, control strategies such as the effective use of hygiene barriers, hand washing, and boot disinfection, the development of appropriate standard operating procedures to minimize risk factors; staff education; incentives to maintain biosecurity at the highest level; and well-designed and well-located farms would all contribute to the reduction of flock positivity (Butzler, 2004; Snelling et al., 2005).

The use of different antimicrobial treatments based on chlorine, sodium chlorite, cetylpyridinium chloride, chlorine dioxide, ozone, peroxyacids, and trisodium phosphate would help to control microbial populations during poultry processing. Furthermore, *Campylobacter* is relatively sensitive to low-dose radiation treatment and could readily be eliminated from poultry meat products by this method (Butzler, 2004). Appropriate precautions in the handling, cooking, and preparation of different foods of animal origin will further reduce the risk of infection (Butzler, 2004).

2.7 *CLOSTRIDIUM BOTULINUM*

2.7.1 The Organism

Clostridium botulinum is an anaerobic, gram-positive, spore-forming rod that causes botulism. Foodborne botulism is a severe neurological disease affecting both humans and animals, and is characterized by paralysis caused by a neurotoxin (BoNT) produced by this microorganism and by *Clostridium baratti* (type E) and *Clostridium butyricum* (type F) (Sharma and Whiting, 2005). Seven serotypes (A to G) of *C. botulinum* have been classified by immunological differences in the BoNT they produce, as well as by the reaction of each strain to specific antisera. The seven serotypes are taxonomically divided into four distinct phenotypic groups (I to IV). However, the serotypes A, B, E, and F, which account for almost all cases of human botulism, could be categorized into groups I and II based on their phenotypic and genotypic characteristics. Strains of group I are proteolytic, have an optimum growth temperature range of 35 to 40°C, and produce heat-resistant spores and A, B, or F toxins. Strains of group II are nonproteolytic, have an optimum growth temperature range of 18 to 25°C, but are capable of growing at refrigerated temperatures and produce spores with lower resistance to heat and B, E, or F toxins (Sharma and Shukla, 2005; Sharma and Whiting, 2005).

BoNT, which is produced during anaerobic growth of *C. botulinum,* is the most poisonous substance in the world, with an estimated ingested human toxic dose of 1 ng/kg body mass. The main occurring forms of botulism are foodborne botulism, wound botulism, and infant botulism. A food may contain viable spores but not yet contain BoNT, because growth is required for toxin production (Sharma and Shukla, 2005; Sharma and Whiting, 2005)

2.7.2 The Illness

Foodborne botulism is a rare disease that results from the consumption of food contaminated with preformed BoNT or after microbial colonization of the gastrointestinal tract and secretion of the neurotoxin. Symptoms of botulism include blurred vision, drooping eyelids, slurred speech, difficulty swallowing, dry mouth, muscle weakness, and descending flaccid muscle paralysis. In foodborne botulism, symptoms generally appear 18 to 36 h following ingestion of contaminated food, and persons with these symptoms require immediate specialized treatment (Lund and Peck, 2001; Sharma and Shukla, 2005).

2.7.3 Contamination of Foods

C. botulinum is widely distributed in soils and sediments of lakes and oceans. The majority of foods are likely to contain spores of *C. botulinum*; for example, it has been isolated from fish, meat, vegetables, fruits, honey, mushrooms, cheese, and nuts (Lund and Peck, 2001; Sharma and Whiting, 2005).

C. botulinum type E is most often associated with cases of fish and seafood contamination, whereas types A and B are associated with soil contamination of foods (Lund and Peck, 2001; Sharma and Whiting, 2005). The heat-resistant spores are capable of surviving for up to 2 h at 100°C, and can survive in foods that are incorrectly or minimally processed under anaerobic conditions. The most common cause of botulism is the consumption of home-canned foods prepared under inappropriate conditions (Lund and Peck, 2001; Sharma and Shukla, 2005).

2.7.4 Prevention and Control

Although BoNT is heat labile and is rapidly inactivated by heating (at 85°C or higher for at least 5 min), a single case of human botulism is considered an outbreak due to its extreme lethality. Control measures to prevent foodborne botulism include acidification, reduction of moisture level, proper thermal processing, and the use of preservatives (Lund and Peck, 2001).

2.8 *CLOSTRIDIUM PERFRINGENS*

2.8.1 The Organism

Clostridium perfringens causes several diseases in humans and animals. In particular, gas gangrene, food poisoning, and necrotic enteritis affect humans. The bacterium is a gram-positive, anaerobic, spore-forming rod whose spores are common contaminants of a variety of foods. This bacterium is able to produce various toxins and enzymes responsible for the associated diseases (Heredia and Labbé, 2001).

C. perfringens is classified into five toxinotypes (A, B, C, D, and E) based on the production of four major toxins (alpha, beta, epsilon, and iota toxins). Only a small fraction (1 to 5%) of all *C. perfringens* isolates, belonging primarily to type A, are capable of producing an enterotoxin responsible for food poisoning (Brynestad and Granum, 2002).

The organism exhibits growth at a temperature range of 15 to 50°C, with an optimal of 37 to 45°C, and with growth reported at temperatures as low as 6°C. Generation times for enterotoxin-positive *C. perfringens* strains grown between 41 and 46°C can be less than 8 min in autoclaved ground beef (Heredia and Labbe, 2001). The ability to form heat-resistant spores and the wide temperature range in which *C. perfringens* can grow are features that allow the bacteria to multiply and survive in different food situations (Brynestad and Granum, 2002; Heredia and Labbé, 2001).

2.8.2 The Illness

Foodborne diseases caused by *C. perfringens* include food poisoning (the most common) and necrotic enteritis caused by enterotoxin-positive *C. perfringens* type A strains and *C. perfringens* type C strains, respectively. Food poisoning can result from ingestion of a large number (10^6 to 10^7) of vegetative cells. Symptoms, which are characterized by abdominal pain, nausea, and diarrhea, start about 6 to 24 h after consumption of contaminated food and last about 24 h. Typically, symptoms are relatively mild, but death may occasionally occur (Brynestad and Granum, 2002; Heredia and Labbé, 2001).

2.8.3 Contamination of Foods

This organism is commonly found in soil and dust, in the intestinal tract of humans and animals, in spices, and on the surfaces of vegetable products, as well as in other raw and processed foods (Brynestad and Granum, 2002; Heredia and Labbé, 2001). *C. perfringens* is also frequently found in meat and poultry products, generally through fecal contamination of carcasses, contamination from other ingredients, and/or post-processing contamination.

Foods that have been linked to *C. perfringens* foodborne illness include roast beef, turkey, meat-containing Mexican foods, and other meat dishes (Brynestad and Granum, 2002; Heredia and Labbé, 2001). For growth the organism requires more than a dozen amino acids and several vitamins that are typically present in meat.

C. perfringens food poisoning is not a reportable disease; however, the Centers for Disease Control and Prevention estimates that 250,000 cases of *C. perfringens* type A food poisoning occur annually in the United States. In Norway in the 1990s, this organism was registered as the most common cause of food poisoning; similarly, the prevalence in other countries, such as Japan and the UK, is also high (Brynestad and Granum, 2002; Heredia and Labbé, 2001). Deaths are not common, but do occur in the elderly and debilitated (Heredia and Labbé, 2001).

2.8.4 Prevention and Control

Improper cooling of food has been identified as an important factor associated with *C. perfringens* food poisoning. As cooked foods cool, they can pass through the entire range of growth of the bacterium, thereby allowing germination and outgrowth of contaminant *C. perfringens* spores into vegetative cells, which can multiply rapidly to reach high numbers. Therefore, rapid cooling of cooked foods is crucial to prevent proliferation of this pathogen (Heredia and Labbé, 2001).

This pathogen is of concern in retail food service, where large volumes of food are prepared in advance and cooled before reheating for service. The U.S. Department of Agriculture Food Safety Inspection Service (USDA-FSIS) draft compliance guidelines for ready-to-eat meat and poultry products state that such products should be cooled at a rate sufficient to prevent more than a 1-log increase in *C. perfringens* cells (Brynestad and Granum, 2002; Heredia and Labbé, 2001). These federal guidelines also state that cooling from 54.4°C to 26.6°C (130°F to 80°F) should take no longer than 1.5 h, and that cooling from 26.6°C to 4.4°C (80°F to 40°F) should take no longer than 5 h. Additional guidelines allow for the cooling of certain cured cooked meats from 54.4°C to 26.7°C (130°F to 80°F) in 5 h, and from 26.7°C to 7.2°C (80°F to 45°F) in 10 h (Brynestad and Granum, 2002; Heredia and Labbé, 2001).

2.9 *ESCHERICHIA COLI*

2.9.1 The Organism

Escherichia coli are facultatively anaerobic gram-negative bacteria that are naturally present in humans and animals as part of the intestinal microflora. Some strains are, however, able to cause disease ranging from mild to cholera-like diarrhea and may lead to potentially fatal complications such as hemolytic uremic syndrome (HUS).

On the basis of pathogenic features, the most important diarrheagenic *E. coli* are classified into at least six distinct groups: enteropathogenic *E. coli* (EPEC), enterotoxigenic *E. coli* (ETEC), enterohemorrhagic *E. coli* (EHEC), enteroinvasive *E. coli* (EIEC), diffuse-adhering *E. coli* (DAEC), and enteroaggregative *E. coli* (EAEC) (Nataro and Kaper, 1998). Of these, only the first four groups have been implicated in food or waterborne illness (Feng and Weagant, 2002).

2.9.2 The Illness

EPEC is the most widespread of the diarrheagenic *E. coli* and is a major cause of human infantile diarrhea predominantly in less developed countries, but with increasing frequency in industrialized areas. EPEC infection results in an acute or persistent watery, nonbloody, or mucoid diarrhea, often accompanied by fever and vomiting. These pathogens colonize the small intestine, induce the degeneration of epithelial microvilli, and adhere intimately to the host cell, originating lesions that result in a reduction in the absorptive capacity of the intestinal mucosa. The disease ranges from a fulminating diarrhea to a subclinical infection, presumably depending on host factors. Most infants with diarrhea caused by EPEC recover uneventfully if water and electrolyte disturbances are corrected promptly (Clarke et al., 2002; Nataro and Kaper, 1998).

EHEC, also referred to as Shiga toxin–producing *E. coli* (STEC), are responsible for serious human infections such as uncomplicated diarrhea, hemorrhagic colitis, and HUS. These strains are known to produce Shiga toxin 1 (Stx1) and Shiga toxin 2 (Stx2), which resemble those of *Shigella dysenteriae* (Betts, 2000; Feng and Weagant, 2002). In addition, other virulence-associated factors include a pO157 plasmid, which encodes hemolysin and the enterocyte effacement locus containing the intimin gene (*eaeA*) (Betts, 2000; Feng and Weagant, 2002). Although serotype O157:H7 is the one that has been implicated most frequently in foodborne outbreaks worldwide, more than 100 STEC serotypes (e.g., members of the O26, O91, O103, O111, O118, O145, and O166 serogroups) are known to cause human illnesses, including HUS (Betts, 2000; Feng and Weagant, 2002).

The incubation period of EHEC diarrhea is usually 3 to 4 days, although incubation times as long as 5 to 8 days or as short as 1 to 2 days have been described in some outbreaks (Betts, 2000; Feng and Weagant, 2002). Initial symptoms include nonbloody diarrhea and crampy abdominal pain; fever and vomiting occur in many patients. After 1 or 2 days, the diarrhea appears bloody and abdominal pain increases and could last between 4 and 10 days. In most patients, the bloody diarrhea will resolve, but in some patients the illness will progress to HUS, which is characterized by hemolytic anemia, thrombocytopenia, and renal failure, with important mortality in children (Nataro and Kaper, 1998).

EIEC consists of 11 known serogroups (O28a, O28c, O29, O112, O124, O136, O143, O144, O152, O164, and O167), which are based on serological characteristics. To cause disease in healthy humans, an infectious dose of 10^6 cells or greater is necessary. The infection occurs as watery diarrhea or dysentery, the latter manifesting as blood, mucus, and leukocytes in the stool, tenesmus, and fever (Nataro and Kaper, 1998).

ETEC is one of the main etiologic agents of diarrhea in infants and travelers. ETEC strains have the ability to produce enterotoxins, either heat-labile toxin (LT is very similar in size, sequence, antigenicity, and function to the cholera toxin) or heat-stable toxin (ST), or both, and surface adhesins known as colonization factors (Feng and Weagant, 2002; Nataro and Kaper, 1998). The infective dose for ETEC in otherwise healthy adults is estimated to be at least 10^8 CFU, but the young, the elderly, and the infirm may be susceptible to lower levels. The illness is characterized by watery diarrhea with little or no fever (Feng and Weagant, 2002; Nataro and Kaper, 1998).

2.9.3 Contamination of Foods

E. coli has growth and survival characteristics very similar to those of other enteric organisms. It survives freezing at −20°C and can survive chill storage, being able to grow at a minimum temperature of 6.5°C. *E. coli* O157:H7 does not have unusual resistance to heat and also tolerates salt levels similar to those of other typical pathogens [e.g., it can grow at a water activity as low as 0.95 (equivalent to 8% salt)]. Pathogenic and nonpathogenic strains of *E. coli* have equally remarkable levels of resistance to extreme acid stress. Survival of *E. coli* O157:H7 in low-pH foods such as mayonnaise, apple cider, orange juice, and fermented sausages and dairy products has been reported (Betts, 2000). *E. coli* normally live in the intestines of warm-blooded animals and may contaminate a wide variety of foods in different ways, including contaminated hands, contaminated fomites serving as vehicles, bowel rupture during evisceration, indirect contamination with polluted water, and handling and packaging of finished products. Food vehicles such as cheese, salmon, yogurt, fruit salad, cantaloupe, cake, vegetables, salami, and most notably, ground beef have been involved in outbreaks (Betts, 2000; Nataro and Kaper, 1998). Transmission of EPEC is fecal–oral, with contaminated hands, contaminated weaning foods or formula, or contaminated fomites serving as vehicles. EPEC has been isolated from dust and aerosols, suggesting potential airborne transmission.

Cattle serve as a main reservoir for *E. coli* O157:H7 strains. Other species, such as horses, deer, sheep, goats, pigs, cats, dogs, chickens, gulls, birds, and flies, have also been reported to be sources of these organisms (Nataro and Kaper, 1998). Most human STEC infections have been traced to consumption of contaminated undercooked foods of bovine origin such as ground beef and raw milk. Other sources of infection include manure-contaminated vegetables, raw milk, some dairy products, mayonnaise, delicatessen food, lamb, venison, deer jerky, cured salami, contaminated water, cross-contamination, and direct contact (Clarke et al., 2002; Feng and Weagant, 2002; Nataro and Kaper, 1998).

Documented EIEC outbreaks are usually foodborne or waterborne, although person-to-person transmission does occur (Feng and Weagant, 2002; Nataro and Kaper, 1998). ETEC infections occur commonly in underdeveloped countries and tend to be clustered in warm, wet months, when multiplication of ETEC in food and water is most efficient. Outbreaks have been associated with raw vegetables, Mexican-style foods, water, and soft cheeses (Nataro and Kaper, 1998).

2.9.4 Prevention and Control

Food pasteurization processes for chilled foods (e.g., 70°C for 2 min) designed to eliminate *Listeria* spp. should also control this organism. As described earlier, this organism can survive in acidic environments; however, careful choice of level and type of acid in combination with appropriate storage conditions and antimicrobial treatments can provide an effective control strategy (Betts, 2000).

In-plant applications have shown effectiveness for decontamination, evidenced by a reduction in the percentage of carcass samples being positive from pre-evisceration to post-processing. Furthermore, effective sanitation strategies have to be applied to reduce the prevalence of this microorganism in the plant (Betts, 2000; Nataro and Kaper, 1998).

2.10 *LISTERIA*

2.10.1 The Organism

Listeria monocytogenes is a ubiquitous gram-positive foodborne pathogen that causes a high fatality rate, particularly in high-risk groups, including elderly and immunocompromised persons as well as pregnant women and their neonates. In the United States, this organism accounts for less than 1% of cases of foodborne illnesses but approximately 28% of deaths from bacterial foodborne illnesses (Kathariou, 2002; Vazquez-Boland et al., 2001).

The genus *Listeria* contains six species: *L. monocytogenes*, *L. innocua*, *L. seeligeri*, *L. welshimeri*, *L. ivanovii*, and *L. grayi*. Only the hemolytic species *L. monocytogenes*, *L. ivanovii*, and *L. seeligeri* are associated with human pathogenicity, although *L. monocytogenes* is the only species that has been involved in known foodborne outbreaks of listeriosis (Cocolin et al., 2002). *L. monocytogenes* has been differentiated into 13 serotypes; however, only four of these serotypes (1/2a, 1/2b, 1/2c, and 4b), have been reported to cause a large majority of human listeriosis cases worldwide (Cocolin et al., 2002).

The genus *Listeria* consists of facultative anaerobic rods of 0.4 by 1 to 1.5 μm that do not form spores, have no capsule, and are motile at 10 to 25°C. *Listeria* can grow over a wide range of temperatures (−1.5 to 45–50°C) and pH ranges (4.3 to 9.6), survive freezing, and are relatively resistant to heat (Cocolin et al., 2002; Kathariou, 2002; Vazquez-Boland et al., 2001). *L. monocytogenes* is able to tolerate high concentrations of salt and has the ability to mount an adaptive acid tolerance response that allows bacterial cells previously exposed to moderately acidic conditions to withstand extreme acid exposure. Furthermore, cross protection has been observed in this microorganism; for example, increased resistance of *L. monocytogenes* to heating at 56°C has been demonstrated following exposure of cells to starvation conditions, ethanol, acid, and H_2O_2 (Vazquez-Boland et al., 2001).

2.10.2 The Illness

Several virulence factors of *L. monocytogenes* have been identified, including hemolysin (listeriolysin O), two distinct phospholipases, a protein (ActA), several internalins, and others (Kathariou, 2002). The primary mode of transmission of this pathogen to humans is the consumption of contaminated food. Although large numbers of *L. monocytogenes* have been detected in foods responsible for epidemic and sporadic cases of listeriosis (typically, 10^6), levels of contamination as low as 10^2 to 10^4 cells per gram of food have also been implicated. Symptoms usually appear about 20 h after the ingestion of heavily contaminated food in cases of gastroenteritis, whereas the incubation period for an invasive form of the illness is generally 20 to 30 days. Listeriosis is usually a very severe disease, and clinical features of systemic listeriosis include late-term spontaneous abortion, prenatal infection, meningitis, encephalitis, septicemia, and gastroenteritis. The disease has a mean mortality rate in humans of 20 to 30% or higher despite early antibiotic treatment (Vazquez-Boland et al., 2001).

2.10.3 Contamination of Foods

L. monocytogenes is widely distributed in the natural environment and has been isolated from a variety of sources, including surface water, soil, sewage, vegetation, feces of humans and animals, food-processing plants, and is often considered ubiquitous in nature. Listeriosis has been associated with contaminated vegetables, milk, meat, poultry, fish, and seafood products. Examples of contaminated products include, but are not limited to, mushrooms, vegetable rennet, coleslaw, corn salad, soft cheese, raw milk, hot dogs, pork tongue in jelly, turkey frankfurters, chicken, sausages, cold-smoked salmon, shrimp, crab, smoked mussels, and smoked cod roe (Cocolin et al., 2002; Kathariou, 2002; Vazquez-Boland et al., 2001).

2.10.4 Prevention and Control

Refrigerated ready-to-eat foods are of concern since such products are typically not heated prior to consumption. Some of these foods can support growth of *L. monocytogenes*. There is currently zero tolerance of this bacterium for ready-to-eat foods in the United States, but the European Union regulations have established a limit of 100 CFU/g for ready-to-eat foods unable to support the growth of *L. monocytogenes*. According to numerous studies in different food-processing plants, the primary source of food product contamination before release to consumers appears to be the processing environment (Kathariou, 2002). Common sites of *L. monocytogenes* contamination include filling and packing equipment, conveyors, chill solutions, slicers, dicers, shredders, and blenders (Cocolin et al., 2002; Kathariou, 2002; Vazquez-Boland et al., 2001). Furthermore, *Listeria* has the ability to form biofilms which allow the cells to survive stressing and sanitizing agents. Usually, the presence of any *Listeria* species in food is an indicator of poor hygiene (Cocolin et al., 2002).

The ubiquitous distribution in nature and food-processing environments, the possibility of cross-contamination during processing of foods, and the ability to form biofilms, grow at low temperatures, and survive stressing conditions are characteristics that should be taken into account to devise an appropriate method to control this microorganism in the final product.

2.11 *PLESIOMONAS SHIGELLOIDES*

2.11.1 The Organism

Plesiomonas shigelloides is a facultatively anaerobic gram-negative rod, is non-spore-forming, measures 0.1 to 1.0 μm by 2 to 3 μm, and belongs to the family Enterobacteriaceae (Fernández-Escartin and García, 2001). The bacterium has a temperature range for growth from 8 to 44°C with an optimum of 30 to 37°C. The bacterium grows at pH 5.0 to 8.0 and tolerates a maximum concentration of 5% NaCl. Several potential virulence factors have been described for *P. shigelloides*, such as cytotoxins, enterotoxin, endotoxin, adhesins, and invasiveness (Santos et al., 1999).

2.11.2 The Illness

Plesiomonas has been implicated in several outbreaks of gastroenteritis. The illness can present as simple watery diarrhea, as dysentery-like (feces with blood, mucus, and leukocytes), or as cholera-like. Ill persons can also exhibit symptoms such as nausea, vomiting, abdominal pain, fever, chills, and migraine headaches. The incubation period lasts between 24 and 50 h, and the duration of symptoms ranges from 1 to 9 days.

2.11.3 Contamination of Foods and Control

Foods involved in outbreaks of gastroenteritis caused by *Plesiomonas* include shellfish (crab, shrimp, and oyster), fish, and contaminated water. The microorganism will not grow at 5°C or at 50°C, and pasteurization will destroy the bacterium. Consumption of raw seafood should be avoided, especially for immunocompromised or debilitated persons (Fernández-Escartin and García, 2001).

2.12 *SALMONELLA*

2.12.1 The Organism

Salmonellosis is one of the leading causes of foodborne diseases throughout the world. The genus *Salmonella* is divided into two species, *S. enterica* and *S. bongori*. To date, more than 2500 serovars of *S. enterica* have been identified, and most serovars have the potential to infect a wide variety of animal species and humans (D'Aoust, 2001).

Serovars of *S. enterica* can differ in host specificity as well as in clinical and epidemiological characteristics. For example, the serovar Typhi only infects humans, whereas the serovars Typhimurium and Enteritidis infect a wide range of hosts, including humans, rodents, and poultry. Serovars also display distinct routes of transmission. Typhimurium and Enteritidis both infect poultry; however, Typhimurium is more likely to be transmitted to humans through chicken meat; Enteritidis is mostly transmitted to humans through chicken eggs. Furthermore, geographic variation of predominant serovars is observed. *S. enterica* serovar Typhimurium is among the serovars most commonly associated with human salmonellosis in most European countries and in the United States (Clavijo et al., 2006).

Salmonella is a gram-negative mesophilic bacterium that can grow at refrigeration temperatures (4 to 10°C), with rapid growth between 25 and 43°C, although it is usually sensitive to temperatures above 55°C. *Salmonella* grows actively in the pH range 3.6 to 9.5 and optimally at nearly neutral pH values (D'Aoust, 2001).

Salmonella can survive in nuts or low-a_w foods for long periods. For example, when inoculated onto pecan halves, the organism survived for at least 32 weeks after contamination, and survived in peanut butter for more than 24 weeks. The organism can die rapidly on eggshells during storage, but survival is enhanced by low temperatures, especially when relative humidity is low. Survival and growth of *Salmonella* has been reported in low-acid foods such as apple juice and tomato core tissue (Shachar and Yaron, 2006).

2.12.2 The Illness

S. enterica is implicated in two main clinical syndromes in humans: enterocolitis and enteric fever. The most common and characteristic disease caused by *S. enterica* in humans is self-limited enterocolitis. It appears 8 to 72 h following exposure to nontyphoid salmonellae, with remission within 4 to 5 days following the onset of disease. Enterocolitis is usually characterized by severe abdominal pain, diarrhea, vomiting, and fever. Enteric fever is an acute gastrointestinal disease which is originated by the invasion of *S.* Typhi or *S.* Paratyphi into human host tissues. Symptoms include watery diarrhea, prolonged and spiking fever, nausea, and abdominal pain, which appear 7 to 28 days following exposure to the infectious agent.

Very young, very old, and immunocompromised individuals are particularly susceptible to *Salmonella* infections, which can degenerate into serious systemic infections. In these patients, mortality rates may increase by up to 40% (D'Aoust, 2001).

2.12.3 Contamination of Foods

Infections with *S. enterica* continue to be an important public health problem worldwide despite numerous legislative and educational initiatives to improve food hygiene. Because of its ubiquity in the environment and ability to colonize animals used in the human food chain, diseases caused by this bacterium are difficult to eradicate. The worldwide emergence of multi-drug-resistant phenotypes among *Salmonella* serotypes enhances the problem. *Salmonella* is frequently present in the gastrointestinal tracts of cattle, pigs, poultry, and other animal species and is transferred to humans via the food chain. Common contaminated foods associated with *Salmonella* infections in humans include poultry, poultry products, eggs and egg products, pork, beef, milk and milk products, seafood, fresh fruits, and vegetables.

2.12.4 Prevention and Control

Prevention of secondary spread from ill person to foods is important in the home or commercial setting. The intermittent shedding of viable salmonellae in the stools of chronic carriers potentiates secondary human infections and cross-contamination of foods. Airborne, hand-to-surface, or surface-to-surface transmission of *Salmonella* can also occur, and a chronic carrier state can follow the acute phase of the disease. Thus, food handlers require special attention if suspected infection occurs.

2.13 *SHIGELLA*

2.13.1 The Organism

Dysentery caused by *Shigella* species is one of the common infectious diseases in developing countries and in travelers to tropical countries. *Shigella* are gram-negative, nonmotile, non-spore-forming, rod-shaped bacteria. The genus is divided into four species or serotypes: *S. dysenteriae, S. flexneri, S. boydii,* and *S. sonnei*, representing subgroups A, B, C, and D, respectively.

Shigella spp. can survive at a low pH for several hours and in acidic foods for extended periods. *S. flexneri* is able to survive at 48°C for at least 11 days in carrot salad (pH 2.2 to 2.9), potato salad (pH 3.3 to 4.4), and coleslaw (pH 4.1 to 4.2), and for up to 20 days in crab salad (pH 4.4 to 4.5) (Zaika, 2002). Adaptation of cells in glucose or mild acid prior to introduction into an acidic environment can enhance survival compared with that of cells that are not adapted (Chan and Blaschek, 2005).

2.13.2 The Illness

After a low infective dose, on the order of 10 to 100 cells, *Shigella* can cause acute inflammatory colitis, which in its worst case is characterized by intestinal cramps, bloody diarrhea (also known as dysentery), and neurologic symptoms, such as lethargy, confusion, severe headache, and convulsions. *S. dysenteriae* causes the most severe symptoms, *S. boydii* and *S. flexneri* produce mild to severe symptoms, and *S. sonnei* brings about mild symptoms. The most severe forms can lead to a mortality rate of 10 to 30% in children under 5 years of age during outbreaks in developing countries.

2.13.3 Contamination of Foods

Shigella spp. can be transmitted by contaminated food and water and through person-to-person contact. Several foodborne shigellosis outbreaks have been associated with the consumption of contaminated vegetable products, including lettuce, parsley, green onion, cilantro, unpasteurized orange juice, salads, and dips. Furthermore, *Shigella* can contaminate several kinds of foods; including raw vegetables, milk, poultry, and some dairy products (Zaika, 2002).

2.13.4 Prevention and Control

Shigellosis outbreaks have been attributed to foods that have been subjected to hand processing or preparation, received limited heat treatment, or have been served raw. Therefore, special care has to be taken on production standards; the personal hygiene of food handlers; the microbiological quality of water used to wash vegetables, fruits, or other kinds of foods; and appropriate conditions for storage or distribution (Chan and Blaschek, 2005).

2.14 *STAPHYLOCOCCUS AUREUS*

2.14.1 The Organism

Staphylococcus aureus is a ubiquitous bacterium that produces a wide variety of exoproteins that contribute to infections in humans and animals, which range from mild to severe and life threatening. *S. aureus* is a common cause of foodborne poisoning worldwide which results from the ingestion of heat-stable enterotoxins produced in foods by enterotoxigenic *S. aureus* (Dinges et al., 2000).

Staphylococcus species are aerobes or facultative anaerobes, gram-positive, nonmotile cocci. Growth of *S. aureus* ranges from 7 to 47.8°C, with an optimum temperature of 35°C. The pH range for growth is between 4.5 and 9.3, with the optimum between pH 7.0 and 7.5. The bacterium is also highly salt tolerant, resistant to nitrites, and capable of growth at a_w values as low as 0.83 under ideal conditions (Bennett, 2005).

S. aureus produces many enzymes and toxins, which include four hemolysins (alpha, beta, gamma, and delta), nucleases, proteases, lipases, hyaluronidase, and collagenase. Some strains produce one or more additional exoproteins, which include toxic shock syndrome toxin 1, the staphylococcal enterotoxins, the exfoliative toxins, and leukocidin. Of these, the enterotoxins, which are potent emetic agents, pose the greatest risk to consumer health. Although many different enterotoxins have been reported to be produced by *S. aureus*, eight are well recognized (types A, B, C1, C2, C3, D, E, and H) (Bennett, 2005; Dinges et al., 2000). Enterotoxins of *S. aureus* are stable at a heat treatment of 100°C for 30 min, a treatment that readily kills the microorganism (Bennett, 2005; Dinges et al., 2000).

2.14.2 The Illness

In order to cause foodborne illness, *S. aureus* must be present in large enough numbers to produce sickening amounts of enterotoxin(s). The signs and symptoms of staphylococcal food poisoning can occur when foods containing approximately 10^5 to 10^8 cells per gram or milliliter or enterotoxin (100 ng) are ingested (Bennett, 2005; Dinges et al., 2000).

Staphylococcal food poisoning is manifested clinically as emesis with or without diarrhea. The illness is acute, with onset occurring 1 to 7 h after ingestion of toxin-contaminated foods. Nausea and possible abdominal cramping result in vomiting and diarrhea; other symptoms may include retching, sweating, headache, dehydration, marked prostration, muscular cramping, and a drop in blood pressure. Body temperature may be above or below normal, and in extreme cases, blood and mucus may be observed in feces and vomitus. Usually, the disease is self-limiting, although death has been reported (Bennett, 2005; Dinges et al., 2000).

2.14.3 Contamination of Foods

S. aureus is a ubiquitous bacterium, being both a human and a zoonotic commensal. A wide variety of foods will support the growth of enterotoxigenic staphylococci. These items may become contaminated during preparation, and toxin will form if these foods are subsequently mishandled prior to consumption. Foods that are incriminated in staphylococcal food poisoning include beef; ham; pork; cooked sausage; chicken; turkey; egg products; tuna; canned lobster bisque; potato salad; canned mushrooms; macaroni; bakery products such as cream-filled pastries, cream pies, and chocolate éclairs; sandwich fillings; boiled goat's milk; spray-dried milk; and other dairy products.

2.14.4 Prevention and Control

Poor personal hygiene, contaminated equipment, and improper holding temperatures are important factors contributing to *S. aureus* outbreaks (Lamb et al., 2002). Food handlers could contaminate foods via the skin, nose, and mouth; therefore, proper hygiene is essential. Cross contamination should be avoided, and foods must be maintained at proper temperature (either refrigerated or heated) to prevent proliferation of the organisms and production of heat-stable enterotoxins (Bennett, 2005). Currently, traditional methods involving good manufacturing practices, thermal processing, and refrigeration are used to control *S. aureus*.

2.15 *VIBRIO*

2.15.1 The Organism

The newly proposed family *Vibrionaceae* comprises only the genus *Vibrio*, with 63 species. These are gram-negative, curved, usually motile rods, which are mesophilic, chemoorganotrophic, have a facultative fermentative metabolism, and are found in aquatic habitats and in association with eukaryotes (Thompson et al., 2004). *V. cholerae*, *V. parahaemolyticus*, and *V. vulnificus* are serious human pathogens of this family.

V. cholerae is subdivided into over 200 serogroups, based on the somatic O antigen. However, only serogroup O1 and the recently emerged O139 have been associated with severe disease and cholera pandemics. The O1 serogroup is divided into two biotypes, classical and El Tor, which can be differentiated by use of assays of hemolysis, hemagglutination, phage, polymyxin B sensitivity, the Voges–Proskauer reaction, or by means of detecting biotype-specific genes. Each of the O1 biotypes can be further subdivided into two major serotypes, Ogawa and Inaba (Sack et al., 2004; Thompson et al., 2004).

A *V. parahaemolyticus* serotyping system based on lipopolysaccharide (O) and capsular (K) antigens has been useful for epidemiological purposes. At least 12 O groups and 65 K groups have been recognized, and antisera for all of these groups are commercially available. Three biotypes (biogroups) of *V. vulnificus*, designated 1, 2, and 3, have been established based on characteristics such as indole production, host specificity, serotype, and genetic subtyping.

2.15.2 The Illness

V. cholerae causes cholera, a severe disease resulting from the ingestion of food or water contaminated with the organism. An infectious dose of around 10^8 bacteria is needed to cause severe cholera in healthy volunteers. The bacteria must pass through and survive the gastric acid barrier of the stomach, then adhere and colonize the intestine and produce cholera toxin, a potent enterotoxin that causes the severe watery diarrhea characteristic of the disease. Other virulence factors that may contribute to virulence include a toxin-coregulated pilus, accessory colonization factors, outer membrane proteins, hemolysins, and hemagglutinins. The primary site of *V. cholerae* colonization is the small intestine. Symptoms usually appear about 18 h to 5 days following ingestion of contaminated food or water, and include watery diarrhea and vomiting. The most distinctive feature of cholera is the painless purging of voluminous stools resembling rice water. In adults with severe cholera, the rate of diarrhea may reach 500 to 1000 mL/h, leading to severe dehydration. Death occurs if inappropriate rehydration and treatment are provided (Sack et al., 2004; Thompson et al., 2004). *V. parahaemolyticus* is capable of causing gastroenteritis. Typical clinical signs include diarrhea, abdominal pain, nausea, vomiting, headache, fever, and chills, with incubation periods ranging from 4 to 96 h. A thermostable direct hemolysin and a thermostable direct hemolysin-related hemolysin are considered the important virulence factors of this pathogen. Other toxins, proteases, cytolysins, and pili may also play a role as virulence factors in *V. parahaemolyticus*.

V. vulnificus is capable of causing severe and often fatal infections in susceptible persons. *V. vulnificus* causes two distinct disease syndromes, primary septicemia and necrotizing wound infections. Among healthy people, it normally causes vomiting, diarrhea, and abdominal pain; but among certain immunocompromised persons, the microorganism can infect the bloodstream, causing septic shock that is fatal in about 50% of cases. A capsular polysaccharide is the primary virulence factor in pathogenesis and is thought to play an inflammatory role within the human body (Thompson et al., 2004).

2.15.3 Contamination of Foods

Vibrios are highly abundant in aquatic environments, including estuaries, marine coastal waters and sediments, and aquaculture settings worldwide (Thompson et al.,

2004). The seasonality of infections, which occur mainly during the warmer months, suggests that water temperature may be an important factor in the epidemiology of *Vibrio* infection. It has been shown that warm environmental temperatures favor rapid growth of vibrios (Sack et al., 2004). Vibrios survive and multiply in association with zooplankton and phytoplankton. Within the marine environment they attach to surfaces provided by plants, green algae, copepods, crustaceans, and insects. Raw or undercooked seafood and contaminated water are the usual vehicles for transmission of vibrios, and oysters, shrimp, clam, mussels, and fish are common sources of infection (Sack et al., 2004; Thompson et al., 2004).

2.15.4 Prevention and Control

Personal hygiene and appropriate food preparation contribute greatly in preventing the occurrence and reducing the severity of outbreaks. Measures such as providing a safe water supply, improving sanitation, cooking high-risk foods (especially seafood), and providing health education would help to control the diseases caused by vibrios.

2.16 *YERSINIA*

2.16.1 The Organism

The yersiniae are gram-negative bacteria that belong to the family Enterobacteriaceae. They consist of 11 species, three of which are pathogenic to humans: *Yersinia pestis, Y. pseudotuberculosis,* and *Y. enterocolitica.*

Y. enterocolitica is a gram-negative, facultative anaerobic foodborne pathogen that has the ability to grow at refrigeration temperatures and survive repeated freezing and thawing, which is a concern for food safety (Bowman et al., 2007). This bacterium has a temperature range for growth usually between 4 and 42°C, but growth has been observed at temperatures as low as −2°C. Growth of *Y. enterocolitica* in foods stored at refrigeration temperatures (e.g., chicken and beef stored at 0 to 1°C or pasteurized milk held at 4°C) has also been reported.

2.16.2 The Illness

After consumption of contaminated food or water with enteropathogenic *Y. pseudotuberculosis* or *Y. enterocolitica,* the organisms pass into the small intestine, where they can translocate across the intestinal epithelium at sites of lymphoid tissue in the gut known as Peyer's patches. Both enteropathogens then migrate to the mesenteric lymph nodes and are subsequently found in the liver and spleen, where they replicate extracellularly. This originates a rapid inflammation, which gives rise to the symptoms that are associated with gastroenteritis. The disease can range from a self-limiting gastroenteritis to a potentially fatal septicemia.

Clinical manifestations include abdominal pain, fever, diarrhea, nausea, and vomiting persisting for 5 to 14 days, occasionally lasting for several months. The importance of *Y. pseudotuberculosis* as a causative agent of human infections worldwide is lower than that of *Y. enterocolitica* (Bowman et al., 2007; Niskanen et al., 2002).

2.16.3 Contamination of Foods

Yersinia is widely distributed in nature and in animal hosts; however, swine serve as a major host for human pathogenic strains (Annamalai and Venkitanarayanan, 2005). Although pork and pork products are considered to be the primary vehicles of *Y. enterocolitica* infection, drinking water and a variety of other foods, including milk, dairy products, beef, lamb, seafood, cheese, tofu, raw vegetables, fresh produce, and seafood, have also been implicated (Annamalai and Venkitanarayanan, 2005; Bowman et al., 2007).

2.16.4 Prevention and Control

Y. enterocolitica is one of the foodborne pathogens that have a wide temperature range of growth, particularly at low temperatures. Hence, contamination of refrigerated foods by the microbe could represent a significant health hazard.

2.17 MYCOTOXINS AND FUNGI

Most mycotoxins of concern are produced by three genera of fungi: *Aspergillus*, *Penicillium*, and *Fusarium*. However, a mycotoxin can be produced by several members of different genus. Here, the most important characteristics of major mycotoxins that contaminate foods are described.

2.17.1 Aflatoxins

Aflatoxins can be produced by four species of *Aspergillus*: *A. flavus*, *A. parasiticus*, *A. nomius*, and *A. pseudotamarii*. Four major aflatoxins, B_1, B_2, G_1, and G_2, plus two additional metabolic products, M_1 and M_2, are significant as direct contaminants of foods and feeds (CAST, 2003).

These metabolites have been implicated in carcinogenicity, mutagenicity, teratogenicity, hepatotoxicity, and aflatoxicosis. Epidemiological studies provide evidence of the carcinogenicity of aflatoxins to humans. Aflatoxicosis is the major syndrome associated with aflatoxins, and the liver is the primary target organ in different animal species. Acute aflatoxicosis follows high to moderate consumption, which provokes fatty, pale, and decolorized livers, derangement of normal blood clotting mechanisms, resulting in hemorrhages, reduction in total serum proteins of the liver, accumulation of blood in the gastrointestinal canal, glomerular nephritis, and lung congestion (Humpf and Voss, 2004).

These fungi invade and grow in a vast array of food and agricultural commodities, and the resulting contamination with aflatoxins often makes these products unfit for consumption (García and Heredia, 2006). Aflatoxins have been found in many foods of animal and plant origin, including cornmeal, peanuts, Brazil nuts, pistachio nuts, cottonseeds, oilseeds, pumpkin seeds, wheat, cassava, rice, cocoa, bread, macaroni, copra, figs, sausage, meat pies, cooked meat, milk, cheese, and eggs. Among these products, frequent preharvest contamination of corn, cotton, peanuts, and tree nuts are of the most concern, because of the level of contamination and consumption by the population of these commodities as food and feed for animals (Bathnagar and García, 2001; García and Heredia, 2006).

Strategies for reducing aflatoxin contamination include development of resistant hybrid corn, control of insect populations in the field to avoid plant injury, nixtamalization (alkaline cooking), and extrusion procedures.

2.17.2 Deoxynivalenol

Deoxynivalenol (DON or vomitoxin) is produced by species such as *F. graminearum* and *F. culmorum*. It can be a significant contaminant of wheat, barley, corn, commercial cattle feed, mixed feed, and oats (CAST, 2003). The LD_{50} values range from 50 to 70 mg/kg body weight. DON exhibits biological effects at very low concentrations, and exposure to as little as 0.1 mg/kg body weight per day may have an adverse effect on the immune response of many animals (CAST, 2003).

Contamination with DON occurs primarily in the field prior to harvesting. An extrusion cooking procedure has been reported to be effective to reduce or eliminate the presence of deoxynivalenol contamination. However, this method is not effective at removing FB_1 when it is also present. Extrusion cooking is therefore an appropriate treatment for deoxynivalenol-contaminated maize in places where, because of the prevailing conditions, these are the only toxins present (García and Heredia, 2006).

2.17.3 Fumonisins

Fumonisins are produced by *Fusarium verticillioides* (syn., *moniliforme*) and *F. proliferatum*. Of the more than 15 fumonisin isomers that have been described so far, fumonisins B_1, B_2, and B_3 are the most abundant. These toxins have been associated epidemiologically and experimentally with equine leucoencephalomalacia, pulmonary edema in swine, and human esophageal cancer (García and Heredia, 2006). Fumonisins are considered to be risk factors for cancer and possibly neural tube defects in some heavily exposed populations.

These metabolites occur primarily in corn and corn-based foods and feeds worldwide. Cleaning corn to remove damaged or moldy kernels reduces fumonisins in foods. Fumonisins are water soluble, and nixtamalization (cooking in alkaline water) lowers the fumonisin content of food products if the cooking liquid is discarded. Baking, frying, and extrusion cooking of corn at high temperatures also reduces fumonisin concentrations in foods, with the amount of reduction achieved depending on cooking time, temperature, recipe, and other factors (Humpf and Voss, 2004).

2.17.4 Ochratoxin

Ochratoxin A is a nephrotoxic secondary metabolite produced by *Penicillum verrucosum* in temperate climates, and *Aspergillus alutaceus, A. carbonarius,* and *A. niger* in hot climates. Ochratoxin A contamination is recognized as a potential human health hazard and has become a more significant public health concern since its classification as a possible human carcinogen, and its association with disorders such as Balkan nephropathy, a human kidney disease. Furthermore, immunosuppressive, teratogenic, and genotoxic activities have been demonstrated (García and Heredia, 2006).

The toxin is found primarily in stored cereal grains, such as barley, rye, wheat, corn, oats, and feeds, although natural occurrence in dry beans, moldy peanuts, coffee, raisins, grapes, dried fruits, nuts, olives, cheese, tissues of swine, sausage, fish, and wine has also been reported (Bathnagar and Garcia, 2001).

2.17.5 Patulin

This mycotoxin has frequently been found in damaged apples, apple cider, apple and pear juices, and other foods. Although the occurrence of patulin in these products is due primarily to *Penicillium* species, *Aspergillus clavatus* and other fungi have the ability to produce it, and could also account for its occurrence. The compound is toxic and produces tumors in rats when injected subcutaneously, but there are no published toxicological or epidemiological data to indicate whether consumption of patulin is harmful for humans. Although it is found in several food products, such as moldy feed and wheat, the major concern is its occurrence in apples and apple products (Bathnagar and García, 2001).

2.17.6 T-2 Toxin

T-2 toxin is produced primarily by *Fusarium sporotrichioides* and also by *F. poae,* and occurs rarely on cereals such as wheat and maize. These fungi are essentially saprophytic; therefore, they would not be associated with human foods except under exceptional circumstances. The toxin is considered to have played a role in large-scale human poisonings in Siberia during this century. T-2 toxin causes outbreaks of hemorrhagic disease in animals and has been associated with alimentary toxic aleukia in humans (García and Heredia, 2006).

2.17.7 Zearalenone

Zearalenone is a secondary metabolite produced by *Fusarium graminearum, F. culmorum, F. equiseti,* and *F. crookwellese*, species that are common contaminants of cereal crops worldwide (García and Heredia, 2006). Zearalenone may be an important etiologic agent of intoxication in young children or fetuses exposed to this estrogenic compound, which results in premature thelarche, pubarche, and breast enlargement (CAST, 2003). These types of endocrine disrupters have recently received much public attention and are widely believed to reduce male fertility in humans and in wildlife populations (García and Heredia, 2006).

It has been determined that the reduced form of zearalenone, zearalenol, has increased estrogenic activity; in fact, both zearalenol and zearalenone have been patented as oral contraceptives (García and Heredia, 2006). Zearalenone production is favored by high humidity and has been found in corn, moldy hay, and pelleted and commercial feed. It may also cooccur with DON in grains such as wheat, barley, oats, and corn (CAST, 2003).

2.18 *CRYPTOSPORIDIUM*

2.18.1 The Organism

Cryptosporidium is a protozoan parasite that causes waterborne outbreaks. Although *C. parvum* and *C. hominis* are the most prevalent species causing disease in humans, infections by *C. felis*, *C. meleagridis*, *C. canis*, and *C. muris* have also been reported (Anonymous, 2004). The transmissible stage of *C. parvum* is the oocyst, which when carried in the feces of humans and companion or domestic animals and wildlife can contaminate surface water (Kniel and Jenkins, 2005).

2.18.2 The Illness

Ingestion of relatively few oocysts can result in an acute self-limited gastrointestinal illness that lasts 1 to 2 weeks in previously healthy persons or indefinitely in those who are immunocompromized. The incubation period after ingestion is about 3 to 11 days, and clinical manifestations range from asymptomatic infections to severe, life-threatening illness. The symptoms include a secretory type of watery diarrhea, vomiting, fever, nausea, anorexia, malaise, abdominal pain, and weight loss (Anonymous, 2004; Casemore, 1990).

2.18.3 Contamination of Foods

Most human infections are probably due to *C. parvum;* infection with this species is also common in livestock animals, especially cattle and sheep, although pigs, goats, and horses can also be infected. Sporulated oocysts are excreted by the infected host through feces and possibly through other routes, such as respiratory secretions.

Transmission of *Cryptosporidium* occurs mainly through contact with contaminated water (e.g., drinking or recreational water) (Anonymous, 2004). Outbreaks of cryptosporidiosis have been associated with different foods, including inadequately pasteurized milk and raw milk, apple cider, basil, green onions, cold chicken salad, raw sausages, and tripe (Anonymous, 2004; Casemore, 1990).

2.18.4 Prevention and Control

This protozoan parasite is a serious issue for the water and fresh produce industry, since contamination via contaminated irrigation waters may occur. Furthermore, food can be contaminated with feces from food handlers who are excreting oocysts.

Of special interest are those foods that are not cooked or heated after handling (Casemore, 1990). Thermal treatments have been very effective for inactivation of protozoan parasites.

High concentrations of salt, glycerol, sucrose, or ethanol have a significant negative effect on oocyst survival. Carbonation, low pH, and alcohol content have been shown to decrease the viability of *C. parvum* oocysts in beverages; membrane filtration, ultraviolet light, high pressure, and irradiation are techniques to control this parasite in foods (Erickson and Ortega, 2006).

2.19 *CYCLOSPORA*

2.19.1 The Organism

Cyclospora is a protozoan that causes cyclosporiasis. *Cyclospora* species are found in humans, insectivores, and other animals; however, *Cyclospora cayatanensis* is the only species of this genus found in humans (Erickson and Ortega, 2006).

2.19.2 The Illness

Cyclosporiasis results after ingestion of contaminated food or water. Ingested oocysts excyst in the gastrointestinal tract and free the sporozoites, which invade the epithelial cells of the small intestine (Erickson and Ortega, 2006). Symptoms of the illness include frequent watery stools, flulike symptoms, and other gastrointestinal complaints, such as flatulence and burping. Anorexia and weight loss are also common. If untreated, symptoms may last for a few days to a month or longer and may follow a relapsing course (Werker, 1997).

2.19.3 Contamination of Foods

Potential sources of infection include fruits and vegetables such as fresh raspberries, lettuce, and basil that could be contaminated with feces of ill persons (Erickson and Ortega, 2006; Werker, 1997).

2.19.4 Prevention and Control

Washing fresh fruit and vegetables using potable water may reduce the likelihood of transmission of the parasite, and commercial freezing and pasteurization inactivate *Cyclospora* oocysts. Good agriculture and handling practices should also be applied to reduce the risk of contamination (Werker, 1997).

2.20 *ENTAMOEBA*

2.20.1 The Organism

Amebiasis is caused by *Entamoeba histolytica,* a protozoan that is 10 to 60 μm in length and moves through via an extension of fingerlike pseudopods (Kucik et al.,

2004). The two stages in the *E. histolytica* life cycle are cysts and trophozoites. Infective cysts are spheres about 12 μm in diameter and can be spread via the fecal–oral route by contaminated food and water or by oral–anal sexual practices.

2.20.2 The Illness

Ingested cysts hatch into trophozoites in the small intestine and move down the digestive tract to the colon. Ameba trophozoites then become cysts that are passed in the stool and can survive for weeks in a moist environment. Infection follows ingestion of viable cysts, with a clinical incubation of a few days to many months (commonly, 2 to 6 weeks). Dysentery with bloody or mucoid diarrhea can occur and in some cases will spread through the bloodstream to the liver, lung, and brain. Most infections, however, are asymptomatic or produce only mild bowel disturbance (Casemore, 1990; Kucik et al., 2004).

2.20.3 Contamination of Foods

Transmission occurs via the fecal–oral route, usually by poor hygiene of food handlers, poor water quality, or by the use of crop fertilization with human waste. The prevalence of amebiasis in Asia, Africa, and Latin America is important. Approximately 10% of the world's population is infected, yet 90% of infected persons are asymptomatic (Casemore, 1990; Kucik et al., 2004).

2.20.4 Prevention and Control

Proper sanitation and hygiene practices are important for avoiding contamination by cysts, and disinfection of water and good agriculture practices are also important. In addition, thermal treatments have been very effective for inactivation of protozoan parasites (Erickson and Ortega, 2006; Kucik et al., 2004).

2.21 *GIARDIA*

2.21.1 The Organism

The common protozoan *Giardia lamblia* is a flagellate protozoan that is an important human pathogen. It is a pear-shaped, binucleate, flagellated organism with trophic (feeding) and cystic (resting) stages. *Giardia* is possibly the most common parasite infection of humans worldwide (Casemore, 1990; Kucik et al., 2004).

2.21.2 The Illness

The life cycle of *Giardia* consists of two stages: the fecal–orally transmitted cyst and the disease-causing trophozoite. Infection can result after ingestion of at least 10 to 25 cysts through contaminated water or food, or by person-to-person contact. Infection may be asymptomatic or result in a broad spectrum of symptoms. After an incubation period of 1 to 2 weeks, symptoms may include nausea, vomiting, malaise, flatulence, abdominal cramps, diarrhea, steatorrhea, fatigue, and weight loss (Casemore, 1990).

2.21.3 Contamination of Foods

Infected persons can excrete cysts intermittently in the stools for weeks or months. Cysts can be found in sewage effluents, in surface waters, and in some potable water supplies. Foodborne transmission can occur with ingestion of raw or undercooked foods. Food-associated outbreak cases have been associated with consumption of cysts of *Giardia*-contaminated salmon and cream cheese dip, cold noodle salad, and fruit salad (Casemore, 1990).

2.21.4 Prevention and Control

Giardiasis is zoonotic, and cross-infectivity among beaver, cattle, dogs, rodents, and bighorn sheep ensures a constant reservoir. Personal hygiene is important to prevent spread from asymptomatic carriers, and includes careful hand washing before preparing meals and after going to the bathroom by food handlers. *Giardia* is resistant to the chlorine levels in normal tap water and survives well in cold mountain streams, but is susceptible to heat and probably to prolonged freezing, although ice used in drinks has been implicated as the source of infection in some cases (Casemore, 1990; Kucik et al., 2004).

2.22 *ANISAKIS SIMPLEX*

2.22.1 The Organism

Anisakis simplex is a nematode parasite that belongs to the Anisakidae family. These nematodes are known to cause a disease referred to as anisakinosis, anisakiasis, or anisakidosis in humans. The life cycle of *Anisakis* involves larval stages with several intermediary hosts and the adult stage, during which the worm parasitizes the stomachs of marine mammals (Lunestad, 2003).

2.22.2 The Illness

Humans can be infected by eating raw or undercooked fish or seafood that contains the third-stage larvae of *A. simplex*. The larvae usually penetrate the gastric wall, causing acute abdominal pain, nausea, diarrhea, and vomiting within a few minutes to several hours (gastric anisakiasis). The organism occasionally penetrates the peritoneal cavity or other visceral organs to cause eosinophilic granuloma. Allergic reactions may accompany or dominate the clinical manifestations (Lunestad, 2003).

2.22.3 Contamination of Foods

The disease has been reported frequently from the Netherlands, Japan, Korea, France, and the United States (Lunestad, 2003). Raw or lightly salted or marinated fish has been involved as the cause of disease in these countries (Lunestad, 2003).

2.22.4 Prevention and Control

Cooking or freezing of all products from fish that are to be eaten raw are useful to reduce the transmission of the nematode. For freezing, a core temperature of at least −20°C for at least 24 h has to be obtained prior to consumption (Lunestad, 2003). Apparently, the antigens produced by anisakid larvae are thermoresistant, and common prophylactic methods (cooking or freezing) may therefore not prevent allergic reactions among consumers.

2.23 *ASCARIS*

2.23.1 The Organism

Ascaris lumbricoides and *A. suum* are very closely related and are capable of cross-infecting both humans and pigs (Brownell and Nelson, 2006). *A. lumbricoides* is a helminth that causes ascariasis, a major public health problem in developing tropical countries.

2.23.2 The Illness and Contamination of Foods

Eggs of the organism can be ingested via water, food, or hands contaminated with human feces. Symptoms of pneumonitis with coughing, wheezing, pulmonary infiltrates, and fever occur after the eggs hatch in the small intestine and the larvae travel to the respiratory system. Gastrointestinal symptoms include abdominal pain, nausea, and vomiting, with vomitus sometimes containing worms. The adult worms are more than 20 cm in length, hence are easily seen in stool. Worms may also emerge from the nose or mouth as a result of coughing or vomiting. After passage in stool, eggs mature and become infective in 5 to 10 days; they may remain so for up to 2 years (Roberts and Kemp, 2001).

2.23.3 Prevention and Control

Ascariasis is among the most common helminthic infections worldwide (about a fourth of the world's population), and the global infection burden has been estimated to be approximately 1.5 billion people. Ascariasis leads to a host of physical and mental disabilities, including cognitive and societal impairment, higher susceptibility to infection, decreased responsiveness to vaccination, and malnutrition, which impairs the development of several hundred million children in developing countries (Brownell and Nelson, 2006; Jackson, 2001).

The control of ascariasis is hindered by the strong resistance of *Ascaris* eggs to inactivation. Chemicals and treatments that inactivate most pathogens (strong acids and bases, oxidants, reductants, protein-disrupting agents, and surface-active agents) have been proven ineffective against *Ascaris*; however, *Ascaris* eggs can be inactivated in minutes by temperatures above 60°C, although they can survive for more than 1 year at 40°C (Brownell and Nelson, 2006).

2.24 *DIPHYLLOBOTHRIUM LATUM*

Diphyllobothriasis is an intestinal infection caused by the fish tapeworm *Diphyllobothrium latum*. Infective larvae of the organism reside in the muscles of trout, salmon, pike, and sea bass, and contaminated raw seafood is a common cause of the disease (Nawa et al., 2005). After being ingested, the larvae (plerocercoids) attach to the mucosa of the small intestine, where they become adult worms about 5 to 10 m in length. The disease is regularly observed in northern Europe, northern America, and Japan.

2.25 *TAENIA*

2.25.1 The Organism

Taenia solium and *Taenia saginata* are important causes of zoonotic diseases in humans. Bovine cysticercosis is caused by the larval stage of the human tapeworm *T. saginata,* and porcine cysticercosis is produced by *T. solium* (Rodriguez-Canul et al., 2002; Geysen et al., 2007).

2.25.2 The Illness and Contamination of Foods

Human infection with *T. saginata* occurs after eating raw or undercooked meat containing viable cysticerci, and transmission to animals occurs upon contamination of food or water by feces of infected humans. Infection with *T. saginata* in humans is often mild and may continue for years without recognizable symptoms, however, when present, symptoms include abdominal pains, headache, and increased appetite (Geysen et al., 2007).

T. solium is transmitted between humans, who carry the adult worm in the intestine, and pigs, which carry the parasite in its larval (cyst or metacestode) stage in muscle tissue (Rodriguez-Canul et al., 2002). Infection of humans by *T. solium* occurs after the ingestion of undercooked infected pork meat. Although the pathogenicity of adult *T. solium* organisms in humans is asymptomatic, infection with the parasite's eggs can lead to massive metacestode infection. In humans, cysts can lodge in the central nervous system and cause neurocysticercosis, a serious problem causing severe and irreversible neurological disturbances. It is considered that neurocysticercosis is responsible for up to 25% of all cases of epilepsy in tropical areas (Rodriguez-Canul et al., 2002).

2.25.3 Prevention and Control

Cysticercosis by *T. solium* is endemic to most developing countries and is seen increasingly in industrialized countries because of immigration. *T. saginata* also remains a major problem in some cattle-raising areas of the world. To control the parasite, good farming practices are necessary, including avoiding contact of animals with human feces (Rodriguez-Canul et al., 2002). Pork meat has to be inspected and appropriate sanitation in slaughterhouses applied. Temperatures higher than 65°C have to be applied to damage *T. solium* metacestodes in pork and pork products, and in the case of *T. saginata*, freezing and proper heat treatment kill the parasite. A generalized infection of a carcass with *T. saginata* causes it to be declared unfit for human consumption; however, lightly infected carcasses are not condemned provided long-term storage at low temperatures (−10°C for 10 days) is used (Geysen et al., 2007).

2.26 *TRICHINELLA SPIRALIS*

2.26.1 The Organism

Several nematode species of the genus *Trichinella* can cause trichinellosis in humans. *T. spiralis,* which is found in many carnivorous and omnivorous animals, and *T. pseudospiralis,* found in mammals and birds, are distributed throughout the world. *T. nativa* is found in arctic and near-arctic regions and infects bears and mammals; *T. nelsoni* is present in equatorial Africa in felid predators and scavenger animals; and *T. bitovi* is present in Europe and western Asia in carnivores but not in domestic swine (Forbes et al., 2003).

2.26.2 The Illness and Contamination of Foods

Clinical trichinellosis in humans is associated with the consumption of tissues (usually, from pork or the meat of horses or certain carnivores) containing more than 1 larva per gram of tissue. The disease is usually asymptomatic or mildly symptomatic; heavy infection can cause myalgias, periorbital edema, eosinophilia, and in rare cases, death (Forbes et al., 2003).

2.26.3 Prevention and Control

Time–temperature combinations for the freezing and cooking of meat are used to kill *T. spiralis,* a freeze-sensitive nematode. Larvae in pork may be rendered noninfective by heating to a temperature of 77°C. Freezing at −15°C for 3 weeks, as in a home freezer, will generally kill larvae in meat; however, *T. nativa*, which is freeze tolerant, can survive in tissues stored frozen for months or years.

2.27 HEPATITIS A AND E VIRUSES

2.27.1 The Organism

The hepatitis A (HAV) and E (HEV) viruses can cause hepatitis in humans. HAV can originate hepatitis A, a liver disease that in rare cases, may cause death in humans.

Hepatitis A is a common form of acute viral hepatitis in many parts of the world. HAV is a RNA virus in the family Picornaviridae. HAV are small, nonenveloped spherical viruses measuring between 27 and 32 nm in diameter. HEV is situated in the caliciviruses group (Koopmans et al., 2002).

2.27.2 The Illness

Hepatitis A is relatively self-limiting, although it lasts up to several months. It is an acute infection of the liver, with fever, nausea, headache, abdominal discomfort, and jaundice. The virus enters via the intestinal tract, and is transported to the liver following a viremic stage in which virus is shed via the bile (Koopmans et al., 2002). Among children younger than 6 years of age, most infections are asymptomatic, and children with symptoms rarely develop jaundice. Among older children and adults, infection is usually symptomatic, with jaundice occurring in the majority of patients (Chancellor et al., 2006; Koopmans et al., 2002). HEV has only relatively recently been established as a cause of waterborne hepatitis outbreaks. The primary source for HEV infection appears to be fecally contaminated water. The virus is endemic over a wide geographic area, primarily in countries with inadequate sanitation where HAV is endemic as well (e.g., southeast Asia, Indian subcontinent, Africa), but not as widespread as HAV. HEV outbreaks have a higher attack rate of clinical disease in persons from 15 to 40 years of age compared with other groups, higher overall case fatality rates (0.5 to 3%), and an unusually high death toll in pregnant women (15 to 20%)(Koopmans et al., 2002).

2.27.3 Contamination of Foods

HAV is transmitted by the fecal–oral route, either by direct contact with a person infected with hepatitis A virus or by ingestion of food or water that has been contaminated with the virus (Chancellor et al., 2006). The majority of foodborne outbreaks of hepatitis A typically occur when food is contaminated by an infected food-service worker at the point of sale or service (Chancellor et al., 2006). In outbreak situations, up to 20% of cases are due to secondary transmission. Waterborne outbreaks are unusual but have been reported in association with drinking fecally contaminated water and swimming in contaminated swimming pools and lakes. A wide variety of foods have been involved in these outbreaks, including shellfish, sandwiches, dairy products, baked products, desserts, fruits, vegetables, and salads (Chancellor et al., 2006; Koopmans et al., 2002).

2.27.4 Prevention and Control

Hepatitis A virus can remain infectious on environmental surfaces for at least one month, and outbreaks of hepatitis A caused by foods contaminated during harvesting or processing have been reported. To reduce the risk of contamination of shellfish, strict control of the quality of growing waters can prevent contamination. This includes control of waste disposal by commercial and recreational boats. The contamination of food products such as produce with HAV can occur at multiple steps throughout the farm-to-table food product chain, including cultivation, harvest, processing, and handling. Good handling practices are therefore very important in preventing foodborne viral infection, and include frequent handwashing and wearing gloves (Chancellor et al., 2006: Koopmans et al., 2002). In addition, heating foods (such as shellfish) to temperatures higher than 85°C for 1 min and disinfecting surfaces with a 1 : 100 solution of sodium hypochlorite in tap water will inactivate HAV (Koopmans et al., 2002).

2.28 NOROVIRUS

2.28.1 The Organism

Norovirus (NV) (formerly called Norwalk-like virus, NLV) is the most widely recognized agent of outbreaks of foodborne and waterborne viral gastroenteritis (Koopmans et al., 2002). Noroviruses are a genetically diverse group of RNA viruses belonging to the family Caliciviridae (Parashar and Monroe, 2001). Human caliciviruses are small, nonenveloped spherical viruses measuring between 28 and 35 nm (Koopmans et al., 2002).

2.28.2 The Illness

After infection with fewer than 100 viral particles and an incubation period of 1 to 3 days, infected persons may develop fever, diarrhea, nausea and vomiting, and headache as prominent symptoms. A large number of organisms are present in stools and vomitus. The illness is generally considered mild and self-limiting, lasting 1 to 3 days. NLV infections are highly contagious, resulting in a high rate of transmission to contacts (Chancellor et al., 2006; Koopmans et al., 2002).

2.28.3 Contamination of Foods

Outbreaks of NLV gastroenteritis (not only foodborne) are common in institutions such as nursing homes and hospitals. Many of the sporadic cases in the community are spread by person-to-person contact, while outbreaks are often associated with the ingestion of food or water contaminated by the virus. It has been shown that food handlers play an important role in the etiology of NLV outbreaks. Infected food handlers may transmit infectious viruses during the incubation period and after recovery from illness (Chancellor et al., 2006). In addition, several waterborne outbreaks of NLV have been described, by both direct (e.g., consumption of tainted water) and indirect (e.g., via washed fruits, by swimming or canoeing in recreational waters) contact (Koopmans et al., 2002). Outbreaks of foodborne disease have been associated with consumption of uncooked and cooked shellfish, ice, water, bakery products, various types of salads, and cold foods (Chancellor et al., 2006; Koopmans et al., 2002).

2.28.4 Prevention and Control

It is important to prevent contamination of harvesting waters with human feces. In addition, exclusion of suspected or ill food handlers, maintenance of strict personal hygiene, and good handling practices are required to minimize the risk of contamination (Chancellor et al., 2006; Koopmans et al., 2002).

REFERENCES

Annamali T, Venkitanarayanan K (2005): Expression of major cold shock proteins and genes by *Yersinia enterocolitica* in synthetic medium and foods. *J Food Prot*. 68:2454–2458.

Anonymous (2004): Cryptosporidiosis (*Cryptosporidium* spp.): a CDC review. *J Environ Health*. 67:52.

Bathnagar D, García S (2001): *Aspergillus*. In: Labbé RG, García S (Eds.). *Guide to Food-borne Pathogens*. Wiley, New York, pp. 35–50.

Bennett RW (2005): Staphylococcal enterotoxin and its rapid identification in foods by enzyme-linked immunosorbent assay-based methodology. *J Food Prot*. 68:1264–1270.

Betts GD (2000): Controlling *E. coli* O157. *Nutr Food Sci*. 30:183.

Bowman AS, Glendening C, Wittum TE, Lejeune JT, Stich RW, Funk JA (2007): Prevalence of *Yersinia enterocolitica* in different phases of production on swine farms. *J Food Prot*. 70:11–16.

Brownell SA, Nelson KL (2006): Inactivation of single-celled *Ascaris suum* eggs by low-pressure UV radiation. *Appl Environ Microbiol*. 72:2178–2184.

Brynestad S, Granum PE (2002): *Clostridium perfringens* and foodborne infections. *Int J Food Microbiol*. 74:195–202.

Butzler JP (2004): *Campylobacter*, from obscurity to celebrity. *Clin Microbiol Infect*. 10:868.

CAST (Council for Agricultural Science and Technology) (2003): *Mycotoxins: Risks in Plant, Animal, and Human Systems*. Task Force Report 139. CAST, Ames, IA.

Casemore D (1990): Foodborne illness: foodborne protozoal infection. *Lancet*. 336:1427.

Chan YC, Blaschek HP (2005): Comparative analysis of *Shigella boydii* 18 foodborne outbreak isolate and related enteric bacteria: role of rpoS and adiA in acid stress response. *J Food Prot*. 68:521–527.

Chancellor DD, Tyagi S, Bazaco MC, et al. (2006): Green onions: potential mechanism for hepatitis A contamination. *J Food Prot*. 69:1468–1472.

Clarke SC, Haigh RO, Freestone PPE, Williams PH (2002): Enteropathogenic *Escherichia coli* infection: history and clinical aspects. *Brt J Biomed Sci*. 59:123–127.

Clavijo RI, Loui C, Andersen GL, Riley LW, Lu S (2006): Identification of genes associated with survival of *Salmonella enterica* serovar Enteritidis in chicken egg albumen. *Appl Environ Microbiol*. 72:1055–1064.

Cocolin L, Rantsiou K, Lacumin L, Cantoni C, Comi G (2002): Direct identification in food samples of *Listeria* spp. and *Listeria monocytogenes* by molecular methods. *Appl Environ Microbiol*. 68:6273–6282.

Corry JK, Martin GL, Sortor BV (2004): Common intestinal parasites. *Am Fam Physician*. 69:1161–1168.

D'Aoust JY (2001). *Salmonella*. In: Labbé RG, García S (Eds.). *Guide to Food-borne Pathogens*. Wiley, New York, pp. 163–192.

Daskalov H (2006): The importance of *Aeromonas hydrophila* in food safety. *Food Control*. 17:474–483.

Dierick K, Coillie EV, Swiecicka I, et al. (2005): Fatal family outbreak of *Bacillus cereus*–associated food poisoning. *J Clin Microbiol*. 43:4277–4279.

Dinges MM, Orwin PM, Schlievert PM (2000): Exotoxins of *Staphylococcus aureus*. *Clin Microbiol Rev*. 13:16–34.

Erickson MC, Ortega YR (2006): Inactivation of protozoan parasites in food, water, and environmental systems. *J Food Prot*. 69:2786–2808

Feng P, Weagant S (2002): Diarrheagenic *Escherichia coli*. In: *Bacteriological Analytical Manual* online. http://www.cfsan.fda.gov/;ebam/bam-toc.html. Accessed February 2008.

Fera MT, Maugeri TL, Gugliandolo C, Beninati M, Giannone E (2004): Detection of *Arcobacter* spp. in the coastal environment of the Mediterranean sea. *Appl Environ Microbiol*. 70:1271–1276.

Fernández-Escartin E, García S (2001): Miscellaneous agents: *Brucella, Aeromonas, Plesiomonas* and b-hemolytic streptococci. In: Labbé RG, García S (Eds.). *Guide to Food-borne Pathogens*. Wiley, New York, pp. 295–314.

Forbes LB, Parker S, Scandrett WB (2003): Comparison of a modified digestion assay with trichinoscopy for the detection of *Trichinella* larvae in pork. *J Food Prot*. 66:1043–1046.

Fosse J, Seegers H, Magras C (2008): Foodborne zoonoses due to meat: a quantitative approach for a comparative risk assessment applied to pig slaughtering in Europe. *Vet Res*. 39, E-pub ahead of print.

García S, Heredia N (2006): Mycotoxins in Mexico: epidemiology, management, and control strategies. *Mycopathology*. 162:255–264.

Geysen D, Kanobana K, Victor B, Rodriguez-Jean de Borchgrave R, Brandt J, Dorny P (2007): Validation of meat inspection results for *Taenia saginata* cysticercosis by PCR—restriction fragment length polymorphism. *J Food Prot*. 70:236–240.

Heredia NL, Labbé RG (2001): Clostridium perfringens. In: Labbé RG, García S (Eds.). *Guide to Food-borne Pathogens*. Wiley, New York, pp. 133–142.

Humpf HU, Voss KA (2004): Effects of thermal food processing on the chemical structure and toxicity of fumonisin mycotoxins. *Mol Nutr Food Res*. 48:255–269.

Jackson GJ (2001): Parasites. In: Labbé RG, García S (Eds.). *Guide to Food-borne Pathogens*. Wiley, New York, pp. 285–294.

Kathariou S (2002): *Listeria monocytogenes* virulence and pathogenicity, a food safety perspective. *J Food Prot*. 65:1811–1829.

Kniel KE, Jenkins MC (2005): Detection of *Cryptosporidium parvum* oocysts on fresh vegetables and herbs using antibodies specific for a *Cryptosporidium parvum* viral antigen. *J Food Prot*. 68:1093–1096.

Koopmans M, Bonsdorff CHV, Vinje J, de Medici D, Monroe S (2002): Foodborne viruses. *FEMS Microbiol Rev*. 26:187–205.

Kucik CJ, Martin GL, Sortor BV (2004): Common intestinal parasites. *Am Fam Physician*. 69 (5):1161–1168.

Lamb JL, Gogley JM, Thompson MJ, Solis DR, Sen S (2002): Effect of low-dose gamma irradiation on *Staphylococcus aureus* and product packaging in ready-to-eat ham and cheese sandwiches. *J Food Prot*. 65:1800–1805.

Lehner A, Tasara T, Stephan R (2005): Relevant aspects of *Arcobacter* spp. as potential foodborne pathogen. *J Food Microbiol*. 102:127–135.

Lund BM, Peck MW (2001): Clostridium botulinum. In: Labbé RG, García S (Eds.). *Guide to Food-borne Pathogens*. Wiley, New York, pp. 69–85.

Lunestad BT (2003): Absence of nematodes in farmed Atlantic salmon (*Salmo salar* L.) in Norway. *J Food Prot*. 66:122–124.

Mead PS, Slutsker L, Dietz V, et al. (1999): Food-related illness and death in the United States. *Emerg Infect Dis*. 5:607–625.

Miller WG, Mandrell RE (2005): Prevalence of *Campylobacter* in the food and water supply: incidence, outbreaks, isolation and detection. In: Kettley JM, Konkel ME (Eds.). Campylobacter: *Molecular and Cellular Biology*. Horizon Bioscience, Norfolk, UK, pp. 101–164.

Nataro JP, Kaper JB (1998): Diarrheagenic *Escherichia coli*. *Clin Microbiol Rev*. 11:142–201.

Nawa Y, Hatz C, Blum J (2005): Sushi delights and parasites: the risk of fishborne and foodborne parasitic zoonoses in Asia. *Clin Infect Dis*. 41:1297–1303.

Niskanen T, Fredriksson-Ahomaa M, Korkeala H (2002): *Yersinia pseudotuberculosis* with limited genetic diversity is a common finding in tonsils of fattening pigs. *J Food Prot*. 65:540–545.

Parashar UD, Monroe SS (2001): Norwalk-like viruses as a cause of foodborne disease outbreaks. *Rev Med Virol*. 11:243–252.

Prouzet-Mauleon V, Labadi L, Bouges N, Menard A, Megraud F (2006): *Arcobacter butzleri*: underestimated enteropathogen. *Emerg Infect Dis* 12 (2):307–309.

Rajkovic A, Uyttendaele M, Ombregt SA, Jaaskelainen E, Salkinoja-Salonen M, Debevere J (2006): Influence of type of food on the kinetics and overall production of *Bacillus cereus* emetic toxin. *J Food Prot*. 69:847–852.

Rasko DA, Altherr MR, Han CS, Ravel J (2005): Genomics of the *Bacillus cereus* group of organisms. *FEMS Microbiol Rev*. 29:303–329.

Roberts A, Kemp C (2001): Ascariasis. *J Am Acad Nurse Pract*. 13:55–57.

Rodriguez-Canul R, Argaez-Rodriguez F, Pacheco de la Gala D, et al. (2002): *Taenia solium* metacestode viability in infected pork after preparation with salt pickling or cooking methods common in Yucatan, Mexico. *J Food Prot*. 65:666–669.

Sack DA, Sack RB, Nair GB, Siddique AK (2004): Cholera. *Lancet*. 363:223–233.

Santos JA, Gonzalez CJ, Lopez TM, Otero A, Garcia-Lopez ML (1999): Hemolytic and elastolytic activities influenced by iron in *Plesiomonas shigelloides*. *J Food Prot*. 62:1475–1477.

Shachar D, Yaron S (2006): Heat tolerance of *Salmonella enterica* serovars Agona, Enteritidis, and Typhimurium in peanut butter. *J Food Prot*. 69:2687–2691.

Sharma SK, Shukla HD (2005): *Clostridium botulinum*: a bug with beauty and weapon. *Crit Rev Microbiol*. 31:11–18.

Sharma SK, Whiting RC (2005): Methods for detection of *Clostridium botulinum* toxin in foods. *J Food Prot*. 68:1256–1263.

Snelling WJ, Matsuda M, Moore JE, Dooley JSG (2005): Under the microscope *Campylobacter jejuni*. *Lett Appl Microbiol*. 41:297–302.

Tantillo G, Di Pinto A, Vergara A, Buonavoglia C (2001): Polymerase chain reaction for the direct detection of *Brucella* spp. in milk and cheese. *J Food Prot*. 64:164–167.

Thompson FL, Lida T, Swings J (2004): Biodiversity of vibrios. *Microbiol Mol Biol Rev*. 68:403–431.

Vandenberg O, Dediste A, Houf K, et al. (2004): *Arcobacter* species in humans. *Emerg Infect Dis*. 10:1863–1867.

Vazquez-Boland JA, Kuhn M, Bereche P, et al. (2001): *Listeria* pathogenesis and molecular virulence determinants. *Clin Microbiol Rev*. 14:584–640.

Werker DH (1997): Cyclosporiasis: another emerging pathogen comes ashore. *Can Med Assoc J*. 157:295.

Zaika LL (2002): Effect of organic acids and temperature on survival of *Shigella flexneri* in broth at pH 4. *J Food Prot*. 65:1417–1421.

PART II

EMERGING ISSUES

CHAPTER 3

CRONOBACTER GEN. NOV. (*ENTEROBACTER*) *SAKAZAKII*: CURRENT KNOWLEDGE AND FUTURE CONSIDERATIONS

GENISIS IRIS DANCER and DONG-HYUN KANG

3.1 INTRODUCTION

(Enterobacter) sakazakii is a gram-negative rod that causes severe illness in human infants, including necrotizing enterocolitis, septicemia, and meningitis. In 2008 the genus *Cronobacter* was proposed to accommodate (*E*). *sakazakii*, which is referred to here as (*E*). *sakazakii* gen. nov. until formal acceptance of the new genus (Iversen et al., 2008). Advances in supportive care have decreased the mortality rates of infections caused by (*E*). *sakazakii*, but survivors of meningitis face severe neurological sequelae. Most cases occur in infants less than 28 days old, and premature or low-birth-weight infants are especially susceptible, probably due to impaired immune response compared to full-term infants and adults. Adults have been infected with (*E*). *sakazakii*, but no cases of adult meningitis have been reported, and nearly all adults infected had underlying disease such as cancer. Antibiotic therapy against (*E*). *sakazakii* is effective, although recent evidence suggests that antibiotic resistance may be increasing.

Contaminated commercial infant formula powders have been implicated in several outbreaks and are suspected to be the main vehicle for (*E*). *sakazakii* infections. In a study of powdered infant formula around the world, 14% of samples were positive for (*E*). *sakazakii*, although none of the samples had more than 1 CFU/g. Controversy exists regarding the potential for (*E*). *sakazakii* to survive infant formula powder processing, but the ability of stationary-phase cells of (*E*). *sakazakii* to survive osmotic stress and drying for extended periods of time has been documented. Although (*E*). *sakazakii* has been isolated from a wide variety of sources, including food-manufacturing plants, indicating that it is widespread, the natural reservoir for (*E*).

Microbiologically Safe Foods, Edited by Norma Heredia, Irene Wesley, and Santos García

sakazakii is unknown. The ability to adhere to surfaces, including rubber, silicon, polycarbonate, and stainless steel, may explain the persistence of (*E*). *sakazakii* on infant formula preparation equipment and in food-manufacturing environments.

Traditionally, identification of (*E*). *sakazakii* required several steps, taking up to 7 days for positive identification. Recently, selective differential media have been developed, shortening the process by several days. Conventional and real-time PCR (polymerase chain reaction) methods have also been developed but do not yet have official approval. Isolation and detection techniques will continue to improve as more information becomes available. The full genome has been sequenced (4.36 Mb). In this chapter we seek to summarize current knowledge of (*E*). *sakazakii* and the implications for future research.

3.2 HISTORY OF ILLNESS CAUSED BY (*E*). *SAKAZAKII*

(*E*). *sakazakii* is largely an opportunistic pathogen, infecting primarily infants and, occasionally, immunocompromised or elderly patients. Infants, defined as children less than 1 year of age, and especially infants less than 28 days old, are the primary victims of (*E*). *sakazakii* infections (FAO/WHO, 2004). The well-documented outbreaks have occurred in hospital settings, especially neonatal intensive care units. However, the Centers for Disease Control and Prevention (CDC) has documented cases of (*E*). *sakazakii* bacteremia in infants at home. In infants, there are three main classes of illness associated with (*E*). *sakazakii*: meningitis, an inflammation of the membranes surrounding the brain, bacteremia or the more serious sepsis, and necrotizing enterocolitis (NEC).

The first outbreak of neonatal meningitis attributed to (*E*). *sakazakii* occurred in 1958, long before its recognition as a species (Urmenyi and Franklin, 1961). The mortality rate of infants who develop (*E*). *sakazakii*–associated neonatal meningitis is estimated to be 40 to 80% (Iversen and Forsythe, 2003). However, survivors face devastating neurological sequelae, including hydrocephalus, quadriplegia, and delayed neural development (Lai, 2001). The first report of bacteremia associated with (*E*). *sakazakii* was in 1979 (Monroe and Tift, 1979). The first reported outbreak of necrotizing enterocolitis was reported in 2001 (van Acker et al., 2001). The mortality rate for infants who develop NEC caused by (*E*). *sakazakii* is estimated to be 10 to 55%. Since its recognition as a new species, there have been at least 28 outbreaks worldwide, affecting at least 75 infants and causing at least 19 deaths (Iversen and Forsythe, 2003).

In at least four outbreaks, contaminated infant formula (IF) powders were confirmed to be the source of infection (Biering et al., 1989; CDC, 2002; Simmons et al., 1989; van Acker et al., 2001). Contamination of equipment used to prepare IF has caused at least two outbreaks (Block et al., 2002; Noriega et al., 1990). In one case, a blender that caused an outbreak continued to test positive for (*E*). *sakazakii* for 5 months after the initial testing (Block et al., 2002). The ability to survive in dry environments such as IF and on IF preparation equipment seems to be an important factor, enabling (*E*). *sakazakii* to cause disease.

Adults have also been infected with (*E*). *sakazakii*, mainly nosocomially acquired, meaning that the infection was contracted at the hospital rather than being the cause of hospitalization. Approximately 50% of nosocomial infections are caused by species in the genus *Enterobacter* (Leclerc et al., 2001). Cases have included urosepsis (Jimenez and Giménez, 1982), bacteremia (Hawkins et al., 1991), pneumonitis (Lai, 2001), and vaginal and wound infections. No cases of meningitis in adults caused by (*E*). *sakazakii* have been reported. Nearly all adults infected with (*E*). *sakazakii* have serious underlying medical conditions, especially cancers (Lai, 2001).

3.3 INFANT SUSCEPTIBILITY

Among infants infected with (*E*). *sakazakii*, most were less than 28 days old, about half weighed less than 2000 g, and two-thirds were born at less than 37 weeks' gestation, making them premature (FAO/WHO, 2004). Several factors probably contribute to the high susceptibility of such infants to (*E*). *sakazakii* infection. First, the immune system of preterm infants is deficient in several respects compared to full-term infants and adults. Polymorphonuclear leukocytes of preterm infants show impaired antibacterial response to lipopolysaccharide from *E. coli* (Henneke et al., 2003). Expression of interleukin-8 is also lower in preterm infant monocytes than in full-term infant and adult monocytes, which reduces the chemotactic response of neutrophils to the site of infection (Schibler et al., 1993). Finally, low levels of IgG antibodies, low levels of complement, proteins that signal antibody-mediated destruction of bacterial pathogens, and exhaustion of neutrophil storage pools, which phagocytize bacterial pathogens, also increase the susceptibility of preterm infants (Haeney, 1994).

Infants that are fed formula are at especially high risk, not only because IF is the most commonly implicated source of (*E*). *sakazakii*, but because formula-fed infants do not receive the antimicrobial agents found in human breast milk. Numerous epidemiological studies demonstrate that breast-fed infants have fewer infections, especially gastrointestinal and respiratory, than formula-fed infants (Cunningham et al., 1991). The benefits extend to preterm infants, with one study showing that preterm infants fed with donated human breast milk were three times less likely to develop necrotizing enterocolitis than were preterm infants fed with IF (McGuire and Anthony, 2003).

Relatively low levels of stomach acid, the buffering capacity of milk, and the use of high-iron-level infant formulas increase the susceptibility of infants to salmonellosis (Miller and Pegues, 2000) and may also contribute to susceptibility to (*E*). *sakazakii*. Iron is an important nutrient for Enterobacteriaceae. In human body fluids such as serum and breast milk, iron is sequestered by high-affinity iron-binding proteins such as transferrin and lactoferrin (Payne, 1988). However, in infant formula, iron is provided by addition of ferrous sulfate to a level of 12.2 μg/mL.

The level of iron found in IF may be a primary factor in the increased risk of infection for formula-fed infants. Chan (2003) found that addition of iron to human breast milk at levels which mimic that of a commercial breast milk fortifier decreased the zone of inhibition of (*E*). *sakazakii*, *E. coli*, *Staphylococcus*, and group B streptococci from greater than 20 mm to 0 mm when evaluated using the filter method. Chan (2003) concluded that addition of iron or human milk fortifiers containing iron reduces the antimicrobial properties of breast milk.

The addition of iron to both whey and casein-based infant formulas increases colonization of the intestine by clostridia and enterococci (Balmer and Wharton, 1991). In addition, the intestinal microflora of breast milk–fed infants is comprised mainly of bifidobacteria, lactobacilli, and staphylococci, while that of formula-fed infants is predominantly coliforms, enterococci, and bacteroides (Wharton et al., 1994). When mice were orally inoculated with organisms from the feces of human infants fed breast milk, the pH of their intestinal contents was lowered and their risk of *Salmonella* Typhimurium colonization was reduced (Hentges et al., 1992).

The iron-binding protein lactoferrin is present in both human and bovine milk. In the human stomach, lactoferrin is cleaved to generate an antimicrobial peptide known as lactoferricin. However, supplementation of IF with bovine lactoferrin has no effect on the composition of the intestinal microflora of formula-fed infants (Balmer and Wharton, 1991; Wharton et al., 1994). The lack of sufficient acid in the stomach of infants and the buffering capacity of IF may inhibit the cleavage of lactoferrin to lactoferricin.

Excessive iron may also increase the risk of necrotizing enterocolitis. Iron is a known catalyst of free-radical oxidation products, which are thought to play an important role in necrotizing enterocolitis (Raghuveer et al., 2002). When formula is supplemented with recombinant human lactoferrin, a reduction in iron-mediated free-radical generation and lipid peroxidation is observed (Raghuveer et al., 2002).

Clearly, the role of IF in neonatal infections is multifactorial, as it alters intestinal microflora composition compared to that of breast-fed infants, provides high iron availability for invading pathogens, and results in iron-mediated oxidation products, all of which increase the risk of infection.

Another factor that may contribute to infant susceptibility to (*E*). *sakazakii* is the use of prophylactic antibiotics against group B streptococci (GBS). Acquired from the maternal vagina during vaginal birth, GBS is the leading cause of neonatal meningitis in developed countries. Many countries have instituted prophylactic use of antibiotics, generally penicillin and ampicillin, which has lowered the incidence of GBS-associated sepsis by 50 to 80% (Moore et al., 2003). Since the inception of intrapartum antibacterial prophylaxis, concern has arisen that gram-negative bacterial meningitis is increasing as a result (Kaye, 2001). A recent review reports that gram-negative bacterial meningitis is not increased by intrapartum antibacterial prophylaxis, except in the case of preterm, low-birth-weight, and very low-birth-weight infants (Moore et al., 2003). This is precisely the group of infants that are at risk of (*E*). *sakazakii* infection. Although the source of (*E*). *sakazakii* is usually infant formula milk whereas the source for other gram-negative bacterial meningitis is maternal, prophylactic antibiotics may reduce the beneficial microflora obtained from the mother, thus increasing the risk of infection.

The numbers of neonatal infections caused by (*E*). *sakazakii* seems likely to rise as increasing numbers of mothers worldwide choose to feed their infants with powdered

IF. Despite recommendations outlined in the *International Code of Marketing of Breast-Milk Substitutes* by the World Health Organization (WHO, 1981), IF continue to be marketed as a processed food. The problems associated with the use of IF in developing countries include the difficulty of reading and following directions for use of dried IF, the inadequate supply of clean water for reconstitution, the high cost of the product, and poor sanitation. The high cost of IF may lead to improper reconstitution and prolonged storage of prepared formula. In countries where refrigeration is inadequate, these factors compound the risk of (*E*). *sakazakii* infection, as (*E*). *sakazakii* doubles in just 21 min at 37°C and 100 min at 21°C in IF (Iversen et al., 2004b).

Despite the widespread attention received by (*E*). *sakazakii* and the risk it poses to the most vulnerable segment of the world's population, the source and virulence mechanisms of (*E*). *sakazakii* are entirely unknown.

3.4 NOVEL PREVENTION STRATEGIES

A number of novel prevention strategies have been suggested for both specific anti-(*E*). *sakazakii* activity and for improving the safety of IF products. Naturally occurring fatty acids or their monoglycerides can inactivate a wide variety of bacterial pathogens, including *Chlamydia trachomatis* (Bergsson et al., 1998), *Neisseria gonorrhoeae* (Bergsson et al., 1999), *Helicobacter pylori* (Petschow et al., 1996), *Haemophilus influenza* and group B streptococci (Isaacs et al., 1995), *Listeria monocytogenes* and *E. coli* (Nair et al., 2004), and even some viral pathogens such as respiratory syncitial virus (Isaacs et al., 1995). Nair et al. (2004) found that (*E*). *sakazakii* in reconstituted IF can be reduced by greater than 5 log after 24 h of incubation at 4 or 8°C in the presence of 25 and 50 mM monocaprylin. When held at higher temperatures, such as 37°C, 25 and 50 mM monocaprylin reduce (*E*). *sakazakii* by 6 and 4 log, respectively. Other fatty acids and their monoglycerides have not been evaluated for reduction of (*E*). *sakazakii*.

An alternative to addition of free fatty acids or monoglycerides to IF is the addition of lipase to IF. Isaacs et al. (1992) found that addition of lipase to IF releases antibacterial and antiviral fatty acids. However, the effect of addition of lipase to IF against (*E*). *sakazakii* has not been evaluated, and rancid flavors may lead infants to reject IF treated with lipases. In light of the severity of disease associated with (*E*). *sakazakii*, the use of such novel intervention strategies should be reconsidered.

3.5 INFANT FORMULA PROCESSING

Powdered IF is produced using two basic schemes: the dry mix and wet mix methods. In the former, which is not commonly used, individual ingredients are dried, mixed, and packed into cans. The dry mix method is problematic from both quality and safety standpoints. Because the dried components may have different particle sizes and densities, obtaining a homogeneous mix is difficult, which may result in substandard product release or improper nutrient balance when the formula is prepared. The mixing of dry ingredients from many sources creates many more opportunities for contamination, and because there is no heat treatment after the combination of ingredients, a small amount of ingredient may contaminate and destroy a large volume of product. For these reasons, the wet mix method is in more common use today. The wet mix involves mixing the ingredients in a wet phase, pasteurization or other stringent heat-treatment, addition of heat-sensitive materials, and spray drying. Although these treatments theoretically kill all vegetative bacterial cells present prior to spray drying, there may be post–heat treatment contamination from the plant environment. One report suggests that a very small proportion (ca. 0.002%) of *E. coli* may survive the conventional spray-drying process (Chopin et al., 1977). Numerous reports exist of survival of spray drying by *Salmonella*, especially when concentrated milk products are fed into the dryer (Licari and Potter, 1970; McDonough and Hargrove, 1968; Miller et al., 1972). As some studies have found at least some strains of (*E*). *sakazakii* to be more heat tolerant (Edelson-Mammel and Buchanan, 2004) and dry stress tolerant (Breeuwer et al., 2003) than other Enterobacteriaceae, including some strains of *E. coli* and *Salmonella*, the possibility of survival of spray drying by (*E*). *sakazakii* should not be ruled out.

Clearly, a better understanding of (*E*). *sakazakii* would allow greater understanding of how this organism contaminates IF and how to prevent such contamination.

3.6 BIOCHEMICAL CHARACTERIZATION AND TAXONOMY

(*E*). *sakazakii* was first described as a yellow pigment–producing *Enterobacter cloacae* in the 8th edition of *Bergey's Manual of Determinative Bacteriology* (Sakazaki, 1974). At that time, only two species, *E. cloacae* and *E. aerogenes*, were recognized in the genera. Subsequent DNA–DNA hybridization studies showed that the pigment-producing strains were not closely related genetically to the non-pigment-producing strains (Steigerwalt et al., 1976). In 1980, (*E*). *sakazakii* was formally designated as a new species, named in honor of Japanese microbiologist Riichi Sakazaki (Farmer et al., 1980).

(*E*). *sakazakii* is a member of the family Enterobacteriaceae, which can be divided into two main groups based on fermentation characteristics: mixed acid and butanediol fermenters. The mixed acid fermenters include the genera *Escherichia*, *Shigella*, *Salmonella*, *Edwardsiella*, *Proteus*, and *Citrobacter* and produce three acids—lactate, succinate, and acetate—in addition to ethanol, carbon dioxide, and hydrogen, but not butanediol. The butanediol fermenters, which include the genera *Enterobacter*, *Erwinia*, *Hafnia*, *Klebsiella*, *Pantoea*, and *Serratia*, produce small amounts of lactate, succinate, and acetate, with the main products butanediol, ethanol, carbon dioxide, and hydrogen. Another major difference is the proportion of carbon dioxide to hydrogen gas produced: The mixed acid fermenters produce the gases in equal amounts, while the butanediol fermenters produce five times more carbon dioxide than hydrogen gas.

The butanediol fermenters are generally more closely related to one another than to the mixed acid fermenters, having a DNA GC content of 53 to 58%, higher than the mixed acid fermenters. The genus *Enterobacter* is motile, produces ornithine decarboxylase, and ferments both lactose and sorbitol.

(*E*). *sakazakii* can be distinguished from *E. cloacae* on the basis of delayed DNase production, inability to ferment sorbitol or produce phosphoamidase or oxidase, and the ability to produce α-glucosidase, Tween-80 esterase, and a yellow pigment. Muytjens et al. (1984) characterized the enzymatic profiles of 129 strains of (*E*). *sakazakii* and found that all (129/129) (*E*). *sakazakii* produced α-glucosidase, whereas none of the 60 *E. cloacae*, 19 *E. aerogenes*, or 18 *E. agglomerans* strains tested produced the enzyme. Furthermore, none of the (*E*). *sakazakii* strains tested showed phosphoamidase activity, whereas 72% of *E. cloacae*, 89% of *E. agglomerans* (now separated into *Escherichia vulneris* and *Pantoea agglomerans*), and 100% of *E. aerogenes* did.

However, only the inability to ferment sorbitol and the production of α-glucosidase and yellow pigment are currently used for phenotype-based identification systems. The lengthy incubation time necessary for Tween-80 esterase and DNase production limits their use in practical applications. Pigment production has been described as being more pronounced at room temperature than at higher incubation temperatures, but this may be due to the presence of light when plates are incubated on the benchtop rather than to the temperature. Yellow colonies can be produced within 24 h at 37°C if plates are simply exposed to visible light (Guillaume-Gentil et al., 2005), although the U.S. Food and Drug Administration (FDA) recommends incubation for several days at room temperature to observe pigment production. Although DNA–DNA hybridization remains the gold standard for identification of the closely related Enterobacteriaceae, little research was performed after the initial studies by Izard et al. (1983). Their study of 13 (*E*). *sakazakii* strains showed an average of 89 ± 10% homology to one another, but only 40 ± 4% homology to *E. cloacae*. The type strain ATCC 29544 was 95% genetically related to the strain chosen as the standard.

A recent phylogenetic study based on 16S rRNA and *hsp60* gene sequences indicates that (*E*). *sakazakii* is more closely related to *C. koseri* (97.8%) than to *E. cloacae* (97.0%) or *C. freundii* (96.0%) (Iversen et al., 2004c). Although the 16S rRNA gene sequences available may be unsuitable for constructing phylogenetic trees of Enterobacteriaceae, PCR amplification of the gene can successfully discriminate (*E*). *sakazakii* from other Enterobacteriaceae. Lehner et al. (2004) sequenced the entire 16S rRNA gene of 13 strains of (*E*). *sakazakii*, including isolates from fruit powder, infant food, milk, production environments, and humans. Two distinct phylogenetic lineages were discovered, with ATCC 51329 in its own lineage and the type strain ATCC 29544 in another, which contained all of the other isolates. The 13 isolates were 99.4 to 100% identical in sequence to type strain ATCC 29544, which was only 97.9% similar to ATCC 51329. The phylogenetic lineages were based separately on four regions described as polymorphism "hot spots." The taxonomy of the Enterobacteriaceae family is changing as more sophisticated genetic information becomes available.

3.7 ENVIRONMENTAL SOURCES OF (*E*). *SAKAZAKII*

The natural habitat or reservoir of (*E*). *sakazakii* is unknown. Muytjens and Kollee (1990) failed to isolate (*E*). *sakazakii* from surface water, soil, raw cow's milk, cattle, rodents, bird dung, domestic animals, grain, mud, or rotting wood. (*E*). *sakazakii* has been isolated from the midgut of *Stomoxys calcitrants*, a blood-sucking fly that preys on domestic cattle, which may contribute to the contamination of dairy products with (*E*). *sakazakii* (Hamilton et al., 2003). A multiple antibiotic-resistant strain of (*E*). *sakazakii* was isolated from 6 of 12 Mexican fruit flies belonging to a laboratory colony (Kuzina et al., 2001). The Mexican fruit fly, *Anastrepha ludens*, is usually associated with citrus fruits, but the multiple antibiotic resistance observed led the authors to speculate that fruit fly–associated bacteria may exchange genetic information with human or other animal-associated bacteria. Further supporting this hypothesis is a report by Burgos and Varela (2002) of a multiple antibiotic-resistant (*E*). *sakazakii* from the soil on a dairy farm.

Despite the failure of Muytjens and Kollee (1990) to isolate (*E*). *sakazakii* from surface waters, others have been able to do so. (*E*). *sakazakii* was among the most frequently isolated gram-negative rods isolated by Mosso et al. (1994) from mesothermal mineral springs in Spain. A vaginal infection due to (*E*). *sakazakii* in Budapest, Hungary was thought to have originated from warm surface water (26 to 28°C) in which the patient had been bathing (Ongradi, 2002). The occurrence of (*E*). *sakazakii* in warm surface waters is not well documention, but further isolation of (*E*). *sakazakii* from warm surface waters is likely.

Although the natural source of (*E*). *sakazakii* is unknown, it has been found in a wide variety of foods worldwide. In a survey of raw and ready-to-eat foods in restaurants in Valencia, Spain, one sample of raw lettuce was contaminated with (*E*). *sakazakii* (Soriano et al., 2001). Overall, (*E*). *sakazakii* was isolated from only one of the 370 samples, and was not isolated from ready-to-eat lettuce or from raw or ready-to-eat pork, beef, or chicken. (*E*). *sakazakii* was also isolated from a cheese made of raw ewe's milk in Madrid, Spain (Morales et al., 2005) and from a traditional drink in Amman, Jordan (Nassereddin and Yamani, 2005). The drink, called *sous*, is prepared by street-side vendors from the root of *Glycyrirhiza glabra*, sodium bicarbonate, and water. The average pH of the sous drinks sampled was 8.6, and most of the samples were above refrigeration temperatures at the time of purchase. The sample from which (*E*). *sakazakii* was isolated had an Enterobacteriaceae count of 2.8 log CFU/mL, but only one colony was chosen for identification, so the number of (*E*). *sakazakii* in the sample cannot be determined. The wide variety of products from which (*E*). *sakazakii* has been isolated indicates that domestic animals may not be an important source of (*E*). *sakazakii*.

(*E*). *sakazakii* has also been isolated from a wide variety of processing environments. A survey of nine food-processing factories found (*E*). *sakazakii* in 9 to 25% of samples from four milk powder factories, 25% of samples from a chocolate factory, 44% of samples from a cereal factory, 27% of samples from a potato factory, and 23% of samples from a pasta factory but no positive samples in a spice factory (Kandhai et al., 2004). The same study found (*E*). *sakazakii* in five of 16 households.

Despite the lack of information regarding the environmental source of (*E*). *sakazakii*, the prevalence of this organism in human food cannot be ignored. With improved isolation and detection techniques, isolation of (*E*). *sakazakii* from environmental samples may become more common.

3.8 RESISTANCE AND VIRULENCE FACTORS OF (*E*). *SAKAZAKII*

3.8.1 Heat Resistance of (*E*). *sakazakii*

Preliminary studies conducted on reconstituted IF indicated that (*E*). *sakazakii* was one of the most thermotolerant members of Enterobacteriaceae, having a *D*-value of 4.2 min at 58°C (Nazarowec-White and Farber, 1997). Subsequent studies in tryptic soy broth (TSB), IF, and phosphate buffer (PB) have concluded that not all (*E*). *sakazakii* are unusually thermotolerant (Breeuwer et al., 2003; Iversen et al., 2004b). Reported *D*-values at 58°C range from 0.27 to 9.87 min (Table 1). The study by Nazarowec-White and Farber (1997) was performed on pooled isolates of (*E*). *sakazakii*, and some have suggested that one particularly heat-resistant strain was responsible for the high *D*-value. Despite the controversy over heat resistance, all studies have concluded that current milk pasteurization standards are more than sufficient to inactivate (*E*). *sakazakii*.

3.8.2 Osmotic Stress Resistance of (*E*). *sakazakii*

Although (*E*). *sakazakii* is not unusually heat resistant, it is remarkably resistant to osmotic stress and drying when tested in the stationary phase. Drying can be seen as an extreme form of osmotic stress and is important to the survival and persistence of (*E*). *sakazakii* in IF, and presumably also in the environments where such products are manufactured.

At room temperature in brain heart infusion (BHI) broth adjusted to a_w 0.934 by addition of sorbitol, an initial population of (*E*). *sakazakii* 1387-2 of about 7 log was reduced by 1 log over 2 months. Over the same time period, several strains of *Salmonella* were reduced by up to 7 log. Another (*E*). *sakazakii* strain was decreased by 3 to 4 log in just 1 month. In BHI broth adjusted to a_w 0.811 by addition of sorbitol, strains of (*E*). *sakazakii* were reduced by 3 to 4 log after two weeks, whereas strains of *Salmonella*, *Escherichia*, *Klebsiella*, *Citrobacter*, and *Serratia* were reduced by 6 log after two weeks (Breeuwer et al., 2003). One strain of (*E*). *sakazakii* was still detected after four weeks.

The same authors found that when stationary-phase cells of (*E*). *sakazakii* and *E. coli* were air dried at 25°C for 46 days, the log reductions in (*E*). *sakazakii* and *E. coli* were 1 to 1.5 and 4, respectively, indicating that (*E*). *sakazakii* is approximately 1000 times more resistant to air drying than *E. coli*. *Klebsiella* and *Serratia* strains were also much more susceptible than (*E*). *sakazakii* to dry stress. Not surprisingly, Breeuwer et al. (2003) also found exponential-phase (*E*). *sakazakii* to be much more sensitive to osmotic stress and drying. After air drying at 25°C, exponential phase

TABLE 1 Decimal Reduction Times and *z*-Values (± Standard Deviation) for Various Strains of (*E*). *sakazakii*

		D-Value (min) at:				
Medium[b]	Strain	54°C	56°C	58°C	60°C	*z*-Value (°C)
TSB	NCTC 11467[c]	14.9 ± 0.65	2.7 ± 0.08	1.3 ± 0.28	0.9 ± 0.17	5.6 ± 0.13
	823[c]	10.2 ± 3.56	1.2 ± 0.01	1.7 ± 0.38	0.2 ± 0.06	5.6 ± 0.50
IF	NCTC 11467[c]	16.4 ± 0.67	5.1 ± 0.27	2.6 ± 0.48	1.1 ± 0.11	5.8 ± 0.40
	823[c]	11.7 ± 5.80	3.9 ± 0.06	3.8 ± 1.95	1.8 ± 0.82	5.7 ± 0.12
	1387-2[d]	n.t.	n.t.	0.5	n.t.	n.t.
	5 clinical isolates[e]	36.72 ± 6.07	10.91 ± 1.52	5.45 ± 0.46	3.06 ± 0.12	6.02
	5 food isolates[e]	18.57 ± 1.14	9.75 ± 0.47	3.44 ± 0.35	2.15 ± 0.07	5.60
	10 pooled isolates[e]	23.70 ± 2.52	10.30 ± 0.72	4.20 ± 0.57	2.50 ± 0.21	5.82
	ATCC 51329[f]	n.t.	n.t.	0.51 ± 0.00	n.t.	n.t.
	NQ2-Environ[f]	n.t.	n.t.	0.53 ± 0.03	n.t.	n.t.
	NQ3-Environ[f]	n.t.	n.t.	0.57 ± 0.07	n.t.	n.t.
	LCDC 674[f]	n.t.	n.t.	0.62 ± 0.08	n.t.	n.t.
	CDC A3 (1)[f]	n.t.	n.t.	0.63 ± 0.04	n.t.	n.t.
	NQ1-Environ[f]	n.t.	n.t.	0.80 ± 0.02	n.t.	n.t.
	EWFAKRC11NNV1493[f]	n.t.	n.t.	5.13 ± 0.11	n.t.	n.t.
	ATCC 29544[f]	n.t.	n.t.	6.12 ± 0.39	n.t.	n.t.
	SK 90[f]	n.t.	n.t.	7.76 ± 0.26	n.t.	n.t.
	LCDC 648[f]	n.t.	n.t.	9.02 ± 0.35	n.t.	n.t.
	4.01C[f]	n.t.	n.t.	9.53 ± 0.39	n.t.	n.t.
	607[f]	n.t.	21.05 ± 2.65	9.87 ± 0.83	4.41 ± 0.38	5.6
PB	1387-2[d]	7.1	2.4	0.48	n.t.	3.1
	16[d]	6.4	1.1	0.4	n.t.	3.6
	1360[d]	n.t.	n.t.	0.34	n.t.	
	145[d]	n.t.	n.t.	0.27	n.t.	

[a] n.t., not tested.
[b] TSB, tryptic soy broth; IF, infant formula; PB, phosphate buffer.
[c] From Iversen et al. 2004b.
[d] From Breeuwer et al. (2003).
[e] From Nazarowec-White and Farber (1997).
[f] From Edelson-Mammel and Buchanan (2004).

populations were reduced by 2 log in 2 weeks, compared with only 1 to 1.5 log for the stationary-phase cells (Breeuwer et al., 2003). Whereas stationary-phase cells of (*E*). *sakazakii* were able to accumulate intracellular trehalose, exponential-phase (*E*). *sakazakii* were not, and neither exponential- nor stationary-phase *E. coli* were able to accumulate intracellular trehalose.

3.8.3 Growth of (*E*). *sakazakii*

(*E*). *sakazakii* is capable of growth on agar media selective for enteric organisms, including MacConkey, eosin methylene blue, and deoxycholate agar, as well as on nonselective media such as tryptic soy agar. It has been reported that some selective broths do not support the growth of all strains of (*E*). *sakazakii*; 3 of 70 strains from a variety of sources were unable to grow in lauryl sulfate broth or brilliant green bile broth at any temperature between 7 and 57°C after 48 h, although their viability was confirmed in tryptic soy broth (Iversen et al., 2004b). In another study, all 99 strains of (*E*). *sakazakii* tested grew to an optical density (OD) at 620 nm of greater than 0.1 within 48 h at both 30 and 45°C, which the authors characterized as strong growth. Growth in selective broths seems to impair carbohydrate metabolism, especially at high temperatures. At 37°C, fermentation of lactose was observed in 80% of strains in lauryl sulfate tryptose broth and 76% of strains in brilliant green bile broth, but at 44°C only 23% and 11% of strains fermented lactose in these media, respectively (Iversen et al., 2004b). Most important, (*E*). *sakazakii* has a generation time of just 21 min at 37°C and 100 min at 21°C in IF (Iversen et al., 2004b).

(*E*). *sakazakii* was reported to grow in filtered raw winery effluent, pH 7.0, with a doubling time of 90 min at 35°C (Keyser et al., 2003). Winery effluent contains ethanol, hexose sugars, and organic acids such as acetic, citric, lactic, malic, succinic, and tartaric. Growth of (*E*). *sakazakii* in winery effluent under these conditions resulted in 477 mg/L volatile fatty acids (Keyser et al., 2003). An (*E*). *sakazakii* strain isolated from raw ewe's milk also produced large amounts of volatile compounds when grown in pasteurized cow's milk cheeses (Morales et al., 2005). The potential stimulatory or inhibitory effect of volatile compounds produced by (*E*). *sakazakii* on other microorganisms is unknown.

Little research has been performed to determine the optimal parameters of growth for (*E*). *sakazakii*. Iversen et al. (2004b) reported that the optimal temperature was between 37 and 43°C, depending on the growth medium. The maximum temperature for growth of (*E*). *sakazakii* seems to be strain dependent. Iversen et al. (2004a) reported that none of 70 strains showed growth after 24 h in TSB at 47°C, but 37% showed growth after 48 h, whereas Guillaume-Gentil et al. (2005) found that all 15 strains showed growth after 24 h in lauryl sulfate tryptose broth (LST) at 47°C.

Recent research has reported the ability of (*E*). *sakazakii* to survive in environments of low to very low water activity, but the minimum water activity (a_w) for the growth of (*E*). *sakazakii* is unknown. Breeuwer et al. (2003) reported that four strains of (*E*). *sakazakii* grew in BHI adjusted to a_w 0.96 with sodium chloride (1.2 M). Guillaume-Gentil (2005) reported that all 99 strains tested were able to grow in lauryl sulfate tryptose broth containing 0.5 M sodium chloride. Growth at low a_w may be important for environmental persistence.

The minimum pH for growth of (*E*). *sakazakii* is also unknown. Four strains were reported to grow between pH 4.5 and 10 in BHI broth (Breeuwer et al., 2003). Resistance to or growth in low-pH environments may allow (*E*). *sakazakii* to persist in the environment, or survive the acidic conditions of the stomach. Furthermore, the specific growth rate under stress conditions may be of practical importance.

3.8.4 Antibiotic Resistance

Antibiotic resistance of (*E*). *sakazakii* may be increasing. A compilation of antimicrobial susceptibility tests from selected publications can be seen in Table 2. The first comprehensive characterization of antibiotic susceptibility was performed in 1984 (Muytjens et al., 1984) and showed that 195 strains of (*E*). *sakazakii* isolated from a wide variety of sources (blood, cerebral spinal fluid) were susceptible to most of the 29 commonly used antimicrobial agents, showing resistance to only cephalothin and sulfamethoxyzole. (*E*). *sakazakii* was comparatively much more susceptible than *E. cloacae*; half of the minimum inhibitory concentration required to suppress 90% of the *E. cloacae* strains was sufficient to repress 90% of the (*E*). *sakazakii* strains for 25 of the agents tested. More recently, Kuzina et al. (2001) reported that a strain of (*E*). *sakazakii* isolated from the Mexican fruit fly *Anastrepha ludens* was resistant to ampicillin, cephalothin, erythromycin, novobiocin, and penicillin, but sensitive to chloramphenicol, doxycycline, kanamycin, polymyxin, rifampin, streptomycin, and tetracycline. However, two isolates of (*E*). *sakazakii* from rats trapped in densely populated areas of Nairobi, Kenya showed resistance only to sulfomethoxyzole and amoxicillin–clavulanate (Gakuya et al., 2001).

Plasmid-mediated extended spectrum β-lactamases (ESBLs) were first observed in 1983 in an isolate of *Klebsiella pneumoniae* (Knothe et al., 1983). Since then, infections caused by ESBL-producing Enterobacteriaceae have increased alarmingly (Mederios, 1997). Plasmids encoding the ESBL confer resistance to the clinically important expanded-spectrum cephalosporins (third- and fourth-generation cephalosporins), including the monobactam azetronam, cefotaxime, and ceftazidime. A recent study found that of 37 ceftazidime-resistant Enterobacteriaceae isolated from a hospital in Bankok, Thailand, five were strains of (*E*). *sakazakii*, and one of the five strains carried the $bla_{\text{VEB-1}}$ gene, which encodes an ESBL (Girlich et al., 2001). Although the $bla_{\text{VEB-1}}$ gene can be carried on extrachromosomal elements, it also possesses the ability to integrate into the host chromosome, efficiently passing itself to future generations. Movement of the $bla_{\text{VEB-1}}$ ESBL is predominantly conjugal, meaning that it is transferred by direct bacterial contact through a sex pilus rather than through dissemination of ESBL-positive strains (Girlich et al., 2001). This conclusion was reached after observation of extremely high conjugal efficiency between the various Enterobacteriaceae isolates, including (*E*). *sakazakii*, and the receptor *E. coli* strain, between 10^{-3} and 10^{-4} (Girlich et al., 2001). In a study of 139 Enterobacteriaceae bloodstream isolates from a hospital in Hong Kong, only one (*E*). *sakazakii* strain was isolated, and it did not produce an ESBL (Ho et al., 2005).

TABLE 2 Antibiotic Susceptibility of (*E*). *sakazakii* from Clinical and Nonclinical Sources[a]

	Reference[b]											
	1	2	3	4	5	6	7	8	9	10	11	12
Aminoglycosides												
Amikacin	S	—	R	—	S	—	—	S	—	—	S	S
Apramycin	—	—	—	—	—	—	—	—	—	—	S	—
Gentamycin	S	S	S	S	S	S	—	R/S	—	S	S	S
Kanamycin	S	S	—	—	—	S	S	—	R	—	S	S
Lividimycin A	—	—	—	—	—	—	—	—	—	—	S	—
Neomycin	—	—	—	—	—	—	—	—	—	—	S	—
Netilmycin	—	—	—	—	—	—	—	—	—	S	S	—
Ribostamycin	—	—	—	—	—	—	—	—	—	—	S	—
Spectinomycin	—	—	—	—	—	—	—	—	R	—	—	—
Streptomycin	—	—	—	—	—	S	S	—	—	—	S	—
Tobramycin	S	—	R	—	S	—	—	—	R	—	S	S
Antifolates												
Sulfamethoxazole	—	—	—	—	—	—	—	—	—	—	S	—
Trimethoprim	—	—	—	—	—	—	—	—	—	—	S	—
Trimethoprim–sulfamethoxazole	—	—	—	—	S	S	—	S	R	—	S	S
B-lactams												
Penicillins												
Amoxicillin	—	—	—	—	—	—	—	—	—	—	S	—
Amoxicilin–clavulanic acid	—	—	—	—	—	—	—	—	—	—	S	—
Ampicillin	S	S	—	S	S	R/S	R	R	—	R	—	S
Ampicillin–sulbactam	—	—	—	—	—	—	—	—	—	—	S	—
Azloclillin	—	—	—	—	—	—	—	—	—	—	S	—
Benzylpenicillin	—	—	—	—	—	—	—	—	—	—	R	—
Carbenicillin	S	—	—	—	—	—	—	—	—	S	—	—
Mezlocillin	—	—	—	—	—	—	—	—	—	—	S	—
Oxicillin	—	—	—	—	—	—	—	—	—	—	R	—
Penicillin	—	—	—	—	—	—	R	—	—	—	—	—
Pipracillin	—	—	—	—	S	—	—	—	—	—	S	S
Pipracillin–tazobactam	—	—	—	—	—	—	—	R/S	—	—	S	—
Ticarcillin	—	—	—	—	S	—	—	—	—	—	S	S
Ticarcillin–clavulante	—	—	—	—	S	—	—	—	—	—	—	—
Carbapenems												
Imipenem	—	—	—	—	S	—	—	—	—	—	S	S
Imipenem–cilastin	—	—	—	—	—	—	—	S	—	—	S	—
Meropenem	—	—	—	—	—	—	—	—	—	—	S	—

(Continued)

TABLE 2 (*Continued*)

	Reference[b]											
	1	2	3	4	5	6	7	8	9	10	11	12
Cephalosporins[c]												
Cefaclor[2]	—	—	—	—	—	—	—	—	—	—	MS/S	—
Cefazoline[1]	—	—	—	—	MS	—	—	R	—	S	S	R
Cefotaxime[3]	—	S	—	—	S	S	—	R/S	—	—	S	S
Cefoxitin[2]	—	—	R	—	S	—	—	—	—	—	MS/S	—
Ceftazidime[3]	—	—	—	—	—	—	—	R/S	—	—	S	S
Ceftriaxone[3]	—	—	—	—	S	—	—	—	—	—	S	S
Cefuroxime[2]	—	S	—	—	S	—	—	—	—	—	S	—
Cephalothin[1]	MS	—	—	—	R	R/S	R	—	—	—	—	—
Loracarbef[2]	—	—	—	—	—	—	—	—	—	—	S	—
Moxalactam[3]	—	S	—	S	—	—	—	—	—	—	—	—
Monobactams												
Aztreonam	—	—	—	—	—	—	—	—	—	—	S	—
Lincosamides												
Clindamycin	—	—	—	—	—	—	—	—	—	R	R	—
Lincomycin	—	—	—	—	—	—	—	—	—	—	R	—
Macrolides												
Azithromycin	—	—	—	—	—	—	—	—	—	—	R/MS	—
Clarithromycin	—	—	—	—	—	—	—	—	—	—	R	—
Erythromycin	—	—	—	—	—	—	R	—	—	MS	R	—
Roxithromycin	—	—	—	—	—	—	—	—	—	—	R	—
Quinolones												
Ciprofloxacin	—	—	—	—	S	—	—	—	—	—	S	S
Enoxicin	—	—	—	—	—	—	—	—	—	—	S	—
Fleroxacin	—	—	—	—	—	—	—	—	—	—	S	—
Nalidixic acid	—	—	—	S	—	—	—	R	—	R	—	—
Norfloxacin	—	—	—	—	—	—	—	—	—	—	S	—
Ofloxicin	—	—	—	—	—	—	—	R/S	—	S	S	S
Pefloxacin	—	—	—	—	—	—	—	R	—	—	S	S
Pipemidic acid	—	—	—	—	—	—	—	—	—	—	S	—
Sparfloxacin	—	—	—	—	—	—	—	—	—	—	S	—
Streptogramins												
Dalfopristin	—	—	—	—	—	—	—	—	—	—	R	—
Dalfopristin–quinupristin	—	—	—	—	—	—	—	—	—	—	R	—
Sulfonamides	—	—	—	—	—	R	—	—	R	—	—	—
Tetracyclines												
Doxyclicline	—	—	—	—	—	—	S	—	—	—	S	—
Minocycline	—	—	—	—	—	—	—	—	—	—	S	—
Tetracycline	—	—	—	S	S	S	S	—	R	S	S	S

TABLE 2 (*Continued*)

	Reference[b]											
	1	2	3	4	5	6	7	8	9	10	11	12
Other antibiotics												
Chloramphenicol	S	S	—	S	—	R/S	S	—	R	—	S	S
Fosfomycin	—	—	—	—	—	—	—	—	—	—	R	—
Furadantin	—	—	—	—	—	—	—	—	—	R	—	—
Fusidic acid	—	—	—	—	—	—	—	—	—	—	R	—
Nitrofurantoin	—	—	—	—	—	—	—	—	—	—	S	—
Novobiocin	—	—	—	—	—	—	R	—	—	—	—	—
Polymyxin	—	—	—	—	—	S	S	—	—	—	—	—
Rifampicin	—	—	—	—	—	—	—	—	—	—	R	—
Rifampin	—	—	—	—	—	—	S	—	R	—	—	—

[a] S, susceptible; R, resistant; MS, mildly susceptible.

[b] 1, Monroe and Tift (1979); 2, Muytjens et al. (1986); 3, Arseni et al. (1987); 4, Willis and Robinson (1988); 5, Hawkins et al. (1991); 6, Nazorowec-White and Farber (1999); 7, Kuzina et al. (2001); 8, Lai (2001); 9, Girlich et al. (2001); 10, Ongradi (2002); 11, Stock and Wiedemann (2002); 12, Block et al. (2002).

[c] 1, First generation; 2, Second generation; 3, Third generation; 4, Fourth generation.

Unfortunately, because (*E*). *sakazakii* is rarely isolated in hospitals, it is difficult to estimate accurately the prevalence of ESBL carriage. Due to the intergenus conjugal nature of ESBL plasmid transfer, increased carriage of ESBL by (*E*). *sakazakii* can be expected in the future.

The trend in antibiotic resistance among isolates of (*E*). *sakazakii* is not surprising and may reflect the increasing antibiotic resistance among Enterobacteriaceae rather than a species-specific trend. However, the antibiotic resistance profiles from hospital isolates of (*E*). *sakazakii* may not be representative of isolates that contaminate IF and other foods.

3.8.5 Virulence Factors of (*E*). *sakazakii*

To date, only one study has directly examined (*E*). *sakazakii* for virulence characteristics. A total of 18 strains of (*E*). *sakazakii* were examined for the ability to produce enterotoxin via the suckling mouse assay and in a tissue culture assay, and were also assayed for infectivity via oral and interperitoneal routes in the suckling mouse (Pagotto et al., 2003). Of the strains tested, four were positive for enterotoxin via the suckling mouse assay, and three of the four were clinical isolates, indicating that the enterotoxin may be important for infectivity. When suckling mice were challenged orally, all strains were fatal at a dose of 10^8 CFU, and some strains caused death with only 10^7 CFU. When suckling mice where challenged by intraperitoneal injection, the fatal dose ranged from 10^5 to 10^7. The infectious dose of (*E*). *sakazakii* in human infants is still unknown. The contamination level of (*E*). *sakazakii* in IF is generally below 3 CFU/g (Muytjens et al., 1988), yet several outbreaks have occurred in which no temperature abuse or delay in feeding occurred (van Acker et al. 2001; CDC, 2002), so it must be assumed that even very low doses of (*E*). *sakazakii* may be capable of causing disease in human infants (FAO/WHO, 2004).

Iron acquisition is an important contributor to virulence in Enterobacteriaceae. Gram-negative organisms require between 0.2 and 0.02 μg/mL iron, yet free iron levels in human serum are much lower, on the order of 10^{-18} M (Payne, 1988). Iron levels in mammalian serum may be limited even further in the event of infection by enhanced synthesis of transferrin, a serum protein that functions as an iron sequesterer (Beaumeir et al., 1984). The ability of gram-negative bacteria to acquire iron in the host is therefore critical to maintaining infection (Beaumeir et al., 1984). In the environment, iron in the ferrous state is virtually insoluble. Although gram-negative bacteria possess a wide variety of iron acquisition strategies, iron acquisition must be tightly regulated to prevent oxidative damage by free intracellular iron (Touati, 2000). To overcome iron limitation in the host and in the environment, microorganisms can synthesize and secrete siderophores. Siderophores are low-molecular-weight compounds that have high iron affinity. Mokracka et al. (2004) recently surveyed extraintestinal isolates of *Enterobacter* and *Citrobacter* for their ability to produce siderophores. Of two (*E*). *sakazakii* strains examined, both were found to secrete the catacholate siderophore enterobactin, while neither secreted the hydroxymate siderophore aerobactin. Aerobactin has been shown to contribute to virulence in *E. coli* (Johnson, 1991) and *Klebsiella* spp. (Podschun and Ullmann, 1998). Enterobactin contributes less to virulence than other siderophores such as aerobactin, despite having a slightly higher affinity for iron than either aerobactin or human iron-binding proteins. In the host, enterobactin can be rendered ineffective by binding to albumin and IgA (Moore and Earhart, 1981), probably due to the aromatic structure (Konopka and Neilands, 1984). Nonetheless, enterobactin may enhance (*E*). *sakazakii*'s ability to outcompete other bacteria for iron outside the host environment. The importance of enterobactin to the virulence of (*E*). *sakazakii* is unknown.

Hemolytic activity has been postulated to be a mechanism of iron acquisition. Hemolysins are an important bacterial virulence factor (Finlay and Falkow, 1989) by providing iron in vivo (Linggood and Ingram, 1982; Waalwijk et al., 1983), among other functions. Many genera in the family Enterobacteriaceae produce hemolysins and other toxins. A heat-resistant, low-molecular-weight hemolysin was isolated from 7 of 50 clinical strains of *Enterobacter cloacae* and was determined to have a molecular weight below 10 kDa and retained hemolytic activity after heating to 60 and 100°C for 30 min, exposure to pH 2 to 6 for 30 min, or treatment with trypsin (Simi et al., 2003). A hemolysin similar to the shlA of *S. marcescens* has been observed in *Proteus mirablis*. The gene encoding the hemolysin of *P. mirablis* (*hpm*) is 52.1% identical to the shl genes of *Serratia*, but the G + C content is 65% in the *P. mirablis* gene compared with 38% in the *Serratia* gene, reflecting the G + C content of each species' total genomic DNA. This homology suggests an ancestral gene that has diverged in the two species, rather than convergent evolution (Braun and Focareta, 1991). Because the gene encoding these similar hemolysins is ancestral, it is likely that similar hemolysins could be found in any number of closely related bacterial species, including (*E*). *sakazakii*.

3.8.6 Biofilm and Capsule Formation

(*E*). *sakazakii* adheres to latex, silicon, polycarbonate, and to a lesser extent, stainless steel when grown in IF (Iversen et al., 2004b). Biofilm formation in gram-negative organisms has been studied extensively in the genera *Pseudomonas*, *Salmonella*, and *Escherichia*. The biofilm matrices formed by these bacterial genera are largely composed of extracellular polysaccharides (EPSs). One study demonstrated that an encapsulated strain of (*E*). *sakazakii* produced biofilms of a higher cell density than those produced by a nonencapsulated strain (Iversen et al., 2004b).

Interestingly, several studies have shown that capsule expression actually inhibits biofilm formation. Joseph and Wright (2004) reported that expression of capsular polysaccharide by *Vibrio vulnificus* inhibits attachment and biofilm formation, while Schembri et al. (2004) found that capsule formation blocks the function of short bacterial adhesions in *E. coli* K12 and *Klebsiella pneumoniae*. In *K. pneumoniae* there is an inverse relationship between expression of capsule and type 1 fimbriae (Matatov et al., 1999), and expression of capsule down-regulates expression of the CF29K adhesion as well (Favre-Bonte et al., 1999). The relationship between expression of capsular polysaccharide and adhesins such as fimbriae in (*E*). *sakazakii* remains to be elucidated.

The production of cellulose is necessary for biofilm formation in *Salmonella enteritidis* (Solano et al., 2002). Studies by Zogaj et al. (2003) showed a fecal isolate of (*E*). *sakazakii* to produce cellulose but not curli fimbriae. The presence of cellulose synthase, the catalytic subunit of which is encoded by *bcsA* (Solano et al., 2002), was confirmed and expressed constitutively by (*E*). *sakazakii* (Zogaj et al., 2003). Remaining genes in the bacterial cellulose synthase (*bcsABCZ*) operon were intact (Zogaj et al., 2003), including *bcsB*, a regulatory subunit, *bcsC*, an oxidoreductase, and *bcsZ*, an endoglucanase (Solano et al., 2002). Although the fecal isolate of (*E*). *sakazakii* did not produce curli fimbriae, structural genes for curli fimbriae, *csgBA*, and a transcriptional activator, *csgD*, were present and intact (Zogaj et al., 2003).

Cellulose production has been associated with chlorine resistance in *Salmonella enteritidis*; after exposure to 30 ppm NaOCl for 20 min, 75% of wild-type, cellulose-producing *S. enteritidis* survived compared with only 0.3% of cellulose-deficient mutants (Solano et al., 2002). If (*E*). *sakazakii* biofilms are comprised mainly of cellulose, a similar increase in chlorine resistance may be observed.

3.9 CURRENT ISOLATION AND DETECTION TECHNIQUES

A number of media exist for the cultivation and presumptive identification of (*E*). *sakazakii*. However, none of the methods recommended at present have been validated or achieved official regulatory status. To date, the FDA has not established an acceptable limit for (*E*). *sakazakii* in powdered IF. However, the level of (*E*). *sakazakii* in IF is generally quite low, between 0.36 and 66 CFU/100 g (Muytjens et al., 1988), so enrichment is necessary.

The FDA-recommended protocol is based on a three-tube most-probable-number (MPN) method using different sample sizes to allow approximation of the number of (*E*). *sakazakii* present prior to enrichment. Three tubes for each sample size, 100, 10, and 1 g, are prepared. Powdered IF is diluted 1 : 10 with sterile prewarmed water, shaken gently to reconstitute, and incubated at 36°C overnight. From each sample, 10 mL is removed, placed in 90 mL of sterile Enterobacteriaceae enrichment broth, and once again incubated at 36°C overnight. Following the enrichment, 100 μL is spread-plated directly onto violet red bile glucose (VRBG) agar. To ensure isolation of single colonies, a 10-μL loopful of the enrichment is also streaked onto VRBG agar. Plates are incubated at 36°C overnight and five presumptive colonies (slimy purple surrounded by a zone of precipitated bile salts) of (*E*). *sakazakii* are picked and re-streaked onto individual tryptic soy agar (TSA) plates. The current method calls for incubation for 48 to 72 h at 25°C on TSA to allow yellow pigment production. However, a recent report suggests that illumination by white light during incubation at 37°C speeds pigment production, allowing pigmentation to be evaluated after only 24 h (Guillame-Gentil et al., 2005). Yellow colonies on TSA are subjected to the API 20E biochemical test battery, including oxidase testing, to confirm as (*E*). *sakazakii*. Completion of the API 20E requires an additional overnight incubation at 36°C. Following confirmation by the API 20E, MPN is estimated using the FDA BAM guidelines, based on how many tubes of each sample size are positive for (*E*). *sakazakii*.

One disadvantage of this method is the lengthy time necessary for identification of (*E*). *sakazakii*, up to 7 days if pigment production requires 3 days. The use of elevated incubation temperature and illumination speeds pigment production on TSA, shortening the procedure by 24 to 48 h. However, a number of selective and differential media have been developed that allow direct screening of the enrichment for (*E*). *sakazakii*, with presumptive colonies available for API 20E confirmation the day after completion of enrichment.

Oh and Kang (2004) developed a fluorogenic, selective, and differential agar known as OK medium which utilizes the α-glucosidase activity of (*E*). *sakazakii*, which hydrolyzes a variety of chromogenic and fluorogenic substrates. Other studies have demonstrated 4-nitrophenol-α-D-glucopyranoside to be easily diffusible on agar (James et al., 1996; Manafi et al., 1991), so the fluorogenic substrate 4-methylumbelliferyl-α-D-glucoside, which is not easily diffusible, was selected (Oh and Kang, 2004). Tryptone was selected as the nitrogen source, as compared with protease peptone I, protease peptone II, and Bacto peptone, it gave the lowest background fluorescence. The formulation contains bile salts, which select against most gram-positive organisms, as well as ferric citrate/sodium thiosulfate, which allows differentiation between hydrogen sulfide producers, which produce black colonies, and nonproducers, which do not, and agar.

Another fluorogenic agar for (*E*). *sakazakii* was evaluated recently by the Association of Official Analytical Chemists. (Leuschner and Bew, 2004). This preparation is nutrient agar (NA)-based and is supplemented with 4-methylumbelliferyl-α-D-glucoside, but it does not contain selective or differential ingredients. On both fluorogenic agars, colonies of (*E*). *sakzakii* give strong blue fluorescence when illuminated with long-wave ultraviolet light after 24 h of incubation at 37°C. Other bacteria are weakly fluorescent or nonfluorescent.

The first chromogenic selective and differential medium, Druggan–Forsythe–Iverson agar (DFI) also utilizes α-glucosidase activity (Iversen et al., 2004a). This agar is based on the widely available tryptic soy agar, with the addition of sodium deoxycholate, sodium thiosulfate, ferric ammonium citrate, and 5-bromo-4-chloro-3-indolyl-α-D-glucopyranoside as the chromogenic substrate. A commercially available preparation based on this formulation is now available.

For both the original and commercial formulations, hydrolysis of 5-bromo-4-chloro-3-indolyl-α-D-glucopyranoside by the enzyme α-glucosidase results in blue–green pigment which is not diffusible on agar. Colonies of (*E*). *sakazakii* appear as blue–green colonies on pale yellow medium. Hydrogen sulfide producers such as *Salmonella* and some *Citrobacter* appear black on this medium, *Serratia* appears pink, *Escherichia hermanii* appears yellow, and most other Enterobacteriaceae appear white, including *E. cloacae*, which does not produce α-glucosidase. However, *Escherichia vulneris*, *Pantoea agglomerans*, and *Citrobacter koseri* were found to give false positives or entirely blue–green colonies.

The first PCR primer set designed for identification was based on the only available full-length 16S rRNA sequence, from the ATCC type strain 29544 (Keyser et al., 2003). The primers used were 5′-cccgcatctctgcaggattctc-3′ and 5′-ctaataccgcataacgtctacg-3′ and allowed discrimination between the (*E*). *sakazakii* strain and one strain each of *E. cloacae*, *Klebsiella*, *E. aerogenes*, and *E. agglomerans*. However, subsequent sequencing of the 16S rRNA of 13 isolates revealed significant specificity issues with this primer set, with (*E*). *sakazakii* ATCC 51329 testing negative and a strain each of *E. cloacae*, *Serratia liquefaciens*, *S. fucaria*, and *Salmonella* Enteritidis testing positive (Lehner et al., 2004). A new set was developed, 5′-gctytgctgacgagtggcgg-3′ and 5′-atctctgcaggattctctgg-3′, based on new 16S rRNA sequence information from 14 strains of (*E*). *sakazakii* (Lehner et al., 2004). This study also revealed two distinct lineages of (*E*). *sakazakii*, with ATCC 51329 belonging to one lineage and ATCC 29004 and ATCC 29544 belonging to the other.

Recently, the FDA (Seo and Brackett, 2005) developed a real-time PCR assay for the rapid detection of (*E*). *sakazakii* in milk, soy, or cereal-based infant formulas. The primers, 5′-gggatattgtcccctgaaacag-3′ and 5′-cgagaataagccgcgcatt-3′, were targeted toward the macromolecular synthesis operon, which consists of three genes: *rpsU*, *dnaG*, and *rpoD*. The intergenic region between *dnaG* and *rpoD* was chosen for amplification due to variation in length and sequence between species of Enterobacteriaceae. Because this method is based on a 5′ nuclease PCR amplification, which requires 100% homology between the fluorescent probe and the template, it is more specific than standard PCR amplifications. Detection of as few as 100 CFU/mL in reconstituted IF was possible without enrichment. This assay was able to discriminate 58 strains of (*E*). *sakazakii* from 5 strains of *E. cloacae*, 3 strains of *E. agglomerans*, and 2 strains of *E. aerogenes*. Outside the genus *Enterobacter*, the assay was negative for 34 strains of *Salmonella*, 5 strains of *Citrobacter*, 4 strains of *Proteus*, 3 strains of *Escherichia*, 3 strains of *Serratia*, and *Providencia rettgeri*, *Hafinia alvei*, *Leclercia adecarboxylata*, *Listeria monocytogenes*, *Bacillus cereus*, and *Pseudomonas aeruginosa*. When combined with 24 h of incubation at 37°C in Enterobacteriaceae enrichment broth, the real-time PCR assay could detect levels as low as 0.6 CFU/g in the powdered IF sample.

REFERENCES

Arseni A, Malamou-Ladas E, Koutsia C, Xanthou M, Trikka E (1987): Outbreak of colonization of neonates with *Enterobacter sakazakii*. *J Hosp Infect*. 9 (2):143–150.

Balmer SE, Wharton BA (1991): Diet and faecal flora in the newborn: iron. *Arch Dis Child*. 66:1390–1394.

Beaumier DL, Caldwell MA, Holbein BE (1984): Inflammation triggers hypoferremia and de novo synthesis of serum transferrin and ceruloplasmin in mice. *Infect Immun*. 46: 489–494.

Bergsson G, Arnfinnsson J, Karlsson SM, Steingrimsson O, Thormar H (1998): In vitro inactivation of *Chlamydia trachomatis* by fatty acids and monoglycerides. *Antimicrob Agents Chemother*. 42:2290–2294.

Bergsson G, Steingrimsson O, Thormar H (1999): In vitro susceptibilities of *Neisseria gonorrhoeae* to fatty acids and monoglycerides. *Antimicrob Agents Chemother*. 43:2790–2792.

Biering G, Karlsson S, Clark NC, Jonsdottir KE, Ludvigsson P, Steingrimsson O (1989): Three cases of neonatal meningitis caused by *Enterobacter sakazakii* in powdered milk. *J Clin Microbiol*. 27:2054–2056.

Block C, Peleg O, Minster N, et al. (2002): Cluster of neonatal infections in Jerusalem due to unusual biochemical variant of *E. sakazakii*. *Eur J Clin Microbiol*. 21:613–616.

Braun V, Focareta T (1991): Pore-forming bacterial protein hemolysins (cytolysins). *Crit Rev Microbiol*. 18:115–158.

Breeuwer P, Lardeau A, Joosten VN (2003): Desiccation and heat tolerance of *Enterobacter sakazakii*. *J Appl Microbiol*. 95:967–973.

Burgos JM, Varela MF (2002): Multiple antibiotic resistant dairy soil bacteria. Paper A-31. In *Proc. 102nd General Meeting of the American Society for Microbiology*, Salt Lake City, UT, May 19–23.

CDC (Centers for Disease Control and Prevention) (2002): *Enterobacter sakazakii* infections associated with the use of powdered infant formula: Tennessee, 2001. *MMWR Morb Mortal Wkly Rep*. 51:297–300.

Chan, GM (2003): Effects of powdered human milk fortifiers on the antibacterial actions of human milk. *J Perinatol*. 23:620–623.

Chopin A, Mocquot G, Graet YL (1977): Destruction of *Microbacterium lacticum*, *Escherichia coli* and *Staphylococcus aureus* in milk by spray drying. II: Effect of drying conditions. *Can J Micriobiol*. 23:755–761.

Cunningham AS, Jelliffe DB, Jelliffe EF (1991): Breast-feeding and health in the 1980s: a global epidemiologic review. *J Pediatr*. 118:659–666.

Edelson-Mammel SG, Buchanan RL (2004): Thermal inactivation of *Enterobacter sakazakii* in rehydrated infant formula. *J Food Prot*. 67:60–63.

FAO/WHO (Food and Agriculture Organization/World Health Organization) (2004): Draft risk assessment for *E. sakazakii*. http://www.who.int/foodsafety/publications/micro/mra6. Accessed March 2005.

Farmer JJ, Asbury MA, Hickman FW, Brenner DJ, *Enterobacteriaceae* Study Group (1980): *Enterobacter sakazakii*: a new species of "Enterobacteriaceae" isolated from clinical specimens. *Int J Syst Bacteriol.* 30:369–584.

Favre-Bonte S, Joly B, Forestier C (1999): Consequences of reduction of *Klebsiella pneumoniae* capsule expression on interactions of this bacterium with epithelial cells. *Infect Immun.* 67:554–561.

Finlay BB, Falkow S (1989): Common themes in microbial pathogenicity. *Microbiol Rev.* 53:210–230.

Gakuya FM, Kyule MN, Gathura PB, Kariuki S (2001): Antimicrobial resistance of bacterial organisms isolated from rats. *East Afr Med J.* 78:646–649.

Girlich D, Poirel L, Leelaporn A, et al. (2001): Molecular epidemiology of the integron-located VEB-1 extended spectrum β-lactamase in nosocomial enterobacterial isolates in Bangkok, Thailand. *J Clin Microbiol.* 39:175–182.

Guillaume-Gentil O, Sonnard V, Kandhai MC, Marugg JD, Joosten H (2005): A simple and rapid cultural method for detection of *Enterobacter sakazakii* in environmental samples. *J Food Prot.* 68:64–69.

Haeney M (1994): Infection determinants at extremes of age. *J Antimicrob Chemother.* 34 (Suppl A): 1–9.

Hamilton JV, Lehane MJ, Braig HR (2003): Isolation of *Enterobacter sakazakii* from midgut of *Stomoxys calcitrans*. *Emerg Infect Dis.* 9:1355–1356.

Hawkins RE, Lissner CR, Sanford JP (1991): *Enterobacter sakazakii* bacteremia in an adult. *South Med J.* 84:793–795.

Henneke P, Osmers I, Bauer K, Lamping N, Versmold HT, Schumann RR (2003): Impaired CD14-dependent and independent response of polymorphonuclear leukocytes in preterm infants. *J Perinat Med.* 31:176–183.

Hentges DJ, Marsh WW, Petschow BW, Thal WR, Carter MK (1992): Influence of infant diets on the ecology of the intestinal tract of human flora–associated mice. *J Pediatr Gastroenterol Nutr.* 14:146–152.

Ho PL, Shek RHL, Chow KH, et al. (2005): Detection and characterization of extended-spectrum β-lactamases among bloodstream isolates of *Enterobacter* spp. in Hong Kong, 2000–2002. *J Antimicrob Chemother.* 55:326–332.

Isaacs CE, Litov RE, Marie P, Thormar H (1992): Addition of lipases to infant formulas produces antiviral and antibacterial activity. *J Nutr Biochem.* 3:304–308.

Isaacs CE, Litov RE, Thormar H (1995): Antimicrobial activity of lipids added to human milk, infant formula, and bovine milk. *J Nutr Biochem.* 6:362–366.

Iversen C, Forsythe SJ (2003): Risk profile of *Enterobacter sakazakii*, an emergent pathogen associated with infant milk formula. *Trends Food Sci Technol.* 11:443–454.

Iversen C, Druggan P, Forsythe S (2004a): A selective differential medium for *Enterobacter sakazakii*, a preliminary study. *Int J Food Microbiol.* 96:133–139.

Iversen C, Lane M, Forsythe SJ (2004b): The growth profile, thermotolerance and biofilm formation of *Enterobacter sakazakii* grown in infant formula milk. *Lett Appl Microbiol.* 38:378–382.

Iversen C, Mullane N, McCardell B, Tall BD, Lehner A, Fanning S, Stephan R, Joosten H (2008): *Cronobacter* gen. nov., a new genus to accommodate the biogroups of *Enterobacter sakazakii*, and proposal of *Cronobacter sakazakii* gen. nov., comb. nov., *Cronobacter malonaticus* sp. nov., *Cronobacter turicensis* sp. nov., *Cronobacter muytjensii* sp. nov., *Cronobacter dublinensis* sp. nov., *Cronobacter* genomospecies 1, and of three subspecies, *Cronobacter dublinensis* subsp. *dublinensis* subsp. nov., *Cronobacter dublinensis* subsp. *lausannensis* subsp. nov. and *Cronobacter dublinensis* subsp. *lactaridi* subsp. nov. *Int J Syst Evol Microbiol.* 58 (pt 6):1442–1447.

Iversen C, Waddington M, On SL, Forsythe S (2004c): Identification and phylogeny of *Enterobacter sakazakii* relative to *Enterobacter* and *Citrobacter* species. *J Clin Microbiol.* 42:5368–5370.

Izard D, Richard C, Leclerc H (1983): DNA relatedness between *Enterobacter sakazakii* and other members of the genus *Enterobacter*. *Ann Microbiol.* 134A:241–245.

James AL, Perry JD, Ford M, Armstrong L, Gould FK (1996): Evaluation of cyclohexenoesculetin-β-D-galactoside and 8-hydroxyquinoline-β-D-galactoside as substrates for the detection of β-galactosidase. *Appl Environ Microbiol.* 62:3868–3870.

Jimenez E B, Giménez C (1982): Septic shock due to *Enterobacter sakazakii*. *Clin Microbiol Newsl.* 4:30.

Johnson JR (1991): Virulence factors in *Escherichia coli* urinary tract infection. *Clin Microbiol Rev.* 4:80–128.

Joseph LA, Wright AC (2004): Expression of *Vibrio vulnificus* capsular polysaccharide inhibits biofilm formation. *J Bacteriol.* 186:889–893.

Kandhai MC, Reij MW, Gorris LG, Guillaume-Gentil O, Schothorst MV (2004): Occurrence of *Enterobacter sakazakii* in food production environments and households. *Lancet.* 363:39–40.

Kaye D (2001): Gram-negative sepsis in neonates may be rising since start of GBS prophylaxis. *Clin Infect Dis.* 32:i–ii.

Keyser M, Witthuhn RC, Ronquest LC, Britz TJ (2003): Treatment of winery effluent with upflow anaerobic sludge blanket (UASB)–granular sludges enriched with *Enterobacter sakazakii*. *Biotechnol Lett.* 25:1893–1898.

Knothe H, Shah P, Kremery V, Antal M, Mitsushashi S (1983): Transferrable resistance to cefotaxime, cefoxitin, cefamandole and cefuroxime in clinical isolates of *Klebsiella pneumoniae* and *Serratia marcescens*. *Infection.* 11:315–317.

Konopka K, Neilands JB (1984): Effect of serum albumin on siderophore mediated utilization of transferrin iron. *Biochemistry.* 23:2122–2127.

Kuzina LV, Peloquin JJ, Vacek DC, Millar TA (2001): Isolation and identification of bacteria associated with adult laboratory Mexican fruit flies, *Anastrepha ludens* (Diptera: Tephritidae). *Curr Microbiol.* 42:290–294.

Lai KK (2001): *Enterobacter sakazakii* infections among neonates, infants, children, and adults: case reports and a review of the literature. *Medicine.* 80:113–122.

Leclerc H, Mossel DAA, Edberg SC, Struijk CB (2001): Advances in the bacteriology of the coliform group: their suitability as markers of microbial water safety. *Annu Rev Microbiol.* 55:201–234.

Lehner A, Tasara T, Stephan R (2004): 16S rRNA gene based analysis of *Enterobacter sakazakii* strains from different sources and development of a PCR assay for identification. *BMC Microbiol.* 4:43.

Leuschner RG, Bew J (2004): A medium for the presumptive detection of *Enterobacter sakazakii* in infant formula: interlaboratory study. *J AOAC Int.* 87:604–613.

Licari JJ, Potter NN (1970): *Salmonella* survival during spray drying and subsequent handling of skim milk powder. II. Effects of drying conditions. *J Dairy Sci.* 53:871–876.

Linggood MA, Ingram PL (1982): The role of alpha haemolysin in the virulence of *Escherichia coli* for mice. *J Med Microbiol.* 15:23–30.

Manafi M, Kneifel W, Bascomb S (1991): Fluorogenic and chromogenic substrates used in bacterial diagnostics. *Microbiol Rev.* 55:335–348.

Matatov R, Goldhar J, Skutelsky E, et al. (1999): Inability of encapsulated *Klebsiella pneumoniae* to assemble functional type 1 fimbriae on their surface. *FEMS Microbiol Lett.* 179:123–130.

McDonough FE, Hargrove RE (1968): Heat resistance of *Salmonella* in dried milk. *J Dairy Sci.* 51:1587–1591.

McGuire W, Anthony MY (2003): Donor human milk versus formula for preventing necrotizing enterocolitis in preterm infants: systematic review. *Arch Dis Child Fetal Neonatal Ed.* 88:11–14.

Medieros AA (1997): Evolution and dissemination of β-lactamases accelerated by generations of β-lactam antibiotics. *Clin Infect Dis.* 24 (Suppl): S19–S45.

Miller IM, Pegues DA (2000): *Salmonella* species, including *Salmonella typhi*. In Mandell GL, Bennett JE, Mandell RD (Eds.). *Douglas and Bennett's Principles and Practice on Infectious Diseases* 5th ed. Churchill Livingstone, Philadelphia, pp. 23–48.

Miller DL, Goepfert JM, Amundson CH (1972): Survival of salmonellae and *Escherichia coli* during the spray drying of various food products. *J Food Sci.* 37:828.

Mokracka J, Koczura R, Kaznowski A (2004): Yersiniabactin and other siderophores produced by clinical isolates of *Enterobacter* spp. and *Citrobacter* spp. *FEMS Immunol Med Microbiol.* 40:51–55.

Monroe PW, Tift WL (1979): Bacteremia associated with *Enterobacter sakazakii* (yellow-pigmented *Enterobacter cloacae). J Clin Microbiol.* 10:850–851.

Moore DG, Earhart CF (1981): Specific inhibition of *Escherichia coli* ferrienterochelin uptake by a normal human serum immunoglobulin. *Infect Immun.* 31:631–635.

Moore MR, Schrag SJ, Schuchat A (2003): Effects of intrapartum antimicrobial prophylaxis for prevention of group-B-streptococcal disease on the incidence and ecology of early-onset neonatal sepsis. *Lancet Infect Dis.* 3:201–213.

Morales P, Felie I, Fernandez-Garcia E, Nunez M (2005): Volatile compounds produced in cheese by Enterobacteriaceae strains of dairy origin. *J Food Prot.* 67:567–573.

Mosso MA, de la Rosa MC, Vivar C, Medina MR (1994): Heterotrophic bacterial populations in the mineral waters of thermal springs in Spain. *J Appl Bacteriol.* 77:370–381.

Muytjens HL, Kollee LA (1990): *Enterobacter sakazakii* meningitis in neonates: causative role of formula? *Pediatr Infect Dis J.* 9:372–373.

Muytjens HL, van der Ros-van de Repe J (1986): Comparative in vitro susceptibilities of eight *Enterobacter* species, with special reference to *Enterobacter sakazakii*. *Antimicrob Agents Chemother.* 29 (2):367–370.

Muytjens HL, Van Der Ros-Van de Repe J, Van Druten HAM (1984): Enzymatic profiles of *Enterobacter sakazakii* and related species with special reference to the α-glucosidase reaction and reproducibility of the test system. *J Clin Microbiol.* 20:684–686.

Muytjens HL, Roelofs-Willemse H, Jaspar GHJ (1988): Quality of powdered substitutes for breast milk with regard to members of the family Enterobacteriaceae. *J Clin Microbiol.* 26:743–746.

Nair MK, Joy J, Venkitanarayanan KS (2004): Inactivation of *Enterobacter sakazakii* in reconstituted infant formula by monocaprylin. *J Food Prot*. 67:2815–2189.

Nassereddin RA, Yamani MI (2005): Microbiological quality of sous and tamarind, traditional drinks consumed in Jordan. *J Food Prot*. 68:773–777.

Nazarowec-White M, Farber JM (1997): Incidence, survival, and growth of *Enterobacter sakazakii* in infant formula. *J Food Prot*. 60:226–230.

Nazarowec-White M, Farber JM (1999): Phenotypic and genotypic typing of food and clinical isolates of *Enterobacter sakazakii*. *J Med Microbiol*. 48 (6):559–567.

Noreiga FR, Kotloff KL, Martin MA, Schwalbe RS (1990): Nosocomial bacteremia caused by *Enterobacter sakazakii* and *Leuconostoc mesenteroides* resulting from extrinsic contamination of infant formula. *Pediatr Infect Dis J*. 9:447–449.

Oh SW, Kang DH (2004): Fluorogenic selective and differential medium for isolation of *Enterobacter sakazakii*. *Appl Environ Microbiol*. 70:5692–5694.

Ongradi J (2002): Vaginal infection by *Enterobacter sakazakii*. *Sex Transm Infect*. 78:467.

Pagotto FJ, Nazarowec-White M, Bidawid S, Farber JM (2003): *Enterobacter sakazakii*: infectivity and enterotoxin production in vitro and in vivo. *J Food Prot*. 66:370–5.

Payne SM (1988): Iron and virulence in the family Enterobacteriaceae. *Crit Rev Microbiol*. 16:81–111.

Petschow BW, Batema RP, Ford LL (1996): Susceptibility of *Helicobacter pylori* to bactericidal properties of medium-chain monoglycerides and free fatty acids. *Antimicrob Agents Chemother*. 40:302–306.

Podschun R, Ullmann U (1998): *Klebsiella* spp. as nosocomial pathogens: epidemiology, taxonomy, typing methods, and pathogenicity factors. *Clin Microbiol Rev*. 11:589–603.

Raghuveer TS, McGuire EM, Martin SM, et al. (2002): Lactoferrin in the preterm infants' diet attenuates iron-induced oxidation products. *Pediatr Res*. 52:964–972.

Sakazaki R (1974): *Enterobacter cloacae*. In: Buchanan RE, Gibbons NE (eds.). Bergey's Manual of Determinative Bacteriology, 8th ed. Williams & Wilkins, Baltimore. p. 325.

Schembri MA, Dalsgaard D, Klemm P (2004): Capsule shields the function of short bacterial adhesions. *J Bacteriol*. 186:1249–1257.

Schibler KR, Trautman MS, Liechty KW, White WL, Rothstein G, Christensen RD (1993): Diminished transcription of interleukin-8 by monocytes from preterm neonates. *J Leukoc Biol*. 53:399–403.

Seo KH, Brackett RE (2005): Rapid, specific detection of *Enterobacter sakazakii* in infant formula using a real-time PCR assay. *J Food Prot*. 68:59–63.

Simi S, Carbonell GV, Falcón RM, et al. (2003): A low molecular weight enterotoxic hemolysin from clinical *Enterobacter cloacae*. *Can J Microbiol*. 49:479–482.

Simmons BP, Gelfand MS, Haas M, Metts L, Ferguson J (1989): *Enterobacter sakazakii* infections in neonates associated with intrinsic contamination of a powdered infant formula. *Infect Control Hosp Epidemiol*. 10:398–401.

Solano CB, Garcia B, Valle J, et al. (2002): Genetic analysis of *Salmonella enteritidis* biofilm formation: critical role of cellulose. *Mol Microbiol*. 43:793–808.

Soriano JM, Rico H, Molto JC, Mañes J (2001): Incidence of microbial flora in lettuce, meat, and Spanish potato omelette from restaurants. *Food Microbiol*. 18:159–163.

Steigerwalt AG, Fanning GR, Fife-Asbury MA, Brenner DJ (1976): DNA relatedness among species of *Enterobacter* and *Serratia*. *Can J Microbiol*. 22:121–137.

Stock I, Wiedemann B (2002): Natural antibiotic susceptibility of *Enterobacter amnigenus*, *Enterobacter cancerogenus*, *Enterobacter gergoviae* and *Enterobacter sakazakii* strains. *Clin Microbiol Infect*. 8 (9):564–578.

Touati D (2000): Iron and oxidative stress in bacteria. *Arch Biochem Biophys*. 373:1–6.

Urmenyi AM, Franklin AW (1961): Neonatal death from pigmented coliform infection. *Lancet*. 1:313–315.

van Acker J, de Smet F, Muyldermans G, Bougatef A, Naessens A, Lauwers S (2001): Outbreak of necrotizing enterocolitis associated with *Enterobacter sakazakii* in powdered milk formula. *J Clin Microbiol*. 39:293–297.

Waalwijk C, MacLaren DM, de Graaff J (1983): In vivo function of hemolysin in the nephropathogenicity of *Escherichia coli*. *Infect Immun*. 42:245–249.

Wharton BA, Balmer SE, Scott PH (1994): Faecal flora in the newborn: effect of lactoferrin and related nutrients. *Adv Exp Med Biol*. 357:91–98.

WHO (World Health Organization) (1981): International Code of Marketing of Breast-Milk Substitutes. WHO, Geneva, Switzerland.

Willis J, Robinson JE (1988): *Enterobacter sakazakii* meningitis in neonates. *Pediatr Infect Dis J*. 7 (3):196–199.

Zogaj X, Bokranz W, Nimtz M, Römling U (2003): Production of cellulose and curli fimbriae by members of the family Enterobacteraceae isolated from the human gastrointestinal tract. *Infect Immunol*. 71:4151–4158.

CHAPTER 4

PRION DISEASES

DEBBIE MCKENZIE and JUDD AIKEN

4.1 INTRODUCTION

The foodborne epidemic of bovine spongiform encephalopathy (BSE) in Great Britain, its subsequent detection in Europe, Japan, and North America, and the link between BSE and an emerging human form of the disease, variant Creutzfeldt–Jakob disease (vCJD), have focused considerable attention on prion diseases. The more recent expansion of chronic wasting disease (CWD) in captive and free-ranging cervids in North America has further increased concerns regarding these diseases. These inevitably fatal neurological disorders, also referred to as transmissible spongiform encephalopathies (TSEs), share several hallmark characteristics, including spongiform degeneration in the central nervous system, accumulation of a structurally abnormal form of a brain protein (the prion protein, PrP) in infected animals, and lack of an antibody response. Uncertainty over the number of humans currently infected with vCJD, extreme resistance of the infectious agent to inactivation, lack of a cure or even a preclinical diagnosis, and uncertainty over the mode of transmission of both BSE and CWD make these diseases particularly vexing.

The biology of prion diseases is different from that of other infectious agents. These differences include their ability to resist traditional sterilization methods, their extended preclinical phase, and difficulties in diagnosis of the disease. These characteristics have had tragic consequences, including the exposure of the cattle population in Great Britain to contaminated feed and the transmission of the resulting bovine disease to humans. One somewhat paradoxical trait is that (with the notable exception of CWD) prion diseases are not readily transmissible. Ingestion of contaminated food is the most common means of transmission, yet experimental infection via the oral route is not a particularly efficient means of infection. With respect to vCJD, the source of infection (e.g., meat, milk, processed bovine products) is not yet clear.

Microbiologically Safe Foods, Edited by Norma Heredia, Irene Wesley, and Santos García

TABLE 1 Animal and Human Prion Diseases

Species	Prion Disease	Source of Infection
Sheep	Scrapie	Acquired, maternal
Cattle	Bovine spongiform encephalopathy	Contaminated feed
Mink	Transmissible mink encephalopathy	Contaminated feed
Cats	Feline spongiform encephalopathy	BSE-infected tissue or meat-and-bone meal
Deer and elk	Chronic wasting disease	Origin unknown; self-sustaining
Human	Kuru	Ritualistic cannibalism
	Creutzfeldt–Jakob Disease	
	Iatrogenic	Infection
	Sporadic	Unknown
	Familial	PrP gene mutation
	Variant CJD	Infection, source BSE
	Gerstmann–Straussler–Scheinker syndrome	PrP gene mutation
	Fatal familial insomnia	
	Familial	PrP gene mutation
	Sporadic	Unknown

4.2 TRANSMISSIBLE SPONGIFORM ENCEPHALOPATHIES

TSEs have been identified in a number of species (Table 1) and include scrapie in sheep and goats, BSE, transmissible mink encephalopathy (TME), feline spongiform encephalopathy (FSE), and CWD. The human diseases include kuru, maintained by ritualistic cannibalism, and CJD, which has sporadic, acquired, and two familial forms, Gerstmann–Straussler–Scheinker syndrome (GSS) and fatal familial insomnia (FFI). All TSEs have been transmitted experimentally to a number of species, ranging from nonhuman primates to rodents. Each of these diseases has its unique set of characteristics, including range of species that can be infected.

4.2.1 Scrapie

Scrapie is a disease of sheep and, rarely, goats that has been recognized for at least 250 years. The term *scrapie* is derived from the pronounced rubbing and scratching of the skin, which occurs in infected sheep 2 to 5 years old; the incubation period appears to be approximately 1 year. Clinical manifestation of scrapie is characterized by ataxia and recumbancy. Scrapie has a worldwide distribution, with the notable exception of Australia and New Zealand, due to aggressive scrapie eradication programs in those countries. The disease is maintained and disseminated by horizontal transmission. Placentas from scrapie-infected animals contain high levels of infectivity and may be a source of transmission. Epidemiologic studies have not provided any link between scrapie in sheep and CJD in humans.

4.2.2 Transmissible Mink Encephalopathy

Transmissible mink encephalopathy is a rare disease observed only in ranch-raised mink. It was first described in Wisconsin in 1947 and has since been observed in Ontario, Finland, Germany, and Russia. The incubation period of natural TME is 7 to 12 months, with clinical symptoms that include hyperexcitability and ultimately, motor incoordination. Exposure is via contaminated foodstuffs, although the source, once believed to be sheep scrapie, is not clear.

4.2.3 Chronic Wasting Disease

CWD is an emerging TSE in captive and free-ranging cervids that was originally described in, and limited to, captive mule deer and elk in Wyoming and Colorado. It has now also been detected in free-ranging (wild) white-tailed deer, mule deer, elk, and moose. Distribution of the disease is limited primarily to North America, with free-ranging cervids in nine American states and two Canadian provinces and captive cervids in eight states and two provinces testing positive for the disease. Due to the inadvertent importation of infected elk, Korea has also reported CWD in farm-raised elk. Clinical signs of CWD include emaciation and a reduced fear of humans. The origin and mode of transmission of CWD is unknown, but the mortality rates within a given captive population can be very high (>90% of all animals at one facility). CWD is unique among the TSEs in that it is the only contagious agent transmitted laterally. Contamination of the environment via body fluids as well as by decomposing carcasses increases the risk for perpetuating the disease within the cervid populations and, possibly, transmission to other species.

4.2.4 Bovine Spongiform Encephalopathy

Bovine spongiform encephalopathy was first identified in the United Kingdom in 1985. BSE is a foodborne infection thought to be caused by the survival of infectivity in cooked animal offal that was incorporated into commercial diets of cattle in Great Britain. Although the primary mode of transmission appears to be via the oral–dietary route, there is an increased risk of infection in the offspring of clinically infected cattle. BSE reached epidemic proportions in the UK during the late 1980s and early 1990s, with approximately 200,000 cattle testing positive for the disease. In addition to devastating British agriculture, BSE appears to have been the source of a novel feline form of the disease (FSE), a natural infection of goats (different from scrapie), and a new human disease of unknown scope, variant CJD.

First documented in 1986, the initial cases of BSE occurred in 1985, although it was probably cycling in cattle prior to that time. The disease peaked in January 1993, with approximately 1000 new cases documented weekly. There have been almost 181,000 documented cases of BSE in Great Britain (Fig. 1). This is an underestimate of the total number of infected cattle, as animals in the preclinical stages of disease would not necessarily been identified. The decline in cases beginning in 1993 is attributed to the 1988 ban on the inclusion of meat-and-bone meal in cattle feed. Due

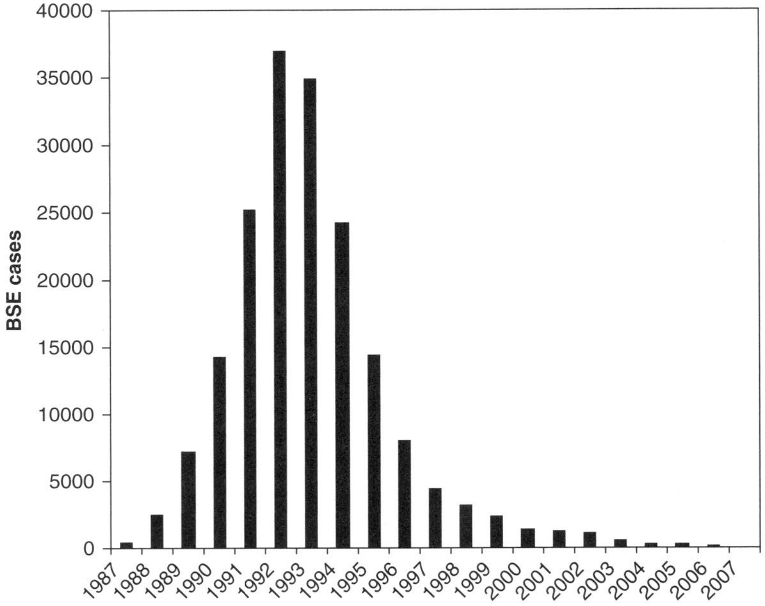

FIG. 1 Bovine spongiform encephalopathy epidemic in the United Kingdom. The decline in cases in cattle that began in 1993 is attributed to the 1988 ban on mammalian meat-and-bone meal supplements. (Data derived from the OIE website, http://www.oie.int/eng/info/en_esbru.htm. The number of positive animals for 2007 is as of 3/31/07.)

to the approximate 5-year incubation period, the effects of the ban were not observed until after the mid-1990s.

Although BSE originated in the UK, it has also been detected in most European countries, probably due to movement of contaminated meat-and-bone meal and/or preclinically affected cattle. In all cases, the number of infected animals is small (hundreds of cases per year). Several cases of BSE have been reported in the United States and Canada. Both countries have instituted feed bans that prohibit the feeding of mammalian protein to ruminant animals.

BSE has infected humans, probably through the consumption of BSE-infected meat (discussed below). Also of concern to the agricultural community and to food safety is whether BSE is transmissible to other food animals. BSE has been observed in a number of different zoo animals as well as in domestic cats and humans. Although naturally occurring BSE has not been documented in sheep (surveillance has been expanded in Europe to include such a possibility), sheep have been infected experimentally with BSE agent. Sheep genotypes that are resistant to scrapie infection have been infected successfully with the BSE agent, raising concerns that BSE could move into sheep populations. Although there is no known association of consumption of scrapie-infected sheep with human disease, it is not known whether the same host restriction will occur if sheep are infected with BSE.

4.2.5 Human TSEs

Human TSEs are primarily sporadic in origin. Sporadic CJD accounts for 90 to 95% of the reported cases of CJD, affecting one person in a million per year. The disease generally occurs in people over 50 years of age, although cases have been reported in persons in their early teens to late 80s. The etiology of sporadic CJD is unknown, and there is no link between scrapie in sheep and sporadic CJD. Familial TSEs (GSS, familial CJD, and FFI) are autosomal dominant disorders that have been linked to specific mutations in the *PrP* gene and that occur at an incidence of one person per 10 million per year. Two factors have contributed to iatrogenic CJD: the presence of CJD titer in preclinical patients and the resistance of these disease agents to inactivation. Iatrogenic CJD has been documented primarily by exposure to central nervous system tissue from infected persons, specifically dura mater, corneal transplants, and cadaveric pituitary growth hormone treatment.

Kuru is a human TSE of the Fore cultural group of Papua New Guinea. The disease was perpetuated by ritualistic cannibalism, which at its height infected approximately 1% of the population. The incidence of kuru has declined dramatically since the cessation of cannibalism in the late 1950s; however, due to the long incubation periods that characterize all TSEs, a few cases still occur.

Variant CJD (vCJD) is an emerging TSE, with the first cases diagnosed in 1996. vCJD can be distinguished from sporadic and familial (genetic) forms of CJD based on clinical, biochemical, and rodent transmission studies. Whereas sporadic CJD affects people in their 50s to 60s, vCJD has, to date, been a disease of teens and young adults. Biological and biochemical studies have tightly linked vCJD with BSE. It is assumed that consumption of beef products is the source of the infection. Recent reports of iatrogenic transmission of vCJD via blood products increases the concern that the number of people infected with vCJD may continue to increase (Peden et al., 2005). Uncertainties over the length of the incubation period, route of infection, and number of people exposed to contaminated bovine products have resulted in very disparate estimates of the future course of this TSE.

4.2.6 Emerging TSEs

Increased TSE surveillance, particularly in the European Union (EU), has identified a number of previously unrecognized TSEs in both cattle and sheep. An unusual form of scrapie, Nor98, was first described in Norway in 1998. Although there is no evidence of lateral or vertical transmission, the host range is unknown. Nor98 affects older animals and has been identified in sheep genotypes thought to be resistant to scrapie infection. Several non-BSE cattle TSEs have also been described recently, primarily a disease referred to as bovine amyloidotic spongiform encephalopathy (BASE). Identification of BASE relies on molecular strain typing and pathological examination of brains from old cows. It is not clear whether this is a new TSE disease or if it has been present but not detected in populations. This TSE differs from BSE in that the cattle affected have PrP plaques in their brains. This disease was first described in Italy and has been observed subsequently in France and Germany.

4.3 NATURE OF THE ILLNESS CAUSED

Prion diseases are inevitably fatal, inducing a progressive neurologic dysfunction after a long preclinical phase. Typical pathological features include spongiform vacuolation, accumulation of PrP^{Sc}, astrocytosis, often accompanied by the accumulation of amyloid plaques. A unique characteristic of all prion diseases is the extended preclinical stage of the disease followed by a short clinical phase. The overall incubation periods are long, taking months to develop in mink, years to develop in sheep, deer, and cattle, and years to decades in humans. The consequences of the long preclinical stage include the inability to diagnose animals and humans in the early stages of the disease, resulting in iatrogenic transmission of CJD, transmission of vCJD via blood transfusion, and inadvertent movement of infected farm-raised cervids. A distinguishing feature of all the TSEs is the deposition of PrP^{Sc}.

Incubation periods of TSEs can vary depending on the strain of TSE agent, host species, route of infection, and dose of inoculum. The incubation period of naturally occurring BSE ranges from 2 to 8 years. Clinical signs of BSE initially involve changes in the animal's temperament, with increased nervousness or aggressiveness. During the 2- to 6-month clinical period, the disease develops into an obvious lack of coordination (ataxia), difficulty in rising, and loss of weight. The initial clinical signs of scrapie occur 2 to 5 years after infection, and the changes in temperament are usually followed by the animals rubbing against enclosures. As the disease progresses, the animals affected exhibit a loss of coordination, weight loss, and gait abnormalities.

Although initial diagnosis of human prion diseases can be difficult in the early stages of clinical disease, these diseases are clinically distinct from each other. GSS is typified by chronic progressive ataxia and terminal dementia and has a clinical duration of 2 to 10 years. FFI initially presents as insomnia followed by ataxia and dementia. Sporadic CJD affects persons in their 50s to 60s. Death occurs within 6 months of the onset of the clinical stage, which presents as a rapidly progressive multifocal dementia and, often, ataxia. vCJD clinically presents as a psychiatric disturbance, with depression being a predominant feature. The clinical course that develops includes ataxia and dementia and is observed primarily in teenagers and young adults. The clinical course is more extended than classical CJD, with vCJD being about 1 year.

4.4 PATHOGENESIS

The pathogenesis of prion diseases can vary depending on the host species and strain of the agent. All TSEs replicate in nervous tissue and exhibit the highest levels of titer and accumulation of the abnormal form of the prion protein (PrP^{Sc}) in the brain and spinal cord. For example, in hamsters infected experimentally with hamster-adapted strains of scrapie and TME, the titer in the brain reaches levels of 10^9 LD_{50} per gram at the terminal stage of the disease process. Infectivity accumulates in the brain and in other tissues throughout the preclinical phase of the disease, such that considerable titer is present long before the onset of clinically recognizable disease.

Sheep scrapie and cervid CWD are unique among TSEs because epizootics can be sustained by horizontal (animal-to-animal) transmission. Routes of natural transmission have not yet been determined, but available evidence suggests that an environmental reservoir of infectivity contributes to the maintenance of these diseases in the affected populations. The oral route of infection appears to be the most likely route for both scrapie and CWD transmission. The oral route of infection has been well described in sheep (Jeffrey and Gonzales, 2004); the agent enters via the alimentary tract, accumulates in the gut-associated lymphoid tissue, particularly in the germinal centers innervated by the sympathetic fibers, and in the myenteric and submucuosal plexuses. The infection then moves to the central nervous system (CNS) via the sympathetic and parasympathetic nerves to the interomediolaterial columns of the spinal cord and into the dorsal nucleus of the vagus nerve in the obex region of the medulla oblongata.

Although less is known about the uptake of infectious agent in CWD-infected cervids, the first tissues involved are the tonsils and the GALT (Sigurdson et al., 1999). PrP^{Sc} is then detected in the enteric nervous system, followed by involvement of the central nervous system at the vagal nucleus and the thoracic spinal cord. Oral inoculation of pooled CWD-positive mule deer brains into mule deer fawns resulted in an early accumulation of CWD-associated PrP in the lymph tissues draining the oral and intestinal mucosa. Lymphoid cells associated with PrP^{CWD} in the tonsils were characterized from clinical and preclinical mule deer. PrP was shown to colocalize, through the use of dual immunofluorescent staining, with the extracellular regions around follicular dendritic cells and B-cells.

Studies characterizing the disease-associated PrP isoform in various tissues from CJD and vCJD patients determined that PrP^{Sc} is readily detectable in lymphoreticular tissues from vCJD and not detectable in sporadic CJD. This is probably due to the oral source of the vCJD infection and suggests a greater potential of iatrogenic transmission of vCJD.

Of particular concern to the safety of food is the deposition and accumulation of PrP^{Sc} and infectivity in tissues where PrP^{Sc} and infectivity are normally not observed in the infected host. A number of different research groups have now demonstrated that infectious agent and/or PrP^{Sc} accumulate in tissues that are inflamed. For example, although PrP^{Sc} is not usually observed in mammary tissues, sheep that are infected with scrapie and have mastitis have significant levels of PrP^{Sc} in the mammary glands. Although the infectious agent has not been identified in milk from scrapie-infected animals, the presence of PrP^{Sc} in mammary lymphoid follicles along with the shedding of macrophages into the milk of sheep with mastitis suggests that this may be a route of horizontal infection within flocks (Ligios et al., 2005). A similar observation has been made in TSE-infected animals that have chronic kidney diseases; PrP^{Sc} is detected in the kidneys, raising the possibility that the agent is or could be shed in the urine of these animals.

4.5 CHARACTERISTICS OF THE AGENT

The unusual biology of the TSEs has influenced how these disorders have been described. Based on their long incubation periods and transmissibility, TSEs were originally described as unconventional or "slow" viruses. The extreme resistance of these agents to ionizing and gamma irradiation combined with the inability to isolate a TSE-specific microorganism prompted speculation that there existed a non–nucleic acid mode of replication. In 1968, a mathematician, J.S. Griffith, proposed three means by which a protein could have self-replicating properties. One of Griffith's models involved the interaction of two proteins having the same primary amino acid sequence, yet differing structurally. In the late 1970s, two groups independently identified brain homogenate fractions that were enriched for infectivity. The detergent extraction and centrifugation steps resulted in the formation of fibular structures referred to as scrapie-associated fibrils in 1981 and as similarly structured prion rods in 1982. Biochemical characterization of the highly infectious preparations identified a protease-resistant protein termed the prion protein. This glycoprotein had a molecular weight of 33 to 35 kDa (in the absence of protease treatment). Treatment with mild protease (50 to 100 μg/mL of proteinase K) reduced the molecular weight to 27 to 30 kDa. Characterization of the gene encoding the prion protein quickly led to the realization that the prion protein was not unique to an undiscovered microorganism but was expressed in uninfected animals and encoded by a single-copy nuclear gene. The difference between the infection-associated and uninfected forms of the protein involved the structure of the two otherwise identical proteins (Table 2). The disease-associated form, in addition to being resistant to proteinase digestion, was found to have more beta sheet structure than the form of the protein expressed in uninfected animals. In 1982, Stanley Prusiner formally proposed the prion hypothesis that identified Griffith's hypothetical protein as the prion protein and defined prions as "small proteinaceous particles which are resistant to inactivation by most procedures that modify nucleic acids" (Prusiner, 1982). Prusiner proposed that the interaction of the prion protein (disease-associated form) with the normal cellular form resulted

TABLE 2 Prion Protein Nomenclature

	Protease Sensitivity	Description
PrP^{C}	Sensitive	Normal isoform of the prion protein
PrP^{Sc}	Resistant	Disease-associated isoform of the prion protein
PrP-sen	Sensitive	Refers to protease digestion characteristics of PrP, often in the absence of transmission data
PrP-res	Resistant	Refers to protease digestion characteristics of PrP, often in the absence of transmission data
Prion rods	Resistant	Structures produced upon detergent extraction of infected tissue; highly infectious, comprised primarily of PrP^{Sc}
Scrapie-associated fibrils	Resistant	Very similar to prion rods

in the conversion of the normal form to the disease form, increasing the amount of abnormal form and thus the level of infectious agent.

The *PrP* gene is highly conserved among mammalian species. Human PrP is a glycoprotein of 253 amino acids. All PrP proteins are cell surface glycoproteins expressed primarily in neurons but also in astrocytes and other cells. PrP^C is synthesized in the endoplasmic reticulum and transported through the Golgi toward the cell surface. Like other GPI-anchored proteins, PrP^C is located primarily in cholesterol-rich, detergent-resistant microdomain complexes of the plasma membrane (rafts). Cell culture studies have demonstrated that once in the membrane, some PrP molecules are released into the extracellular space, while most are internalized into an endocytic compartment. The normal function of the protein is not known. There is some evidence, based on a metal-binding domain present in the N-terminal region of the polypeptide and the binding of copper to synthetic peptides, that PrP^C is a metalloprotein. PrPC may also have a role in protecting a cell against apoptosis and oxidative damage (for a review, see Westergard et al., 2007). The generation of transgenic mice lacking the prion gene ($PrP^{-/-}$) demonstrated that PrP^C is not an essential gene. When the $PrP^{-/-}$ mice are infected with mouse-adapted scrapie, they do not accumulate PrP^{Sc}, develop spongiform lesions, or replicate infectivity.

PrP^{Sc} represents a conformational variant of PrP^C. In contrast to PrP^C, PrP^{Sc} forms insoluble aggregates with a β-sheet content characteristic of an amyloidogenic protein polymer. PrP^{Sc} assembles into fibrils both in vivo and in vitro, is resistant to heat, radiation, and conventional disinfectants such as alcohol and formalin, and is partially resistant to digestion with proteinase K (PK). In most cases, PK digestion removes 60 to 70 amino acid residues from the N-terminus, generating PrP27-30, the protease-resistant core of PrP^{Sc}.

Although during the course of a TSE infection, the conversion of PrP^C to PrP^{Sc} has been well documented, the molecular mechanism by which the conversion occurs is not yet known. Models for the generation of PrP^{Sc} are based on an autocatalytic process involving the interaction of PrP^C with PrP^{Sc}. The most experimentally relevant model is the nucleation-dependent polymerization model. In this model, infectious PrP^{Sc} is an ordered aggregate (probably a small oligomer consisting of 14 to 28 PrP^{Sc} molecules) that acts as a seed. Upon binding to the seed, PrP^C acquires the conformation of the PrP^{Sc} subunits in the oligomer (Silveira et al., 2005).

4.5.1 TSE Strains

TSE strains have the unique distinction of being employed historically as evidence of the existence of an essential nucleic acid as the infectious agent and, more recently, also being used to support the protein-only (prion) hypothesis.

Different strains of TSEs can adapt and/or exist in a given host species. Although the first TSE strains identified were in goats infected with scrapie, the majority of TSE strains have been characterized in rodent models. It is estimated that 20 different prion strains have been produced upon transmission of TSEs to rodents. Strains are defined by a number of characteristics, the most easily identified being incubation period and clinical symptoms. Strain-specific histopathological differences (e.g., brain location of spongiform changes, number and size of spongiform changes) have led to the development of lesion profile analysis, which measures the extent and distribution of spongiform degeneration in the central nervous system. Lesion profiling, in which nine standard areas of the brain are assigned a score based on the intensity of vacuolation, provides a quantitative assessment of spongiform degeneration. The migration pattern of PrP^{Sc} on PAGE (polyacrylamide gel electrophoresis) has also proven to be a useful tool to distinguish TSEs. Human TSEs can be classified based on PK digestion products of PrP^{Sc} as the migration of PrP^{Sc} bands representing different degrees of PrP glycosylation. Defining the ratio of di-, mono-, and nonglycosylated forms of PrP^{Sc} is referred to as a glycoform profile.

A strong link between TSE strain and PrP^{Sc} structure was identified by Richard Marsh and colleagues. The investigators passaged TME into hamsters and after numerous passages identified two stable hamster-adapted strains (Bessen and Marsh, 1994). The strains, referred to as Hyper (HY) and Drowsy (DY), were easily distinguished by differences in both incubation period and clinical symptoms. Animals infected with the HY strain exhibited hyperexcitability and cerebellar ataxia at 65 days post-inoculation (dpi), while those infected with the DY strain presented with lethargy at 168 dpi with no hyperexcitability or cerebellar ataxia. The PK-resistant forms of PrP^{HY} and PrP^{DY} migrate differently on SDS (sodium dodecyl sulfate)-PAGE, with all three isoforms (diglycosylated, monoglycosylated, and nonglycosylated) of PrP^{DY} migrating with a 1- to 2-kDa lower molecular weight than that of the isoforms generated in a HY infection. These qualitative differences in the proteolytic degradation pattern of the two proteins having identical primary sequences strongly suggest that different second or tertiary conformations exist between HY and DY. These differences have been confirmed by a number of different studies, including FTIR and circular dichroism.

4.5.2 Interspecies Transmission

The ability of a TSE agent to infect a new host is one of the most critical concerns with respect to food safety and is referred to as the species barrier effect. Sheep scrapie exhibits a relatively high species barrier and is not readily transmitted to other species (other than goats). BSE, on the other hand, has a relatively low species barrier and has readily been transmitted, both experimentally and naturally, to a number of new hosts. Transmission of a TSE to a new host species is an inefficient process, resulting in a significantly longer incubation period in the new host species compared to the original host species. Subsequent passage in the new host species results in the reduction and eventual stabilization of the incubation. For example, the mink TSE agent, TME, has limited pathogenicity in ferrets, with clinical symptoms occurring after an extended incubation period of approximately 24 months. A second passage (ferret to ferret) results in a reduction of the incubation period to 18 months, while a third passage results in a 4-month incubation period that is stable upon further ferret passage. Ferret-adapted TME (4-month incubation period) has limited pathogenicity in mink, requiring about a 24-month incubation period. A similar adaptation of agent to a new host is occurring with the infection of humans via blood transfusions from preclinical vCJD patients; incubation periods are shorter than observed with the BSE-to-human infection.

The apparent strong sheep-to-bovine species barrier may have been overcome in a similar manner. Scrapie-infected sheep were rendered and the meat-and-bone meal by-products included as a supplement to cattle rations. The physicochemical stability that characterizes these infectious agents resulted in the scrapie agent surviving the heat treatment present in the rendering process. Cattle fed scrapie-infected meat-and-bone meal were then rendered and included in meat-and-bone meal supplements, thus recycling infectivity in the cattle population of Great Britain.

It is a rather unique characteristic of the BSE agent that it transmits readily to numerous other species. Experimentally, BSE has been transmitted, in addition to cattle, to a number of species, including mice, mink, sheep, goats, marmosets, and macaque monkeys. It is this weak species barrier that has led to the emerging vCJD epidemic.

4.6 EPIDEMIOLOGY

The TSE landscape has shifted considerably over the past 20 years, from CJD being an extremely rare and relatively unknown disease and scrapie being an agricultural nuisance and of veterinary interest, to the outbreak of the agriculturally disastrous BSE epidemic and the realization that BSE can and has been transmitted to humans. The expanding CWD epizootic also increases the risk that the CWD agent will move into new species.

4.6.1 Human TSEs

The epidemiology of human prion diseases encompasses three forms: sporadic, familial, and acquired. CJD (sporadic) has an incidence of approximately one person per million per year worldwide. It occurs in persons in their fifth to sixth decades of life and has a worldwide distribution. The familial forms of CJD and GSS are even rarer, affecting one person per 10 million per year.

vCJD is clearly an emerging disease. Not surprisingly given the BSE link, almost every case has occurred in the UK. As of this writing (July 2007), there have been 170 cases in Great Britain (Fig. 2), one in Ireland, and two in France. Currently, the majority of vCJD cases have been restricted to people who are homozygous for methionine at position 129 in the prion protein. Cases have been observed in people who are heterozygous (methionine/valine) at this same position. It is not yet known whether homozygosity (valine) at this PrP codon will provide resistance to infection or just longer incubation periods. Although the number of vCJD cases has declined over the past 4 to 5 years, it is not clear whether the number of cases has peaked or if these cases have just represented the most susceptible persons. Given the uncertainty about a number of the risk factors (e.g., precise route of infection, amount of BSE agent that entered the human food chain), it is not possible to predict the future prevalence of this disease.

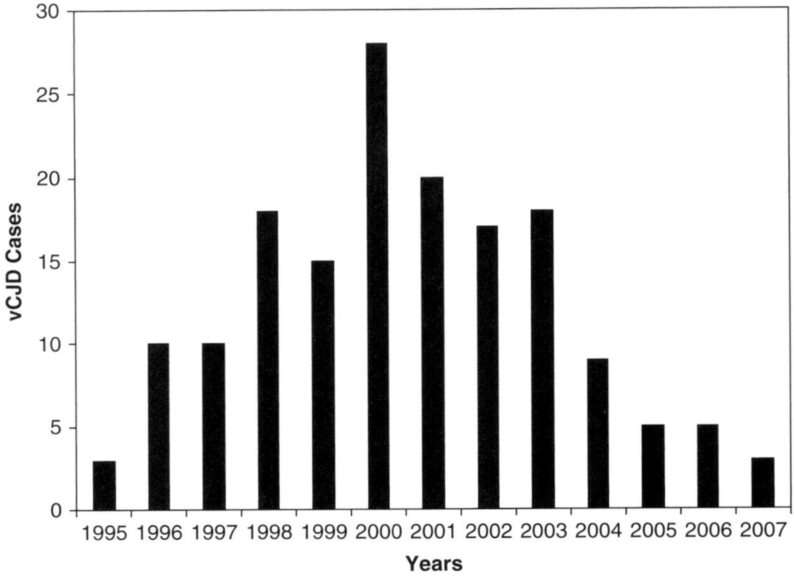

FIG. 2 Number of vCJD human cases in Great Britain. (Data derived from http://www.cjd.ed.ac.uk/figures.htm. The 2007 data include cases to August.)

4.6.2 Chronic Wasting Disease

As mentioned above, the range and prevalence of CWD has been increasing annually in the United States and Canada. Like sheep scrapie, CWD epizootics can be maintained by horizontal transmission from infected to naive animals, and transmission is mediated, at least in part, by an environmental reservoir of infectivity (Johnson et al., 2007). The presence of an environmental reservoir affects several epidemiological factors, including contact rate (the frequency with which animals come in contact with the disease agent), duration of exposure (time period over which animals come in contact with the agent), and the efficiency of transmission (the probability that an exposed individual contracts the disease). It has been hypothesized that soil can serve as a reservoir for CWD. Deer and other ruminants ingest hundreds of grams of soil daily. Experimentally, infectious agent bound to soil is more transmissible than unbound agent. Soil can be contaminated with CWD agent via the decomposition of infected carcasses, shedding of agent through the alimentary system, burial of carcasses, and perhaps via urine and saliva.

4.7 PRP^{SC} DETECTION

One of the greatest challenges in the prion field is the need to develop accurate and highly sensitive methods of assaying for TSE infection. Traditional detection and/or verification of a TSE infection involved the histological examination of the brain for evidence of spongiform degeneration typically combined with animal bioassays to determine transmissibility. The identification of the disease-associated form of the prion protein and the generation of PrP antibodies facilitated Western blot and immunohistochemical approaches to the detection of PrP^{Sc}-containing tissue. It should be noted, however, that antibodies specific to the disease-associated form of the prion protein, although described in the literature, are not yet commercially available. The most accurate diagnosis occurs in animals and humans during the clinical stages of the disease through examination of the central nervous system. Brains of infected animals during the clinical phase of the disease contain the highest level of spongiform degeneration and the greatest accumulation of PrP^{Sc}. The earlier the stage of infection, the more difficult these diseases are to diagnose.

Western blot analysis involves the treatment of tissue homogenates with mild levels of PK (50 to 100 μg/mL for 1 to 2 hours). PrP^{C}, the only PrP isoform in uninfected tissue, is digested completely, whereas PrP^{Sc} exhibits resistance to the digestion (Fig. 3). A portion of the N-terminal region of the PrP^{Sc} isoform is cleaved during digestion, resulting in a smaller protease-resistant core of about 27 to 30 kDa (Fig. 3).

Within the past several years, a number of other assays have been developed for the detection of prion infectivity/PrP^{Sc}. A number of companies have developed ELISA assay for the rapid detection of PrP^{Sc}, and these assays are now used routinely to screen for BSE and CWD in national laboratories in the United States, Canada, and the EU. A more sensitive test is the conformation-dependent immunoassay, which uses antibodies to distinguish between PrP^{C} and PrP^{Sc}. As PrP^{Sc}-specific antibodies become available, the utility of this method of detection will increase.

Two novel approaches to detection of the TSE agent have also been developed recently. The first of these, the scrapie cell assay, uses neuroblastoma cells that have

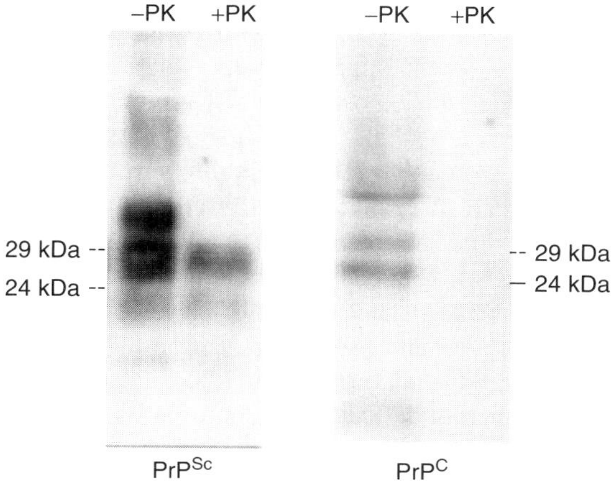

FIG. 3 Proteinase K sensitivity of PrP obtained from brain homogenate from an infected animal (left panel) and with PrP^{C} (right panel) that is not associated with infectivity.

been selected due to their high rate of infectibility by TSE agents (Klohn et al., 2003). After infection and splitting of the cell cultures, the samples are spotted onto an ELISAPOT and detected by immunoreactivity with antibodies to PrP. Although this method appears to be as sensitive as animal bioassay when used with a specific strain of mouse-adapted scrapie agent, it has not been readily adapted for use with other TSE agents. The second novel approach is a protein amplification reaction, similar in principle to PCR reactions. In this approach, developed by Claude Soto, small amounts of PrP^{Sc} or infected tissue extracts are mixed with brain homogenate from uninfected animals, sonicated, and then incubated; this cycle is repeated a large number of times and generates significant levels of PrP^{Sc}, which can then be detected using conventional methods (such as Western blot of ELISA). This method, referred to as protein misfolding cyclical amplification (PMCA), has been instrumental in identifying PrP^{Sc} in biological samples such as blood from CWD-infected deer (Soto et al., 2005).

4.8 PHYSICAL MEANS OF DESTRUCTION OF THE ORGANISM

One of the most challenging areas of prion disease research involves development of treatments that inactivate the infectious agent. The extreme physicochemical stability of the prion disease agent is the underlying cause of the BSE epidemic, the iatrogenic transmission of CJD via contaminated surgical instruments, and probably the spread of CWD.

The resistance of these agents to inactivation has been recognized for decades. The resistance of scrapie to formalin during the preparation of a vaccine resulted in the accidental transmission of scrapie in the 1930s. Standard autoclaving (121°C for 15 min) does not eliminate infectivity.

Many of the inactivation studies have been performed in the laboratory of David Taylor (for a review, see Taylor, 2000). Chemical methods of inactivation, including ethanol, formaldehyde, glutaraldehyde, and hydrogen peroxide, which exhibit efficacy in the sterilization and decontamination of microorganisms, are of little practical use with prion diseases. One-hour exposure to NaOCl solution containing 20,000 ppm of Cl_2 is suitable for inactivating TSE agents. It should be noted that there are TSE strain differences in inactivation. Richard Kimberlin and colleagues determined that autoclaving one mouse-adapted strain (strain 139A) for 2 h at 126°C resulted in its inactivation, whereas a second strain (strain 22A) was not inactivated (Taylor, 2000).

Chemical denaturation of infectious preparations results in a reduction of infectivity and concomitant decline in the amount of protease-resistant PrP. Our group has shown that both infectivity and the abnormal form of the protein can be regenerated upon dilution of the denaturant. It should be emphasized that the preceding experiments were performed under carefully controlled laboratory conditions. The study does emphasize the need to ensure destruction of the protein during inactivation treatments.

The UK government advisory committee recommends 134 to 137°C for 18 min or a series of successive cycles of 134 to 137°C for a minimum of 3 min per cycle for autoclaving CJD. The Office International des Épizooties recommends the following treatment for the inactivation of TSEs in meat-and-bone meal containing ruminant proteins: (1) reduction of particle size to 50 mm prior to heating, and (2) raw material being subjected to saturated steam conditions to a temperature of 133°C or above for 20 min.

This resistance to inactivation may contribute to the lateral transmission of CWD. Several lines of evidence suggest that cervids shed CWD agent through feces, saliva, and urine. TSE agents bind avidly to soil and can persist in the soil for at least 3 years. Since deer (and a number of other species) ingest large quantities of soil, it is likely that the environment serves as a reservoir of infectivity.

4.9 PREVENTION AND CONTROL MEASURES

4.9.1 Animal TSEs

With scrapie, control measures involve primarily the eradication not only of the affected animals but also of their associated flocks. Despite eradication efforts, scrapie remains a self-sustaining disease of sheep throughout the world. Scrapie eradication programs have been successful in Australia but not in the United States.

The unusual (for TSEs) transmission characteristics of CWD have resulted in CWD being a rapidly emerging disease and suggest that its eradication will be very difficult. Experimental animal transmission studies with CWD indicate a "typical" species barrier, suggesting that CWD would not be a health risk to humans. The identification of CWD agent in skeletal muscle of infected deer is of concern, however, as it suggests that it will be possible for humans to consume infected tissue (Angers et al., 2006). Reduction of the number of infected animals on the landscape is also very important, as the combination of the high numbers of deer shedding agent into the environment, the persistence of the agent in the environment, and the subsequent enhanced transmissibility of soil-bound agent into hosts will perpetuate the epidemic.

Being a foodborne disease, BSE has declined dramatically as a result of the ban on feeding ruminant meat-and-bone meal to cattle. There is little evidence of cattle-to-cattle transmission of BSE. It is, therefore, argued that strict adherence to the feed ban will result in its elimination.

4.9.2 vCJD

The lack of treatment for these diseases has focused efforts to minimize further transmission of vCJD. It is believed that the dramatic decline in BSE, coupled with the exclusion of bovine brain or nervous tissue in human food mandated by the British government in 1995, has reduced tremendously and/or eliminated further BSE-to-human transmission. The greatest concern is the unknown number of infected humans who are at a preclinical stage of the disease. Several cases of vCJD have now been identified in which the source of the infectious agent appears to be blood transfusions, the blood having been donated by people preclinical for vCJD. The incubation periods are shorter, probably due to adaptation of the agent to the human host (i.e., as described earlier, repeated passage within the same host species usually results in a shorter incubation period). In the United States there are restrictions on donating blood if the person has visited or lived in Great Britain.

Estimates of the total number of potential cases of vCJD range from a few dozen to hundreds of thousands of people. There are currently too many unknowns (e.g., route of infection, number of people exposed, effectiveness of CNS exclusion from meat, levels of infectivity present) to provide an accurate assessment of the future incidence of the disease. Given the long incubation periods that characterize these diseases, however, we can expect additional vCJD cases to occur for decades to come.

4.9.3 Food Safety

The risk to humans from BSE is still emerging. Clearly, humans can be infected with BSE; the route of exposure is unclear but appears to be through the ingestion of contaminated beef or beef by-products. Risk to humans can be decreased by surveillance and testing of all high-risk cattle.

The risk to humans from CWD is currently unknown. There have been no documented cases of human TSE from the consumption of CWD-infected deer or exposure to CWD during processing of infected deer. The number of people potentially exposed to CWD is very low compared to the number of people thought to be exposed to BSE-infected meat; hence, it is too early to conclude that there is no risk of human disease from consumption of CWD-infected venison.

The CDC currently recommends that no part of any animal infected with a TSE should enter the human food chain.

REFERENCES

Angers RC, Browning SR, Seward TS, et al. (2006): Prions in skeletal muscles of deer with chronic wasting disease. *Science*. 311:1117.

Bessen RA, Marsh RF (1994): Distinct PrP properties suggest the molecular basis of strain variation in transmissible mink encephalopathy. *J Virol*. 68:7859–7868.

Jeffrey M, Gonzales L (2004): Pathology and pathogenesis of bovine spongiform encephalopathy and scrapie. *Curr Top Microbiol Immunol*. 284:65–97.

Johnson CJ, Pedersen JA, Chappell RJ, McKenzie D, Aiken JM (2007): Oral transmissibility of prion disease is enhanced by binding to soil particles. *Pub Libr Sci Pat*. 6:e93

Klohn PC, Stoltze L, Flechsig E, Enari M, Weissmann C (2003): A quantitative, highly sensitive cell-based infectivity assay for mouse scrapie prions. *Proc Natl Acad Sci*. 30:1166–1171.

Ligios C, Sigurdson CJ, Santucciu C, et al. (2005): PrP^{Sc} in mammary glands of sheep affected by scrapie and mastitis. *Nat Med*. 11:1137–1138.

Peden AJ, Ritchie DL, Ironside JW (2005): Risks of transmission of variant Creutzfeldt–Jakob disease by blood transfusion. *Folia Neuropathol*. 43:271–278.

Prusiner SB (1982): Novel proteinaceous infectious particles cause scrapie. *Science*. 216:136.

Sigurdson CJ, Williams ES, Miller MW, Spraker TR, O'Rourke KI, Hoover EA (1999): Oral transmission and early lymphoid tropism of chronic wasting disease PrPres in mule deer fawns (*Odocoileu hemionus*). *J Gen Virol*. 80:2757–2764.

Silveira JR, Raymond GJ, Hughson AG, et al. (2005): The most infectious prion protein particles. *Nature*. 437:257–261.

Soto C, Anderes L, Suardi S, et al. (2005): Pre-symptomatic detection of prions by cyclic amplification of protein misfolding. *FEBS Lett*. 31:638–642.

Taylor DM (2000): Inactivation of transmissible degenerative encephalopathy agents: a review. *Vet J*. 159:10–17.

Westergard L, Christensen HM, Harris DA (2007): The cellular prion protein (PrP^C): its physiological function and role in disease. *Biochem Biophys Acta*. 1772:629–644.

CHAPTER 5

AVIAN INFLUENZA A (H5N1): POTENTIAL THREAT TO FOOD SAFETY

JAMES MARK SIMMERMAN and PETER K. BEN EMBAREK

5.1 INTRODUCTION

Influenza viruses belong to the family Orthomyxoiviridae and have three types: influenza A, B and C. Influenza types A and B viruses are known to cause most human disease; only type A viruses have been documented to cause human pandemics. Influenza virions are enveloped particles of spherical or slightly elongated dimensions measuring 80 to 120 nm in diameter. The genome consists of single-stranded, negative-sense RNA in eight gene segments that code for 10 proteins (Wright and Webster, 2001).

The major surface glycoproteins are the hemagglutinin (HA) and neuraminidase (NA). While the transmission and pathogenesis of human influenza viruses is a polygenic trait, HA and NA play pivotal roles. Sixteen different HAs (differing by at least 30% in their nucleotide homology) and nine different NA subtypes have been identified. Of these, only viruses with combinations of HA 1-3 and NA 1-2 were known to cause severe disease in humans until the occurrence H5N1 infection in humans in 1997. Specific antibody against HA is protective, but minor antigenic changes occur frequently, and new strains can infect and cause disease in persons who have antibody against other related but antigenically distinct strains. Antibody to NA may help modify disease severity. Briefly, neuraminidase promotes the release of virus from infected cells, inhibits the aggregation of new virions, and facilitates their spread to other respiratory tract cells (Colman, 1994). Hemagglutinin mediates receptor binding and membrane fusion of influenza virus and is the primary target for infectivity-neutralizing antibodies (Skehel and Wiley, 2000). While the determinants of viral tropism and receptor specificity are polygenic, hemagglutinin is believed to be the key molecule in terms of species specificity, antibody response, and pathogenesis.

The receptor specificity of HA is an important determinant of the ability of H5N1 viruses to cross the species barrier (Suzuki et al., 2000). Human influenza viruses bind

Microbiologically Safe Foods, Edited by Norma Heredia, Irene Wesley, and Santos García

preferentially to cells with sialic acid receptors containing α-2,6-galactose linkages, while avian viruses bind preferentially those containing α-2,3-galactose linkages (Stephenson et al., 2003). However there is evidence that even a single amino acid substitution in the *HA* gene can significantly alter receptor specificity of avian H5N1 viruses, providing them with the ability to bind to receptors optimal for human influenza viruses (Gambaryan et al., 2006). The pandemic implications of such a mutation are significant, as the H1N1 virus that caused a massive pandemic in 1918 was also of avian origin and acquired a preference for the α-2,6-galactose receptors (Glaser et al., 2005; Taubenberger et al., 2005; Tumpey, 2005). However, another study employing a comparative ferret model and plasmid-based reverse genetic methods to generate H5N1 reassortant viruses demonstrated the complexity of the genetic basis for transmissibility of influenza viruses. Neither human influenza H3N2 surface proteins nor human influenza virus internal proteins were sufficient for a 1997 H5N1 virus to develop pandemic characteristics, even after serial passages in ferrets (Maines et al., 2006). Close monitoring of the genetic evolution and receptor binding preference of H5N1 viruses is a public health priority.

The presence of multiple basic amino acids at the HA cleavage site is characteristic of highly pathogenic avian strains (Claas et al., 1998; Subbarao et al., 1998). While the current H5N1 viruses have been found to possess this predictor for increased pathogenicity, it is interesting to note that the 1918 pandemic H1N1 virus did not (Tumpey, 2005). Since its identification in humans in 1997, the H5N1 virus has undergone rapid evolution, demonstrated by development of multiple genotypes (Guan et al., 2002), antigenic changes (WHO, 2005d), increased pathogenicity and extrapulmonary disease (Govorkova et al., 2005; Liu et al., 2005; Maines et al., 2005), an extended host range (Kuiken et al., 2004; Thanawongnuwech et al., 2005), increasing numbers of human clusters (Olsen et al., 2005b), and development of resistance to antiviral medications that inhibit the M2 ion channel [(adamantanes) (Bright et al., 2005; Guan and Chen, 2005). In addition, one report has documented the development of resistance to the neuraminidase inhibitor oseltamivir, another of the influenza antiviral medications (Le et al., 2005). The latter developments are of potential public health importance, as antiviral medications are key public health tools to combat a future pandemic (Ferguson et al., 2005; Hayden, 2001; Longini et al., 2005).

5.2 EMERGENCE OF H5N1 AVIAN INFLUENZA

Wild waterfowl, gulls, and shorebirds are the natural reservoir for influenza type A viruses, and viruses representing all 16 subtypes of hemagglutinin (HA) and nine subtypes of neuraminidase (NA) have been isolated from these species (Stallknecht et al., 1990; Suarez and Schultz-Cherry, 2000). Until the emergence of highly pathogenic avian influenza (HPAI) H5N1, influenza A viruses in waterfowl were considered to be in evolutionary stasis, causing mainly asymptomatic infections (Hulse-Post et al., 2005; Suarez, 2000; Webster et al., 1992, 1995). In contrast, many influenza A virus subtypes have been documented to cause symptomatic infection in marine mammals, horses, pigs, cats, and dogs (Crawford et al., 2005; Kaye and Pringle, 2005; Liu et al., 2003; Swayne and Suarez, 2000). Until the 1997 outbreak of H5N1 in Hong

Kong among domestic poultry and 18 human cases, however, only subtypes H1–3 had been associated with severe disease in humans (Mounts et al., 1997; Shortridge et al., 1998). Concerns for spread among poultry, human health, and the potential for emergence of an influenza pandemic virus prompted the culling of millions of poultry in Hong Kong and the implementation of extensive measures to prevent further spread (Sims et al., 2003).

Due to their low-fidelity polymerase and segmented genome, influenza A viruses are characterized by extreme genetic variability (Lin et al., 2004; Wu and Yan, 2005). In addition, cross-species transmission events appear to accelerate the rates of mutations (Guan et al., 2003; Li et al., 2004; Webster, 1997). Across much of Asia, it is common practice to both raise and market multiple bird and other animal species in close proximity to humans, creating an ideal environment for the development of new influenza virus reassortants potentially capable of causing disease in humans (Choi et al., 2005; Kung et al., 2003; Peiris et al., 2001; Webster, 2004). In addition, large-scale agribusinesses that maintain production facilities in many Asian countries may also facilitate the international dissemination of avian influenza virus strains (Kwon et al., 2005; Thomas et al., 2005). Finally, the interaction of wild migratory waterfowl with domestic ducks and chickens may also have contributed to the geographic spread of the H5N1 virus (Hubalek, 2004; Krauss et al., 2004; Ligon, 2005; Liu et al., 2005). In fewer than 10 years since the virus was identified in Hong Kong, it has become endemic in much of East Asia and in 2005 and 2006 spread to Europe, the Near East, Africa, and most of Asia (Information, 2005; Lee et al., 2005).

The precursor to the H5N1 virus identified in Hong Kong in 1997 was first detected in geese in Guangdong province of China in 1996 (A/Goose/Guangdong/1/96-like). Despite extensive control measures, new H5N1 reassortants emerged and caused outbreaks among birds in Hong Kong in 2000 and 2001, and were linked to two human deaths in 2002 (Guan et al., 2002; Peiris et al., 2004; Sturm-Ramirez et al., 2004). In 2001, H5N1 viruses were isolated from live wet poultry markets in Vietnam (Nguyen et al., 2005). In 2003, highly pathogenic avian influenza (HPAI) H5N1 viruses caused massive mortality among poultry in large commercial poultry farms in Thailand, Cambodia, China, Indonesia, Japan, Laos, South Korea, and Vietnam (Harper et al., 2004; Tiensin et al., 2005). As of February 2004, 23 human H5N1 cases and 18 deaths had been reported in Vietnam and Thailand (WHO, 2004a). By 2007, Cambodia, China, Djibouti, Egypt, Indonesia, Iraq, and Turkey had joined the list of countries reporting human fatalities. H5N1 is now considered endemic among poultry in East and Southeast Asia. Infection and culling have resulted in the deaths of more than 200 million poultry, with devastating economic losses to large agribusinesses and to small farmers (FAO, 2005).

5.3 EPIDEMIOLOGY OF HUMAN H5N1 INFECTION

Each new human infection with avian influenza A (H5N1) virus represents an important opportunity to advance what is known about the epidemiology of this novel pathogen. Human influenza is transmitted principally through droplets of respiratory secretions, fomite and aerosol transmission may also occur. While the routes of transmission for H5N1 have not been established definitively, most patients have had direct exposure to infected birds, including butchering, consuming incompletely cooked or raw poultry products, and handling fighting cocks or other poultry commonly being reported (Beigel et al., 2005; Chotpitayasunondh et al., 2005). Such exposures suggest that pharyngeal or gastrointestinal inoculation of the virus may be an important method of transmission. Importantly, while chickens infected with H5N1 rapidly develop symptoms that can signal a risk for potential human exposure, domestic ducks can remain apparently healthy while continuing to excrete virus (Chen et al., 2004; Sturm-Ramirez et al., 2005). And although viral replication is greatly reduced, vaccinated chickens may also excrete virus (Swayne et al., 2001). These findings have implications for widespread human exposures in Asia, where duck husbandry is very common or in countries where large-scale poultry vaccination is used.

No sustained human-to-human transmission of H5N1 infection has occurred to date. Such transmission is a necessary feature of a pandemic and necessitates continued vigilance to look for evidence of efficient transmission. Although transmission directly from infected poultry explains most cases to date, small clusters of human cases have been reported, raising the possibility of limited person-to-person transmissions (Kandun et al., 2006; Olsen et al., 2005b).

In Hong Kong in 1997, neutralizing antibodies to H5N1 were found in 6 of 51 household contacts, one with no clear history of exposure to poultry (Katz et al., 1999). In Thailand, probable transmission from a severely ill child to a family member who provided intensive and prolonged nursing care was reported (Ungchusak et al., 2005). Documenting human-to-human transmission is complicated by the high frequency of potential confounding exposures to poultry or a contaminated environment, delays in the initiation of epidemiologic investigations, and limited availability of clinical specimens of adequate quality. To date, no evidence of sustained person-to-person transmission of H5N1 virus has been identified, but rapid investigation of H5N1 cases is needed to identify and attempt to contain such an event promptly should it occur.

Mild or asymptomatic H5N1 virus infection appears to be uncommon. In Hong Kong, 8 (3.7%) of 217 exposed health care workers and 2 (0.7%) of 309 unexposed health care workers had mild or asymptomatic infections with evidence of serologic conversion (Bridges et al., 2000). Another study among Hong Kong poultry workers found that 10% had serological evidence of prior infection (Bridges et al., 2002). However, a serosurvey of case contacts and persons with presumably intense exposures in rural Cambodia in 2005 did not support the widespread occurrence of mild or asymptomatic disease (Vong et al., 2006). Early identification of an expanded spectrum of illness with H5N1 infection is of public health importance, as it may represent a key change toward a virus with increased pandemic potential.

5.4 CLINICAL PRESENTATION AND LABORATORY DIAGNOSIS

Most clinical descriptions of H5N1 are from patients hospitalized with severe pneumonia. The incubation period for H5N1 ranges from 2 to 8 days, with a median of 4 days (Beigel et al., 2005; Bridges et al., 2002, Olsen et al., 2005b; Tran et al., 2004).

This appears to be longer than for human influenza viruses, for which the incubation period is 1 to 4 days with a median of 2 days (Cate, 1987). Most H5N1-infected patients present with high fever and systemic influenza-like symptoms, such as nausea, headache, and myalgia. Upper respiratory symptoms are not always present. A few case reports have documented atypical syndromes, including patients whose primary symptoms are gastrointestinal (Apisarnthanarak et al., 2004) or neurological (de Jong et al., 2005). Diarrhea is common and may precede the onset of respiratory symptoms by several days (Apisarnthanarak et al., 2004). Clinically significant lymphopenia and mild to moderate thrombocytopenia are common laboratory findings (Tran et al., 2004). Lower respiratory tract symptoms are usually found on admission to the hospital, with dyspnea developing in a median of 5 days from onset of illness in one group of patients in Thailand (Chotpitayasunondh et al., 2005). A variety of radiographic abnormalities usually follows closely after the onset of dyspnea, including diffuse, multifocal, or patchy infiltrates, interstitial infiltrates, or lobular consolidation. Pleural effusions are less common. In many patients, the clinical course worsens over several days, with the onset of acute respiratory distress syndrome (ARDS) and the characteristic diffuse "ground-glass" infiltrates on chest x-ray. Death is commonly preceded by multiorgan failure (Beigel et al., 2005; Chan, 2002; Chotpitayasunondh et al., 2005).

Laboratory diagnosis is complicated by the difficulty in obtaining properly collected and well-maintained clinical specimens. H5N1 infection has often not been suspected until late in the course of illness or even after death (Ungchusak et al., 2005). Isolation of H5N1 virus from respiratory specimens using embryonated hen's eggs or tissue cell culture under enhanced biosafety level 3 (BSL-3) conditions is the "gold standard." Reverse transcriptase– polymerase chain reaction (RT-PCR) testing of respiratory specimens is most frequently used to diagnose H5N1 infection, due to its high sensitivity, speed, and safety. Nasopharyngeal and lower respiratory tract specimens are optimal to detect H5N1 virus (WHO, 2006a). Stool specimens, lung tissue, and blood have tested positive for viral RNA and yielded virus isolates (Beigel et al., 2005; de Jong et al., 2005).

Serologic testing for evidence of H5N1 antibody is limited by a method's technical complexity and the need to use live H5N1 virus under BSL-3 laboratory conditions. When properly timed acute and convalescent serum samples have been collected, the microneutralization assay with confirmatory Western blot assay is highly sensitive and specific (Rowe et al., 1999). The traditional hemagglutination-inhibition test (HI) does not require live virus and effectively detects increases in human influenza antibody in serum. However, the HI is insensitive for the detection of human antibody responses to avian H5 hemagglutinin, even in the presence of high titers of neutralizing antibody after confirmed infection. A modified HI test using horse red blood cells has been developed (Stephenson et al., 2003) and is being field tested in Indonesia. Rapid antigen influenza diagnostic tests are much less sensitive than PCR methods and are not currently recommended for the purpose of detecting H5N1 (Chotpitayasunondh et al., 2005).

In most cases, religious beliefs, social customs, and a scarcity of trained pathologists have prevented postmortem analyses. Early reports have found severe pulmonary injury with histopathological changes of diffuse alveolar damage and hyaline membrane formation similar to pneumonia due to human influenza virus infection (To et al., 2001; Uiprasertkul et al., 2005). Specimens collected during autopsy have yielded evidence of H5N1 virus in the lungs, intestinal tract, and blood (Chutinimitkul et al., 2006; Guarner et al., 2000; Uiprasertkul et al., 2005).

5.5 FOOD SAFETY CONSIDERATIONS

Across East and Southeast Asia, billions of terrestrial and aquatic poultry are raised annually for household consumption, commercial food markets, ornamental collection, and gaming purposes. Poultry husbandry is extremely common in the region. One survey in rural Thailand documented that 74% of households raise at least one type of poultry (Olsen et al., 2005a). In addition, international trafficking in wild Asian birds is an ongoing environmental problem with human health implications (Karesh et al., 2005; Van Borm et al., 2005). These activities result in frequent human exposures as well the distribution of avian influenza viruses across international borders.

In both rural and poor urban settings, multiple avian species and swine are often raised in close proximity to each other, increasing the risk of cross-species transmission and a reassortment event (Ito et al., 1998; Webster and Hulse, 2004). In addition to their economic importance, such practices are often deeply rooted in social and religious customs. For example, the consumption of raw duck blood is considered a delicacy in Vietnam but may constitute a risk for avian influenza infection (CDC, 2005; WHO, 2005b).

While Hong Kong has made substantial progress in controlling avian influenza through farm and market regulations (Kung et al., 2003), most Asian countries lack the human and financial resources required to improve biosecurity significantly in traditional farming and marketing practices. The situation is particularly severe for millions of Asia's poorest citizens, where the loss of poultry to H5N1 infection or culling to control the disease can have serious nutritional consequences. The threat of large-scale poultry culling can also be a significant deterrent for villagers to report poultry outbreaks to veterinary authorities. Further, visibly ill or dead chickens are often butchered and eaten by poor families, a practice that has been implicated in a growing number of fatal human cases (Dinh et al., 2006; Govorkova et al., 2006).

Avian influenza viruses have been reported to cause mild disease and rare human fatalities for many years (Swayne and King, 2003). However, since the 1997 outbreak of HPAI H5N1 in Hong Kong that sickened 18 and killed 6 persons, food safety concerns have greatly increased (Mounts et al., 1999). In contrast to low pathogenic strains that are recovered mainly from the respiratory and gastrointestinal tracts of infected poultry, highly pathogenic H5N1 viruses have been isolated from the brain, blood, bone, breast, and thigh meat (Swayne and Beck, 2005). Domestic cats, tigers, and leopards that consumed uncooked poultry carcasses in laboratory experiments and in a zoo resulted in fatal infections, suggesting that consumption of uncooked meat is a potential risk to humans (Keawcharoen et al., 2004; Kuiken et al., 2004; Thanawongnuwech et al., 2005). Avian influenza viruses including H5N1 have been isolated from live poultry from markets in Hong Kong, Vietnam, Taiwan, Laos, and Korea with a prevalence of up to 3%, depending on the species and season (Boltz et al., 2006; Choi et al., 2005; Liu et al., 2003; Nguyen et al., 2005; Shortridge et al., 1998; Yen, 2001). These studies suggest that there are occupational and consumer risks associated with traditional live markets. Commercially produced poultry are also vulnerable to infection. Highly pathogenic H5N1 virus has been isolated in industrially produced and imported frozen duck meat in Japan and South Korea (Mase et al., 2005; Swayne and Pantin-Jackwood, 2006). Although ill chickens will normally stop laying, H5N1 and other avian influenza viruses have been isolated from the yolk, albumin, and shell surfaces of eggs produced by infected chickens and quail (Swayne and Beck, 2004; WHO, 2005b). H5N1 viruses have also been isolated from privately imported duck and goose eggs during routine checks (Vong et al., 2006). Because infected ducks and geese are often asymptomatic, their eggs may be more likely than chicken eggs to be marketed. Similarly, vaccinated chickens exposed to H5N1 may excrete low levels of virus while experiencing either mild or asymptomatic infection (Swayne et al., 2001). However, correctly administered immunization with high-quality vaccine has been shown to prevent the deposition of HPAI virus in chicken meat (Swayne and Beck, 2005).

Avian influenza viruses retain their infectivity in raw poultry meat, and their viability may be extended by the refrigeration and freezing processes common in the food industry (Mase et al., 2005). At 4°C the virus can remain viable in feces for at least 35 days and up to 23 days in carcasses. At 37°C H5N1 viruses have been shown to remain viable for 6 days in fecal samples (Normaile and Enserink, 2004; Sturm-Ramirez et al., 2005). Although there are differences in environmental survival times between strains, avian influenza viruses excreted by waterfowl into surface water sources can persist for long periods, depending on such factors as pH, salinity, and temperature. Although there is little evidence supporting surface water as a source of human H5N1 infection, caution should be taken avoid oral ingestion, aspiration, or surface contamination of poultry meat with untreated water in affected areas (WHO, 2005b).

In comparison to other viral pathogens that commonly cause foodborne illness, avian influenza viruses are relatively heat sensitive (Swayne, 2006a). The World Health Organization (WHO) and the U.S. Department of Agriculture (USDA) recommend cooking to achieve core temperatures of at least 70°C. If thermometers are not available, no part of the meat should remain pink in color (WHO, 2005b). These recommended cooking temperatures are designed to inactivate common foodborne pathogens such as *Salmonella* and effectively inactivate H5N1 virus. Thermal inactivation studies of H5N1 in chicken meat have demonstrated D_{60}-values (the time at 60°C required to reduce the concentration of H5N1 by 1 log) of 34.1 and 28.6 in chicken breast and thigh meat, respectively. Calculated D_{70}-values were 0.43 and 0.34 in breast and thigh meat, respectively. No viable H5N1 viruses were recovered after 1 at 70°C in chicken meat (Swayne, 2006a). Industry standard pasteurization protocols for liquid egg products have also been shown to inactivate HPAI, while lower-temperature processes were not sufficient to inactive these viruses in dried egg whites (Swayne and Beck, 2004).

Although conventional cooking and pasteurization practices will inactivate H5N1 viruses, the global burden of foodborne diseases such as salmonellosis and campylobacteriosis suggests that consumption of undercooked poultry products is common. Still, the majority of human H5N1 cases to date have been associated with close contact with sick or dead poultry, particularly with the processing of diseased or dead birds (Dinh et al., 2006; Swayne, 2006b). The practice of home slaughtering, defeathering, and eviscerating sick or dead poultry is likely to result in high-dose exposures. Given proper cooking practices, the preparation of infected poultry, rather than its consumption, may then be the principal source of concern.

5.6 GLOBAL RESPONSE

The unprecedented spread and virulence of avian influenza A (H5N1) in poultry and continuing human infections raise concern that a global influenza pandemic could occur. An effective response requires political commitment and transparency and the cooperation of animal and human health authorities at every level. In most countries the capacity of the veterinary health system falls behind that of human public health, and significant efforts will be required to correct this deficit. In much of Asia, H5N1 is now endemic in poultry, and eradication appears unlikely. Coordinated efforts should aim to reduce the amount of virus circulating in domestic poultry flocks and decrease the risk of avian-to-human infection, thereby minimizing the potential for development of an H5N1 strain capable of efficient and sustained human-to-human transmission.

Control of the infection in poultry through improved biosecurity in all farming sectors and enhanced safeguards during distribution and marketing is a priority. In response to massive losses during outbreaks in 2003 and 2004, the commercial poultry sector has taken effective steps to reduce H5N1 infection. However, changing animal husbandry practices in millions of small "backyard" farms in rural and urban settings is a major challenge. Systematic poultry surveillance, accurate laboratory diagnosis, separation of domestic poultry from wild birds, rapid culling of infected flocks, strict movement restrictions, and restocking or adequate financial compensation to farmers are key components of an effective control program (FAO, 2005). Countries that choose to vaccinate poultry as one component of a broader control program must have reliable systems in place to assure vaccine quality and proper administration, to monitor efficacy, and must have long-term funding to sustain the vaccination program.

Public education campaigns to discourage behavior known to be associated with the risk of bird-to-human transmission are essential. Home slaughtering, defeathering, and eviscerating infected poultry, as well as consumption of incompletely cooked poultry, may result in human infections. Therefore, education and incentives to discourage the harvesting of infected poultry and proper food preparation methods are urgently needed. Similarly, family members and health care providers caring for H5N1-infected patients must be educated and equipped with personal protective equipment to reduce the risk of human-to-human transmission. As early symptoms of H5N1 infection are nonspecific, surveillance for H5N1 infection has focused primarily on severe respiratory illness in hospitals. Improving laboratory diagnostic capacity to detect H5N1 virus is essential. Development of a rapid and accurate diagnostic H5N1 test that could be conducted in basic hospital laboratories would represent a major advance. Systematic serological surveys are needed to monitor for mild or asymptomatic illness which could suggest that the virus has become better adapted to humans.

Each new human case merits thorough investigation. Multiple sequential clinical specimens should be collected and viruses submitted promptly to a WHO collaborating laboratory. Molecular analysis of the H5N1 genome is essential to monitor for changes in host affinity, genetic reassortment, antigenic drift, and antiviral resistance, and to ensure that virus strains used to develop vaccine candidates are current (WHO, 2005c). Reverse genetics has been used to develop nonvirulent H5N1 strains for vaccines (Lipatov et al., 2005). Vaccine trials are under way in several countries, and one vaccine has been found to be immunogenic at high doses (Treanor et al., 2007). Clinical research to describe the natural history of illness, better definition of transmission routes, and development of more effective treatment protocols are priorities.

H5N1 avian influenza is a threat to animal and human health worldwide. A long-term, multisector approach with sustained funding is needed to control the disease in poultry and to detect changes that may herald the emergence of a pandemic virus.

REFERENCES

Apisarnthanarak A, Kitphati R, Thongphubeth K, et al. (2004): Atypical avian influenza (H5N1). *Emerg Infect Dis.* 10:1321–1324.

Beigel JH (2005): Avian influenza A (H5N1) infection in humans. *N Engl J Med.* 353:1374–1385.

Boltz DA, Douangngeun B, Sinthasak S, et al. (2006): H5N1 influenza viruses in Lao People's Democratic Republic. *Emerg Infect Dis.* 12 (10).

Bridges, CB, Katz JM, Seto WH, et al. (2000): Risk of influenza A (H5N1) infection among health care workers exposed to patients with influenza A (H5N1), Hong Kong. *J Infect Dis.* 181:344–348.

Bridges CB, Lim W, Hu-Primmer J, et al. (2002): Risk of influenza A (H5N1) infection among poultry workers, Hong Kong, 1997–1998. *J Infect Dis.* 185:1005–1010.

Bright RA, Medina M, Xu X, et al. (2005): Incidence of adamantane resistance among influenza A (H3N2) viruses isolated worldwide from 1994 to 2005: a cause for concern. *Lancet.* 366:1175–1181.

Cate TR (1987): Clinical manifestations and consequences of influenza. *Am J Med.* 82:15–19.

CDC,(Centers for Disease Control and Prevention) (2005): Recent avian influenza outbreaks in Asia and Europe. http://www.cdc.gov/flu/avian/outbreaks/asia.htm. Accessed October 2005.

Chan PK (2002): Outbreak of avian influenza A (H5N1) virus infection in Hong Kong in 1997. *Clin Infect Dis.* 34:S58–S64.

Chen H, Deng G, Li Z, et al. (2004): The evolution of H5N1 influenza viruses in ducks in southern China. *Proc Natl Acad Sci.* 101:10452–10457.

Choi YK, Seo SH, Kim JA, Webby RJ, Webster RG (2005): Avian influenza viruses in Korean live poultry markets and their pathogenic potential. *Virology.* 332:529–537.

Chotpitayasunondh T, Ungchusak K, Hanshaoworakul W, et al. (2005): Human disease from influenza A (H5N1), Thailand, 2004. *Emerg Infect Dis.* 11:201–209.

Chutinimitkul S, Bhattarakosol P, Srisuratanon S, et al. (2006): H5N1 influenza A virus and infected human plasma. *Emerg Infect Dis.* 12:1041–1043.

Claas EC, Osterhaus ADME, Van Beek R, et al. (1998): Human influenza A H5N1 virus related to a highly pathogenic avian influenza virus. *Lancet.* 351:472–477.

Colman PM (1994): Influenza virus neuraminidase: structure, antibodies, and inhibitors. *Protein Sci.* 3:1687–1696.

Crawford PC, Dubovi EJ, Castleman WL, et al. (2005): Transmission of equine influenza virus to dogs. *Science.* 310:482–485.

de Jong MD, Van Cam B, Tu QuiP, et al. (2005): Fatal avian influenza A (H5N1) in a child presenting with diarrhea followed by coma. *N Engl J Med.* 352:686–691.

Dinh PN, Long HT, Kim NT, et al. (2006): Risk factors for human infection with avian influenza A H5N1, Vietnam, 2004. *Emerg Infect Dis.* 12:1841–1847.

FAO (Food and Agriculture Organization) (2005): Avian influenza: a threat to rural livelihoods, agricultural production and human health. http://www.fao.org/newsroom/en/focus/2004/36467/index.html. Accessed March 2008.

Ferguson NM, Cummings DAT, Cauchemez S, et al. (2005): Strategies for containing an emerging influenza pandemic in Southeast Asia. *Nature.* 437:209–214.

Gambaryan A, Tuzikov A, Pazynina G, Bovin N, Balish A (2006): Evolution of the receptor binding phenotype of influenza A (H5) viruses. *Virology.* 344:432–438.

Glaser L, Stevens J, Zamarin D, et al. (2005): A single amino acid substitution in 1918 influenza virus hemagglutinin changes receptor binding specificity. *J Virol.* 79:11533–11536.

Govorkova EA, Rehg JE, Krauss S, et al. (2005): Lethality to ferrets of H5N1 influenza viruses isolated from humans and poultry in 2004. *J Virol.* 79:2191–2198.

Govorkova EA, Webby RJ, Humberd J, Seiler JP, Webster RG (2006): Immunization with reverse-genetics-produced H5N1 influenza vaccine protects ferrets against homologous and heterologous challenge. *J Infect Dis.* 194:59–167.

Guan Y, Chen H (2005): Resistance to anti-influenza agents. *Lancet.* 366:1139–1140.

Guan Y, Peiris JS, Lipatov AS, et al. (2002): Emergence of multiple genotypes of H5N1 avian influenza viruses in Hong Kong SAR. *Proc Natl Acad Sci.* 99:8950–8955.

Guan Y, Peiris JSM, Poon LLM, et al. (2003): Reassortants of H5N1 influenza viruses recently isolated from aquatic poultry in Hong Kong SAR. *Avian Dis.* 47:911–913.

Guarner J, Shieh WJ, Dawson J, et al. (2000): Immunohistochemical and in situ hybridization studies of influenza A virus infection in human lungs. *Am J Clin Pathol.* 114: 227–233.

Harper SA, Fukuda K, Uyeki TM, Cox NJ, Bridges CB (2004): Prevention and control of influenza: recommendations of the Advisory Committee on Immunization Practices (ACIP). *MMWR Morb Mortal Wkly Rep.* 53:1–40.

Hayden FG (2001): Perspectives on antiviral use during pandemic influenza. *Philos Trans R Soc Lond B Biol Sci.* 356:1877–1884.

Hubalek Z (2004): An annotated checklist of pathogenic microorganisms associated with migratory birds. *J Wildl Dis.* 40:639–659.

Hulse-Post DJ, Sturm-Ramirez KM, Humberd J, et al. (2005): Role of domestic ducks in the propagation and biological evolution of highly pathogenic H5N1 influenza viruses in Asia. *Proc Natl Acad Sci*. 102:10682–10687.

Information OD (2005): Highly pathogenic avian influenza in Romania. http://www.oie.int/eng/info/hebdo/a_current.htm#Sec10. Accessed October 20, 2005.

Ito T, Couceiro JNSS, Kelm S, et al. (1998): Molecular basis for the generation in pigs of influenza A viruses with pandemic potential. *J Virol*. 72:7367–7373.

Kandun IN, Wibisono H, Sedyaningsih ER, et al. (2006): Three Indonesian clusters of H5N1 virus infection in 2005. *N Engl J Med*. 355:2186–2194.

Karesh WB, Cook RA, Bennett EL, Newcomb J (2005): Wildlife trade and global disease emergence. *Emerg Infect Dis*. 11:1000–1002.

Katz, JM, Lim W, Bridges CB, et al. (1999): Antibody response in individuals infected with avian influenza A (H5N1) viruses and detection of anti-H5 antibody among household and social contacts. *J Infect Dis*. 180:1763–1770.

Kaye D, Pringle CR (2005): Avian influenza viruses and their implication for human health. *Clin Infect Dis*. 40:108–112.

Keawcharoen J, Oraveerakul K, Kuiken T, et al. (2004): Avian influenza H5N1 in tigers and leopards. *Emerg Infect Dis*. 10:2189–2191.

Krauss S, Walker D, Pryor SP, et al. (2004): Influenza A viruses of migrating wild aquatic birds in North America. *Vector Borne Zoonotic Dis*. 4:177–189.

Kuiken T, Rimmelzwaan G, Riel D, Amerongen G, Baars M, Fouchier AO (2004): Avian H5N1 influenza in cats. *Science*. 306:241.

Kung NY, Guan Y, Perkins NR, et al. (2003): The impact of a monthly rest day on avian influenza virus isolation rates in retail live poultry markets in Hong Kong. *Avian Dis*. 47:1037–1041.

Kwon YK Joh SJ, Kim MC, et al. (2005): Highly pathogenic avian influenza (H5N1) in the commercial domestic ducks of South Korea. *Avian Pathol*. 34:367–370.

Le QM, Kiso M, Someya K, et al. (2005): Avian flu: isolation of drug-resistant H5N1 virus. *Nature*. 437:1108.

Lee CW, Suarez DL, Tumpey TM, Sung HW, Kwon YK, Lee YJ (2005): Characterization of highly pathogenic H5N1 avian influenza A viruses isolated from South Korea. *J Virol*. 79:3692–3702.

Li KS, Guan Y, Wang J, et al. (2003): The quest of influenza A viruses for new hosts. *Avian Dis*. 47:849–856.

Ligon BL (2005): Avian influenza virus H5N1: a review of its history and information regarding its potential to cause the next pandemic. *Semin Pediatr Infect Dis*. 16:326–335.

Lin YP, Gregory V, Bennett M, Hay A (2004): Recent changes among human influenza viruses. *Virus Res*. 103:47–52.

Lipatov AS, Webby RJ, Govorkova EA, Krauss S, Webster RG (2005): Efficacy of H5 influenza vaccines produced by reverse genetics in a lethal mouse model. *J Infect Dis*. 191:1216–1220.

Liu M, He S, Walker D, et al. (2003): The influenza virus gene pool in a poultry market in south central China. *Virology*. 305:267–275.

Liu J, Xiao H, Lei F, et al. (2005): Highly pathogenic H5N1 influenza virus infection in migratory birds. *Science*. 309:1206.

Longini IM, Nizam A, Xu S, et al. (2005): Containing pandemic influenza at the source. *Science*. 309:1083–1087.

Maines TR, Lu XH, Erb SM, et al. (2005): Avian influenza (H5N1) viruses isolated from humans in Asia in 2004 exhibit increased virulence in mammals. *J Virol*. 79:11788–11800.

Maines TR, Chen LM, Matsuoka Y, Chen H, Rowe T (2006): Lack of transmission of H5N1 avian–human reassortant influenza viruses in a ferret model. *Proc Natl Acad Sci*. 103:12121–12126.

Mase M, Eto M, Tanimura N, et al. (2005): Isolation of a genotypically unique H5N1 influenza virus from duck meat imported into Japan from China. *Virology*. 339:101–109.

Mounts AW, Kwon H, Izurieta HS, et al. (1999): Case–control study of risk factors for avian influenza A (H5N1) disease, Hong Kong, 1997. *J Infect Dis*. 180:505–508.

Nguyen DC, Uyeki TM, Jadhao S, et al. (2005): Isolation and characterization of avian influenza viruses, including highly pathogenic H5N1, from poultry in live bird markets in Hanoi, Vietnam, in 2001. *J Virol*. 79:4201–4212.

Normile D, Enserink M (2004): Infectious diseases: avian influenza makes a comeback, reviving pandemic worries. *Science*. 305:321.

Olsen SJ, Laosiritaworn Y, Pattanasin S, Prapasiri P, Dowell SF (2005a): Poultry-handling practices during avian influenza outbreak, Thailand. *Emerg Infect Dis*. 11:1601–1603.

Olsen S, Ungchusak K, Sovann L, et al. (2005b): Family clustering of avian influenza A (H5N1). *Emerg Infect Dis*. 11:1799–1801.

Peiris JSM, Guan Y, Markwell D, Ghose P, Webster RG, Shortridge KF (2001): Cocirculation of avian H9N2 and contemporary "human" H3N2 influenza A viruses in pigs in southeastern China: potential for genetic reassortment? *J Virol*. 75:9679–9686.

Peiris JSM, Yu WC, Leung CW, et al. (2004): Re-emergence of fatal human influenza A subtype H5N1 disease. *Lancet*. 363:617–619.

Rowe T, Abernathy RA, Hu-Primmer J, et al. (1999): Detection of antibody to avian influenza A (H5N1) virus in human serum by using a combination of serologic assays. *J Clin Microbiol*. 37:937–943.

Shortridge KF, Zhou NN, Guan Y, et al. (1998): Characterization of avian H5N1 influenza viruses from poultry in Hong Kong. *Virology*. 252:331–342.

Sims LD, Ellis TM, Dyrting K, Peiris M, Guan Y, Shortridge KF (2003): Avian influenza in Hong Kong 1997–2002. *Avian Dis*. 47:832–838.

Skehel JJ, Wiley DC (2000): Receptor binding and membrane fusion in virus entry: the influenza hemagglutinin. *Annu Rev Biochem*. 69:531–569.

Stallknecht DE, Shane SM, Zwank PJ, Senne DA, Kearney MT (1990): Avian influenza viruses from migratory and resident ducks of coastal Louisiana. *Avian Dis*. 34:398–405.

Stephenson I, Wood JM, Nicholson KG, Zambon MC (2003): Sialic acid receptor specificity on erythrocytes affects detection of antibody to avian influenza haemagglutinin. *J Med Virol*. 70:391–398.

Sturm-Ramirez KM, Ellis T, Bousfield B, et al. (2002): Reemerging H5N1 influenza viruses in Hong Kong in 2002 are highly pathogenic to ducks. *J Virol*. 78:4892–4901.

Sturm-Ramirez KM, Hulse-Post DJ, Govorkova EA, et al. (2005): Are ducks contributing to the endemicity of highly pathogenic H5N1 influenza virus in Asia? *J Virol*. 79: 11269–11279.

Suarez DL (2000): Evolution of avian influenza viruses. *Vet Microbiol*. 74:15–27.

Suarez DL, Schultz-Cherry S (2000): Immunology of avian influenza virus: a review. *Dev Comp Immunol.* 24 (2–3): 269–283.

Subbarao K, Klimov A, Katz J, et al. (1998): Characterization of an avian influenza A (H5N1) virus isolated from a child with a fatal respiratory illness. *Science.* 279:393–396.

Suzuki Y, Ito T, Suzuki T, et al. (2000): Sialic acid species as a determinant of the host range of influenza A viruses. *J Virol.* 74:11825–11831.

Swayne DE (2006a): Microassay for measuring thermal inactivation of H5N1 high pathogenicity avian influenza virus in naturally infected chicken meat. *Int J Food Microbiol.* 108:268–271.

——— (2006b): Occupational and consumer risks from avian influenza viruses. *Dev Biol (Basel).* 124:85–90.

Swayne DE, Beck JR (2004): Heat inactivation of avian influenza and Newcastle disease viruses in egg products. *Avian Pathol.* 33:512–518.

——— (2005): Experimental study to determine if low-pathogenicity and high-pathogenicity avian influenza viruses can be present in chicken breast and thigh meat following intranasal virus inoculation. *Avian Dis.* 49:81–85.

Swayne DE, King DJ (2003): Avian influenza and Newcastle disease. *J Am Vet Med Assoc.* 222:1534–1540.

Swayne DE, Pantin-Jackwood M (2006): Pathogenicity of avian influenza viruses in poultry. *Dev Biol (Basel).* 124:61–67.

Swayne DE, Suarez DL (2000): Highly pathogenic avian influenza. *Rev Sci Tech.* 19:463–482.

Swayne DE, Beck JR, Perdue ML, Beard CW (2001): Efficacy of vaccines in chickens against highly pathogenic Hong Kong H5N1 avian influenza. *Avian Dis.* 45:355–365.

Taubenberger JK, Reid AH, Lourens RM, Wang R, Jin G, Fanning TG (2005): Characterization of the 1918 influenza virus polymerase genes. *Nature.* 437:889–893.

Thanawongnuwech R, Amonsin A, Tantilertcharoen R, et al. (2005): Probable tiger-to-tiger transmission of avian influenza H5N1. *Emerg Infect Dis.* 11:699–701.

Thomas ME, Bouma A, Ekker HM, Fonken AJM, Stegeman JA, Nielen M (2005): Risk factors for the introduction of high pathogenicity avian influenza virus into poultry farms during the epidemic in the Netherlands in 2003. *Prev Vet Med.* 69:1–11.

Tiensin T, Chaitaweesub P, Songserm T, et al. (2005): Highly pathogenic avian influenza H5N1, Thailand, 2004. *Emerg Infect Dis.* 11:1664–1672.

To KF, Chan PKS, Chan KF, et al. (2001): Pathology of fatal human infection associated with avian influenza A H5N1 virus. *J Med Virol.* 63:242–246.

Tran TH, Nguyen TL, Luong TS, et al. (2004): Avian influenza A (H5N1) in 10 patients in Vietnam. *N Engl J Med.* 350:1179–1188.

Treanor JD (2007): Influenza—The goal of control. *N Eng J Med.* 14:1439–1441.

Tumpey TM (2005): Characterization of the reconstructed 1918 Spanish influenza pandemic virus. *Science.* 310:77–80.

Uiprasertkul M, Puthavathana P, Sangsiriwut K, et al. (2005): Influenza A H5N1 replication sites in humans. *Emerg Infect Dis.* 11:1036–1041.

Ungchusak K, Auewarakul P, Dowell SF, et al. (2005): Probable person-to-person transmission of avian influenza A (H5N1). *N Engl J Med.* 352:333–340.

Van Borm S, Thomas I, Hanquet G, et al. (2005): Highly pathogenic H5N1 influenza virus in smuggled Thai eagles, Belgium. *Emerg Infect Dis.* 11:702–705.

Vong S, Coghlan B, Mardy S, et al. (2006): Low frequency of poultry-to-human H5N1 virus transmission, southern Cambodia, 2005. *Emerg Infect Dis.* 12 (10).

Webster RG (1997): Influenza virus: transmission between species and relevance to emergence of the next human pandemic. *Arch Virol Suppl.* 13:105–113.

——— (2004): Wet markets: a continuing source of severe acute respiratory syndrome and influenza? *Lancet.* 363:234–236.

Webster RG, Hulse DJ (2004): Microbial adaptation and change: avian influenza. *Rev Sci Tech.* 23:453–465.

Webster RG, Peiris JSM (2004): Genesis of a highly pathogenic and potentially pandemic H5N1 influenza virus in eastern Asia. *Nature.* 430:209–213.

Webster RG, Bean WJ, Gorman OT, Chambers TM, Kawaoka Y (1992): Evolution and ecology of influenza A viruses. *Microbiol Rev.* 56:152–179.

Webster RG, Sharp GB, Claas EC (1995): Interspecies transmission of influenza viruses. *Am J Respir Crit Care Med.* 152:S25–S30.

WHO (World Health Organization) (2004a): Avian influenza A(H5N1). *Wkly Epidemiol Rec.* 79:65–70.

——— (2004b): Cumulative number of confirmed human cases of avian influenza A/(H5N1) reported to WHO. http://www.who.int/csr/disease/avian_influenza/country/cases_table_2005_10_10/en/index.html. Accessed October 2005.

——— (2005a): Avian influenza—cumulative number of cases—update 18. http://www.who.int/ csr/don/2005_05_19/en/index.html. Accessed December 2006.

——— (2005b): *Highly Pathogenic H5N1 Avian Influenza Outbreaks in Poultry and in Humans: Food Safety Implications.* INFOSAN Information Note. WHO, Geneva, Switzerland.

——— (2005c): Global Influenza Program Surveillance Network. Evolution of H5N1 avian influenza viruses in Asia. *Emerg Infect Dis.* 11:1515–1521.

——— (2006a): WHO guidelines for the collection of human specimens for laboratory diagnosis of avian influenza infection. http://www.who.int/csr/disease/avian_influenza/guidelines/humanspecimens/en/index.html. Accessed December 2006.

——— (2006b): Review of latest available evidence on risks to human health through potential transmission of avian influenza (H5N1) through water and sewage. In *Water, Sanitation and Health. Public Health and Environment.* WHO, Geneva, Switzerland.

Wright P, Webster R (2001). *Orthomyxoviruses.* In: Knipe HP (Ed.): *Field's Virology.* Lippincott Williams & Wilkins, Philadelphia, pp. 1533–1579.

Wu G, Yan S (2005): Mutation features of 215 polymerase proteins from different influenza A viruses. *Med Sci Monit.* 11:BR367–BR372.

Yen HL (2001): Influenza surveillance in poultry markets and its interspecies transmission in Taiwan. In *Proc World Congress on Options for the Control of Influenza IV*, Amsterdam, The Netherlands.

PART III

FOOD SAFETY ISSUES AND THE MICROBIOLOGY OF SPECIFIC COMMODITIES

CHAPTER 6

FOOD SAFETY ISSUES AND THE MICROBIOLOGY OF BEEF

ROBIN C. ANDERSON, STEVEN C. RICKE, BWALYA LUNGU,
MICHAEL G. JOHNSON, CHRISTY OLIVER,
SHANE M. HORROCKS, and DAVID J. NISBET

6.1 INTRODUCTION

World demand for high-quality animal protein presents opportunities for growth and expanded trade, which is predicted to increase more than 6% for major beef-producing countries and their beef industries (USDA-FAS, 2006, 2007). Contingent upon increased consumer demand for beef is the production of high-quality, microbiologically safe products. An enhanced stringency of food safety standards has increased the burden for producers and processors to regulate and document their production practices and to implement pathogen control practices. From a food safety standpoint, bacterial pathogens of major concern to beef include enterohemorrhagic *Escherichia coli* (especially *E. coli* O157:H7), *Salmonella*, *Campylobacter*, and *Listeria* (Swartz, 2002). The annual economic loss in 2000 associated with these bacterial pathogens was \$5 to 6 billion (Murphy et al., 2003).

6.2 ENTEROHEMORRHAGIC *ESCHERICHIA COLI* O157:H7 IN BEEF

Pathogenic *E. coli* (see Chapter 2) fall into six major categories: enterotoxigenic, enteroinvasive, enteroaggregative, diffusely adherent, enteropathogenic, and enterohemorrhagic (Feng, 2001). Enterohemorrhagic *E. coli* cause hemorrhagic colitis in humans. The disease typically manifests after a 3- to 4-day incubation period as a severe diarrhea that progresses within 3 days to bloody diarrhea in 90% of cases; acute abdominal cramping and vomiting but rarely fever accompany the disease, which lasts about 2 to 9 days (Feng, 2001; Karch et al., 2005). In about 3 to 7% of total cases and about 15% of cases involving children less than 10 years of age, a complication

Microbiologically Safe Foods, Edited by Norma Heredia, Irene Wesley, and Santos García

of the disease known as hemolytic uremic syndrome (HUS) can result (Feng, 2001; Karch et al., 2005). This syndrome manifests as microangiopathic hemolytic anemia, thrombocytopenia, and intravascular hemolysis and can cause renal failure leading to death in 3 to 5% of cases and to permanent kidney and/or neurological damage in many of the other cases (Feng, 2001; Karch et al., 2005).

Enterohemorrhagic *E. coli* possess a number of virulence attributes, including genes for one or both Shiga toxins (*stx1* and *stx2*), enterohemolysin (*ehxA*), and intestinal adherence factors associated with the locus of enterocyte effacement (LEE), including intimin (*eae*), the translocated intimin receptor (*Tir*), and secreted protein encoded by *EspA, EspB,* and *EspD* (Law, 2000; Nataro and Kaper, 1998). These and, potentially, others traits contribute to the high pathogenicity of this pathogen to humans, as the infectious dose is as low as 10 to 100 cells (Feng, 2001; Karch et al., 2005). Whereas *E. coli* O157:H7 is probably the best known, numerous other EHEC or Shiga toxin–producing serotypes exist (Feng, 2001; Hussein, 2007).

Escherichia coli O157:H7 has been particularly problematic for the beef industry, costing an estimated $2.7 billion loss to the U.S. beef industry alone during the first 10 years since the Jack-in-the-Box outbreak (Kay, 2003). Whereas *E. coli* O157:H7 is estimated to cause a small proportion (0.5% or 62,458 cases) of the total foodborne-caused illnesses in the United States each year (Mead et al., 1999), large outbreaks, with particularly drastic consequences to young children, have attracted media and thus consumer attention to this pathogen. Of the total estimated foodborne-caused hospitalizations, 3% or 1843 are attributed to *E. coli* O157:H7, as are 52 deaths (2.9% of total) (Mead et al., 1999). Large outbreaks associated with the consumption of contaminated ground beef, such as an outbreak affecting 732 people in 1992–1993 in the western United States, of which 55 (mostly children) developed HUS, resulting in the death of four children, have implicated cattle as an important reservoir (Karch et al., 1999). Other ruminants, such as sheep, deer, and goats, can be reservoirs of *E. coli* O157:H7 or Shiga toxin–producing *E. coli*, as can feral and domestic pigs, horses, dogs, seagulls, and house flies (Feng, 2001; Karch et al., 1999, 2005; Naylor et al., 2005). The largest outbreak, due to consumption of radish sprouts served in the school lunch program, occurred in 1996 in Sakai City, Osaka, Japan, and affected more than 8000 people, of which 106 were children, resulting in three deaths (Karch et al., 1999; Michino et al., 1999). Other sources of infections to humans include unpasteurized apple cider or milk, produce, salami, fried potatoes with cheese and spices, potato salad, mayonnaise, yogurt, salmon roe, homemade venison jerky, contact with animals at petting zoos, and contaminated municipal water and swimming pools (Buchanan and Doyle, 1997; Feng, 2001). Interpersonal contact, particularly between family members and attendees of day care centers, has also been documented as a means of *E. coli* O157:H7 transmission (Feng, 2001; Karch et al., 2005).

6.2.1 Prevalence

Human infections peak in summer and early autumn, which coincides with peak fecal shedding by cattle (Bach et al., 2002b; Karch et al., 1999; Naylor et al., 2005;

Rasmussen and Casey, 2001; Renter and Sargeant, 2002); however, considerable variation in prevalence exists between and even within geographic regions. Practically all cattle herds in the United States contain at least some animals colonized by *E. coli* O157:H7, although animal prevalence rates can vary from 0 to >30%, with prevalence being similar in beef and dairy cattle (Bach et al., 2002b; Elder et al., 2000; Rasmussen and Casey, 2001; Renter and Sargeant, 2002). In general, prevalence rates have been found to be higher in the years following the implementation of more sensitive detection methods, such as immunomagnetic separation, than in years before the use of such methods (Gansheroff and O'Brien, 2000; Naylor et al., 2005). More recently, for instance, Khaitsa et al. (2007) reported prevalence as high as 80% in feedlot cattle. In their study, three stages of infection, pre-epidemic, epidemic, and post-epidemic, were observed, and the incidence of shedding was most frequent and the duration of fecal shedding was longest during the epidemic stage.

Prevalence rates in an examination of Finnish cattle were reported to be 1.3% of total cattle tested and ranged from 0 to 6.9%, depending on the abattoir (Lahti et al., 2003). In the United Kingdom, 7.5% of cattle at slaughter yielded *E. coli* O157:H7-positive fecal specimens, and 40% of the farms had at least one animal testing positive for the pathogen (Omisakin et al., 2003). Prevalence rates reported are: Brazil, 1.5%; Japan, 1.8%; Australia, 1.9%; and Scotland, 25% (Naylor et al., 2005). In the Netherlands, prevalence rates from two studies reported that 10.6% of slaughter cattle and from 0.8 to 22.4% of cattle on tested dairy farms were positive for *E. coli* O157 (Heuvelink et al., 1998a, b). *Escherichia coli* O157:H7 was recovered from only one (0.5%) of 200 cattle tested in Argentina, although other Shiga toxin–producing *E. coli* serotypes were isolated from 86 (39%) of these animals (Meichtri et al., 2004). Shiga toxin–producing *E. coli* were isolated on 95% of farms tested between 1993 and 1995 in Spain and from 0 to 100% of the cattle on the farms, with an overall animal prevalence rate of 37% in calves and 27% in cows; however, only 8 (0.7%) of the 1069 cattle tested were positive for *E. coli* O157:H7 (Blanco et al., 2003). From 1993 to 1999 the recovery rate of *E. coli* O157:H7 from 161 calves tested was 0.6%, 0% from 525 cows, 2% from 383 slaughter cattle, and 12% from 471 fed calves, and the authors concluded that these rates were similar to those found elsewhere in Europe and North America (Blanco et al., 2003).

Conedera et al. (2001) reported that *E. coli* O157 was isolated from approximately 4% of 341 dairy calves in one survey and was isolated from 10.7% of a total of 1293 rectal swabs collected from between 92 and 59 animals over an 11- to 15-month period, with peaks as high as 23.7% in summer months. In a Norwegian study, only two of 197 cattle herds had *E. coli* O157:H7-positive fecal specimens (Vold et al., 1998), and *E. coli* O157 was recovered from only 1.25% of 240 (120 dairy and 120 beef) cattle in Mexico (Callaway et al., 2004). Up to 35% of dairy cows shed *E. coli* O157:H7, with nearly twice as many lactating as nonlactating cows shedding *E. coli* O157:H7 (Fitzgerald et al., 2003). Neither parity nor number of days in the milking cycle affected shedding of *E. coli* O157:H7 (Fitzgerald et al., 2003).

6.2.2 Gastrointestinal and Pen Ecology

Most *E. coli* are commensal inhabitants of the gastrointestinal tract and because they are common constituents of excreted feces, often finding their way into water, soil, and sediment (Durso et al., 2004), they have been used extensively as indicators of fecal contamination of food or water (Feng, 2001). Feces, manure, feed, feed bunks, drinking water, and house flies harbor *E. coli* O157:H7 (Alam and Zurek, 2004; Bach et al., 2002b; Duffy, 2003; LeJune et al., 2001; Lynn et al., 1998; Rice and Johnson, 2000), and these sources are thought to play a large role in the dissemination of the organism throughout the herd. In pen environments, exposure and reexposure to these various inoculum sources as well as by animal-to-animal contact probably contribute to the apparently cyclic and transient infection and reinfection of cattle by *E. coli* O157:H7 (Rasmussen and Casey, 2001; Renter and Sargeant, 2002).

In nonfasted cattle, generic *E. coli* are typically present at higher concentrations than *E. coli* O157:H7. For instance, generic *E. coli* were present at about 10^3 to 10^4 CFU/mL in ruminal contents and approximately 10^5 to 10^7 CFU/g in feces (Anderson et al., 2002, 2005; Fegan et al., 2004). By comparison, concentrations of *E. coli* O157:H7 in calves experimentally inoculated with 2×10^{11} CFU did not persist, declining rapidly from an initial high of about 10^4 to 10^5 CFU/mL ruminal fluid 2 h post-inoculation to levels detectable by enrichment only by 3 days post-inoculation (Grauke et al., 2002). *Escherichia coli* O157:H7 concentrations in the feces of these experimentally inoculated calves were first detected 6 h after inoculation and then declined from a high of approximately 10^5 CFU/g achieved 1 day post-inoculation to levels detectable by enrichment only by day 7 post-inoculation (Grauke et al., 2002). Similarly, Buchko et al. (2000) observed that experimentally inoculated *E. coli* O157:H7 populations were rapidly depleted from the rumen of steers but recovered from feces for up to 67 days post-inoculation, thereby indicating that the lower gastrointestinal tract is a more important colonization site than the rumen. In naturally colonized animals, fecal concentrations of *E. coli* O157:H7 in feedlot cattle averaged 1.6×10^3 CFU/g (Cobbold et al., 2007), with fecal specimens containing concentrations higher than that being a rare occurrence (Fegan et al., 2004).

Considerable attention has been directed to the hypothesis that a certain proportion of cattle may shed high numbers of these pathogens (Naylor et al., 2003). It is suspected that even a few of these super-shedding animals within a herd, those shedding more than 10^3 or 10^4 CFU Shiga toxin–producing *E. coli* per gram of feces (depending on the study) may be of greater importance than overall population prevalence per se (Cobbold et al., 2007; Low et al., 2005; Naylor et al., 2003; Omisakin et al., 2003). For instance, Omisakin et al. (2003) reported that while only 9% of 44 infected animals presented to slaughter were found to shed more than 10^4 *E. coli* O157 per gram of feces, these few animals accounted for more than 96% of the total *E. coli* O157 burden shed by all infected animals. Moreover, Ogden et al. (2004) reported that concentrations of *E. coli* O157 in feces of high-shedding animals is greater in the summer than the winter, and this may contribute to the high seasonal rate of human infections. The higher rate of *E. coli* O157 shedding observed in the summer months has not yet been explained fully, although a recent hypothesis by Edrington et al. (2006a) proposed that hormonal changes associated with longer daylight intervals may be contributing. It is now thought that *E. coli* O157:H7 super-shedders harbor the organisms primarily within a 1- to 15-cm segment of the rectum just proximal to the rectal–anal junction and that this site may be a site of true colonization and attachment (Low et al., 2005; Naylor et al., 2003).

Numerous studies have examined the effect of diet, ionophores, and fasting on fecal *E. coli* O157:H7 shedding, with mixed results (Wells et al., 2009). Diez-Gonzalez et al. (1998) reported that feeding a 90% concentrate diet increased concentrations of generic *E. coli* populations 100-fold compared to concentrations in cattle fed a timothy hay diet. Moreover, the *E. coli* recovered from the concentrate-fed cattle were considerably more resistant to acid shock, purportedly due to increased exposure to higher volatile fatty acid concentrations that resulted from the feeding of more readily fermentable substrates (Diez-Gonzalez et al., 1998). Acid resistance is considered by some to increase the virulence of gut pathogens such as *E. coli* O157:H7 by promoting their ability to survive low-pH, high-gastric acid conditions in the human stomach (Price et al., 2000). Others also found that feeding diets high in forage reduced *E. coli* concentrations or shedding (Callaway et al., 2003b; Gilbert et al., 2005; Gregory et al., 2000; Jordan and McEwen, 1998), but this concept has been challenged. For instance, Hovde et al. (1999) found that experimentally inoculated cattle fed grain or medium- to low-quality hay shed similar concentrations of *E. coli* O157:H7 and that acid resistance of the *E. coli* O157:H7 recovered was unaffected by the diet. Moreover, they reported that the forage-fed cattle shed detectable levels of *E. coli* O157:H7 longer (39 to 42 days) than did grain-fed cattle, which shed the inoculated strain an average of 4 days (Hovde et al., 1999). Van Baale et al. (2004) also observed that cattle fed roughage shed higher numbers of *E. coli* O157:H7 and for longer duration than cattle fed a grain diet. Diets containing barley rather than corn have also been shown to significantly support increased shedding of *E. coli* O157:H7, with one study reporting an increase in prevalence from 38.2% or 50% in steers fed either an 85% cracked corn or 70% : 15% barley/cottonseed diet to 63.2% in steers fed an 85% barley diet (Buchko et al., 2000). In a subsequent study, however, *E. coli* O157:H7 shedding rates in cattle decreased from 2.4% to 1.3%, and concentrations shed decreased only from 3.3 $\log_{10}$ to 3.0 $\log_{10}$ CFU per gram of feces for cattle fed corn or barley finishing diets, respectively (Berg et al., 2004). Thus, the actual impact of such marginal differences on ultimate carcass safety is questionable in the latter study.

Fasting or feed deprivation conditions often associated with transportation of cattle to slaughter have long been considered to promote gut environments more favorable to *E. coli* by reducing concentrations of inhibitory volatile fatty acids produced during fermentation of feedstuffs (Brownlie and Grau, 1967; Grau et al., 1969; Rasmussen et al., 1993; Wolin, 1969). However, results to date have been conflicting, with some studies suggesting that gut *E. coli* concentrations were increased following a fast (Brownlie and Grau, 1967; Grau et al., 1969) and others finding that fasting had no or mixed effects on ruminal or fecal concentrations of *E. coli*, despite having the expected effect on pH and volatile fatty acid concentrations (Anderson et al., 2002; Cray et al., 1998; Harmon et al., 1999). Moreover, Minihan et al. (2003) found no effect of shipping or lairage on fecal prevalence of *E. coli* O157 in two cohorts of cattle in Ireland, with prevalences of 18, 13, and 12%, respectively in one cohort and 1.7, 1.7, and 0%, respectively, in the other. Additionally, Barham et al. (2002) observed that respective prevalence of *E. coli* O157 in feces and on hides decreased from 9.5% and 18% before shipping to 5.5% and 4.5%, after shipping, suggesting that feed deprivation does not necessarily promote favorable conditions for growth of *E. coli*. In the study by Anderson et al. (2002), fasting did result in decreased VFA concentrations and a neutralization of the pH in the bovine rumen, but total culturable anaerobes were also decreased, implying that while depletion of nutrients available to support growth probably occurred, it affected the total microbial population. Under such conditions it was reasoned that *E. coli* populations would be no more capable than other indigenous anaerobes of competing for limiting nutrients (Anderson et al., 2002). It is reasonable to speculate, however, that upon refeeding, should such an event occur, *E. coli* may propagate more rapidly than populations of slower-growing anaerobes.

Ionophore antibiotics are commonly fed in beef cattle production systems to improve the efficiency of animal production, and because the timing of their implementation coincides approximately with the first occurrence of human *E. coli* O157:H7 infections, their potential effects on *E. coli* O157:H7 prevalence and shedding have been evaluated (Bach et al., 2002a; Callaway et al., 2003a). In vitro, the ionophore monensin had no inhibitory effect on the growth of *E. coli* O157:H7 when applied at concentrations equivelant to levels fed to feedlot cattle (Bach et al., 2002a) or 10-fold higher (Edrington et al., 2003c). These results were not unexpected, however, as ionophores are typically more effective against gram-positive than against gram-negative bacteria. However, Bach et al. (2002a) noted that because of the differential effects of monensin against gram-positive and gram-negative bacteria, they could not discount the possibility that monensin may indirectly open a niche for *E. coli* O157:H7. Numerous other studies, however, have clearly shown that *E. coli* O157:H7 prevalence and shedding were not increased in ruminants fed monensin or other ionophores (lasalocid, laidlomycin propionate, or bambermycin) (Callaway et al., 2003a; Dargatz et al., 1997; Edrington et al., 2003b, 2006b; Garber et al., 1995; Van Baale et al., 2004).

6.3 *SALMONELLA* IN BEEF

Consumption of food and food products derived from meat- and egg-producing animals is believed to be the main source of foodborne salmonellosis in the United States, with an annual cost ranging in the billions (Bryan, 1980, 1981; Frenzen et al., 1999; St. Louis et al., 1988; Todd, 1989). Symptoms of the disease in humans usually occur over 8 to 72 h and include abdominal pain, nausea, and watery diarrhea (D'Aoust, 2001). Enteriditis, Typhimurium, and Typhi are the three main serotypes isolated worldwide (Herikstad et al., 2002). *Salmonella enterica* serotypes Typhimurium and Dublin are considered to be the primary host-adapted serotypes to cattle, with Dublin being the causative biotype for bovine bacteremia (Rabsch et al., 2002). However, other serotypes, such as Enteriditis, which has been thought to be most associated with chicken eggs, have also been isolated from beef in foodborne outbreaks (Patrick et al., 2004; St. Louis et al., 1988), and more recently, infection by *Salmonella* serovar Newport in people consuming beef has raised concern as to its possible emergence as a prominent foodborne pathogen (Gupta et al., 2003).

6.3.1 Factors That Influence the Spread of *Salmonella*

Foodborne *Salmonella* spp. are generally widespread in agricultural environments. In a recent study of 18 farms from five states, *Salmonella* serovars were recovered from beef, dairy, poultry, and swine farms (Rodriguez et al., 2006). *Salmonella* have also been recovered at different stages during beef slaughter (Stolle, 1981). In addition to the pre- and post-processing facilities, other routes of transmission have been identified, but only a few have been characterized in detail. Within an animal house, airborne routes have been extensively characterized as a potential route for transmission of *Salmonella* in poultry (Holt et al., 1998; Kwon et al., 1999, 2000a). However, outdoor airborne transmission of pathogens is also possible, and depending on proximity can originate from agricultural or municipal sources (Pillai et al., 1996; Pillai and Ricke, 2002). For cattle feedlots it has been suggested that airborne dust is a potential route not only for the transmission of pathogens, but can predispose susceptibility to bacterial and viral infections (MacVean et al., 1986; Wilson et al., 2002). However, Wilson et al. (2002) recovered lower microbial numbers in feedlot dust than those from previous reports from intensively housed farm animals. Animal feed sources of *Salmonella* have been well documented (Maciorowski et al., 2004, 2006b, 2007; Ricke et al., 2005). Animal by-product ingredients have received the most focus as a reservoir for *Salmonella* (Maciorowski et al., 2004), but contamination can occur at any stage of feed processing, including recontamination after thermal processing (Jones and Ricke, 1994; Maciorowski et al., 2006a, 2007; Ricke, 2005). When Bender et al. (1997) fed *Salmonella* artificially contaminated meat-and-bone meal to fistulated dairy cows, *Salmonella* could be recovered from rumen contents, feces, and mesenteric lymph nodes.

Unlike that found with *E. coli*, transportation of cattle has been reported in numerous studies to predispose animals to increased shedding of *Salmonella*. For instance, Corrier et al. (1990) reported that *Salmonella*-prevalence calves shipped from Tennessee to west Texas increased 0 to 1.5% immediately upon arrival at the feedlot and increased further to 8% after 30 days in the feedlot. In cattle shipped to slaughter, respective prevalence levels of *Salmonella* in feces and on hides increased from 18% and 6% before transport to 46% and 89% at the packing plant (Barham et al., 2002). Others have also observed increased prevalence of *Salmonella* on hides following shipment of cattle to slaughter, (Beach et al., 2002; Reicks et al., 2007). Beach et al. (2002) reported that hide contamination by *Salmonella* increased significantly following transportation to slaughter in both adult and feedlot cattle, from 19.8% to 52.2% and 18% to 56%, respectively. They also reported that while fecal *Salmonella* prevalence increased from 1% to 21% in adult cows shipped to slaughter, the prevalence in feedlot cattle was unaffected (3% vs. 5% before and after shipping, respectively). The authors speculated that high-energy diets fed to the feedlot cattle and their higher

Campylobacter colonization status (>60% vs. <8% in adult cattle) may have contributed to the lack of a transportation effect on fecal shedding of *Salmonella* in these cattle.

6.3.2 *Salmonella* and Rumen Ecology

Part of the variability in *Salmonella* occurrence in beef animals lies with the susceptibility of the rumen environment to *Salmonella* survival. It is traditionally believed that the full-fed ruminant animals possess a rumen considered to be hostile to pathogens such as *Salmonella*, due to the high levels of fermentation (Chambers and Lysons, 1979). However, several factors can mitigate this hostility. Feed deprivation can lead to increased numbers of *Salmonella* in cattle (Brownlie and Grau, 1967; Grau et al., 1969), and in poultry, removal of feed has led to a gut environment much more conducive to expression of virulence genes and subsequent invasion of internal organs (Dunkley et al., 2007; Durant et al., 1999a). Volatile fatty acids (VFAs) are considered to be inhibitory to *Salmonella* growth, but this inhibition is dependent on concentration and degree of acidity (Cherrington et al., 1991; Goepfert and Hicks, 1969; McHan and Shotts, 1993). However, induction of acid tolerance can provide protection against organic acids (Baik et al., 1996) and influence virulence response (Durant et al., 1999b, 2000a–c; Lawhon et al., 2002). Exposure to VFAs at neutral pH can induce resistance to inorganic acids as well as high osmolarity and reactive oxygen (Greenacre et al., 2003; Kwon and Ricke, 1998; Kwon et al., 2000b). Several biological agents exist in the rumen that can directly or indirectly lyse or destroy bacteria, including bacteriophages, bacteriocins, and protozoans. Although anaerobic protozoans typically prey on rumen bacteria, using them as a nutrient source, it has recently been shown that *Salmonella* can survive in these protozoans, and these survivors are more invasive in tissue culture, resulting in *Salmonella* exhibiting a hyperinvasive phenotype (Carlson et al., 2007; Rasmussen et al., 2005).

6.4 *LISTERIA* IN BEEF

The annual economic loss in 2000 associated with foodborne *Listeria monocytogenes* was estimated at $2.3 billion (wwww.ers.usda.gov). During the period October 1, 1993 to September 30, 1998, microbial contamination of food and cosmetic products was the leading cause for recalls, accounting for a total of 1370 recalls (36% of all products recalled). *Listeria monocytogenes* accounted for the greatest number of food products recalled. Nearly two-thirds of all product recalls due to *L. monocytogenes* contamination were dairy products, pastries, salads, or sandwiches (Wong et al., 2000).

6.4.1 Ecology of *Listeria*

Ruminants are often fed forage that is contaminated with *L. monocytogenes* and frequently shed this organism in their feces. Zundel and Bernard (2006) reported that in *Listeria*-free sheep that had been inoculated with *L. monocytogenes*, this pathogen spread throughout the entire volume of the forestomachs within 4 h and through the entire gastrointestinal tract within 24 h. These sheep shed *L. monocytogenes* for 10 days. *Listeria* persisted for at least 14 days in rumen digest and retropharyngeal lymph nodes and at relatively high levels of about 10^4 CFU/g in palatine tonsils. They concluded that *L. monocytogenes* translocates throughout the digestive tract of asymptomatic sheep, with the exception of the gallbladder, and that brief and low-level fecal excretion of *L. monocytogenes* is concomitant with transitory asymptomatic infection in sheep.

Fenlon (1985) reported that silage containing low levels of oxygen was contaminated with *L. monocytogenes*, whereas silage kept under strict anaerobic conditions with a consistently low pH did not include any *Listeria*. In silage, the strictly anaerobic conditions coupled with the predominance of lactic acid bacteria that reduce the pH results in conditions that are unfavorable for *L. monocytogenes* growth. Damaged silage bags with high amounts of oxygen also did not support *L. monocytogenes* growth, and *L. monocytogenes* was probably outcompeted by aerobic microorganisms. However, the conditions in the silage bales that contained low amounts of oxygen restricted aerobic species, and limited acid production by the lactics allowed the proliferation of *L. monocytogenes*. Therefore, farmers feeding silage to their animals need to take into account the atmospheric status of their silage, as this could be a source of *L. monocytogenes* for susceptible and asymptomatic animals. Microaerophilic conditions in silage may allow the persistence and further dissemination of *L. monocytogenes* in the farm environment.

In addition to the persistence of *L. monocytogenes* observed in bovine manure-amended soil, Nightingale et al. (2004) showed that the bovine farm ecosystem maintains a high prevalence of *L. monocytogenes*, including subtypes linked to human listeriosis cases and outbreaks. It also appears that cattle contribute to amplification and dispersal of *L. monocytogenes* into the farm environment.

6.4.2 Dissemination Factors of *Listeria*

The prevalence of *L. monocytogenes* in bovine and other farm ecosystems presents a challenge to the food industry, where zero tolerance of *L. monocytogenes* on RTE foods is mandated. Not only could beef processing plants be contaminated with *L. monocytogenes* from raw bovine products, but some of these *L. monocytogenes* may persist within the plant environment and thus recontaminate processed RTE beef products.

Control of *L. monocytogenes* in preharvest environments remains elusive. This is due partially to the persistence of the organism in the environment. In a study conducted by Dowe et al. (1997), soil type apparently influenced the survival of *L. monocytogenes*, with sandy soil having the worst long-term prospects for survival. Soils with greater absorption of moisture showed marked *L. monocytogenes* growth. Therefore, moisture levels may also be the most influential abiotic factor in determining *L. monocytogenes* levels. *L. monocytogenes* increased from low inoculum levels but decreased from high inoculum levels and also reached higher levels more rapidly in autoclaved soil. Multiplication of *L. monocytogenes* in these soils strengthens the hypothesis that this environment is a key reservoir for the organism. Interestingly, this pathogen thrives in the presence of some natural background flora. The presence of reduced microbial competitors in soil amended with solid chicken manure also supported higher populations of *L. monocytogenes* than did soils amended with either liquid hog manure or inorganic nitrogen–phosphorus–potassium fertilizer. It appears that low levels of *L. monocytogenes* such as those shed in fecal matter may provide adequate inoculum to establish a population of *L. monocytogenes* in soil.

In conclusion, *L. monocytogenes* routes of contamination both pre- and post-harvest are better understood, but developing effective control measures for all potential sites of contamination remains difficult. Future work is needed to develop more understanding of this organism when present in low-oxygen and anaerobic environments and how this may influence growth, survival, and pathogenesis.

6.5 *CAMPYLOBACTER* IN BEEF

Campylobacter spp. are now estimated to be the leading bacterial cause of food-borne illness in several developed countries. In the United States it causes 1,963,141 illnesses, 10,539 hospitalizations, and 99 deaths annually (Mead et al., 1999) at an estimated cost of $1,215,300,000 annually (USDA-ERS, 2008). After a 1- to 7-day incubation period, campylobacteriosis involves symptoms such as abdominal cramps, mild to severe inflammatory diarrhea, and bloody stools, which typically last for 2 to 3 days (Ketley, 1997). Campylobacteria can also infrequently cause post-infection complications associated with acquiring immune-mediated neuropathies—Guillain–Barré syndrome or Miller–Fisher syndrome (Jacobs et al., 1998; Nachamkin et al., 1998; Rees et al., 1995; Salloway et al., 1996)—and may potentially contribute to the development of inflammatory bowel diseases such as Crohn's disease (Lamhonwah et al., 2005).

Campylobacter are small, curved-to-spiral-shaped, flagellated gram-negative rods ranging from 0.5 to 8 μm in length and 0.2 to 0.5 μm wide (Penner, 1988). The genus *Campylobacter* is made up of 17 species (Foster et al., 2004; On, 2001); however, in the United States, about 99% of *Campylobacter* infections are caused by *C. jejuni* (CDC, 2005). *Campylobacter coli* is recognized as the next most prevalent food-poisoning species and is estimated to have been responsible for approximately 26,000 cases of intestinal inflammatory responses in 2000 (Gillespie et al., 2002; Tam et al., 2003). These *Campylobacter* appear well adapted to survive and colonize within the digestive tracts of warm-blooded hosts, and while conditions that include a microaerobic atmosphere and temperatures ranging between 37 and 42°C are optimal for growth (Altekruse et al., 1999), *Campylobacter* are capable of surviving on countertops for several days, and transmission to food during preparation in kitchens has been reported (Luber et al., 2006).

6.5.1 Prevalence

Campylobacter jejuni and *C. coli* are natural colonizers of the gastrointestinal tracts of domestic and feral animals and are generally asymptomatic in food production animals (Stanley and Jones, 2003). Despite early reports of their isolation from cattle (Garcia et al., 1985; Manser and Dalziel, 1985; Munroe et al., 1983), *Campylobacter* have been recognized primarily as important foodborne pathogens in poultry and unpasteurized dairy products (Butzler and Oosterom, 1991). For instance, *C. jejuni* has been recovered at isolation rates as high as 98% from retail poultry products (Altekruse et al., 1999) and 12.3% from bulk tank milk samples (Oliver et al., 2005). Nevertheless, *Campylobacter* are known to be present on dairy farms, with prevalence being higher in lactating cows (42.9%) than in cull cows (30.3%) (Wesley et al., 2000). A recent study reported that prevalence was higher in calves than in cows and higher on smaller than on larger farms in Wisconsin (Sato et al., 2004). This study also reported that prevalence rates were similar (29.1% and 26.7%, respectively) on the conventional and antimicrobial-free dairy farms studied (Sato et al., 2004).

With respect to beef cattle, Garcia et al. (1985) found *C. jejuni* to present more often in steers (55%) than in cows (22%) or bulls and heifers (each at 40%). Conversley, Bae et al. (2005) reported a higher prevalence rate of *C. jejuni* in cow–calf operations (47.1%) than in calf rearing, in a feedlot operation (23.8% and 31.6%, respectively), or in dairy operations (31.2%). Length of time within a feedlot appears to affect colonization status as prevalence of *C. jejuni* in fed cattle increased during feeding from 1.6% to as high as 63% near the finishing period (Besser et al., 2005). Prevalence rates in slaughter cattle, as determined via culture of rectal swabs collected before and after transit, were similar in feedlot cattle (64% to 68%, respectively) and adult cattle (6% to 7%, respectively), thus indicating that transportation had little effect on colonization status (Beach et al., 2002). Hide contamination as determined via a culture of swabs taken at the animals' hindquarter region, decreased during transit from 25% to 13% *Campylobacter*-positive samples in the feedlot cattle but were similar for the adult cattle (1% to 2%, respectfully) (Beach et al., 2002). In cattle, prevalence rates in general have been higher for *C. jejuni* than for *C. coli* (Bae et al., 2005; Harvey et al., 2005; Inglis and Kalischuk, 2003; Inglis et al., 2004), although Bae et al. (2005) found that *C. coli* prevalence was nearly equivalent to that of *C. jejuni* (20% vs. 23.8%, respectfully) in calf-rearing operations. *Campylobacter* prevalence in feedlot cattle has been found in at least one study to be much higher than that of *Salmonella* (Beach et al., 2002). Studies elsewhere have reported *Campylobacter* prevalences in beef cattle to be 24.8% in Northern Ireland (Madden et al., 2007), 53.9% in northeastern Italy (Pezzotti et al., 2003), 31.1% in Finland (Hakkinen et al., 2007), 26% in southwestern Norway (Johnsen et al., 2006), 10.2% in Switzerland (Al-Saigh et al., 2004), and 58% for feedlot cattle and 2% for pasture cattle in Australia (Bailey et al., 2003). Unlike that observed with dairy cattle, beef cattle do not appear to exhibit increased *Campylobacter*-colonization status during the summer months (Stanley et al., 1998).

6.5.2 Gastrointestinal Ecology

Garcia et al. (1985) sampled multiple internal viscera for *C. jejuni* and *C. coli* and successfully recovered *C. jejuni* serotypes from the gallbladder, large intestine, small intestine, liver, and lymph nodes. The gallbladder mucosal tissue and bile have been found to be good sites for *Campylobacter* colonization (Garcia et al., 1985; Saito et al., 2005) and *Campybacter*-positive liver samples have been recovered from 12% of beef cows sampled and 54.2% of Japanese oxen sampled, with most isolates identified as *C. jejuni* (Kramer et al., 2000). In one study, *Campylobacter* were readily recovered from fecal specimens of feedlot steers but not from ruminal contents of the same animals (Gutierrez-Bañuelos et al., 2007). *Campylobacter jejuni* and *C. coli* are generally asymptomatic in most colonized cattle; however, cases of diarrhea and gastroenteritis in calves have been reported, and this may be one rational for increased antibiotic use within farms and feedlots (Stanley and Jones, 2003).

6.6 CONTROL OF FOODBORNE PATHOGENS IN BEEF

A number of technologies have been developed to reduce contamination of carcasses by foodborne pathogens during slaughter and processing (Castell-Perez and Moreira, 2004; Keeton and Eddy, 2004). The meat industry has generally adopted a multiple-hurdle approach encompassing the training of food handlers in effective hygiene and implementation of postharvest interventions such as hot water and organic acid rinses, steam pasteurization, chemical dehairing, steam vaccuming, and irradiation (Acuff et al., 1987; Belk, 2001; Cherrington et al., 1991; Dickson, 1992; Dorsa, 1997; Farkas, 1998; Hardin et al., 1995; Koohmaraie et al., 2005; Micheals et al., 2004; Ricke, 2003; Ricke et al., 2005). Interventions such as these are intended to minimize contamination of meat products by foodborne pathogens. For instance, despite its ubiquitous dissemination in animals, *Listeria* is considered primarily a food safety risk post-harvest, and subsequently, a wide variety of chemical and physical interventions have been examined and/or proposed (Tompkin, 2002). More recently, Dimitrijevic et al. (2006) demonstrated that several nitro-based compounds decreased growth rates of *L. monocytogenes* during anaerobic culture and aerobic 4°C storage over 4 months.

In the red meat industry, hide removal and evisceration are particularly important critical control points, as these processes have been proposed as most likely to result in the contamination of carcasses (Pearce et al., 2004; Ryan, 2007; Tergney and Bolton, 2006). For beef processors in the United States, the efficacy of post-harvest interventions must be extremely high since *E. coli* O157:H7 is classified as an adulterant by the Food and Drug Administration, which applies a zero tolerance for the pathogen in ground meat (USDA-FSIS, 2004). However, despite Herculean efforts by packers and processors, current post-harvest interventions are not infallible, as product recalls and outbreaks of human foodborne disease continue to occur. In a risk assessment conducted by Cassin et al. (1998), the concentration of *E. coli* O157:H7 in feces of animals at slaughter was the greatest risk factor associated with *E. coli* O157:H7 foodborne illness from the consumption of hamburgers, suggesting that reducing carriage within animals pre-harvest may be beneficial. Moreover, other risk assessments have indicated that pre-harvest interventions would reduce human exposure to pathogens (Hynes and Wachsmuth, 2000; Vugia et al., 2003). Consequently, considerable research has been directed toward the development of interventions that can reduce the incidence and concentrations of foodborne pathogens in food animals during on-farm rearing; however, minimizing the spread of foodborne pathogens via on-farm measures remains elusive.

On-farm food safety undoubtedly begins with good animal husbandry and farm management, including effective sanitation practices (Collins and Wall, 2004; OIE, 2006). Contaminated feed and poor-quality silages have long been recognized as a potential source of pathogens to livestock operations, with many of the pathogens surviving for several months in dry feeds (Crump et al., 2002; Davis et al., 2003; Fenlon and Wilson, 2000; Lynn et al., 1998; Nightingale et al., 2004; Wilkinson, 1999). Consequently, considerable focus has been directed toward eliminating these sources of infection, particularly *Salmonella,* in animal and poultry feeds (Ha et al., 1998a, b; Juven et al., 1984). The addition of organic acids to repress *Salmonella* in feeds has been the primary set of antimicrobial compounds examined particularly for poultry feed (Hinton and Linton, 1988; Khan and Katamay, 1969; Maciorowski et al., 2004, 2006a).

Once a foodborne pathogen has been ingested by the animal, however, it becomes more difficult to minimize and/or eliminate these pathogens from a complex ecosystem such as the rumen or lower gastrointestinal area without disruption of more beneficial microflora. Antibiotics can be effective as feed supplements, such as has been shown with the use of neomycin to reduce bovine carriage of *E. coli* O157:H7 (Elder et al., 2003; Loneragan and Brashears, 2005), but uncontrolled use may promote the emergence of resistant foodborne pathogen strains of risk to human therapies (Cox et al., 2007).

Considerable research aimed at developing safe chemical feed or water supplements to reduce the incidence, survivability, and virulence of microbial pathogens in the gut of food animals during all stages of production is under way. For instance, the use of an experimental chlorate product to specifically target respiratory nitrate reductase enzymes possessed by *E. coli* and *Salmonella* has recently been investigated. It was hypothesized that an experimental product containing chlorate (ECP) may selectively kill nitrate-respiring *Salmonella* and *E. coli*, which also reduce chlorate to cytotoxic chlorite (Pichinoty and Piéchaud, 1968; Stewart, 1988) without harming beneficial gut bacteria (Anderson et al., 2000). In support of this hypothesis, *Salmonella* serovar Typhimurium DT104 and *E. coli* O157:H7, but not total culturable anaerobes, were reduced more than 10,000-fold during in vitro incubation of buffered ruminal fluid supplemented with 1.25 and 5 mM active chlorate ion (Anderson et al., 2000). Several studies have since demonstrated that intraruminal, drinking water, or feed administration of ECP significantly reduced fecal *E. coli* concentrations (Anderson et al., 2002, 2005; Callaway et al., 2002; Fox et al., 2005). Evidence from these studies indicated that an experimental chlorate product designed to bypass the rumen so as to enhance delivery of the active ion to the lower gut increased bactericidal efficacy in the lower gut (Anderson et al., 2005; Edrington et al., 2003a; Fox et al., 2005). Whereas studies testing ECP against *Salmonella* in cattle have yet to be done, numerous studies have shown significant reductions in *Salmonella* colonization in the alimentary tract of broilers, turkeys, and pigs (Anderson et al., 2001a, b; 2004; Byrd et al., 2003; Moore et al., 2006; Patchanee et al., 2007).

Another potential supplemental feeding strategy involves the administration of select nitroalkanes (i.e., 2-nitropropanol, 2-nitroethane, and 2-nitroethanol) that have been shown to exhibit inhibitory activity against *E. coli* O157:H7, *Listeria*, *Campylobacter*, and *Yersinia* in vitro (Anderson et al., 2007; Horrocks et al., 2007; Jung et al., 2004a). Moreover, the nitroalkanes were shown to reduce *Salmonella* colonization effectively in the gut of broilers (Jung et al., 2004b), and *Salmonella* and *Campylobacter* colonization in pigs (Jung et al., 2003), and to synergistically enhance the bactericidal activity of chlorate against *Salmonella* Typhimurium (Anderson et al., 2006c, 2007). Their efficacy has not yet been demonstrated in cattle (Gutierrez-Bañuelos et al., 2007). An attractive aspect of the nitroalkanes is that these compounds have been shown to be potent inhibitors of enteric methanogenesis (Anderson et al., 2006a; Gutierrez-Bañuelos et al., 2007) as well as against *Listeria* spp. (Dimitrijevic et al., 2006). Thus, the potential could be used to reduce economic and environmental costs associated with ruminal methane production and *Listeria* spp. should the latter be recognized as a preharvest problem. Similarly, the medium-chain fatty acid laurate and its glycerol monoester, monolaurin, also inhibit ruminal methanogenesis and *Listeria* (Božic et al., 2007a, b). The bactericidal effects of laurate and monolaurin probably result from a disruption of the cell wall of gram-positive or gram-positive-type organisms, which includes many ruminal bacteria that contribute to digestion, and thus their use as feed additives throughout the feeding. Additionally, their assimilation into intramuscular or subcutaneous fat may be undesirable from a human health perspective. However, it is not unreasonable to suspect that their use during the last day or several days before slaughter may significantly reduce gut carriage of *Listeria* with minimal effects on production efficiency or fat accretion. Another preharvest food safety strategy that captures economic benefits for livestock producers is the commercial dietary supplement, Tasco-14 (a preparation of the marine seaweed *Ascophyllum nodosum*), which has positive effects on carcass quality and product shelf life (Braden et al., 2007). When fed to feedlot cattle at 2% of the diet dry matter, Tasco-14 reduced incidence of *E. coli* O157-positive on hide swabs by more than 30% and feces by more than 9% (Braden et al., 2004). Fecal samples from the Tasco-14 supplement cattle also had less *Salmonella* than did nonsupplement cattle at the end of the feeding period (Braden et al., 2004).

Biocontrol methods employing the use of lytic bacteriophages are presently receiving much research emphasis as potential strategies to reduce the carriage of foodborne pathogens, being spurred on by the recent approval of an anti-*Listeria* phage spray for processed meat and poultry (Joerger, 2003; Strauch et al., 2007). Kudva et al. (1999) reported anti-*E. coli* O157:H7 lysis by specific bacteriophages and application of lytic bacteriophages to the rectoanal junction of experimentally inoculated cattle significantly lowered concentrations of *E. coli* O157:H7 recovered from this site (Sheng et al., 2006). Raya et al. (2006) reported 2-log-unit reductions in *E. coli* O157:H7 in sheep by 2 days post-administration. Lysis by bacteriophages specific for *Salmonella* and *Campylobacter* has been attempted with mixed success in poultry. In broliers, Wagenaar et al. (2005) reported 3-log reductions of *C. jejuni* by 3 days post-phage administrion, and Loc Carrillo et al. (2005) reported 0.5- to

5-log reductions of *C. jejuni* within 5 days of treatment. Phage therapy to broilers has been shown to reduce colinization by the *Salmonella* serovar Enteritidis by 0.3 to 3.5 log units (Fiorentin et al., 2005; Sklar and Joerger, 2001).

Preventing initial establishment and colonization of *Salmonella* in the animal would appear to be the optimal approach. Generation of antibodies either as a feed amendment or via a genetically engineered plant or grain that can be fed has some merit but may be cost prohibitive (Berghman et al., 2005). Beneficial probiotic and competitive cultures, the latter named for their purported ability to exclude by outcompeting the pathogen, have been used successfully in poultry to limit colonization in the gut (Anderson et al., 2006b). These approaches, however, have typically involved young birds with a minimal microflora present prior to introduction of the probiotic (Nisbet et al., 1994, 1996a, b), and thus this type of intervention in theory might prove to be more difficult to establish in the more complex ruminant ecosystem, where functionality of competitiveness is less well understood (Ricke and Pillai, 1999). Nevertheless, beneficial effects of administering probiotic lactic acid or nonpathogenic colicin-producing *E. coli* bacteria on reducing the incidence of shedding of *E. coli* O157:H7 in cattle and on hides have been reported (Brashears et al., 2003a, b; Elam et al., 2003; Schamberger et al., 2004; Younts-Dahl et al., 2004; Zhoa et al., 1998, 2003).

Immunizing young animals such as calves offers the opportunity to use the animal's immune system to ward off future systemic infections after exposure to foodborne pathogens later in life (Mastroeni et al., 2000). Parenteral vaccinations of young calves against *S.* Typhimurium using an auxotrophic-attenuated live strain limited the clinical signs expressed in calves exposed to the virulent version of the strain (van der Walt et al., 2001). Vaccination of cattle with components of the type III secretory system has been shown to help reduce shedding of *E. coli* O157:H7 in cattle. Potter et al. (2004) reported that vaccination reduced both the incidence (15 vs. 57 incidents of shedding out of 112 possible incidents over 14 days by vaccinated or nonvaccinated cattle, respectively; $n = 8$ per group) and concentration of *E. coli* O157:H7 shedding (6.25 vs. 81.25 CFU/g of feces for vaccinated and nonvaccinated cattle, respectively). In a subsequent study, however, vaccination with the type III immunogens was ineffective in reducing prevalence of *E. coli* O157:H7 (Van Donkersgoed et al., 2005). Thus, it is clear that a more in-depth understanding of the factors that influence virulence response of foodborne *Salmonella* and enterohemorrhagic *E. coli* in beef cattle is needed. Given the broad host range and multiple serotypes of foodborne pathogens, the development of multivalent vaccines against *Salmonella* and possibly against enterohemorhaggic *E. coli* may be needed to achieve better effectiveness (Wallis, 2001). In the case of *Salmonella*, for instance, pathogenesis requires multiple genes for complete virulence expression and can be regulated by a number of environmental factors, including anaerobiosis and VFA (Durant et al., 2000b; Ernst et al., 1990; Francis et al., 1992; Lucas and Lee, 2000; Marcus et al., 2000; Singh et al., 2000). Complete sequencing of foodborne pathogens coupled with implementation of newer molecular screening tools such as transposon footprinting and microarray analysis should further delineate virulence responses (De Keersmaecker et al., 2005; Hayashi et al., 2001; Kwon and Ricke, 2000, Kwon et al., 2002; Lucchini et al., 2001; Marchal et al., 2004; McClelland et al., 2001; Parkhill et al., 2000) and enable the construction of optimal genetic vaccine constructs.

Effective control of foodborne pathogens will also potentially rely on sensitive and rapid detection during the early states of their establishment in the beef environment. A myriad of cultural, immunological, and molecular methods have been employed for detection and identification of pathogens in various environments and sample matrices (see Chapter 27) (Bettelheim and Beutin, 2003; Gasanov et al., 2005; Gracias and McKillip, 2004; Kulkarni et al., 2002; Maciorowski et al., 2006b; Petrenko and Sorokulova, 2004; Ricke, 2005). Molecular detection using polymerase chain reaction approaches have been successful but are limited by their inability to distinguish nonviable from viable cells in feed (Maciorowski et al., 2000, 2005). Newer approaches that involve direct measurement of gene expression would resolve some of these issues. To illustrate, application of microarray technology provides an opportunity to screen rapidly for specific strains of *Salmonella* (Goldschmidt, 2006; Maciorowski et al., 2005; Nutt et al., 2004). However, standardization of these as well as conventional cultural methodologies between laboratories remains a problem (Gracias and McKillip, 2004; Malorny et al., 2003).

6.7 CONCLUSIONS

Enterohemorrhagic *E. coli, Salmonella, Listeria*, and *Campylobacter* remain foodborne pathogens of significance to the beef industry. The annual economic loss in 2000 associated with these foodborne pathogens was estimated at $5 to 6 billion (Murphy et al., 2003). Considerable research has yielded important information pertaining to the epidemiology and ecology of these pathogens in cattle, and progress has been made toward the development of interventions to minimize their carriage in animals. Preharvest interventions such as the seaweed preparation, Tasco-14, and probiotic mixtures of lactic acid bacteria are Generally Recognized as Safe (GRAS) within the United States and with such status they are commercially available. An anti-*E. coli* O157:H7 vaccine for cattle has been approved by the Canadian Food Inspection Agency for use in Canada. Interventions employing chlorate or nitrocompounds await regulatory approval from agencies such as the U.S. Food and Drug Administration. Challenges remain for the beef industry; however, as issues that extend well beyond the pathogens discussed in this chapter, including the emergence of existing and new pathogens, the emergence and spread of antimicrobial-resistant bacteria and environmental issues come to the forefront.

REFERENCES

Acuff GR, Vanderzant C, Savell JW, Jones DK, Griffin DB, Ehlers JG (1987): Effect of acid decontamination of beef subprimal cuts on the microbiological and sensory characteristics of steaks. *Meat Sci.* 19:217–226.

Alam MJ, Zurek L (2004): Association of *Escherichia coli* O157:H7 with houseflies on a cattle farm. *Appl Environ Microbiol.* 70:7578–7580.

Al-Saigh H, Zweifwl C, Blanco J, et al. (2004): Fecal shedding of *Escherichia coli* O157:H7, *Salmonella*, and *Campylobacter* in Swiss cattle at slaughter. *J Food Prot.* 67:679–684.

Altekruse SE, Stern NJ, Fields PI, Swerdlow DL (1999): *Campylobacter jejuni*: an emerging foodborne pathogen. *Emerg Infect Dis.* 5:28–35.

Anderson RC, Buckley SA, Kubena LF, Stanker LH, Harvey RB, Nisbet DJ (2000): Bactericidal effect of sodium chlorate on *Escherichia coli* O157:H7 and *Salmonella* Typhimurium DT104 in rumen contents in vitro. *J Food Prot.* 63:1038–1042.

Anderson RC, Buckley SA, Callaway TR, et al. (2001a): Effect of sodium chlorate on *Salmonella* Typhimurium concentrations in the weaned pig gut. *J Food Prot.* 64:255–258.

Anderson RC, Callaway TR, Buckley SA, et al. (2001b): Effect of oral sodium chlorate administration on *Esherichia coli* O157:H7 in the gut of experimentally infected pigs. *Int J Food Microbiol.* 71:125–130.

Anderson RC, Callaway TR, Anderson TJ, Kubena LF, Keith NK, Nisbet DJ (2002): Bactericidal effect of sodium chlorate on *Escherichia coli* concentrations in bovine ruminal and fecal concentrations in vivo. *Microb Ecol Health Dis.* 14:24–29.

Anderson RC, Hume ME, Genovese KJ, et al. (2004): Effect of drinking water administration of experimental chlorate ion preparations on *Salmonella enterica* serovar Typhimurium colonization in weaned and finished pigs. *Vet Res Commun.* 28:179–189.

Anderson RC, Carr MA, Miller RK, et al. (2005): Effects of experimental chlorate preparations as feed and water supplements on *Escherichia coli* colonization and contamination of beef cattle and carcasses. *Food Microbiol.* 22:439–447.

Anderson RC, Carstens GE, Miller RK, et al. (2006a): Effect of oral nitroethane and 2-nitropropanol administration on methane-producing activity and volatile fatty acid production in the ovine rumen. *Bioresource Technol.* 97:2421–2426.

Anderson RC, Genovese KJ, Harvey RB, Callaway TR, Nisbet DJ (2006b): Havest food safety applications of competitive exclusion cultures and probiotics. In: Goktepe I, Juneja VK, Ahmedna M (Eds.). *Probiotics in Food Safety and Human Health.* Taylor & Francis, New York, pp. 273–284.

Anderson RC, Jung YS, Genovese KJ, et al. (2006c): Low level nitrate or nitroethane preconditioning enhances the bactericidal effect of suboptimal experimental chlorate treatment against *Escherichia coli* and *Salmonella* Typhimurium but not *Campylobacter* in swine. *Foodborne Pathol Dis.* 3:461–465.

Anderson RC, Jung YS, Oliver CE, et al. (2007): Effects of nitrate or nitro-supplementation, with or without added chlorate, on *Salmonella enterica* serovar Typhimurium and *Escherichia coli* in swine feces. *J Food Prot.* 70:308–315.

Bach SJ, McAllister TA, Veira DM, Gannon VPJ, Holley RA (2002a): Effect of monensin on survival and growth of *Escherichia coli* O157:H7 in vitro. *Can Vet J.* 43:718–719.

——— (2002b): Transmission and control of *Escherichia coli* O157:H7: a review. *Can J Anim Sci.* 82:475–490.

Bae W, Kaya KN, Hancock DD, Call DR, Park YH, Besser TE (2005): Prevalence and antimicrobial resistance of thermophilic *Campylobacter* spp. from cattle farms in Washington State. *Appl Environ Microbiol.* 71:169–174.

Baik HS, Bearson S, Dunbar S, Foster JW (1996): The acid tolerance response of *Salmonella typhimurium* provides protection against organic acids. *Microbiology.* 142:3195–3200.

Bailey GD, Vanselow BA, Hornitzky MA, et al. (2003): A study of the foodborne pathogens: *Campylobacter, Listeria, Yersinia,* in faeces from slaughter-age cattle and sheep in Australia. *Commun Dis Intell.* 27:249–257.

Barham AR, Barham BL, Johnson AK, Allen DM, Blanton JR Jr, Miller MF (2002): Effects of the transportation of beef cattle from the feedyard to the packing plant on prevalence levels of *Escherichia coli* O157 and *Salmonella. J Food Prot.* 65:280–283.

Beach JC, Murano EA, Acuff GR (2002): Prevalence of *Salmonella* and *Campylobacter* in beef cattle from transport to slaughter. *J Food Prot.* 65:1687–1693.

Belk KE (2001): Beef decontamination technologies. In: *Beef Facts, Beef Safety.* National Cattlemen's Beef Association, Washington, DC, pp. 1–8.

Bender JB, Sreevatsan S, Robinson RA, Otterby D (1997): Animal by-products contaminated with *Salmonella* in the diets of lactating dairy cows. *J Dairy Sci.* 80:3064–3067.

Berg J, McAllister T, Bach S, Stilborn R, Hancock D, LeJune J (2004): *Escherichia coli* O157:H7 excretion by commercial feedlot cattle fed either barley- or corn-based finishing diets. *J Food Prot.* 67:666–671.

Berghman LR, Abi-Ghanem D, Waghela SD, Ricke SC (2005): Antibodies: An alternative for antibiotics. *Poult Sci.* 84:660–666.

Besser TE, LeJune JT, Rice DH, et al. (2005): Increasing prevalence of *Campylobacter jejuni* in feedlot cattle through feeding period. *Appl Environ Microbiol.* 71:5752–5758.

Bettelheim KA, Beutin L (2003): Rapid laboratory identification and characterization of verocytotoxigenic (Shiga toxin producing) *Escherichia coli* (VTEC/STEC). *J Appl Microbiol.* 95:205–217.

Blanco J, Blanco M, Blanco JE, et al. (2003): Verotoxin-producing *Escherichia coli* in Spain: prevalence, serotypes, and virulence genes of O157:H7 and non-O157 VTEC in ruminants, raw beef products, and humans. *Exp Biol Med.* 228:345–350.

Božic AK, Anderson RC, Carstens GE, Nisbet DJ (2007a): In vitro effects of the methane-inhibitors nitroethane, 2-nitro-1-propanol, lauric acid, and lauricidin® on select populations of Gram-positive bacteria. In *Proc. Symposium on Veterinary Medicine, Animal Husbandry and Economy in Animal Health and Food Safety Production,* Herceg Novi, Montenegro, p. 153.

Božic AK, Anderson RC, Ricke SC, et al. (2007b): Comparison of select methane-inhibitors on ruminal methane production in vitro. In *Proc. Symposium on Veterinary Medicine, Animal Husbandry and Economy in Animal Health and Food Safety Production,* Herceg Novi, Montenegro, p. 23.

Braden KW, Blanton JR Jr, Allen AG, Pond KR, Miller MF (2004): *Ascophyllum nodosum* supplementation: a preharvest intervention for reducing *Escherichia coli* O157:H7 and *Salmonella* spp. in feedlot steers. *J Food Prot.* 67:1824–1828.

Braden KW, Blanton JR Jr, Montgomery JL, van Santen E, Allen AG, Miller MF (2007): Tasco supplementation: effects on carcass characteristics, sensory attributes, and retail shelf-life. *J Anim Sci.* 85:754–768.

Brashears MM, Galyean ML, Loneragan GH, Mann JE, Killinger-Mann K (2003a): Prevalence of *Escherichia coli* O157:H7 and performance by beef feedlot cattle given *Lactobacillus* direct-fed microbials. *J Food Prot.* 66:748–754.

Brashears MM, Jaroni D, Trimble J (2003b): Isolation, selection and characterization of lactic acid bacteria for a competitive exclusion product to reduce shedding of *Escherichia coli* O157:H7 in cattle. *J Food Prot.* 66:355–363.

Brownlie LE, Grau FH (1967): Effect of food intake on growth and survival of Salmonellas and *Escherichia* in the bovine rumen. *J Gen Microbiol.* 46:125–134.

Bryan FL (1980): Foodborne diseases in the United States associated with meat and poultry. *J Food Prot.* 43:140–150.

——— (1981): Current trends in foodborne salmonellosis in the U.S. and Canada. *J Food Prot.* 44:394–402.

Buchanan RL, Doyle MP (1997): Foodborne disease significance of *Escherichia coli* O157:H7 and other enterohemorrhagic *E. coli*. *Food Technol.* 51:69–76.

Buchko SJ, Holley RA, Buchko SJ, Olson WO, Gannon VPJ, Veira DM (2000): The effect of different grain diets on fecal shedding of *Escherichia coli* O157:H7 by steers. *J Food Prot.* 63:1467–1474.

Butzler J, Oosterom J (1991): *Campylobacter*: pathogenicity and significance in foods. *Int J Food Microbiol.* 12:1–8.

Byrd JA, Anderson RC, Callaway TR, et al. (2003): Effect of experimental chlorate product administration in the drinking water on *Salmonella* Typhimurium contamination of broilers. *Poult Sci.* 82:1403–1406.

Callaway TR, Anderson RC, Genovese KJ, et al. (2002): Sodium chlorate supplementation reduces *E. coli* O157:H7 populations in cattle. *J Anim Sci.* 80:1683–1689.

Callaway TR, Edrington TS, Rychlik JL, et al. (2003a): Ionophores: their use as ruminant growth promotants and impact on food safety. *Curr Issues Intest Microbiol.* 4:43–51.

Callaway TR, Elder RO, Keen JE, Anderson RC, Nisbet DJ (2003b): Forage feeding to reduce preharvest *Escherichia coli* populations in cattle: a review. *J Dairy Sci.* 86:852–860.

Callaway TR, Anderson RC, Tellez G, et al. (2004): Prevalence of *Escherichia coli* O157 in cattle and swine in central Mexico. *J Food Prot.* 67:2274–2276.

Carlson SA, Sharma VK, McCuddin ZP, Rasmussen MA, Franklin SK (2007): Involvement of a *Salmonella* genomic island 1 gene in the rumen protozoan-mediated enhancement of invasion for multiple-antibiotic-resistant *Salmonella enterica* serovar Typhimurium. *Infect Immun.* 75:792–800.

Cassin MH, Lammerding AM, Todd ECD, Ross W, McColl RS (1998): Quantitative risk assessment for *Escherichia coli* O157:H7 in ground beef hamburgers. *Int J Food Microbiol.* 41:21–44.

Castell-Perez M, Moreira RG (2004): Decontamination systems. In: Beier RC, Pillai SD, Phillips TD (Eds.). *Preharvest and Post Harvest Food Safety: Contemporary Issues and Future Directions*. Blackwell Publishing, Ames, IA, pp. 337–347.

CDC (Centers for Disease Control and Prevention) (2005): *Campylobacter* infections. http://www.cdc.gov/ncidod/dbmd/diseaseinfo/campylobacter_g.htm. Accessed May 2007.

Chambers PG, Lysons RJ (1979): The inhibitory effect of bovine rumen fluid on *Salmonella* Typhimurium. *Res Vet Sci.* 26:273–276.

Cherrington CA, Hinton M, Mead GC, Chopra I (1991): Organic acids: chemistry, antibacterial activity and practical applications. *Adv Microb Physiol.* 32:87–108.

Cobbold RN, Hancock DD, Rice DH, et al. (2007): Rectoanal junction colonization of feedlot cattle by *Escherichia coli* O157:H7 and its association with supershedders and excretion dynamics. *Appl Environ Microbiol* 73:1563–1568.

Collins JD, Wall PG (2004): Food safety and animal production systems: controlling zoonosis at farm level. *Rev Sci Tech Off Int Epizoot.* 23:685–700.

Conedera G, Chapman PA, Marangon S, Tisato E, Dalvit P, Zuin A (2001): A field study of *Escherichia coli* O157 ecology on a cattle farm in Italy. *Int J Food Microbiol.* 66:85–93.

Corrier DE, Purdy CW, DeLoach JR (1990): Effects of marketing stress on fecal excretion of *Salmonella* spp. in feeder calves. *Am J Vet Res.* 51:866–869.

Cox LA Jr, Popken DA, Carnevale R (2007): Quantifying human health risks from animal antimicrobials. *Interfaces.* 37:22–38.

Cray WC Jr, Casey TA, Bosworth BT, Rasmussen MA (1998): Effect of dietary stress on fecal shedding of *Escherichia coli* O157:H7 in calves. *Appl Environ Microbiol.* 64: 1975–1979.

Crump JA, Griffin PM, Angulo FJ (2002): Bacterial contamination of animal feed and its relationship to human foodborne illness. *Clin Infect Dis.* 35:859–865.

D'Aoust JY (2001): *Salmonella*. In: Labbé RG, García S (Eds.). *Guide to Food-borne Pathogens.* Wiley, New York, pp. 163–191.

Dargatz DS, Wells SJ, Thomas LA, Hancock DD, Garber LP (1997): Factors associated with the presence of *Escherichia coli* O157 in feces of feedlot cattle. *J Food Prot.* 60:466–470.

Davis MA, Hancock DD, Rice DH, et al. (2003): Feedstuffs as a vehicle of cattle exposure to *Escherichia coli* O157:H7 and *Salmonella enterica*. *Vet Microbiol.* 95:199–210.

De Keersmaecker SCJ, Marchal K, Verhoeven TLA, Engelen K, Vanderleyden J, Detweiler CS (2005): Microarray analysis and motif detection reveal new targets of the *Salmonella enterica* serovar Typhimurium HilA regulatory protein, including *hilA* itself. *J Bacteriol.* 187:4381–4391.

Dickson JS (1992): Acetic acid action on beef tissue surfaces contaminated with *Salmonella typhimurium*. *J Food Sci.* 57:297–301.

Diez-Gonzalez F, Callaway TR, Kizoulis MG, Russell JB (1998): Grain feeding and the dissemination of acid-resistant *Escherichia coli* from cattle. *Science.* 281:1666–1668.

Dimitrijevic M, Anderson RC, Callaway TR, et al. (2006): Inhibitory effect of select nitrocompounds on growth and survivability of *Listeria monocytogenes* in vitro. *J Food Prot.* 69:1061–1065.

Dorsa WJ (1997): New and established carcass decontamination procedures commonly used in the beef-processing industry. *J Food Prot.* 60:1146–1151.

Dowe MJ, Jackson ED, Mori JG, Bell CR (1997): *Listeria monocytogenes* survival in soil and incidence in agricultural soils. *J Food Prot.* 60:1201–1207.

Duffy G (2003): Verocytotoxigenic *Escherichia coli* in animal faeces, manures and slurries. *J Appl Microbiol.* 94:94S–103S.

Dunkley KD, McReynolds JL, Hume ME, et al. (2007): Molting in *Salmonella* Enteritidis–challenged laying hens fed alfalfa crumbles. I: *Salmonella* Enteritidis colonization and virulence gene *hilA* response. *Poult Sci.* 86:1633–1639.

Durant JA, Corrier DE, Byrd JA, Stanker LH, Ricke SC (1999a): Feed deprivation affects crop environment and modulates *Salmonella enteritidis* colonization and invasion of Leghorn hens. *Appl Environ Microbiol.* 65:1919–1923.

Durant JA, Lowry VK, Nisbet DJ, Stanker LH, Corrier DE, Ricke SC (1999b): Short-chain fatty acids affect cell-association and invasion of HEp-2 cells by *Salmonella typhimurium*. *J Environ Sci Health Pt B.* 34:1083–1099.

——— (2000a): Late logarithmic *Salmonella typhimurium* HEp-2 cell association and invasion response to short-chain volatile fatty acid addition. *J Food Saf.* 20:1–11.

——— (2000b): Short-chain fatty acids alter HEp-2 cell association and invasion by stationary growth phase *Salmonella typhimurium*. *J Food Sci*. 65:1206–1209.

Durant JA, Corrier DE, Ricke SC (2000c): Short-chain volatile fatty acids modulate the expression of the *hilA* and *invF* genes of *Salmonella* Typhimurium. *J Food Prot*. 63: 573–578.

Durso LM, Smith D, Hutkins RW (2004): Measurements of fitness and competition in commensal *Escherichia coli* and *E. coli* O157:H7 strains. *Appl Environ Microbiol*. 70: 6466–6472.

Edrington TS, Callaway TR, Anderson RC, et al. (2003a): Reduction of *E. coli* O157:H7 populations in sheep by supplementation of an experimental sodium chlorate product. *Small Ruminant Res*. 49:173–181.

Edrington TS, Callaway TR, Bischoff KM, et al. (2003b): Effect of feeding the ionophores monensin and laidlomycin propionate and the ionophore bambermycin to sheep experimentally infected with *Esherichia coli* O157:H7 and *Salmonella typhimurium*. *J Anim Sci*. 81:553–560.

Edrington TS, Callaway TR, Varey PD, et al. (2003c): Effects of the antibiotic ionophores monensin, lasalocid, laidlomycin propionate and bambermycin on *Salmonella* and *E. coli* O157:H7 in vitro. *J Appl Microbiol*. 94:207–213.

Edrington TS, Callaway TR, Ives SE, et al. (2006a): Seasonal shedding of *Escherichia coli* O157:H7 in ruminants: a new hypothesis. *Foodborne Pathog Dis*. 3:413–421.

Edrington TS, Looper ML, Duke SE, et al. (2006b). Effect of ionophore supplementation on the incidence of *Escherichia coli* O157:H7 and *Salmonella* and antimicrobial susceptibility of fecal coliforms in stocker cattle. *Foodborne Pathog Dis*. 3:284–291.

Elam NA, Gleghorn JF, Rivera JD, et al. (2003): Effects of live cultures of *Lactobacillus acidophilus* (strains NP45 and NP51) and *Propionibacterium freudenreichii* on performance, carcass, and intestinal characteristics, and *Escherichia coli* strain O157 shedding of finishing beef steers. *J Anim Sci*. 81:2686–2698.

Elder RO, Keen JE, Siragusa GR, Barkocy-Gallagher GA, Koohmaraire M, Laegreid WW (2000): Correlation of enterohemorrhagic *Escherichia coli* O157 prevalence in feces, hides, and carcasses of beef cattle during processing. *Proc Natl Acad Sci*. 97:2999–3003.

Elder RO, Keen JE, Edrington T, Callaway T, Anderson R, Nisbet D (2003): Intervention to reduce fecal shedding of enterohemmorrhagic *Escherichia coli* O157:H7 in fed beef cattle. In *Proc. 5th International Symposium on Shiga Toxin (Verocytotoxin)-producing* Escherichia coli *infections, Edinburgh, UK*, p. 94.

Ernst RK, Dombroski DM, Merrick JM (1990): Anaerobiosis, type 1 fimbriae, and growth phase are factors that affect invasion of HEp-2 cells by *Salmonella typhimurium*. *Infect Immun*. 58:2014–2016.

Farkas J (1998): Irradiation as a method for decontaminating food: a review. *Int J Food Microbiol*. 44:189–204.

Fegan N, Vanderlinde P, Higgs G, Desmarchelier P (2004): The prevalence and concentration of *Escherichia coli* O157 in faeces of cattle from different production systems at slaughter. *J Appl Microbiol*. 97:362–370.

Feng P (2001): *Escherichia coli*. In: Labbé RG, García S (Eds.). *Guide to Foodborne Pathogens*. Wiley, New York, pp. 143–162.

Fenlon DR (1985): Wild birds and silage as reservoirs of *Listeria* in the agricultural environment. *J Appl Bacteriol*. 59:537–543.

Fenlon DR, Wilson J (2000): Growth of *Escherichia coli* O157 in poorly fermented laboratory silage: a possible environmental dimension in the epidemiology of *E. coli* O157. *Lett Appl Microbiol.* 30:118–121.

Fiorentin L, Vieira ND, Barioni W Jr (2005): Oral treatment with bacteriophages reduces the concentration of *Salmonella* Enteritidis PT4 in caecal contents of broilers. *Avian Pathol.* 34:258–263.

Fitzgerald AC, Edrington TS, Looper ML, et al. (2003): Antimicrobial susceptibility and factors affecting the shedding of *E. coli* O157:H7 and *Salmonella* in dairy cattle. *Lett Appl Microbiol.* 37:392–398.

Foster G, Holmes B, Steigerwalt AG, et al. (2004): *Campylobacter insulaenigrae* sp. nov., isolated from marine mammals. *Int J Syst Evol Microbiol.* 54:2369–2373.

Fox JT, Anderson RC, Carstens GE, et al. (2005): Effect of nitrate adaption on the bactericidal activity of an experimental chlorate product against *Escherichia coli* in cattle. *Int J Appl Res Vet Med.* 3:76–80.

Francis CL, Starnbach MN, Falkow S (1992): Morphological and cytoskeletal changes in epithelial cells occur immediately upon interaction with *Salmonella typhimurium* grown under low-oxygen conditions. *Mol Microbiol.* 6:3077–3087.

Frenzen PD, Riggs TL, Buzby JC, et al. (FoodNet Working Group) (1999): *Salmonella* cost estimate update using FoodNet data. *Food Rev.* 22:10–15.

Gansheroff LJ, O'Brien AD (2000): *Escherichia coli* O157:H7 in beef cattle presented for slaughter in the U.S.: higher prevalence rates than previously estimated. *Proc Natl Acad Sci.* 97:2959–2961.

Garber LP, Wells SJ, Hancock DD, et al. (1995): Risk factors for fecal shedding of *Escherichia coli* O157:H7 in dairy calves. *J Am Vet Med Assoc.* 207:46–49.

Garcia MM, Lior H, Stewart RB, Ruckerbauer GM, Trudel JRR, Skljarevski A (1985): Isolation, characterization, and serotyping of *Campylobacter jejuni* and *Campylobacter coli* from slaughter cattle. *Appl Environ Microbiol.* 49:667–672.

Gasanov U, Hughes D, Hansbro PM (2005): Methods for the isolation and identification of *Listeria* spp. and *Listeria monocytogenes*: a review. *FEMS Microbiol Rev.* 29:851–875.

Gilbert RA, Tomkins N, Padmananabha J, Gough JM, Krause DO, McSweeney CS (2005): Effect of finishing diets on *Escherichia coli* populations and prevalence of enterohaemorrhagic *E. coli* virulence genes in cattle faeces. *J Appl Microbiol.* 99:885–894.

Gillespie IA, O'Brien SJ, Frost JA, et al. (2002): A case–case comparison of *Campylobacter coli* and *Campylobacter jejuni* infection: a tool for generating hypotheses. *Emerg Infect Dis.* 8:937–942.

Goepfert JM, Hicks R (1969): Effect of volatile fatty acids on *Salmonella typhimurium. J Bacteriol.* 97:956–958.

Goldschmidt MC (2006): The use of biosensor and microarray techniques in the rapid detection and identification of salmonellae. *J AOAC Int.* 89:530–537.

Gracias KS, McKillip JL (2004): A review of conventional detection and enumeration methods for pathogenic bacteria in food. *Can J Microbiol.* 50:883–890.

Grau FH, Brownlie LE, Smith MG (1969): Effects of food intake on numbers of salmonellae and *Escherichia coli* in rumen and faeces of sheep. *J Appl Bacteriol.* 32:112–117.

Grauke LJ, Kudva IT, Yoon JW, Hunt CW, Williams CJ, Hovde CJ (2002): Gastrointestinal tract location of *Escherichia coli* O157:H7 in ruminants. *Appl Environ Microbiol.* 68:2269–2277.

Greenacre EJ, Brocklehurst TF, Waspe CR, Wilson DR, Wilson PDG (2003): *Salmonella enterica* serovar Typhimurium and *Listeria monocytogenes* acid tolerance response induced by organic acids at 20°C: optimization and modeling. *Appl Environ Microbiol*. 69: 3945–3951.

Gregory NG, Jacobson LH, Nagle TA, Muirhead RW, Leroux GJ (2000): Effect of preslaughter feeding system on weight loss, gut bacteria, and the physiochemical properties of digesta in cattle. *NZ J Agric Res*. 43:351–361.

Gupta A, Fontana J, Crowe C, et al. (2003): Emergence of multidrug-resistant *Salmonella enterica* serotype Newport infections resistant to expanded-spectrum cephaloporins in the United States. *J Infect Dis*. 188:1707–1716.

Gutierrez-Bañuelos H, Anderson RC, Carstens GE, et al. (2007): Zoonotic bacterial populations, gut fermentation characteristics and methane production in feedlot steers during oral nitroethane treatment and after the feeding of an experimental chlorate product. *Anaerobe*. 13:21–31.

Ha SD, Maciorowski KG, Kwon YM, Jones FT, Ricke SC (1998a): Indigenous feed microflora and *Salmonella typhimurium* marker strain survival in poultry mash diets containing varying levels of protein. *Anim Feed Sci Technol*. 76:23–33.

——— (1998b): Survivability of indigenous feed microflora and a *Salmonella typhimurium* marker strain in poultry mash treated with buffered propionic acid. *Anim Feed Sci Technol*. 75:145–155.

Hakkinen M, Heiska H, Hänninen M (2007): Prevalence of *Campylobacter* spp. in cattle in Finland and antimicrobial susceptibilities of bovine *Campylobacter jejuni* strains. *Appl Environ Microbiol*. 73:3232–3238.

Hardin MD, Acuff GR, Lucia LM, Oman JS, Savell JW (1995): Comparison of methods for decontamination from beef carcass surfaces. *J Food Prot*. 58:368–374.

Harmon BG, Brown CA, Tkalcic S, et al. (1999): Fecal shedding and rumen growth of *Escherichia coli* O157:H7 in fasted calves. *J Food Prot*. 62:574–579.

Harvey RB, Hume ME, Droleskey RE, et al. (2005): Further characterization of *Campylobacter* isolated from U.S. dairy cows. Foodborne Pathog Dis. 2:182–187.

Hayashi T, Makino K, Ohnishi M, et al. (2001): Complete genome sequence of enterohemorrhagic *Escherichia coli* O157:H7 and genomic comparison with a laboratory strain K-12. *DNA Res*. 8:11–22.

Herikstad H, Motarjemi Y, Tauxe RV (2002): *Salmonella* surveillance: a global survey of public health serotyping. *Epidemiol Infect*. 129:1–8.

Heuvelink AE, Van Der Biggelaar FLAM, De Boer E, et al. (1998a): Isolation and characterization of verocytotoxin-producing *Escherichia coli* O157 strains from Dutch cattle and sheep. *J Clin Microbiol*. 36:878–882.

Heuvelink, AE, Van Den Biggelaar FLAM, Zwartkruis-Nahuis JTM, et al. (1998b): Occurrence of verocytotoxin-producing *Escherichia coli* O157 on Dutch dairy farms. *J Clin Microbiol*. 36:3480–3487.

Hinton M, Linton AH (1988): Control of *Salmonella* infection in broiler chickens by the acid treatment of their feed. *Vet Rec*. 123:416–421.

Holt PS, Mitchell BW, Gast RK (1998): Airborne horizontal transmission of *Salmonella enteriditis* in molted laying chickens. *Avian Dis*. 42:45–52.

Horrocks SM, Jung YS, Huwe JK, et al. (2007): Effects of short-chain nitrocompounds against *Campylobacter jejuni* and *Campylobacter coli* in vitro. *J Food Sci*. 72:M50–M55.

Hovde CJ, Austin PR, Cloud KA, Williams CJ, Hunt CW (1999): Effect of cattle diet on *Escherichia coli* O157:H7 acid resistance. *Appl Environ Microbiol.* 65:3233–3235.

Hussein HS (2007): Prevalence and pathogenicity of Shiga toxin–producing *Escherichia coli* in beef cattle and their products. *J Anim Sci.* 85 (E Suppl): E63–E72.

Hynes NA, Wachsmuth IK (2000): *Escherichia coli* O157:H7 risk assessment in ground beef: a public health tool. In *Proc. 4th International Symposium and Workshop on Shiga Toxin (Verocytotoxin)-Producing* Escherichia coli *Infections*, Kyoto, Japan, p. 46.

Inglis GD, Kalischuk LD (2003): Use of PCR for direct detection of *Campylobacter* species in bovine feces. *Appl Environ Microbiol.* 69:3435–3447.

Inglis GD, Kalischuk LD, Busz HW (2004): Chronic shedding of *Campylobacter* species in beef cattle. *J Appl Microbiol.* 97:410–420.

Jacobs BC, Rothbarth PH, Van Der Meche FG, et al. (1998): The spectrum of antecedent infections in Guillain-Barré syndrome: a case–control study. *Neurology.* 51:1110–1115.

Joerger RD (2003): Alternatives to antibiotics: bacteriocins, antimicrobial peptides and bacteriophages. *Poult Sci.* 82:640–647.

Johnsen G, Zimmerman K, Lindstedt B-A, Vardund T, Herikstad H, Kapperud G (2006): Intestinal carriage of *Campylobacter jejuni* and *Campylobacter coli* among cattle from south-western Norway and comparative genotyping of bovine and human isolates by amplified-fragment length polymorphism. *Acta Vet Scand.* 48:4. Published online June 6, 2006.

Jones FT, Ricke SC (1994): Researchers propose tentative HACCP plan for feed manufacturers. *Feedstuffs.* 66:32, 36–38, 40–42.

Jordan D, McEwen SA (1998): Effect of duration of fasting and a short-term high-roughage ration on the concentration of *Escherichia coli* biotype 1 in cattle feces. *J Food Prot.* 61:531–534.

Jung YS, Anderson RC, Genovese KJ, et al. (2003): Reduction of *Campylobacter* and *Salmonella* in pigs treated with a select nitrocompound. In *Proc. 5th International Symposium on the Epidemiology and Control of Foodborne Pathogens in Pork*, Hersonissos, Crete, pp. 205–207.

Jung YS, Anderson RC, Callaway TR, et al. (2004a): Inhibitory activity of 2-nitropropanol against select food-borne pathogens in vitro. *Lett Appl Microbiol.* 39:471–476.

Jung YS, Anderson RC, Edrington TS, et al. (2004b): Experimental use of 2-nitropropanol for reduction of *Salmonella* Typhimurium in the ceca of broiler chicks. *J Food Prot.* 67:1045–1047.

Juven BJ, Cox NA, Bailey JS, Thomsen JE, Charles OW, Shutze JV (1984): Survival of *Salmonella* in dry food and feed. *J Food Prot.* 47:445–448.

Karch H, Bielaszewska M, Bitzan M, Schmidt H (1999): Epidemiology and diagnosis of Shiga toxin–producing *Escherichia coli* infections. *Diagn Microbiol Infect Dis.* 34:229–243.

Karch H, Tarr PI, Bielaszewska M (2005): Enterohaemorrhagic *Escherichia coli* in human medicine. *Int J Med Microbiol.* 295:405–418.

Kay S. (2003): $2.7 billion, the cost of *E. coli* O157:H7. *Meat Poult.* February, pp. 26–34.

Keeton JT, Eddy SM (2004): Chemical methods for decontamination of meat and poultry. In: Beier RC, Pillai SD, Phillips TD (Eds.). *Preharvest and Post Harvest Food Safety: Contemporary Issues and Future Directions.* Blackwell Publishing, Ames, IA, pp. 319–336.

Ketley JM (1997): Pathogenesis of enteric infection by *Campylobacter. Microbiology.* 143:5–21.

Khaitsa ML, Smith DR, Stoner JA, et al. (2007): Incidence, duration, and prevalence of *Escherichia coli* O157:H7 fecal shedding by feedlot cattle during the finishing period. *J Food Prot.* 66:1972–1977.

Khan M, Katamay M (1969): Antagonistic effect of fatty acids against *Salmonella* in meat and bone meal. *Appl Microbiol.* 17:402–404.

Koohmaraie M, Arthur TM, Bosilevac JM, Guerini M, Shackelford SD, Wheeler TL (2005): Post-harvest interventions to reduce/eliminate pathogens in beef. *Meat Sci.* 71:79–91.

Kramer JM, Frost JA, Bolton FJ, Wareing DRA (2000): *Campylobacter* contamination of raw meat and poultry at retail sale: identification of multiple types and comparison with isolates from human infection. *J Food Prot.* 63:1654–1659.

Kudva IT, Jelacic S, Tarr PI, Youderian P, Hovde CJ (1999): Biocontrol of *Escherichia coli* O157 with O157-specific bacteriophages. *Appl Environ Microbiol.* 65:3767–3773.

Kulkarni SP, Lever S, Logan JMJ, Lawson AJ, Stanley J, Shafi MS (2002): Detection of *Campylobacter* species: a comparison of culture and polymerase chain reaction based methods. *J Clin Pathol.* 55:749–753.

Kwon YM, Ricke SC (1998): Induction of acid resistance of *Salmonella typhimurium* by exposure to short-chain fatty acids. *Appl Environ Microbiol.* 64:3458–3463.

——— (2000): Efficient amplification of multiple transposon-flanking sequences. *J Microbiol Methods.* 41:195–199.

Kwon YM, Woodward CL, Peña J, Corrier DE, Pillai SD, Ricke SC (1999): Comparison of methods for processing litter and air filter matrices from poultry houses to optimize polymerase chain reaction detection of *Salmonella typhimurium*. *J Rapid Methods Automat Microbiol.* 7:103–111.

Kwon YM, Woodward CL, Corrier DE, Byrd JA, Pillai SD, Ricke SC (2000a): Recovery of a marker strain of *Salmonella typhimurium* in litter and aerosols from isolation rooms containing infected chickens. *J Environ Sci Health Pt B.* 35:517–525.

Kwon YM, Park SY, Birkhold SG, Ricke SC (2000b): Induction of resistance of *Salmonella typhimurium* to environmental stresses by exposure to short-chain fatty acids. *J Food Sci.* 65:1037–1040.

Kwon YM, Kubena LF, Nisbet DJ, Ricke SC (2002): Functional screening of bacterial genome for virulence genes by transposon footprinting. In: Clark VL, Pavoil PM (Eds.). *Methods in Enzymology: Bacterial Pathogenesis,* Part C, Vol. 358. Academic Press, San Diego, CA, pp. 141–152.

Lahti E, Ruoho O, Rantala L, Hänninen M, Honkanen-Buzalski T (2003): Longitudinal study of *Escherichia coli* O157 in a cattle finishing unit. *Appl Environ Microbiol.* 69:554–561.

Lamhonwah A, Ackerley C, Onizuka R, et al. (2005): Epitope shared by functional variant of organic cation/carnitine transporter, OCTN1, *Campylobacter jejuni* and *Mycobacterium paratuberculosis* may underlie susceptibility to Crohn's disease at 5q31. *Biochem Biophys Res Commun.* 337:1165–1175.

Law D (2000): Virulence factors of *Escherichia coli* O157 and other Shiga toxin–producing *E. coli*. *J Appl Microbiol.* 88:729–745.

Lawhon SD, Maurer R, Suyemoto M, Altier C (2002): Intestinal short-chain fatty acids alter *Salmonella typhimurium* invasion gene expression and virulence through BarA/SirA. *Mol Microbiol.* 46:1451–1464.

LeJune JT, Besser TE, Hancock DD (2001): Cattle water troughs as a reservoir of *Escherichia coli* O157. *Appl Environ Microbiol.* 67:3053–3057.

Loc Carrillo CL, Attebury RJ, El-Shibiny A, et al. (2005): Bacteriophage therapy to reduce *Campylobacter jejuni* colonization of broiler chickens. *Appl Environ Microbiol.* 71:6554–6563.

Loneragan GH, Brashears MM (2005): Pre-harvest interventions to reduce carriage of *E. coli* O157 by harvest-ready feedlot cattle. *Meat Sci.* 71:72–78.

Low JC, McKendrick II, McKechnie C, et al. (2005): Rectal carriage of enterohemorrhagic *Escherichia coli* O157 in slaughtered cattle. *Appl Environ Microbiol.* 71:93–97.

Luber P, Brynestad S, Topsch D, Scherer K, Bartelt E (2006): Quantification of *Campylobacter* species cross-contamination during handling of contaminated fresh chicken parts in kitchens. *Appl Environ Microbiol.* 72:66–70.

Lucas RL, Lee CA (2000): Unravelling the mysteries of virulence gene regulation in *Salmonella typhimurium*. *Mol Microbiol.* 36:1024–1033.

Lucchini S, Thompson A, Hinton JCD (2001): Microarrays for microbiologists. *Microbiology.* 147:1403–1414.

Lynn TV, Hancock DD, Besser TE, et al. (1998): The occurrence and replication of *Escherichia coli* in cattle feeds. *J Dairy Sci.* 81:1102–1108.

Maciorowski KG, Pillai SD, Ricke SC (2000): Efficacy of a commercial polymerase chain reaction–based assay for detection of *Salmonella* spp. in animal feeds. *J Appl Microbiol.* 89:710–718.

Maciorowski KG, Jones FT, Pillai SD, Ricke SC (2004): Incidence, sources, and control of food-borne *Salmonella* spp. in poultry feeds. *World's Poult Sci J.* 60:446–457.

Maciorowski KG, Pillai SD, Jones FT, Ricke SC (2005): Polymerase chain reaction detection of foodborne *Salmonella* spp. in animal feeds. *Crit Rev Microbiol.* 31:45–53.

Maciorowski KG, Herrera P, Kundinger MM, Ricke SC (2006a): Animal production and contamination by foodborne *Salmonella*. *J Verbr Lebensm.* 1:197–209.

Maciorowski KG, Herrera P, Jones FT, Pillai SD, Ricke SC (2006b): Cultural and immunological detection methods for *Salmonella* spp. in animal feeds: a review. *Vet Res Commun.* 30:127–137.

Maciorowski KG, Herrera P, Jones FT, Pillai SD, Ricke SC (2007): Effects of poultry and livestock feed contamination with bacteria and fungi. *Anim Feed Sci Technol.* 133: 109–136.

MacVean DW, Franzen DK, Keefe TJ, Bennett BW (1986): Airborne particle concentration and meteorologic conditions associated with pneumonia incidence in feedlot cattle. *Am J Vet Res.* 47:2676–2682.

Madden RH, Murray KA, Gilmour A (2007): Carriage of four bacterial pathogens by beef cattle in Northern Ireland at time of slaughter. *Lett Appl Microbiol.* 44:115–119.

Malorny B, Tassios PT, Radstrom P, Cook N, Wagner M, Hoorfar J (2003): Standardization of diagnostic PCR for the detection of foodborne pathogens. *Int J Food Microbiol.* 83: 39–48.

Manser PA, Dalziel RW (1985): A survey of campylobacter in animals. *J Hyg (Cambridge).* 95:15–21.

Marchal K, De Keersmaecker S, Monsieurs P, et al. (2004): *In silico* identification and experimental validation of PmrAB targets in *Salmonella typhimurium* by regulatory motif detection. *Genome Biol.* 5:R9.1–R9.20.

Marcus SL, Brumell JH, Pfeifer GG, Finlay BB (2000): *Salmonella* pathogenicity islands: big virulence in small packages. *Microbes Infect.* 2:145–156.

Mastroeni P, Chabalgoity JA, Dunstan SJ, Maskell DJ, Dougan G (2000): *Salmonella*: immune responses and vaccines. *Vet J.* 161:132–164.

McClelland M, Sanderson KE, Spieth J, et al. (2001): Complete genome sequence of *Salmonella enterica* serovar Typhimurium LT2. *Nature.* 413:852–856.

McHan F, Shotts EB (1993): Effect of short-chain fatty acids on the growth of *Salmonella typhimurium* in an in vitro system. *Avian Dis.* 37:396–398.

Mead PS, Slutsker L, Dietz V, et al. (1999): Food-related illness and death in the United States. *Emerg Infect Dis.* 5:607–625.

Meichtri L, Miliwebsky E, Gioffré A, et al. (2004): Shiga toxin–producing *Escherichia coli* in healthy young beef steers from Argentina: prevalence and virulence properties. *Int J Food Microbiol.* 96:189–198.

Micheals B, Keller C, Blevins M, et al. (2004): Prevention of food worker transmission of foodborne pathogens: risk assessment and evaluation of effective hygiene intervention strategies. *Food Serv Technol.* 4:31–49.

Michino H, Araki K, Minami S, et al. (1999): Massive outbreak of *Escherichia coli* O157:H7 infection in schoolchildren in Sakai City, Japan, associated with consumption of white radish sprouts. *Am J Epidemiol.* 150:787–796.

Minihan D, O'Mahony M, Whyte P, Collins JD (2003): An investigation on the effect of transport and lairage on the fecal shedding prevalence of *Escherichia coli* O157 in cattle. *J Vet Med.* 50:378–382.

Moore RW, Byrd JA, Knape KD, et al. (2006): The effect of an experimental chlorate product on *Salmonella* recovery of turkeys when administered prior to feed and water withdrawal. *Poult Sci.* 85:2101–2105.

Munroe DL, Prescott JF, Penner JL (1983): *Campylobacter jejuni* and *Campylobacter coli* serotypes isolated from chickens, cattle, and pigs. *J Clin Microbiol.* 18:877–881.

Murphy RY, Duncan LK, Driscoll KH, Marcy JA, Beard BL (2003): Thermal inactivation of *Listeria monocytogenes* on ready-to-eat turkey breast meat products during postcook in-package pasteurization with hot water. *J Food Prot.* 66:1618–1622.

Nachamkin I, Allos BM, Ho T (1998): *Campylobacter* species and Guillain–Barré syndrome. *Clin Microbiol Rev.* 11:555–567.

Nataro JP, Kaper JB (1998): Diarrheagenic *Escherichia coli*. *Clin Microbiol Rev.* 11:142–201.

Naylor SW, Low JC, Besser TE, et al. (2003): Lymphoid follicle dense mucosa at the terminal rectum is the principal site of colonization of *Escherichia coli* O157:H7 in the bovine host. *Infect Immun.* 71:1505–1512.

Naylor SW, Gally DL, Low JC (2005): Enterohaemorrhagic *E. coli* in veterinary medicine. *Int J Med Microbiol.* 295:419–441.

Nightingale KK, Schukken YH, Nightingale CR, et al. (2004): Ecology and transmission of *Listeria monocytogenes* infecting ruminants and in the farm environment. *Appl Environ Microbiol.* 70:4458–4467.

Nisbet DJ, Ricke SC, Scanlan CM, Corrier DE, Hollister AG, DeLoach JR (1994): Inoculation of broiler chicks with a continuous-flow derived bacterial culture facilitates early native cecal bacterial colonization and increases resistance to *Salmonella typhimurium*. *J Food Prot.* 57:12–15.

Nisbet DJ, Corrier DE, Ricke SC, Hume ME, Byrd JA II, DeLoach JR (1996a): Maintenance of the biological efficacy in chicks of a cecal competitive-exclusion culture against *Salmonella* by continuous-flow fermentation. *J Food Prot.* 59:1279–1283.

——— (1996b): Cecal propionic acid as a biological indicator of the early establishment of a microbial ecosystem inhibitory to *Salmonella* in chicks. *Anaerobe*. 2:345–350.

Nutt JD, Woodward CL, Kubena LF, Nisbet DJ, Kwon YM, Ricke SC (2004): Potential for rapid in vitro assays to measure foodborne *Salmonella* virulence in foods: a review. *J Rapid Methods Automat Microbiol*. 12:234–246.

Ogden ID, MacRae M, Strachan NJC (2004); Is the prevalence and shedding concentrations of *E. coli* O157 in beef cattle in Scotland seasonal? *FEMS Microbiol Lett*. 233:297–300.

OIE (Office International des Epizooties Animal Production Food Safety Working Group) (2006). Guide to good farming practices for animal production food safety. *Rev Sci Tech Off Int Epizoot*. 25:823–836.

Oliver SP, Jayarao BM, Almeida RA (2005): Foodborne pathogens in milk and the dairy farm environment: food safety and public health implications. *Foodborne Pathog Dis*. 2:115–129.

Omisakin F, MacRae M, Odgen ID, Strachan NJC (2003): Concentration and prevalence of *Escherichia coli* O157 in cattle feces at slaughter. *Appl Environ Microbiol*. 69: 2444–2447.

On SLW (2001): Taxonomy of *Campylobacter, Arcobacter, Helicobacter* and related bacteria: current status, future prospects and immediate concerns. *J Appl Microbiol*. 90:1S–15S.

Parkhill J, Wren BW, Mungall K, et al. (2000): The genome sequence of the food-borne pathogen *Campylobacter jejuni* reveals hypervariable sequences. *Lett Nature*. 403:665–668.

Patchanee P, Crenshaw TD, Bahnson PB (2007): Oral sodium chlorate, topical disinfection, and younger weaning age reduce *Salmonella enterica* shedding in pigs. *J Food Prot*. 70:1798–1803.

Patrick ME, Adcock PM, Gomez TM, et al. (2004): *Salmonella* Enteriditis infections, United States, 1985–1999. *Emerg Infect Dis*. 10:1–7.

Pearce RA, Bolton DJ, Sheridan JJ, McDowell DA, Blair IS, Harrington D (2004): Studies to determine the critical control points in pork slaughter hazard analysis and critical control point systems. *Int J Food Microbiol*. 90:331–339.

Penner JL (1988): The genus *Campylobacter*: a decade of progress. *Clin Microbiol Rev*. 1:157–172.

Petrenko VA, Sorokulova IB (2004): Detection of biological threats: a challenge for directed molecular evolution. *J Microbiol Methods*. 58:147–168.

Pezzotti G, Serafin A, Luzzi I, Mioni R, Milan M, Perin R (2003): Occurrence and resistance to antibiotics of *Campylobacter jejuni* and *Campylobacter coli* in animals and meat in northeastern Italy. *Int J Food Microbiol*. 82:281–287.

Pichinoty F, Piéchaud M (1968): Recherche des nitrate-réductases bactéreriennes A et B: méthodes. *Ann Inst Pasteur*. 114:77–98.

Pillai SD, Ricke SC (2002): Bioaerosols from municipal and animal wastes: background and contemporary issues. *Can J Microbiol*. 48:681–696.

Pillai SD, Widmer KW, Dowd SE, Ricke SC (1996): Occurrence of airborne bacterial pathogens and indicators during land application of sewage sludge. *Appl Environ Microbiol*. 62:296–299.

Potter AA, Klashinsky S, Li Y, et al. (2004): Decreased shedding of *Escherichia coli* O157:H7 by cattle following vaccination with type III secreted proteins. *Vaccine*. 22:362–369.

Price SB, Cheng C, Kaspar CW, et al. (2000): Role of rpoS in acid resistance and fecal shedding of *Escherichia coli* O157:H7. *Appl Environ Microbiol*. 66:632–637.

Rabsch W, Andrews HL, Kingsley RA, et al. (2002): *Salmonella enterica* serotype Typhimurium and its host-adapted variants. *Infect Immun.* 70:2249–2255.

Rasmussen MA, Casey TA (2001): Environmental and food safet aspects of *Escherichia coli* O157:H7 infections in cattle. *Crit Rev Microbiol.* 27:57–73.

Rasmussen MA, Cray WC Jr, Casey TA, Whipp SC (1993): Rumen contents as a reservoir of enterohemorrhagic *Escherichia coli*. *FEMS Microbiol Lett.* 114:79–84.

Rasmussen MA, Carlson SA, Franklin SK, McCuddin ZP, Wu MT, Sharma VK (2005): Exposure to rumen protozoa leads to enhancement of pathogenicity of and invasion by multiple-antibiotic-resistant *Salmonella enterica* bearing SGI1. *Infect Immun.* 73:4668–4675.

Raya RR, Varey P, Ooot RA, et al. (2006): Isolation and characterization of a new T-even bacteriophage, CEV1, and determination of its potential to reduce *Escherichia coli* O157:H7 levels in sheep. *Appl Environ Microbiol.* 72:6405–6410.

Rees JH, Soudain SE, Gregson NA, Hughes RAC (1995): *Campylobacter jejuni* infection and Guillain–Barré syndrome. *N Engl J Med.* 333:1374–1379.

Reicks AL, Brashears MM, Adams KD, Brooks JC, Blanton JR, Miller MF (2007): Impact of transportation of feedlot cattle to the harvest facility on the prevalence of *Escherichia coli* O157:H7, *Salmonella*, and total aerobic microorganisms on hides. *J Food Prot.* 70:17–21.

Renter DG, Sargeant JM (2002): Enterohemorrhagic *Escherichia coli* O157: epidemiology and ecology in bovine production environments. *Anim Health Res Rev.* 3:83–94.

Rice EW, Johnson CH (2000): Survival of *Escherichia coli* O157:H7 in dairy cattle drinking water. *J Dairy Sci.* 83:2021–2023.

Ricke SC (2003): Perspectives on the use of organic acids and short chain fatty acids as antimicrobials. *Poult Sci.* 82:632–639.

——— (2005): Ensuring the safety of poultry feed. In: Mead GC (Ed.): *Food Safety Control in the Poultry Industry*. Woodhead, Cambridge, UK, pp. 174–194.

Ricke SC, Pillai SD (1999): Conventional and molecular methods for understanding probiotic bacteria functionality in gastrointestinal tracts. *Crit Rev Microbiol.* 25:19–38.

Ricke SC, Kundinger MM, Miller DR, Keeton JT (2005): Alternatives to antibiotics: chemical and physical antimicrobial interventions and foodborne pathogen response. *Poult Sci.* 84:667–675.

Rodriguez A, Pangloli P, Richards HA, Mount JR, Draughon FA (2006): Prevalence of *Salmonella* in diverse environmental farm samples. *J Food Prot.* 69:2576–2580.

Ryan JH (2007): On-line real time aid to the verification of CCP compliance in beef slaughter HACCP systems. *Food Control.* 18:689–696.

Saito S, Yatsuyanagi J, Harata S, et al. (2005): *Campylobacter jejuni* isolated from retail poultry meat, bovine feces and bile, and human diarrheal samples in Japan: comparison of serotypes and genotypes. *FEMS Immunol Med Microbiol.* 45:311–319.

Salloway S, Mermael LA, Seamans M, et al. (1996): Miller–Fisher syndrome associated with *Campylobacter jejuni* bearing lipopolysaccharide molecules that mimic human GD_3. *Infect Immun.* 64:2945–2949.

Sato K, Bartlett PC, Kaneene JB, Downes FP (2004): Comparison of prevalence and antimicrobial susceptibilities of *Campylobacter* spp. isolates from organic and conventional dairy herds in Wisconsin. *Appl Environ Microbiol.* 70:1442–1447.

Schamberger GP, Phillips RL, Jacobs JL, Diez-Gonzalez F (2004): Reduction of *Escherichia coli* O157:H7 populations in cattle by addition of colicin E7–producing *E. coli* to feed. *Appl Environ Microbiol.* 70:6053–6060.

Sheng H, Knecht HJ, Kudva IT, Hovde CJ (2006): Application of bacteriophages to control intestinal *Escherichia coli* O157:H7 levels in ruminants. *Appl Environ Microbiol.* 72:5359–5366.

Singh RD, Khullar M, Ganguly NK (2000): Role of anaerobiosis in virulence of *Salmonella typhimurium*. *Mol Cell Biochem.* 215:39–46.

Sklar IB, Joerger RD (2001): Attempts to utilize bacteriophage to combat *Salmonella enterica* serovar Enteritidis infection in chickens. *J Food Saf.* 21:15–29.

St Louis ME, Morse DL, Potter ME, et al. (1988): The emergence of grade A eggs as a major source of *Salmonella enteriditis* infections. *JAMA.* 259:2103–2107.

Stanley K, Jones K (2003): Cattle and sheep farms as reservoirs of *Campylobacter*. *J Appl Microbiol.* 94:104S–130S.

Stanley KN, Wallace JS, Currie JE, Diggle PJ, Jones K (1998): The seasonal variation of thermophilic campylobacters in beef cattle, dairy cattle and calves. *J Appl Microbiol.* 85:472–480.

Stewart V (1988): Nitrate respiration in relation to facultative metabolism in enterobacteria. *Microbiol Rev.* 52:190–232.

Stolle A (1981): Spreading of *Salmonella* during cattle slaughtering. *J Appl Bacteriol.* 50:239–245.

Strauch E, Hammerl JA, Hertwig S (2007): Bacteriophages: new tools for safer food? *J Verbr Lebensm.* 2:138–143.

Swartz MN (2002): Human diseases caused by foodborne pathogens of animal origin. *Clin Infect Dis.* 34 (Suppl 3): S111–S122.

Tam CC, O'Brien SJ, Adak GK, Meakins SM, Frost JA (2003): *Campylobacter coli*: an important foodborne pathogen. *J Infect.* 47:28–32.

Tergney A, Bolton DJ (2006): Validation studies on an online monitoring system for reducing faecal and microbial contamination on beef carcasses. *Food Control.* 17:378–382.

Todd ECD (1989): Preliminary estimates of costs of foodborne diseases in the United States. *J Food Prot.* 52:595–601.

Tompkin RB (2002): Control of *Listeria monocytogenes* in the food-processing environment. *J Food Prot.* 65:709–725.

USDA-ERS (U.S. Department of Agriculture–Economic Research Service) (2008): Economics of foodborne disease: other pathogens. http://www.ers.usda.gov/briefing/foodsafety/economic.htm. Accessed May 2008

USDA-FAS (U.S. Department of Agriculture–Foreign Agricultural Service) (2006): Livestock and Poultry; World Markets and Trade. Circular Series DL&P 2-06. http://www.fas.usda.gov/dlp/circular/2006/2006%20Annual/Livestock&Poultry.pdf. Accessed May 2007

——— (2007): Livestock and Poultry; World Markets and Trade. Circular Series DL&P 1-07. http://www.fas.usda.gov/dlp/circular/2007/livestock_poultry_04-2007.pdf. Accessed May 2007

USDA-FSIS (U.S. Department of Agriculture–Food Safety and Inspection Service) (2004): Microbiological testing program and other verification activities for *Escherichia coli* O157:H7 in raw ground beef products and raw ground beef components and beef patty components. http://www.fsis.usda.gov/OPPDE/rdad/FSISDirectives/10.010.1.pdf. Accessed May 2007.

Van Baale MJ, Sargeant JM, Gnad DP, DeBay BM, Lechtenberg KF, Nagaraja TG (2004): Effect of forage or grain diets with or without monensin on ruminal persistence and fecal *Escherichia coli* O157:H7 in cattle. *Appl Environ Microbiol.* 70:5336–5342.

Van Der Walt ML, Vorster JH, Steyn HC, Greeff AS (2001): Auxotrophic, plasmid-cured *Salmonella enterica* serovar *Typhimurium* for use as a live vaccine in calves. *Vet Microbiol.* 80:373–381.

Van Donkersgoed J, Hancock D, Rogan D, Potter AA (2005): *Escherichia coli* O157:H7 vaccine field trial in 9 feedlots in Alberta and Saskatchewan. *Can Vet J.* 46:724–728.

Vold L, Johansen KB, Kruse H, Skjerve E, Wasteson Y (1998): Occurrence of shigatoxigenic *Escherichia coli* O157 in Norwegian cattle herds. *Epidemiol Infect.* 120:21–28.

Vugia D, Hadler J, Chaves S, et al. (2003): Preliminary FoodNet data on the incidence of foodborne illnesses—selected sites, United States, 2002. *MMWR Morb Mortal Wkly Rep.* 52:340–343.

Wagenaar JA, Van Bergen MAP, Muellar MA, Wassenaar TM, Carlton RM (2005): Phage therapy reduces *Campylobacter jejuni* colonization in broilers. *Vet Microbiol.* 109:275–283.

Wallis TS (2001): *Salmonella* pathogenesis and immunity: we need effective multivalent vaccines. *Vet J.* 161:104–106.

Wells JE, Shackelford SD, Berry ED, Kalchayanand N, Guerini MN, Varel VH, Arthur TM, Bosilevac JM, Freetly HC, Wheeler TL, Ferrell CL, Koohmaraie M (2009): Prevalence and level of *Escherichia coli* O157:H7 in feces and on hides of feedlot steers fed diets with or without wet distillers grains with solubles. *J Food Prot.* (in press).

Wesley IV, Wells SJ, Harmon KM, et al. (2000): Fecal shedding of *Campylobacter* and *Arcobacter* spp. in dairy cattle. *Appl Environ Microbiol.* 66:1994–2000.

Wilkinson JM (1999): Silage and animal heath. *Nat Toxins.* 7:221–232.

Williams JE, Benson ST (1978): Survival of *Salmonella typhimurium* in poultry feed and litter at three temperatures. *Avian Dis.* 22:742–747.

Wilson SC, Morrow-Tesch J, Straus DC, et al. (2002): Airborne microbial flora in a cattle feedlot. *Appl Environ Microbiol.* 68:3238–3242.

Wolin MJ (1969): Volatile fatty acids and the inhibition of *Escherichia coli* growth by rumen fluid. *Appl Microbiol.* 17:83–87.

Wong S, Street D, Delgado SL, Klontz KC (2000): Recalls of foods and cosmetics due to microbial contamination reported to the US Food and Drug Administration. *J Food Prot.* 63:1113–1116.

Younts-Dahl SM, Galyean ML, Loneragan GH, Elam NA, Brashears MM (2004): Dietary supplementation with *Lactobacillus*- and *Propionibacterium*-based direct-fed microbials and prevalence of *Escherichia coli* O157 in beef feedlot cattle and on hides at harvest. *J Food Prot.* 67:889–893.

Zhoa T, Doyle MP, Harmon BG, Brown CA, Mueller POE, Parks AH (1998): Reduction of carriage of enterohemorrhagic *Escherichia coli* O157:H7 in cattle by inoculation with probiotic bacteria. *J Clin Microbiol.* 36:641–647.

Zhoa T, Tkalcic S, Doyle MP, Harmon BG, Brown CA, Zhoa P (2003): Pathogenicity of enterohemorrhagic *Escherichia coli* in neonatal calves and evaluation of fecal shedding by treatment with probiotic *Escherichia coli*. *J Food Prot.* 66:924–930.

Zundel E, Bernard S (2006): *Listeria monocytogenes* translocates throughout the digestive tract in asymptomatic sheep. *J Med Microbiol.* 55:1717–1723.

CHAPTER 7

FOOD SAFETY ISSUES AND THE MICROBIOLOGY OF MILK AND DAIRY PRODUCTS

MANSEL W. GRIFFITHS

7.1 INTRODUCTION

The history of milk consumption parallels that of human beings, beginning many thousands of years ago with the oldest known civilizations. People probably began domesticating animals between 8000 and 5000 B.C., and cattle were first used as sources of food in Asia or northeast Africa. The earliest record documenting the use of cow's milk is a 5000-year-old mosaic frieze discovered in a temple in the Euphrates Valley near Babylon depicting men milking cows and milk being poured through a crude strainer into stone jars.

Milk and milk products are also mentioned in the Bible and in early Hindu writings. The use of milk in religious ceremonies and as a medicine has been documented by the Ancient Greeks, Romans, and Egyptians. The Vikings carried large supplies of butter on their sea voyages, and Marco Polo, in the thirteenth century, wrote that the Tartar armies enjoyed a fermented form of mare's milk. When Christopher Columbus landed in the New World in 1492, he is quoted as saying: "It was wonderful to see . . . land for cattle, although they have none."

Descriptions of diseases associated with milk also go back to ancient times with the incidence of an illness similar to brucellosis being described in the Bible in Genesis. However, milk infections were first documented properly in 1857, when Dr. M. W. Taylor of Penrith, England reported an outbreak of typhoid among his patients. At around this time, Louis Pasteur started his work on fermentation. Subsequently, Emperor Napoleon III asked him to investigate spoilage problems, which were causing considerable economic losses to the wine industry. Pasteur went to a vineyard in Arbois in 1864 to study this problem, where he demonstrated that wine spoilage was caused by microorganisms that could be killed by heating the wine to 55°C

Microbiologically Safe Foods, Edited by Norma Heredia, Irene Wesley, and Santos García

for several minutes. Pasteur subsequently applied this process to milk. In honor of Pasteur, the heating of milk to destroy pathogens has been termed *pasteurization*, and it has become the cornerstone of the modern dairy industry.

Despite arguments over the nutritional status of milk, it is still an important part of our diet and is a valuable source of calcium, protein, vitamins, and possibly beneficial fatty acids such as conjugated linoleic acid. However, the components that make milk a nourishing drink for humans can also be utilized for growth by bacteria. It is therefore imperative to understand the microbiology of milk, especially when new production and processing systems are introduced. In this chapter the microbiology of milk and milk products at all points along the value chain is reviewed briefly, and issues related to the safety of dairy products are identified.

7.2 MICROFLORA OF RAW MILK

7.2.1 Production of Milk

In the majority of developed countries, cows are milked by machine and the milk is transferred to refrigerated bulk storage tanks, where it is held prior to transportation to processing facilities. The implementation of refrigerated storage has resulted in a dramatic change in the microflora of raw milk, due to microbial selection and adaptation. The dynamic changes in the bacterial population in milk associated with refrigeration have been monitored by molecular methods such as temporal temperature gel electrophoresis (TTGE) and denaturing gradient gel electrophoresis (DGGE) (Lafarge et al., 2004). Considerable evolution of bacterial populations was found during storage of milk at 4°C with the emergence of psychrotrophic bacteria such as *Listeria* spp. or *Aeromonas hydrophila* within 24 h as opposed to the 48 h found using cultural methods. It has also been suggested that the stage of growth of psychrotrophic contaminants may play a role in their subsequent ability to grow in stored milk, with cells in the stationary phase of growth being better adapted to rapid growth in milk (Rowe et al., 2003).

Undoubtedly, the introduction of refrigerated bulk tanks, as well as adoption of pasteurization, have had a significant impact on the incidence and nature of milk-borne illness (Fig. 1). In developed countries during the mid-twentieth century, before widespread use of pasteurization and refrigeration, the main agents of bacterial infection associated with milk were *Mycobacterium tuberculosis*, *Brucella abortus*, and *Staphylococcus aureus* (Jayaro et al., 2001). However, by the end of the century these were no longer predominant, and they had been replaced by agents that were able to survive or even grow at refrigeration temperatures, such as *Campylobacter jejuni* and *Salmonella* spp., *Listeria*, and *Yersinia* (Phillips and Griffiths, 1990).

Undoubtedly, other factors also contributed to this change, including herd eradication programs to control tuberculosis. The result is that milk and dairy products are among the safest foods to eat, and they are now responsible for only 2 to 6% of outbreaks in many developed countries (Table 1). Nevertheless, the dairy industry should not become complacent, as surveys have demonstrated that about 5% of

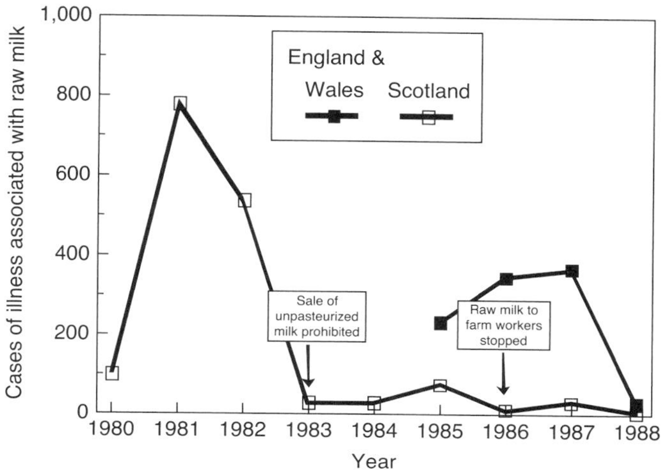

FIG. 1 Effect of regulatory changes on the incidence of milkborne illness in the UK. (Data from Burt and Wellsteed, 1991.)

good-quality milks can contain potentially pathogenic bacteria (Table 2). However, the prevalence of potentially pathogenic bacteria in milk may be underestimated when cultural methods are used to detect their presence. Karns et al. (2005) showed that the prevalence of *Salmonella enterica* in bulk tank milks from U.S. dairies was 2.6% when assayed using conventional culture techniques, but this figure rose to 11.8% when real-time PCR (polymerase chain reaction) was used to analyze the enrichment cultures.

In the middle of this century the main illnesses associated with the consumption of milk were brucellosis and tuberculosis. These have been eradicated as milkborne illnesses in developed countries, mainly through herd certification programs,

TABLE 1 Outbreaks of Milkborne Infectious Intestinal Disease in Various Countries

Country	Period	Percent of Outbreaks Involving Milk or Milk Products
Canada (Ontario)	1997–2001	4.3
England and Wales	1992–2000	1.5
Finland	1983–1990	3
France	1988–1997	6.1
Germany	1993–1996	5.5
Netherlands	1991–1994	5.7
Poland	1992–1996	3.5
United States	1988–1992	2.2

Source: Buyser et al. (2001), Gillespie et al. (2003), Lee and Middleton (2003).

TABLE 2 Incidence (% Positive Samples) of Potential Bacterial Pathogens in Raw Milk from Surveys

Organism	Ontario, Canada[a]	Normandy, France[b]	South Dakota[c]	Raw Milk Surveys (1990–1995)[d]
Aeromonas hydrophila	—	—	—	35.3
Campylobacter jejuni	0.5	1.4	9.2	4.8–12.3
Clostridium perfringens	—	1.4	—	9.3
Listeria monocytogenes	2.7	5.8	4.6	0–15.6
Salmonella spp.	0.2	2.9	6.1	0.1–8.9
Staphylococcus aureus	—	62.0	—	—
Verotoxigenic *E. coli*	0.9	—	3.8	—
Yersinia enterocolitica	—	36.2	6.1	15.1–30.0

[a]From Steele et al. (1997).
[b]From Desmasures et al. (1997).
[c]From Burt and Wellsteed (1991).
[d]From Griffiths (2004).

the installation of refrigerated bulk tanks for collection of milk on farms, and the introduction of pasteurization. The majority of present-day milkborne illnesses are attributable to *Salmonella* spp., *Campylobacter* spp., and *Listeria monocytogenes*, among others, and are associated with the consumption of raw milk or pasteurized milk that has either received inadequate heat treatment or has been contaminated after heating. These epidemiological changes have been brought about by the adoption of new milk production, processing, and distribution practices, some of which were discussed above. Other factors, for example the changing characteristics of microorganisms and demographic changes such as the aging population and increase in numbers of immunocompromised persons, will ensure that problems will continue to arise (Eyles, 1995).

Other pressures have been exerted on governments to relax their requirement for pasteurization. The demand of consumers for "natural" foods, coupled with the upsurge in organic farming, has contributed to the perception that raw milk is nutritionally better and healthier. The irony is that the incidence of salmonellosis, campylobacteriosis, and yersiniosis is more prevalent in rural areas and is partly linked to the consumption of raw milk in these communities.

7.2.2 Contamination from the Udder

Contamination from Udder Infection Milk emerging from the udder of healthy cows is essentially sterile. However, udder infections are common; for example, it has been estimated that about one-third of dairy cattle in the UK suffer from mastitis (Bramley and McKinnon, 1990). The most common agents of mastitis are *Staphylococcus aureus*, *Streptococcus agalactiae*, *Str. uberis*, and *Escherichia coli*. As well as producing visible clinical infection, less acute, subclinical states are often encountered and can only be diagnosed by examination of the milk for characteristic changes, such as elevated somatic cell counts in the milk. The organisms enter the udder by way of the duct at the teat tip, and some, such as *S. aureus*, can colonize the duct. Machine milking may propel the organisms into the teat duct, but this is not the only route of contamination (Bramley and McKinnon, 1990). From the duct the organisms can enter the milk and can contribute significantly to the numbers present in bulk tank samples (Hayes and Boor, 2001). When the microbiological quality of raw milk was investigated over a 5-month period in New York State, it was found that streptococci, staphylococci, and gram-negative bacteria accounted for 69, 3, and 3% of total bacterial count variability, respectively (Zadoks et al., 2004). Bacteriological and strain typing data indicated that control of mastitis-causing species of streptococci was important for improvement of the microbial quality of raw milk.

Whereas the organisms that cause mastitis do not generally grow in refrigerated milk, they are able to survive under these conditions and thus are a public health concern, as staphylococcal enterotoxins and toxic shock syndrome toxin-1 can be pre-synthesised in the udder and secreted into milk in cows and goats suffering from *S. aureus* mastitis (Niskanen et al., 1978; Valle et al., 1991).

The control of mastitis through antibiotic therapy may contribute to the transfer of antibiotic resistance to human pathogens from drug-resistant organisms. However, a U.S. study concluded that there was no trend toward increased antibiotic-resistance among mastitis pathogens isolated from milk samples between 1994 and 2001 (Makovec and Ruegg, 2003). Multiple antibiotic-resistant strains of organisms, including *E. coli*, *Salmonella* spp., and *S. aureus*, have been isolated from raw and pasteurized milk (Diaz de Aguayo et al., 1992).

Contamination from the External Surface of the Udder The external surface of the udder can also contribute to the microbial contamination of milk. Bedding materials, mud, dung, soil, and other matter are all a rich source of microorganisms that can adhere readily to skin. Sanaa et al. (1993) showed that poor cleanliness of cows, inadequate lighting of milking parlors and barns (which may be an indication of neglect of milking hygiene), and incorrect disinfection of towels used to dry the udder were all significant risk factors associated with contamination of raw milk by *L. monocytogenes* on dairy farms.

A reduction in bacterial levels on teats is observed when cows are on pasture, and this led to lower bacterial counts in milk during this period, suggesting that bedding affords the greatest contribution to udder contamination (Griffiths, 2004). The dominant microflora on the teats of cows housed in byres were micrococci, but it has also been estimated that 90% of the spores found in raw milk come from this source (Griffiths, 2004). However, the principal source of psychrotrophic spore-formers (mainly *Bacillus* spp.) in milk appears to be contamination of the teat by the upper layer of soil in pastureland and by feces, but this obviously is not the case for cows that are zero-grazed. There is also a distinct seasonal effect on the incidence of psychrotrophic spore-formers in milk, with the highest levels being observed in late summer and early autumn (Griffiths, 2004). *Clostridium* spores can be introduced into milk from feedstuffs, especially silage, and bedding and silage are also an important source of contamination by *Listeria* spp. and other potential human pathogens, such as *Yersinia enterocolitica* and *Aeromonas hydrophila* (Griffiths, 2004).

7.2.3 Environmental Sources of Contamination

In a modern dairy, milking personnel and aerial contamination are likely to be insignificant sources of microbiological contamination of milk. However, there is increasing concern about the safety of water supplies, and there have been several recent outbreaks of waterborne illness, including a large *E. coli* O157:H7 outbreak at Walkerton in Ontario, Canada (Brown and Hussain, 2003). In this incident, illness was also caused by contamination of the water supply with *Campylobacter jejuni* (Clark et al., 2005). Outbreaks have also been attributed to contamination of water by *Cryptosporidium parvum* (Dawson, 2005; Sharma et al., 2003), and it is known that oocysts of this protozoan can be present in raw milk, albeit at low incidence rates ($<1\%$), but their source is undetermined (Laberge and Griffiths, 1996). Thus, problems may arise when contaminated water is used to rinse and wash equipment.

7.2.4 Contamination from Milking and Storage Equipment

Significant contamination of milk can arise from inadequately sanitized surfaces of milking and milk storage equipment, due to the proliferation of microorganisms in milk residues remaining in crevices, joints, rubber gaskets, and dead ends of badly cleaned milking plants (Murphy and Boor, 2000). The most important contaminants introduced by this route are the gram-negative psychrotrophs, which predominate among the microflora that adhere to stainless-steel milk transfer pipelines and readily form biofilms (Lee Wong, 1998). The only real protection against the introduction of bacteria into the milk supply during milking is adequate sanitation of all the equipment, and the efficacy of sanitation depends largely on the design of the plant and other factors, such as the hardness of the water supply (Griffiths, 2004).

Robotic, or automatic, milking is being introduced in many countries, but research on the impact of this on milk quality is limited. In one study, the bulk milk quality of 98 Danish farms with automatic milking systems was analyzed from 1 year before introduction of automatic milking until 1 year after (Rasmussen et al., 2002). Bulk milk total bacterial counts, anaerobic spore counts, and somatic cell counts (SCCs) increased when automatic milking was introduced, and this was accompanied by an almost twofold increase in the frequency of milk quality failures. These failures were most frequent in the first 3 months after the start of automatic milking. The increase in bacterial counts originated partly from contamination of milk from the teat surface and partly from lack of cleaning of the milking equipment or cooling of the milk. The increase in bulk milk SCCs indicated that milk from cows with high cell counts was not diverted to the same degree during automatic milking as when milking was carried out conventionally. Introduction of a self-monitoring program, including survey of the bulk milk quality, did not reduce the frequency of high total bacterial counts of the bulk milk to the level of conventional milking. However, the program reduced the overall frequency of milk quality failures.

Farm bulk tanks are easier to clean and, consequently, have a much lower bacterial content than the milk pipeline. However, ancillary equipment such as agitators, dipsticks, outlet plugs, and cocks can be difficult to clean and may be a source of contamination (Bramley and McKinnon, 1990). Perhaps the greatest contribution to contamination provided by bulk tanks is the potential growth of bacteria during storage. When the microflora of downgraded Danish bulk tank milk was examined to identify the main causes of increased microbial counts, gram-negative, oxidase-positive bacteria were found in 72% of the samples, coliforms in 20% of samples, and noncoliforms in 49% of samples (Holm et al., 2004). The relative distribution of the microorganisms within the milk samples is shown in Table 3. Microorganisms associated primarily with poor hygiene dominated the microflora in 64% of samples, psychrotrophic bacteria dominated the microflora in 28% of samples, and mastitis bacteria dominated the microflora in 9% of samples. Storage of the bulk tank milk for 48 h instead of 24 h did not affect the proportion of downgraded milk samples. Other surveys have indicated that alternate-day collection has little effect on the bacteriological quality of bulk tank milk, provided that it is cooled rapidly to 4°C or below before addition to the tank (Griffiths, 2004). However, milk from alternate-day collections arriving at a processing site will contain organisms that are entering the

TABLE 3 Occurrence and Number of Microorganisms in Danish Bulk Tank Milk with Counts Above 3.0×10^4 CFU/mL

Type of Microorganism	Identified[a] (% of Samples)	Geometric Mean[b] (CFU/mL)
Gram-negative bacteria		
Oxidase-positive[c]	72	2.5×10^4 (8.0×10^2 to 3.0×10^6)
Oxidase-negative coliforms	20	1.7×10^4 (8.0×10^2 to 2.0×10^5)
Noncoliforms	49	1.3×10^4 (5.0×10^2 to 6.0×10^5)
Gram-positive microorganisms		
Bacillus spp.	9	5.2×10^3 (5.0×10^2 to 8.5×10^4)
Coryneforms	28	8.5×10^3 (4.9×10^2 to 1.9×10^5)
Enterococcus spp.	19	5.0×10^3 (4.8×10^2 to 1.7×10^5)
Lactococcus spp.	32	1.5×10^4 (9.6×10^2 to 3.0×10^6)
Micrococcus spp.	53	1.2×10^4 (6.9×10^2 to 7.0×10^5)
Other gram-positive rods	20	1.0×10^4 (4.9×10^2 to 6.6×10^5)
Staphylococcus aureus	9	5.7×10^3 (4.9×10^2 to 1.7×10^5)
Coagulase-negative *Staphylococcus* spp.	31	8.3×10^3 (9.0×10^2 to 2.5×10^5)
Streptococcus dysgalactiae	19	7.2×10^3 (4.9×10^2 to 8.0×10^5)
Streptococcus uberis	15	3.4×10^4 (1.8×10^3 to 1.4×10^6)
Yeasts	20	5.2×10^3 (4.8×10^2 to 2.2×10^4)

Source: Holm et al. (2004).
[a] If ≥5% of the total population.
[b] Minimum to maximum counts are shown in parentheses.
[c] Approximately 70% *Pseudomonas* spp.

exponential phase of growth, and the amount of time that this milk can subsequently be stored will be affected adversely.

7.2.5 Contamination During Transportation and Storage at the Processing Facility

Milk is usually transported in insulated tanks or in tankers equipped with refrigerated storage. Increases in bacterial count during this stage are due primarily to inadequately cleaned vehicles or growth of bacteria already present in the milk. The latter is dependent on the temperature of the milk and duration of the journey.

Changes in dairy industry practices, such as a shortened workweek and scarcity of milk at certain times of year due to the adoption of quota systems, have led to milk being stored longer before processing. Thus, the temperature at which milk is stored becomes critical and milk should be cooled to, and maintained at 3°C on receipt at the processing plant before storage (Hatt and Wilbey, 1994).

7.2.6 Contamination During Processing

Genotyping has been used increasingly to trace the origins and routes of transmission of microorganisms in food-processing plants. In one such study, randomly amplified polymorphic DNA (RAPD) typing was employed to track sources of contaminants in pasteurized milk (Eneroth et al., 2000). Bacteria recontaminating pasteurized milk exhibited many different RAPD types and were shown to originate primarily from water and air in the filling equipment or in the immediate surroundings. It was also shown that strains of recontaminating flora, which were largely pseudomonads, could persist for prolonged periods in the filling equipment and environment, presumably due to their ability to form biofilms (Austin and Bergeron, 1995; Sharma and Anand, 2002).

7.3 PUBLIC HEALTH CONCERNS FROM DAIRY PRODUCTS

As mentioned earlier in this chapter, milk and milk products continue to be a potential source of foodborne illness, and all sectors of the industry should strive to improve the safety of their products. Management systems to control food safety, such as hazard analysis of critical control points (HACCP), have been implemented at all points along the value chain (McDonald, 2003). Friedhoff et al. (2005) have described the use of simple microbiological criteria, including aerobic mesophilic colony counts, Enterobacteriaceae counts, and in some instances, enumeration of yeast, performed on samples taken during processing in small businesses to verify good manufacturing practices. This verification through monitoring was found to be an attractive alternative to the examination of end products.

Although raw milk is still the most significant source of milkborne illness, outbreaks associated with pasteurized milk continue to occur (Table 4). Illness in several industrialized countries attributable to various dairy products caused by different

TABLE 4 Etiology of Milkborne Outbreaks in England and Wales, 1992–2000, and Their Association with Milk Types

	Number of Outbreaks Associated with Milk Type				
Pathogen	Unpasteurized	Pasteurized[a]	Mixed[b]	Bird-Pecked[c]	Total
EHEC[d]	5	3	1	0	9
Campylobacter spp.	4	1	1	1	7
S. Typhimurium	5	1	0	0	6
S. Enteritidis PT4	0	2	0	0	2
Other salmonellae	0	2	0	0	2
Cryptosporidium	0	1	0	0	1
Total	14	10	2	1	27

Source: Gillespie et al. (2003).
[a] Milk sold as pasteurized.
[b] In one outbreak a mixture of milk sold as pasteurized and milk sold as pasteurized and unpasteurized milk was reported; in a second a mixture of unpasteurized milk and bird-pecked pasteurized milk was reported.
[c] Integrity of package compromised by birds pecking at the seal.
[d] Enterohemorrhagic *Escherichia coli.*

etiological agents has been discussed by Buyser et al. (2001) and a summary of cases linked to dairy products is presented in Table 5.

7.4 MILK AND CREAM

The important pathogens present in raw milk have been reviewed in a publication of the International Dairy Federation (IDF, 1993), and their public health significance has been discussed (Desmarchelier, 2001; Ryser, 2004).

Outbreaks of illness are due to consumption of raw and pasteurized milk contaminated with a variety of organisms, including *E. coli* O157:H7, *Salmonella* spp., *Campylobacter jejuni*, *Yersinia enterocolitica*, and *Listeria monocytogenes*. Some of these outbreaks have involved large numbers of cases, such as that occurring in Illinois in 1983, where contamination of pasteurized milk by *Salmonella* Typhimurium resulted in about 16,000 cases (Sun, 1985), and more recently in Japan, where contamination of low-fat milk made from reconstituted skim milk powder by *Staphylococcus aureus* resulted in more than 13,000 illnesses (Asao et al., 2003). Generally, the outbreaks involving pasteurized products have been shown to result from post-process contamination or a failure in the pasteurization process.

As well as the more common pathogens associated with raw milk, recent attention has focused on the potential of raw milk for the transmission of other organisms. For example, Farrell et al. (1991) have suggested that raw milk may be a vehicle for the transmission of *Borrelia burgdorferi*, the agent responsible for Lyme disease, and it has been shown that the organism can survive for at least 46 days in milk stored at 5°C. Also, *Mycobacterium paratuberculosis*, suspected to be the etiological

TABLE 5 Illness Associated with Milk and Milk Products in Several Industrialized Countries, 1980–1997

		Milk			Cheese and Related Products			Cream, Butter, Yoghurt		
Agent	Number of Outbreaks	Raw/ Unpasteurized	Pasteurized	Unknown	Unpasteurized	Pasteurized	Unknown	Pasteurized	Unknown	Infant Formula, Pasteurized
Staphylococcus aureus	10	2	6	—	3	2	2			
Salmonella	29	6	3	1	11	2	1	1	—	4
L. monocytogenes	14	—	2	—	4	1	4	1	2	
E. coli	11	2	2	2	3	1		1		
Total cases	23,203	1,452	17,275	15	3,134	950	199	36	12	130
Deaths	100	3	22	0	45	20	6	4	0	0

Source: Buyser et al. (2001).

agent of Crohn's disease, has been isolated from 1.6% of raw milk samples and 1.8% of pasteurized milk samples in the UK. The presence of modified atmosphere packaging (MAP) in pasteurized milk has generated speculation that the organism can survive high-temperature, short-time (HTST) pasteurization and prompted calls for the minimum pasteurization temperature to be increased. However, work has shown that current HTST treatments are sufficient to control the organism (Grant, 2005; Griffiths, 2002). Recently, verocytotoxigenic strains of *E. coli*, particularly the serotype *E. coli* O157:H7, have caused severe food-related outbreaks. Although the primary source appears to be inadequately cooked beef burgers, dairy cattle have been shown to be a major reservoir for infection, and cases linked to the consumption of raw milk have been reported (Hussein and Sakuma, 2005). These have included cases among the families of dairy farmers.

It is not only bacterial contamination of milk that causes concern. There have been large outbreaks of cryptosporidiosis, an illness produced by the protozoan *Cryptosporidium parvum* (Laberge and Griffiths, 1996), and it is thought that raw foods, including milk, are a common source of *Toxoplasma gondii* infection (Giaccone et al., 2000). The role of milk in the transmission of foodborne viruses is also uncertain, but it is an area where considerable research is needed (Koopmans and Duizer, 2004; Koopmans et al., 2002).

The markets for extended-shelf-life (ESL) milk are expanding (Henyon, 1999). In Europe, these milks are produced by heat treatment of 127°C for 5 s, followed by nonaseptic packaging. Mayr et al. (2004a) reported that the shelf life of these milks was limited by nonsystematic post-process contamination by non-spore-forming gram positive bacteria present at very low numbers. However, when heat treatment between 100 and 145°C was applied to milk, psychrotrophic *Bacillus* spp. were isolated only from milk processed at temperatures at or below 134°C (Mayr et al., 2004b). *Bacillus licheniformis* was the predominant species isolated from ESL milk following incubation of plates at 30°C, but *B. subtilis* and *B. cereus* were also isolated (Table 6). All these species have been associated with foodborne illness (Griffiths and Schraft, 2002).

TABLE 6 Aerobic Spore-formers in ESL (127°C for 5 s) Milk Isolated at 30°C

Organism	Number of Isolates	Percent
Bacillus licheniformis	470	73
Bacillus subtilis	35	5
Bacillus cereus	26	4
Brevibacillus brevis	18	3
Bacillus pumilus	9	1
Bacillus amyloliquefaciens	8	1
Other *Bacillus* spp.	5	1
Paenibacillus spp.	5	1
Aneurinibacillus spp.	5	1
Unidentifiable	64	10

Source: Mayr et al. (2004b).

Thus, the safety issues associated with ESL milk include the extended storage time at refrigeration temperatures that may allow the psychrotrophic *Bacillus* spp. remaining after the heat treatment to grow; indeed, the temperatures used for ESL may activate the spores of *Bacillus* spp; leading to germination and outgrowth (Guirguis et al., 1983). Because of the lack of competition from other organisms, their growth may be improved and they may become adapted to this "new" niche. This may be important since it is known that *B. subtilis* develops competency (the ability to acquire new genetic material) during growth in milk (Zenz et al., 1998).

Although ultrahigh temperature (UHT, 135°C for 1 to 2 s) milks have not been implicated in milkborne outbreaks, over the last decade a *Bacillus* sp., *B. sporothermodurans*, producing highly heat-resistant spores has emerged which can grow in packaged UHT milk (Lembke et al., 2000). Outbreaks of *B. cereus* infections have occurred due to the consumption of contaminated cream (Ryser, 2004).

7.5 CHEESE AND FERMENTED DAIRY PRODUCTS

Although fermented products have been considered safe due to their high acidity, there have been outbreaks linked to yogurt and cheese. These have included incidents of salmonellosis linked to cheddar cheese, such as that involving *S.* Typhimurium in Canada in 1983, which affected more than 2000 people. Some of the more significant cheese-related outbreaks of salmonellosis are documented in Table 7. Several pathogens, including *Salmonella* and enterohemmorhagic *E. coli*, can survive in hard cheeses for prolonged periods. For example, *S.* Enteritidis has been shown to survive in cheddar cheese for more than 99 days (Fig. 2); *E. coli* O157:H7 survives for 158 days

TABLE 7 Outbreaks of Salmonellosis Linked to Cheese

Year	Cheese	Method of Processing Milk	Country	Serotype	No. of Cases
1982	Accawi	Raw	Canada	Muenster	3
1984	Cheddar	Thermized[a]	Canada	Typhimurium	2700
1985	Vacherin	Raw	Switzerland	Typhimurium	>40
1989	Irish soft cheese	Raw	England	Dublin	42
	Mozzarella	Unknow	United States	Javiana & Orianberg	164
1990	Goat cheese	Raw	France	Paratyphi B	277
1993	Goat cheese	Raw	France	Paratyphi B	273
1995	Doubs	Raw	France & Switzerland	Dublin	>25
1996	Cheddar	Thermized	England	Gold-Coast	84
1997	Mexican style	Raw	United States	Typhimurium	110

[a]Heat treated (unpasteurized).

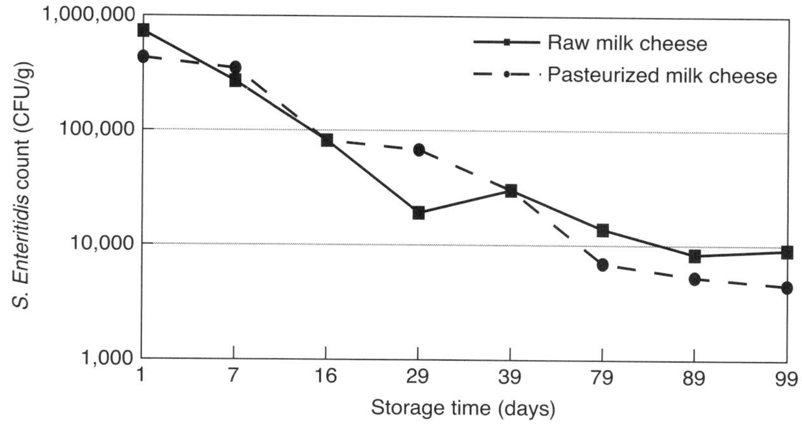

FIG. 2 Survival of *Salmonella* Enteritidis in cheddar cheese. (From Modi et al., 2001.)

when initial numbers were above 10^3 CFU/mL (Reitsma and Henning, 1996). There is also evidence that foodborne pathogens may survive better in products made from pasteurized milk, due to inactivation of antimicrobial compounds by the heat treatment. Marek et al. (2004) have shown that *E. coli* O157:H7 survives significantly better in cheddar cheese whey from pasteurized milk than from raw milk.

The link between *L. monocytogenes* and soft cheese is well recognized, and there have been several outbreaks of listeriosis in which soft cheeses such as Brie have been implicated (Ryser, 2007). This has led to an advisory to pregnant women to avoid consumption of soft cheese.

E. coli O157:H7 has also been shown to be able to survive in yogurt (Shiao and Chen, 2005) and result in illness (Ryser, 2004). In one unusual incident, 27 cases of botulism resulted from the consumption of hazelnut yogurt, which had been prepared using hazelnut puree contaminated with botulinum toxin (Mitchell et al., 1990). Outbreaks of botulism linked to cheese were also reported in the 1990s in Iran and Italy (Ryser, 2004). Currently, there are reports of an outbreak of shigellosis in the Ukraine linked to contaminated kefir, which has resulted in about 380 cases of illness, mainly affecting children.

7.6 ICE CREAM

Foodborne pathogens have been shown to survive in ice cream and produce illness. Arguably the largest foodborne outbreak recorded, which involved almost a quarter of a million people in the United States, was the result of contamination of ice cream mix with *S.* Enteritidis during transportation in a truck that had previously been used to carry liquid egg (Ryser, 2004). Ice cream has also been the vehicle for staphylococcal poisoning. Prior exposure to low temperatures can increase survival of *E. coli* O157:H7 during subsequent freezing (Grzadkoska and Griffiths, 2001). The practical importance of cross-protection, whereby an organism becomes more resistant to subsequent stress following exposure to a sublethal stress, needs to be better understood.

7.7 BUTTER

There have been at least three cases of staphylococcal intoxication linked to butter in the United States in the last 35 years (Ryser, 2004). All were type A. In 1999, an outbreak of listeriosis involving 25 cases caused by *L. monocytogenes* serotype 3a occurred in Finland. An investigation found the outbreak strain in packaged butter served at a hospital and at the source dairy. Recall of the product ended the outbreak (Lyytikainen et al., 2000). The data from this outbreak were used to estimate infectious dose. The highest single dose (7.7×10^4 CFU in one meal) could have been sufficient to cause the listeriosis cases. However, listeriosis cases could have been caused by a prolonged daily consumption of contaminated butter during the hospital stay. The estimated daily dose, based on the hospital kitchen data or the highest detected level in a wholesale sample (11,000 CFU/g), would have varied from 1.4×10^1 to 2.2×10^3 CFU/day or from 2.2×10^4 to 3.1×10^5 CFU/day, respectively (Maijala et al., 2001).

7.8 MILK POWDER

Recently, it has been found that contamination of powdered infant milk formula by *Enterobacter sakazakii* can lead to infant death due to meningitis or neonatal necrotizing enterocolitis (see Chapter 3). Although the rate of infection is low, with only 48 cases of illness due to *E. sakazakii* reported from 1961 to 2003, the severity of the illness makes it of concern to the dairy industry. The organism has been isolated from 35% of environmental samples taken from a dry niche in milk powder production plants and from up to 12% of cans of infant formula. However, the source of this organism remains a mystery (Gurtler et al., 2005). There have been outbreaks due to contamination of infant formula by *B. cereus* (Ryser, 2004), and this has led to the adoption of international standards for the organism in infant formula.

The impact on the industry of a major outbreak of milk-borne disease is arguably best illustrated by the events of June and July 2000, when contamination of milk powder by *S. aureus* enterotoxin occurred in the Snow Brand plant at Taiki, Hokkaido, Japan (Asao et al., 2003). This powder was reconstituted and sold as fluid milk, causing more than 14,000 cases of illness and possibly one death. The contamination was the result of an electrical failure, leading to raw milk being held on the line for 3 h at elevated temperatures, and the organism was subsequently isolated from a valve at their Osaka plant. The outbreak highlighted several deficiencies in hygiene practices at the Snow Brand sites and led to the closure of all of Snow Brand's 21 dairy plants, plunging the company into an economic crisis.

7.9 DETECTION OF MICROORGANISMS IN MILK

Although conventional plate counts will continue to be the main method of assessing quality and safety of dairy products in the short term, the advent of molecular tools has provided us with a new battery of analytical techniques for the detection, enumeration, and identification of microorganisms. Methods such as real- time PCR are revolutionizing the speed and accuracy with which we can detect and enumerate food-borne pathogens (Maukonen et al., 2003). Real-time PCR assays have been described for the detection of *Mycobacterium paratuberculosis*, *Bacillus anthracis*, *Salmonella* spp., *Campylobacter jejuni*, *Listeria monocytogenes*, *Yersinia enterocolitica*, and *E. coli* O157:H7 as well as viruses such as hepatitis A. Commercial systems based on real-time PCR are now in use in the food industry for routine analysis of products. However, advances need to be made in the area of sample preparation before the techniques can be applied directly to foods (Fung, 2002; Malorny et al., 2003).

As well as their use in detection, molecular methods can be used to characterize microorganisms. Dogan and Boor (2003), using ribotyping, were able to show that there were multiple sites of contamination for *Pseudomonas* spp. within processing plants and dairy products and that the ribotype was related to the spoilage potential of the strain. Denaturing gradient gel electrophoresis (DGGE) and temporal temperature gradient electrophoresis (TTGE) can be used to improve our understanding of the ecology of food systems. In these methods, the total DNA is extracted from the sample and a 16S or 28S rRNA gene sequence is amplified using PCR. The bands are then separated by gradient electrophoresis according to their melting temperatures. Using these techniques it is possible to monitor dynamic changes in bacterial populations in raw milk during refrigerated storage, and it allows simultaneous detection of several pathogens that cannot be cultured together (Lafarge et al., 2004). In addition, these techniques can be used to identify bacteria that are difficult to culture. For example, Sabour et al. (2003) have determined the microbial flora associated with the bovine teat canal of beef and dairy cattle using DGGE. They showed that the predominant bacteria present in both types of animal belonged to the classes Clostridia and Bacilli. They also identified novel sequences not corresponding to known bacteria in both groups of animals.

Simple hygiene monitoring tests based on ATP bioluminescence are available commercially, and these have been used successfully to evaluate the cleanliness of milking equipment, bulk tanks and milk tankers (Paez et al., 2003), as well as processing lines (Moore et al., 2001; Oulahal-Lagsir et al., 2000). Methods have also been developed to assess raw milk quality within 2 min (Brovko et al., 1999; Samkutty et al., 2001).

7.10 NOVEL PROCESSING METHODS

Methods such as the addition of CO_2 (Martin et al., 2003), lactic acid bacteria (Griffiths et al., 1991), and lactoperoxidase activation (Seifu et al., 2005) have been used to preserve raw milk, with varying degrees of success. These are generally seen as ways to extend the storage time of the milk before processing. Other nonthermal methods to improve the safety and quality of milk have been investigated. These include the use of pulsed electric fields to cause perturbations in the membrane of cells (Mittal and Griffiths, 2005) and high pressure (Trujillo et al., 2002). However, it is unlikely that any of these processes will be comparable to pasteurization by heat, and work has focused on combinations of nonthermal methods as well as their combination with antimicrobial agents such as bacteriocins (Ross et al., 2003).

Other techniques, such as bactofugation and microfiltration, have found commercial application in the production of ESL milks (Joppen, 2004). Microfiltration, in particular, is gaining widespread acceptance, and recent work has shown that treatments equivalent to bactofugation and microfiltration are able to remove 95 to 99.9% of *Mycobacterium paratuberculosis* cells from suspension (Grant et al., 2005).

Heat pasteurization will continue to be the prime method for the control of milk-borne illness, at least until nonthermal processes such as high pressure and pulsed electric field have been perfected.

7.11 GLOBAL TRADE AND REGULATIONS

The dairy industry is one of the most regulated sectors in developed countries. A detailed discussion of regulations pertaining to the dairy industry is outside the scope of this review; however, international trade in dairy commodities is increasing. In 2004, World Trade Organization negotiations (the Doha Round) resulted in agreements on a framework for reducing agricultural supports, and this will have significant impact on the industry (Suzuki and Kaiser, 2005). Another trend that is having an impact on milk production is the increase in organic farming. This has been particularly noticeable in Europe, where regulations to standardize organic production have been implemented (Rosati and Aumaitre, 2004). The dairy industry is changing in many ways, and developing tools to manage this change will be a prime focus of research worldwide.

REFERENCES

Asao T, Kumeda Y, Kawai T, et al. (2003): An extensive outbreak of staphylococcal food poisoning due to low-fat milk in Japan: estimation of enterotoxin A in the incriminated milk and powdered skim milk. *Epidemiol Infect.* 130:33–40.

Austin JW, Bergeron G (1995): Development of bacterial biofilms in dairy processing lines. *J Dairy Res.* 62:509–519.

Bramley AJ, McKinnon CH (1990): The microbiology of raw milk. In: Robinson RK (Ed.): *Dairy Microbiology*, Vol. 1. Elsevier Applied Science, London, pp. 163–208.

Brovko LY, Froundjian VG, Babunova VS, Ugarova NN (1999): Quantitative assessment of bacterial contamination of raw milk using bioluminescence. *J Dairy Res.* 66:627–631.

Brown RS, Hussain M (2003): The Walkerton tragedy: issues for water quality monitoring. *Analyst.* 128:320–322.

Burt R, Wellsteed S (1991): Food safety and legislation in the dairy industry. *J Soc Dairy Technol.* 44:80–86.

Buyser M-LD, Dufour B, Maire M, Lafarge V (2001): Implication of milk and milk products in food-borne diseases in France and in different industrialised countries. *Int J Food Microbiol.* 67:1–17.

Clark CG, Bryden L, Cuff WR, et al. (2005): Use of the Oxford multilocus sequence typing protocol and sequencing of the flagellin short variable region to characterize isolates from a large outbreak of waterborne Campylobacter sp. strains in Walkerton, Ontario, Canada. *J Clin Microbiol.* 43:2080–2091.

Dawson D (2005): Foodborne protozoan parasites. *Int J Food Microbiol.* 103:207–227.

Desmarchelier PM (2001): Pathogenic microbiological contaminants of milk. *Aust J Dairy Technol.* 56:123.

Desmasures N, Gueguen M (1997): Monitoring the microbiology of high quality milk by monthly sampling over 2 years. *J Dairy Res.* 64:271–280.

Desmasures N, Bazin F, Gueguen M (1997): Microbiological composition of raw milk from selected farms in the Camembert region of Normandy. *J Appl Microbiol.* 83:53–58.

Diaz de Aguayo ME, Duarte ABL, Montes de Oca Canastillo F (1992): Incidence of multiple antibiotic resistant organisms isolated from retail milk products in Hermosillo, Mexico. *J Food Prot.* 55:370–373.

Dogan B, Boor KJ (2003): Genetic diversity and spoilage potentials among Pseudomonas spp. isolated from fluid milk products and dairy processing plants. *Appl Environ Microbiol.* 69:130–138.

Eneroth A, Ahrne S, Molin G (2000): Contamination routes of gram-negative spoilage bacteria in the production of pasteurized milk, evaluated by randomly amplified polymorphic DNA (RAPD). *Int Dairy J.* 10:325–331.

Eyles MJ (1995): Trends in foodborne disease and implications for the dairy industry. *Aust J Dairy Technol.* 50:10–14.

Farrell GM, Yousef AE, Marth EH (1991): Survival of *Borelia burgdorferi* in whole milk, low fat milk, and skim milk at 34°C and in skim milk at 5°C. *J Food Prot.* 54:532–536.

Friedhoff RA, Houben APM, Leblanc JMJ, Beelen JMWM, Jansen JT, Mossel DAA (2005): Elaboration of microbiological guidelines as an element of codes of hygienic practices for small and/or less developed businesses to verify compliance with hazard analysis critical control point. *J Food Prot.* 68:139–145.

Fung DYC (2002): Rapid methods and automation in microbiology. *Comp Rev Food Sci Food Safet.* 1:3–22.

Giaccone V, Colavita G, Miotti-Scapin R (2000): *Toxoplasma gondii* in food: the how and why of an unusual and underestimated foodborne disease. *Ig Mod.* 113:439–452.

Gillespie IA, Adak GK, O'Brien SJ, Bolton FJ (2003): Milkborne general outbreaks of infectious intestinal disease, England and Wales, 1992–2000. *Epidemiol Infect.* 130:461–468.

Grant IR (2005): Zoonotic potential of *Mycobacterium avium* ssp. *paratuberculosis*: the current position. *J Appl Microbiol.* 98:1282–1293.

Grant IR, Williams AG, Rowe MT, Muir DD (2005): Investigation of the impact of simulated commercial centrifugation and microfiltration conditions on levels of *Mycobacterium avium* ssp. *paratuberculosis* in milk. *Int J Dairy Technol.* 58:138–142.

Griffiths MW (2002): Mycobacterium paratuberculosis. In: Blackburn CW, McClure PJ (Eds.). *Foodborne Pathogens: Hazards, Risk Analysis and Control*. Woodhead Publishing, Cambridge, UK, pp. 489–500.

——— (2004): Milk and unfermented milk products. In: Lund BM, Baird-Parker AC, Gould GW (Eds.). *The Microbiological Safety and Quality of Food*, Vol. I. Aspen Publishers, Gaithersburg, MD, pp. 507–534.

Griffiths MW, Schraft H (2002): *Bacillus cereus* Food Poisoning. In: Cliver D (Ed.): *Foodborne Diseases*. Elsevier Science, London, pp. 261–270.

Griffiths MW, Banks JM, McIntyre L, Limond A (1991): Some insight into the mechanism of inhibition of psychrotrophic bacterial growth in raw milk by lactic acid bacteria. *J Soc Dairy Technol*. 44:24–29.

Grzadkowska D, Griffiths MW (2001): Cryotolerance of *Escherichia coli* 0157:H7 in laboratory media and food. *J Food Sci*. 66:1169–1173.

Guirguis AH, Griffiths MW, Muir DD (1983): Sporeforming bacteria in milk. I: Optimisation of heat-treatment for activation of spores of *Bacillus* species. *Milchwissenschaft*. 38:641–644.

Gurtler JB, Kornacki JL, Beuchat LR (2005): *Enterobacter sakazakii*: a coliform of increased concern to infant health. *Int J Food Microbiol*. 104:1–34.

Hatt B, Wilbey A (1994): Temperature control in the cold chain. *J Soc Dairy Technol*. 47:77–80.

Hayes MC, Boor K (2001): Raw milk and fluid milk products. In: Marth EH, Steele JL (Eds.). *Applied Dairy Microbiology*. Marcel Dekker, New York, pp. 59–76.

Henyon DK (1999): Extended shelf-life milks in North America: a perspective, *Int J Dairy Technol*. 52:95–101.

Holm C, Jepsen L, Larsen M, Jespersen L (2004): Predominant microflora of downgraded Danish bulk tank milk. *J Dairy Sci*. 87:1151–1157.

Hussein HS, Sakuma T (2005): *Invited Review:* Prevalence of Shiga toxin–producing *Escherichia coli* in dairy cattle and their products. *J Dairy Sci*. 88:450–465.

IDF (International Dairy Federation) (1993): *Significance of Pathogenic Organisms in Raw Milk*. IDF Bulletin. Document 142. FIL-IDF, Brussels, Belgium.

Jayarao BM, Henning DR (2001): Prevalence of foodborne pathogens in bulk tank milk. *J Dairy Sci*. 84:2157–2162.

Joppen L (2004): Globesity: fighting the fat. *Food Eng Ingred*. 29:44.

Karns JS, Van Kessel JS, McCluskey BJ, Perdue ML (2005): Prevalence of *Salmonella enterica* in bulk tank milk from US dairies as determined by polymerase chain reaction. *J Dairy Sci*. 88:3475–3479.

Koopmans M, Duizer E (2004): Foodborne viruses: an emerging problem. *Int J Food Microbiol*. 90:23–41.

Koopmans M, von Bonsdorff CH, Vinje J, de Medici D, Monroe S (2002): Foodborne viruses. *FEMS Microbiol Rev*. 26:187–205.

Laberge I, Griffiths MW (1996): Prevalence, detection and control of *Cryptosporidium parvum* in food. *Int J Food Microbiol*. 32:1–26.

Lafarge V, Ogier JC, Girard V, et al. (2004): Raw cow milk bacterial population shifts attributable to refrigeration. *Appl Environ Microbiol*. 70:5644–5650.

Lee MB, Middleton D (2003): Enteric illness in Ontario, Canada, from 1997 to 2001. *J Food Prot*. 66:953–961.

Lee Wong AC (1998): Biofilms in food processing environments. *J Dairy Sci.* 81:2765–2770.

Lembke F, Hammer P, Herman L, et al. (2000): *Bacillus sporothermodurans:* a bacillus forming highly heat-resistant spores. *Bull Int Dairy Fed.* 357:3–27.

Lyytikainen O, Autio T, Maijala R, et al. (2000): An outbreak of *Listeria monocytogenes* serotype 3a infections from butter in Finland. *J Infect Dis.* 181:1838–1841.

MacDonald D (2003): Has HACCP failed to deliver? *Int Food Hyg.* 13:11–14.

Maijala R, Lyytikainen O, Autio T, Aalto T, Haavisto L, Honkanen-Buzalski T (2001): Exposure of *Listeria monocytogenes* within an epidemic caused by butter in Finland. *Int J Food Microbiol.* 70:97–109.

Makovec JA, Ruegg PL (2003): Antimicrobial resistance of bacteria isolated from dairy cow milk samples submitted for bacterial culture: 8,905 samples (1994–2001). *J Am Vet Med Assoc.* 222:1582–1589.

Malorny B, Tassios PT, Radstrom P, Cook N, Wagner M, Hoorfar J (2003): Standardization of diagnostic PCR for the detection of foodborne pathogens. *Int J Food Microbiol.* 83:39–48.

Marek P, Mohan Nair MK, Hoagland T, Kumar V (2004): Survival and growth characteristics of *Escherichia coli* O157:H7 in pasteurized and unpasteurized cheddar cheese whey. *Int J Food Microbiol.* 94:1–7.

Martin JD, Werner BG, Hotchkiss JH (2003): Effects of carbon dioxide on bacterial growth parameters in milk as measured by conductivity. *J Dairy Sci.* 86:1932–1940.

Maukonen J, Matto J, Wirtanen G, Raaska L, Mattila-Sandholm T, Saarela M (2003): Methodologies for the characterization of microbes in industrial environments: a review. *J Ind Microbiol Biotechnol.* 30:327–356.

Mayr R, Gutser K, Busse M, Seiler H (2004a): Gram positive non-sporeforming recontaminants are frequent spoilage organisms of German retail ESL (extended shelf life) milk. *Milchwissenschaft.* 59:262–266.

——— (2004b): Indigenous aerobic sporeformers in high heat-treated (127°C, 5s) German ESL (extended shelf life) milk. *Milchwissenschaft.* 59:143–146.

Mitchell E, O'Mahony M, Gilbert RJ, et al. (1990): Two outbreaks of Legionnaires' disease in Bolton Health District. *Epidemiol Infect.* 104:159–170.

Mittal GS, Griffiths MW (2005): Pulsed electric field processing of liquid foods and beverages. In: Sun DW (Ed.): *Emerging Technologies for Food Processing.* Elsevier Academic Press, Amsterdam, The Netherlands, pp. 99–181.

Modi R, Hirvi Y, Hill A, Griffiths MW (2001): Effect of phage on survival of *Salmonella* enteritidis during manufacture and storage of cheddar cheese made from raw and pasteurized milk. *J Food Prot.* 264:927–933.

Moore G, Griffith C, Fielding L (2001): A comparison of traditional and recently developed methods for monitoring surface hygiene within the food industry: a laboratory study. *Dairy Food Environ San.* 21:478–488.

Murphy SC, Boor KJ (2000): Trouble-shooting sources and causes of high bacteria counts in raw milk. *Dairy Food Environ San.* 20:606–611.

Niskanen A, Koiranen L, Roine K (1978): Staphylococcal enterotoxin and thermonuclease production during induced bovine mastitis and the clinical reaction of enterotoxin in udders. *Infect Immun.* 19:493–498.

Oulahal-Lagsir N, Martial-Gros A, Bonneau M, Bum LJ (2000): Ultrasonic methodology coupled to ATP bioluminescence for the non-invasive detection of fouling in food processing equipment: validation and application to a dairy factory. *J Appl Microbiol.* 89:433–441.

Paez R, Taverna M, Charlon V, Cuatrin A, Etcheverry F, da Costa LH (2003): Application of ATP-bioluminescence technique for assessing cleanliness of milking equipment, bulk and milk transport tankers. *Food Prot Trends*. 23:308–314.

Phillips JD, Griffiths MW (1990): Pasteurized dairy products: the constraints imposed by environmental contamination. In Nriagu JO, Simmons MS (Eds.). *Food Contamination from Environmental Sources*, Vol. 23. Wiley, New York, pp. 387–456.

Rasmussen MD, Bjerring M, Justesen P, Jepsen L (2002): Milk quality on Danish farms with automatic milking systems. *J Dairy Sci*. 85:2869–2878.

Reitsma CJ, Henning DR (1996): Survival of enterohemorrhagic *Escherichia coli* O157:H7 during the manufacture and curing of cheddar cheese. *J Food Prot*. 59:460–464.

Rosati A, Aumaitre A (2004): Organic dairy farming in Europe. *Livest Prod Sci*. 90:41–51.

Ross AIV, Griffiths MW, Mittal GS, Deeth HC (2003): Combining nonthermal technologies to control foodborne microorganisms. *Int J Food Microbiol*. 89:125–138.

Rowe MT, Dunstall G, Kilpatrick D, Wisdom GB (2003): Effect of growth phase on the subsequent growth kinetics of psychrotrophic bacteria of raw milk origin. *Int J Dairy Technol*. 56:35–38.

Ryser ET (2004): Public health concerns. In: Marth EH, Steele JL (Eds.). *Applied Dairy Microbiology*. Marcel Dekker, New York, pp. 397–545.

——— (2007). Incidence and behavior of *Listeria monocytogenes* in cheese and other fermented dairy products. In: ET Ryser, Marth EH (Eds.) *Listeria, Listeriosis, and Food Safety*. CRC Press, Boca Raton, FL, pp. 405–502.

Sabour PM, Gill JJ, Gong J, Yu H, Leslie K, Griffiths MW (2003): Comparative molecular analysis of microbial flora associated with the bovine teat canal. In Proc. 19th International Genetics Congress, Melbourne, Australia.

Samkutty PJ, Gough RH, Adkinson RW, McGrew P (2001): Rapid assessment of the bacteriological quality of raw milk using ATP bioluminescence. *J Food Prot*. 64:208–212.

Sanaa M, Poutrel B, Menard JL, Serieys F (1993): Risk factors associated with contamination of raw milk by *Listeria monocytogenes* in dairy farms. *J Dairy Sci*. 76:2891–2898.

Seifu E, Buys EM, Donkin EF (2005): Significance of the lactoperoxidase system in the dairy industry and its potential applications: a review. *Trends Food Sci Technol*. 16:137–154.

Sharma M, Anand SK (2002): Biofilms evaluation as an essential component of HACCP for food/dairy processing industry: a case. *Food Control*. 13:469–477.

Sharma S, Sachdeva P, Virdi JS (2003): Emerging water-borne pathogens. *Appl Microbiol Biotechnol*. 61:424-428.

Shiao ML, Chen J (2005): The influence of an extracellular polysaccharide, comprised of colanic acid, on the fate of *Escherichia coli* O157:H7 during processing and storage of stirred yogurt. *LWT Food Sci Technol*. 38:785–790.

Steele ML, McNab WB, Poppe C, et al. (1997): Survey of Ontario bulk tank raw milk for food-borne pathogens. *J Food Prot*. 60:1341–1346.

Sun M (1985): Desperately seeking *Salmonella* in Illinois. *Science*. 228:829–830.

Suzuki N, Kaiser HM (2005): Impacts of the Doha Round framework agreements on dairy policies. *J Dairy Sci*. 88:1901–1908.

Trujillo AJ, Capellas M, Saldo J, Gervilla R, Guamis B (2002): Applications of high-hydrostatic pressure on milk and dairy products: a review. *Innov Food Sci Emerg Technol*. 3: 295–307.

Valle J, Gomez-Lucia E, Piriz S, Vadillo S (1991): Staphylococcal enterotoxins and toxic shock syndrome toxin-1 (TSST-1) production during induced goat mastitis. *J Food Prot.* 54:267–271.

Zadoks RN, Gonzalez RN, Boor KJ, Schukken YH (2004): Mastitis-causing streptococci are important contributors to bacterial counts in raw bulk tank milk. *J Food Prot.* 67:2644–2650.

Zenz KI, Neve H, Geis A, Heller KJ (1998): *Bacillus subtilis* develops competence for uptake of plasmid DNA when growing in milk products. *Syst Appl Microbiol.* 21:28–32.

CHAPTER 8

FOOD SAFETY ISSUES AND THE MICROBIOLOGY OF POULTRY

IRENE V. WESLEY

8.1 INTRODUCTION

Poultry, including broilers, turkey, duck, and quail, rank in third place among products incriminated in foodborne illness. For the United States, annual per capita poultry consumption (73.5 lb) is highest among the meat groups, exceeding beef (62.4 lb) and pork (46.4 lb) (USDA-ARS, 2007).

In 1996–1998, the U.S. Department of Agriculture (USDA) Food Safety and Inspection Service (FSIS) conducted nationwide microbial baseline surveys of beef, hogs, poultry, and turkey carcasses (Table 1). The data show the highest contamination of poultry carcasses, including broilers and turkeys, with *Campylobacter* (~90%), *Salmonella* (~20%), and *L. monocytogenes*. FSIS baseline of ground products similarly recovered *Salmonella* in ground chicken (44.6%) and in ground turkey (49.9%) meat (USDA-FSIS, continuously updated-b). Performance standards for *Salmonella*, based on these national surveys, are in place with a limit for carcass contamination of 18.2% of turkeys and 20% of broilers. *Campylobacter* performance standards are pending.

Pathogen intervention strategies have reduced human illness and deaths. CDC FoodNet estimates an overall 21% decrease in bacterial foodborne illnesses in the 1996–1999 interval (Fig. 1). *Salmonella* levels in raw poultry have declined since 1990, when approximately 40% of carcasses tested were *Salmonella* positive, to 2000, when less than 10% of carcasses were positive. However, from 2002 to 2005, when 16% of carcasses were positive, FSIS recorded an increase in *Salmonella* in broilers. Because the reduction of human salmonellosis is lagging behind that of other human foodborne infections, in 2007 USDA-FSIS launched an initiative to reduce *Salmonella* in broilers, which included publishing the names of meat plants that have trouble controlling *Salmonella*.

Microbiologically Safe Foods, Edited by Norma Heredia, Irene Wesley, and Santos García

TABLE 1 Summary of Microbiological Baseline Data for Selected Foodborne Bacteria on Carcasses[a]

	Steers/Heifers	Cows/Bulls	Hogs	Turkeys	Broilers
E. coli O157:H7	0.2	0	0	0	0
Campylobacter	4	1.1	31.5	90.3	88.2
Salmonella	1	2.7	8.7	18.5	20
L. monocytogenes	4.1	11.3	7.4	5.9	15

Source: USDA-FSIS (continuously updated-b).
[a]Percent positive samples; n = ca. 2000 each.

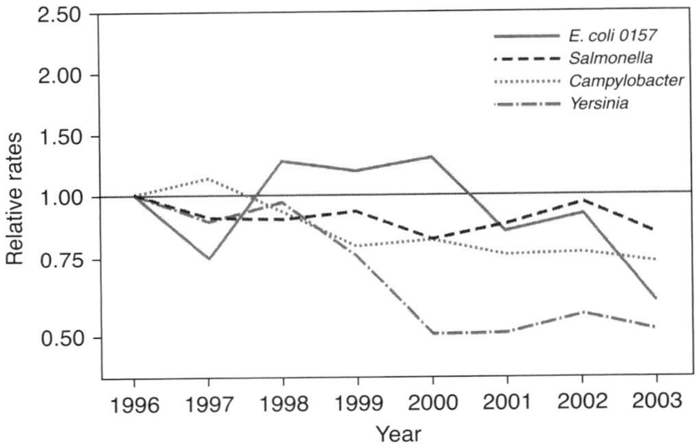

FIG. 1 Relative rates of bacterial foodborne pathogens compared with 1996–1999 baseline period. (From CDC, 2006.)

Federal agencies, in collaboration with the poultry industry, have implemented guidelines to remove contaminated meat and poultry products from commerce. For example, between 2000 and 2001, FSIS requested voluntary recall of approximately 31.5 million pounds of poultry products due to the presence of foodborne pathogens (USDA-FSIS, continuously updated-a).

Although the current emphasis is on pathogen reduction post-harvest at the processing level, clearly, reducing the on-farm prevalence of potential human pathogens will deliver clean birds to the abattoir, which may result in an overall decline in human foodborne illness. In this chapter we address methods to reduce foodborne pathogens from farm to fork: during poultry production, processing, and ultimately at the consumer's table.

8.2 CHARACTERISTICS OF FOODBORNE ILLNESS

Campylobacter and *Salmonella* are the two most important bacterial pathogens incriminated in foodborne illness related to poultry products, while *Listeria monocytogenes* is more frequently associated with contaminated ready-to-eat products, including poultry. *Campylobacter* and *Salmonella* inhabit the intestinal tract of clinically healthy birds. In contrast, in humans, consumption of contaminated undercooked poultry results either in no clinical illness or in nausea, vomiting, diarrhea, fever, dehydration, and headaches. Antimicrobial characteristics of the avian mucosa may underlie this phenomenon (Young et al., 2007).

8.2.1 *Campylobacter*

Campylobacter jejuni (Fig. 2) is the leading cause of human foodborne illness worldwide and infects 1% of the population of Western Europe each year (Humphrey et al., 2007). In the United States, the nearly 2 million human cases account for an estimated $1.2 billion in productivity losses annually. Based on attribution data, contaminated poultry (72%), dairy products (7.8%), and red meats, including beef (4.3%) and pork (4.4%), are vehicles of transmission and acknowledged risk factors (Hoffman et al., 2007; Miller and Mandrell, 2005). However, other factors, such as water, contact with pets, and worldwide travel, are significant. *Campylobacter* resides in protozoans, which may explain its survival in rivers and streams.

Campylobacter grow in low-oxygen environments (5% O_2) and are termed *microaerophiles*. Therefore, growth media incorporate oxygen quenchers, such as blood and activated charcoal. In the laboratory a microaerobic environment is achieved with commercially available special gas packets or incubators (5% CO_2, 85% N_2, 10% CO_2). *C. jejuni* and *C. coli* grow optimally at 42°C (thermotolerant), which coincides with the body temperature of poultry.

Campylobacter replicate in the mucus layer over the intestinal villi of its host, where minimal amounts of oxygen are available. They survive but do not multiply on poultry carcasses or on contact surfaces present in the slaughterhouse or on kitchen cutting boards. Drying and freezing kill *Campylobacter*. Freezing is a major critical

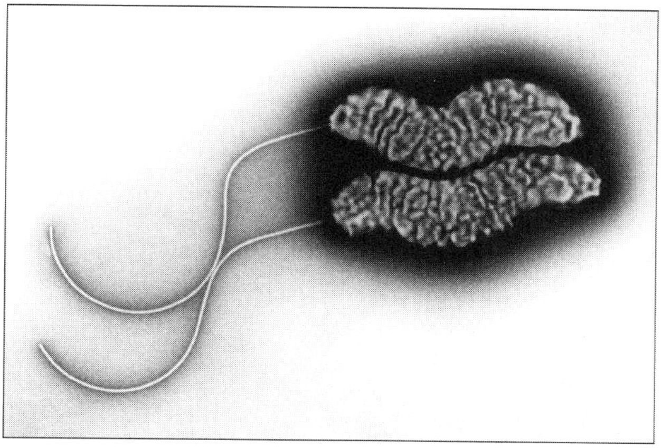

FIG. 2 *Campylobacter*, the leading cause of bacterial foodborne illness, shown with single flagella. (Courtesy of Al Ritchie.)

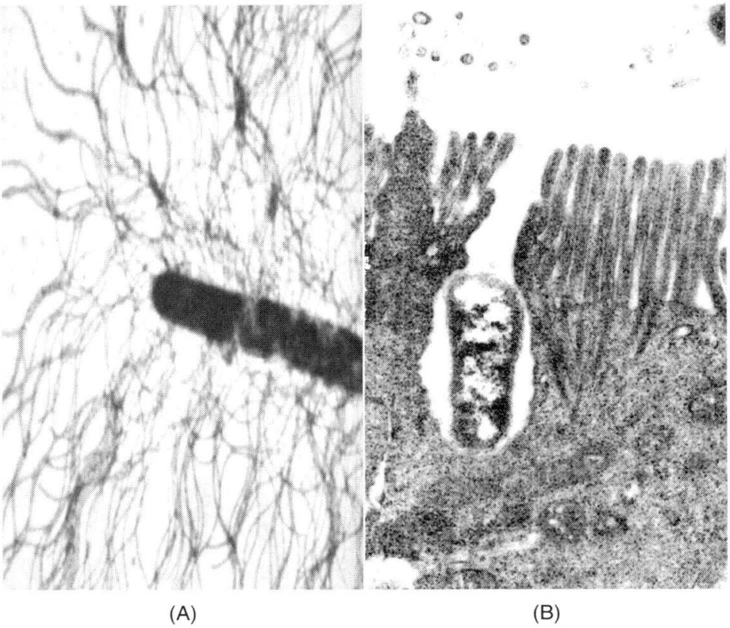

FIG. 3 *Salmonella* with multiple flagella (A) and in the crypts of the intestine (B). (From Meyerholz et al., 2002, with permission.)

control point in carcass processing. Thus, low infectious dose for humans (1000 CFU), coupled with *Campylobacter's* inability to replicate during refrigeration, indicate that even modest reductions during processing and food preparation may alleviate human illness.

8.2.2 *Salmonella*

There are approximately 2500 serotypes of *Salmonella enterica* (Fig. 3). The most common serotypes isolated from turkeys and from broilers between 1997 and 2005 (Morningstar-Flugrad, 2006) and from human clinical cases in 2005 (CDC, 2006) are shown in Table 2.

8.3 APPROACHES TO MAINTAINING PRODUCT QUALITY AND REDUCING THE NUMBER OF MICROORGANISMS

8.3.1 Flock-to-Fork Concept

The FSIS/APHIS Animal Production Technical Analysis Group identified the critical control points of live production (Fig. 4). Good agricultural practices (GAPs) and hazard analysis of critical control points (HACCP) are intervention programs

TABLE 2 ***Salmonella enterica*** **Serotypes Most Frequently Isolated from Turkeys, Broilers, and Human Clinical Cases**

Turkey Isolates, 1997–2005	Percent of Total	Broiler Isolates 1997–2005	Percent of Total	Human Isolates, 2005	Percent of Total
Heidelberg	20.9	Kentucky	35.5	Typhimurium	19
Hadar	16.6	Heidelberg	20.3	Enteritidis	18
Senftenberg	8.1	Typhimurium	6.2	Newport	10
Reading	7.3	Typhimurium var. 5-[a]	4.9	Heidelberg	6
Saint Paul	6.5	Enteritidis	4.3	Javiana	5
Agona	5.0	Hadar	4	I4, (5), 12:i:-, 154	3
Schwarzengrund	4.5	4(s)12:i:-	3.1	Montevideo	2.2
Muenster	3.7	Montevideo	2.7	Muenchen	2
Arizona	2.7	Thompson	2.3	Saintpaul	1.9
Typhimurium	2.5	Schwarzengrund	2.2	Braenderup	1.7

Source: Morningstar-Flugrad (2006), CDC (2006).
[a]Formerly Copenhagen.

designed for poultry to minimize and eliminate bacterial foodborne pathogens in poultry, which are transmitted in feed, water, and *in ovo*. On-farm strategies (e.g., best management practices, good agricultural practices) attempt to minimize pathogens in live birds that enter the slaughter facilities. On-farm intervention programs begin at the breeder farms, continue to the hatcheries, and through grow-out at the poultry farms. The more rigorous mandated HACCP guidelines, which require documentation, are in place at feed mills, slaughter operations, processing facilities, distribution centers, and continue through to retail.

Salmonella is the model used in developing on-farm best management practices (BMPs) since (1) all species of livestock are a source of the organism; (2) *Salmonella* was ranked number one for its impact on human health; (3) there is significant knowledge of salmonellosis compared with other foodborne pathogens; and (4) the poultry industry has a long history of voluntary control and eradication programs for *Salmonella*. Implementation of BMPs and microbiological control technologies against *Salmonella* at food safety control points during live production of turkeys should also control other pathogens (NTF, 1999).

8.3.2 On-Farm Interventions

Breeders Foundation hatcheries supply not only future generations of breeder flocks but are also the ultimate source of meat birds for human consumption. Pathogen reduction begins with procurement of clean pathogen-free breeder stock at the foundation hatchery and requires strict biosecurity, vaccination, and regular surveillance of the breeder flocks for pathogens, especially *Salmonella enteritidis* (Fig. 3). *Salmonella* transmission occurs both by vertical transmission (*in ovo*, hen to progeny) and via the fecal–oral route (horizontal transmission). Because of the known routes of bacterial transmission (through progeny, feed, and water), a clean breeder stock, clean environment, clean source of drinking water, and clean feed are critical during all phases of poultry production.

To maintain potable water, breeder and poultry farms use "closed"-nipple drinker systems to minimize fecal contamination of the drinking water, unlike "open" drinker systems, which used Bell or Plasson drinkers. The use of water sanitizers such as chlorine (2 to 3 ppm) or other organic acid to flush the water system periodically retards bacterial growth.

Hatcheries The high quality of eggs arriving at a multiplier hatchery will minimize problems during the hatching process. Procuring eggs from farms enrolled in the National Poultry Improvement Plan or other industry group ensures egg quality and *Salmonella*-free status. Eggs contaminated during and after the laying process introduce pathogens into the commercial hatchery. Baby chicks or turkey poults are exposed to bacterial contaminants as early as 1 day of age.

Hatchery sanitation utilizing disinfectants and sanitizers retards the growth of pathogens. Stringent microbial monitoring and sampling of the hatchery environment and equipment assures the effectiveness of sanitation standard operating procedures. Evaluation of first-day mortality is a practical indicator of the effectiveness of hatchery intervention programs.

Turkey poults are routinely immunized at the hatchery for Newcastle disease virus, turkey coryza (*Bordetella*), and coccidiosis. Antimicrobial injections (gentamicin) may be given to the day-of-hatch turkey poult to repress bacterial pathogens.

Meat Bird Live production of the meat bird begins at the commercial hatchery with the broiler chick or turkey poult, continues through grow-out, and concludes with the transportation of a market-weight bird to slaughter.

Day-of-hatch turkey poults are delivered to the farm and placed on fresh litter in a clean, fumigated house. The food safety control points to block microbial, chemical, and physical contaminants during turkey production are detailed in Fig. 4. To avoid introduction of pathogens from adult birds, strict biosecurity is in place, with only farm personnel attending the young birds having access to the brooder house. Turkey poults remain in the brooder house until about 3 weeks of age, at which time they are moved to the grower/finisher house. The brooder house is thoroughly cleaned, disinfected, and fresh litter is placed for the next group of turkey poults. A source of clean water and *Salmonella*-free feed will ensure a *Salmonella*-free bird.

Salmonella and *C. jejuni* are commensals of poultry with young birds colonized early in life. Because it can be transmitted vertically *in ovo* from the hen to the chick, *Salmonella* may enter the house with the day-of-hatch birds. Both *Salmonella* and *Campylobacter* gain access to the flock during grow-out via contaminated water, feed, arthropods, rodents, wild birds, via contamination on boots of farm workers, aerosol, and pecking of manure-contaminated litter (Berndtson, 1996; Corry and Atabay, 2001; Jacobs-Reitsma, 2000). The flock may be contaminated with *Campylobacter* by the third week of life. Maternal antibodies may prevent colonization at a younger age (Sahin et al., 2003).

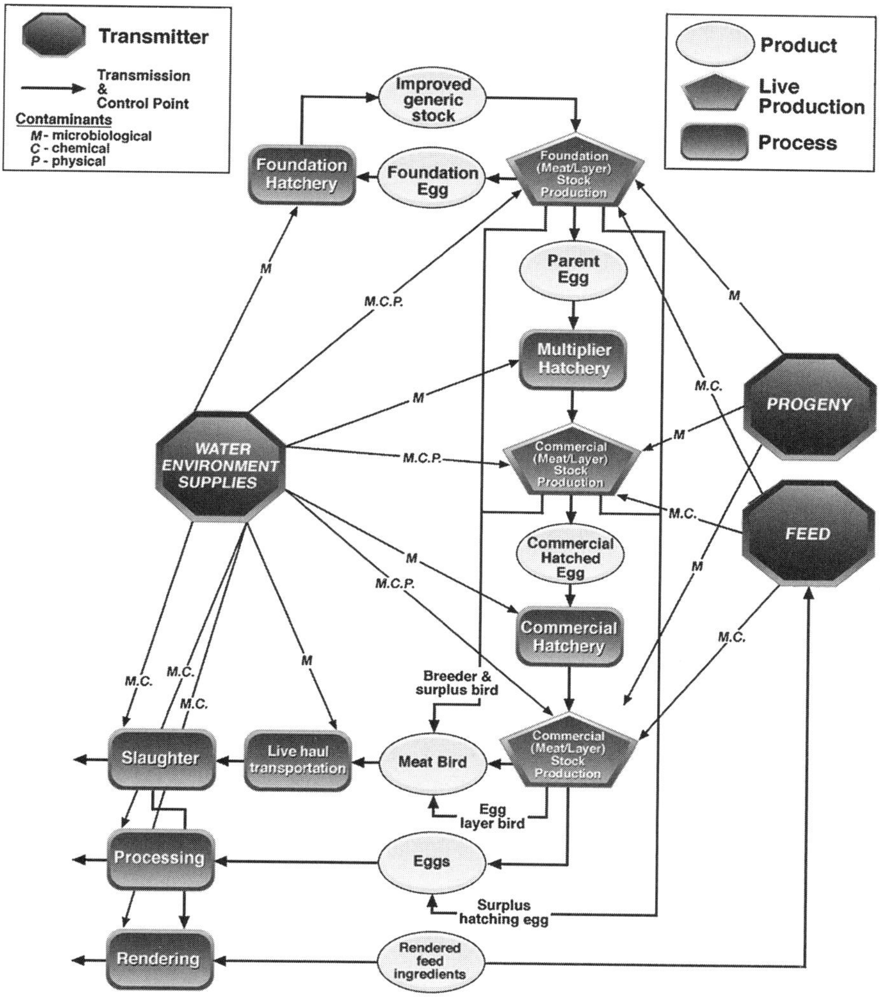

FIG. 4 Animal production flowchart with food safety control points: poultry. USDA-FSIS/APHIS Animal Production Technical Analysis Group (NTF, 1999).

On-farm intervention methods in place for *Salmonella* and *Campylobacter* include regular maintenance of drinkers, biosecurity (e.g., rodent and insect control, restricting house access to farm personnel), routine changing of boots or assignment of boots to individual bird houses (Berndtson, 1996). Improved house ventilation, which dries the litter, has been proposed as a means of reducing *Salmonella* in the flock (Mallinson, 2004). Some flocks may be free of *Salmonella* and *Campylobacter*, while others studies report nearly 100% contamination at market weight. Differences in flock management, especially biosecurity, may explain the prevalence differences.

Vaccination The ideal *Campylobacter* vaccine must confer, at its best, protection for each of the 48 heat-stable Penner and 48 heat-labile Lior antigens as well as the 76 phage types that have been described (Newell et al., 2000). Based on the 66 serotypes and 76 defined phage types employed in routine typing schemes in the United Kingdom, the estimated 5016 different serotype–phage type combinations may overwhelm current vaccine strategies! The short life span of broilers (~6 to 8 weeks) suggests that vaccination of broilers for *Salmonella* and *Campylobacter* may not be cost-effective. Thus, alternatives, such as competitive exclusion have been explored.

Competitive Exclusion Day-old baby chicks are sprayed with the intestinal flora obtained from adult specific pathogen-free (SPF) birds. Introduction of intestinal flora from an adult bird into newly hatched chicks accelerates gut maturation and may increase resistance to *Salmonella* colonization. If *Salmonella* is present in breeder flocks, it may contaminate the outer shell surface. Cox et al. (2000) reported that *Salmonella* penetrates porous egg shells and is ingested by the developing chick *in ovo*, which upon hatching would spread the infection to other birds. Hence, well-characterized microbial competitors of *Salmonella* may represent an effective early on-farm intervention (Bailey et al., 2000). Because it dwells in the mucus film overlying the villi, *Campylobacter* levels in the intestine are not abated by competitive exclusion cultures (Line et al., 1998).

Feed Mill The major steps of feed production and their accompanying critical control points (CCPs) are shown in Fig. 5. Bacterial pathogens may be present in feed ingredients or may be introduced at any number of points in the production and delivery of finished feed to farm bins. Feed formulation, production, and quality control at the feed mill are central to the production of *Salmonella*-free birds. Healthy flocks are more resistant to disease agents during grow-out and arrive at market with a lower risk of infection with pathogens, resulting in a microbiologically safer food for human consumption (NTF, 1999).

Contaminants may enter the feed with the animal, vegetable, liquid, or bagged ingredients. Intervention programs at the feed mill begin with the purchase of high-quality, ideally *Salmonella*-free ingredients, and continue with dry grain storage areas free of rodents and wild birds, high-temperature pelleting, environmental controls (dust, moisture), biosecurity (rodent, insect control), and controlled access of employees (NTF, 1999).

Each feed ingredient supplier should be approved as a reputable source of material of acceptable quality. Ideally, a *Salmonella*-negative specification (specific number of negative samples) could be included in the ingredient-purchasing contract (NTF, 1999).

The pelleting process heats the mash feed (180 to 190°F/82 to 88°C for 45 s), followed by drying with clean air to 12% moisture. Thus, heat-treated, dried pelleted feed reduces the risk of introduction of *Salmonella* and other pathogens into flocks. However, moisture, rodents, dust, and air may recontaminate the finished feed.

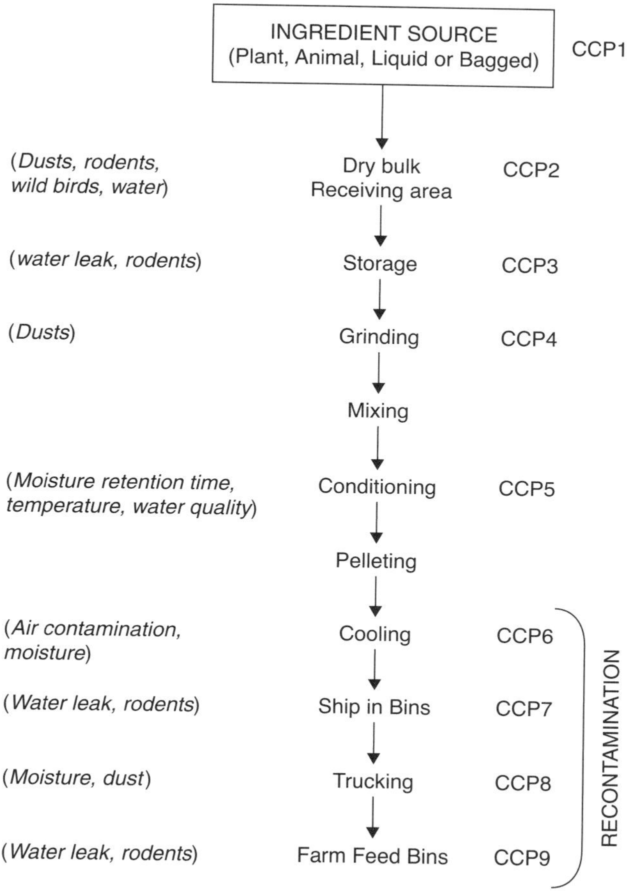

FIG. 5 The major steps of feed production and their accompanying critical control points. (From www.hybridturkeys.com.)

Moisture control within the feed mill prevents the multiplication of pathogens in the ingredients during storage prior to grinding and in the finished product. Dust control blocks cross-contamination of ingredients and in finished feed. Routine cleanup in and around the mill prevents buildup of feed and feed ingredients, which attract wild birds and rodents and support the growth of mold, spoilage organisms, and bacterial pathogens.

Feed Withdrawal To minimize gut rupture, feed is withdrawn from the market-weight bird prior to transport to the slaughterhouse. The National Turkey Federation (1999) has compiled extensive guidelines for humane feed withdrawal, catching, crating, and transport of turkeys to the abattoir. Pathogen-reduction strategies on the farm include feed withdrawal to empty the gut and thus minimize fecal contamination of the carcass. Birds off feed will peck litter and may drink water to excess, increasing the rate of fecal contamination during processing. Inadequate feed withdrawal may result in birds being transported to the slaughter facility with excessive feed and feces in their intestine. An increase in intestinal contents of the caged bird during transportation to and holding at the abattoir increases the probability that the intestine may rupture during the evisceration, thereby contaminating the carcass. However, feed withdrawal, while lowering intestinal contents, decreases volatile fatty acids (increases the intestinal pH), which favor proliferation of *Salmonella* (Hinton et al., 2000a,b), and increases the contamination of the crop with *Salmonella* and *Campylobacter* (Smith and Berrang, 2006).

Crating Personnel chase, crate, and load turkeys onto live-haul trucks. This excites the birds, leading to bruising, scratching, and injury. To prevent transmission of pathogens between farms, loading equipment is disinfected between premises.

Transport Stress due to commingling and crowding further disseminates *Campylobacter* and *Salmonella*. Commingling of birds in crates as well as the crates themselves may transiently infect broilers immediately prior to slaughter. In addition, transport during rainy weather as well as transport stress may predispose to transient infections. An increase in intestinal fluid and a higher rate of fecal contamination during processing are correlated with excessive time on a truck.

Lairage Comfortable holding conditions at the holding areas at the abattoir (lairage) should minimize stress. High bird densities and high temperatures in the transport crates increase defecation and subsequent fecal contamination of the birds. Wind protection in winter and adequate water and ventillation in summer minimize stress during holding.

Feed withdrawal, crating, transport, and lairage at the abattoir have no effect on the prevalence of *Salmonella* in turkeys (Rostagno et al., 2006; Wesley et al., 2005a,b). *Salmonella* prevalence on-farm (33%) was identical to that of birds slaughtered after catching, crating, transport, and lairage at a commercial turkey establishment (33%) (Rostagno et al., 2006). In contrast, these identical perimarketing events were associated with shifts in the population of *Campylobacter jejuni* and *Campylobacter coli* pre- and post-transport (Wesley et al., 2005c).

House Sanitation Between flocks, the vacated turkey house is thoroughly cleaned, disinfected, the upper layer of the litter removed, and clean litter applied (top-dressed). Because of cost, disposal issues, and other considerations, complete litter removal after each flock is not practiced in the United States. However, it has been demonstrated that complete litter removal and fumigation of broiler houses in Sweden eliminated *Campylobacter* (Berndtson, 1996).

8.3.3 In-Plant Interventions

Hazard Analysis Critical Control Points HACCP systems were implemented by large poultry establishments on January 26, 1998. Each phase of current slaughter practices, from shackling to immersion in the chiller tank, provides opportunities for dissemination of microbial foodborne pathogens as well as spoilage organisms (Barbut, 2001; McNamara, 1997).

Dressing After resting (lairage), birds are unloaded from transport crates, shackled, stunned, exsanguinated, and scalded (4 min, 50 to 58°C) to facilitate defeathering (Fig. 6). Scalding may cross-contaminate carcass surfaces. Microbes that survive scalding may be more difficult to remove during later stages of processing, due to the selection of a more robust population. Similarly, the mechanical rubber fingers of the feather picker and equipment used for mechanical evisceration may transfer bacterial foodborne pathogens from one carcass to another. *Salmonella* and *Campylobacter*, which colonize the exposed deep feather follicles, are protected from disinfectants.

Evisceration The vent is opened, internal organs removed, and gizzards, liver, heart, and testicles may be harvested. Whereas the broiler industry has mechanized the evisceration process, turkeys are eviscerated manually.

After evisceration, carcasses pass through a chlorinated spray wash and enter a chlorinated chiller, where body temperatures drop to 40°F (4°C). Addition of chlorine to the chiller reduces *Salmonella* and *Campylobacter* (Corry and Atabay, 2001). However, cooling of carcasses by immersion in chiller may cross-contaminate carcasses. Therefore, critical control points (CCPs) for the chiller water include maintaining effective temperature, pH, antimicrobial concentrations, flow rate, and low levels of organic material. To illustrate, *Listeria* survives in water with low levels of chlorination, as shown in studies in Sweden in which *Listeria* was recovered from 58% of broilers immersed in chiller tanks with inconsistent chlorine levels (2 to 15 ppm) compared with 0% of carcasses in immersed in chiller tanks, which consistently measured 10 ppm of free available chlorine (Loncarevic et al., 1994).

Irradiation, steam pasteurization, and crust freezing are alternatives to immersion of carcasses in the chlorinated chiller (James et al., 2007). Freezing is a major CCP and reduces *Campylobacter* on carcasses originating from known contaminated flocks (Lindqvist and Lindblad, 2008). However, the consumer's preference for fresh, nonfrozen poultry may have resulted in increased cases of campylobacteriosis in Iceland (Stern et al., 2003).

Cross-contamination occurs during processing and may be attributed to (1) spillage of gut ingesta onto the carcass during evisceration, (2) abattoir workers handling of carcasses, (3) contaminated knives, (4) aerosol contamination, and (5) immersion in the chiller. Since birds are shackled upside down during processing, wings (30% *Salmonella* positive) are more readily contaminated than drumsticks (17% *Salmonella* positive) (Plummer et al., 1995). In the United States, line speeds of about 70 to 90 birds per minute will contribute to cross-contamination. The interval from

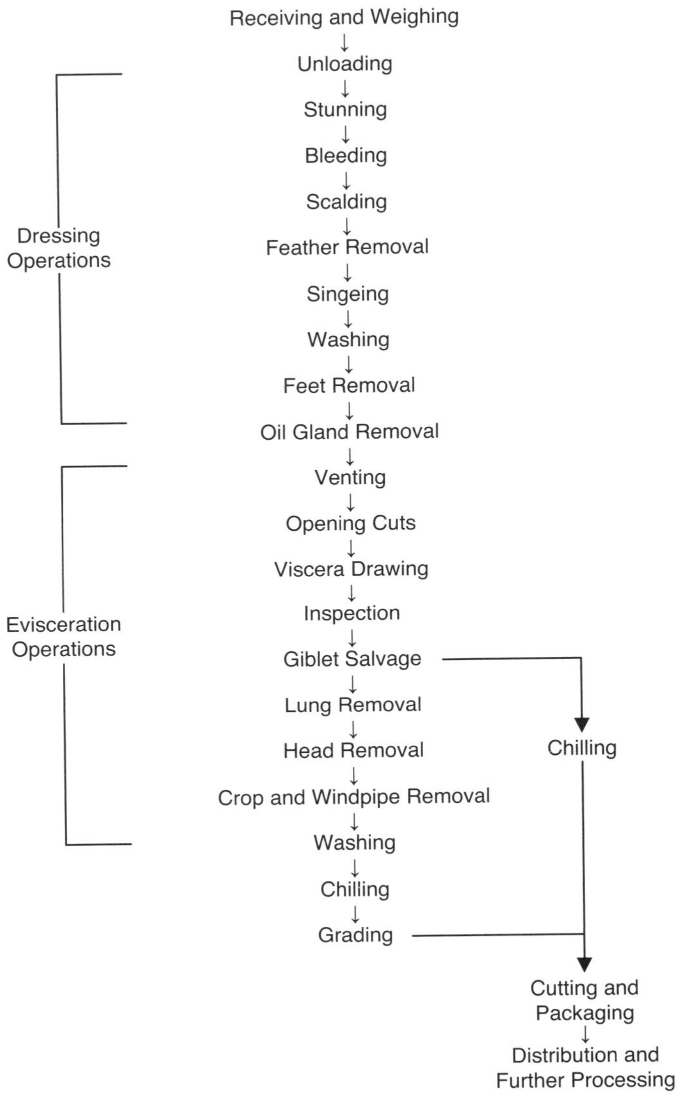

FIG. 6 Poultry processing flowchart. (From Barbut, 2001, with permission.)

time of shackling to exiting the chiller is approximately 3 h for turkeys slaughtered commercially.

Further Processing Cooled carcasses are butchered for retail purchase as fresh meat, frozen, or sent to the cooking area and prepared as precooked or ready-to-eat (RTE) product. To eliminate recontamination of the finished product, some poultry processors deliver the cooked product off-site for slicing. In the past, extensive handling transferred bacterial pathogens, such as *Listeria*, from the plant environment to meat during processing (Genigeorgis et al., 1990). In an earlier evaluation of a turkey frank facility, the post-peeling conveyor belt was contaminated with *L. monocytogenes* of the identical genotype that caused a listeriosis fatality attributed to consumption of turkey franks produced at that site (Wenger et al., 1990). Contamination of cooked products by faulty ventilation systems may have compromised delicatessen meats incriminated in a later multistate listeriosis outbreak. Strict adherence to HACCP plans has significantly reduced post-cooking contamination. Since there is zero tolerance for *L. monocytogenes* in ready-to-eat products, processing plants have implemented state-of-the-art cutting rooms, which rival surgical suites in sanitation for slicing cooked meat to avoid contamination with *L. monocytogenes.*

HACCP in-plant intervention strategies target reduction of spoilage and bacterial foodborne pathogens in RTE products. A program of verification, record maintenance, and contingency planning monitors and controls critical points (Buchanan and Whiting, 1998), especially when it addresses the cooking, smoking, pickling, and canning process. Any deviation in time and temperature control compromises the safety of the RTE poultry product. Microbial testing ensures that all means of contamination have been identified, monitored, and are being controlled (Kvenberg and Schwalm, 2000).

Plant Environment Ventilation, air-handling systems, and worker movements also disseminate foodborne bacterial pathogens. To lower the risk associated with airborne product contamination, air movement is directed from the finished product to the live bird area. In studies of airborne microbes in commercial processing plants, *Campylobacter* were recovered in air samples taken from defeathering (21 CFU/15 ft^3) and evisceration (8 CFU/15 ft^3) areas, but not in air samples collected in postevisceration locations (Whyte et al., 2001). Worker movements are restricted to prevent cross-contamination between evisceration and cutting/packaging areas. Good manufacturing practice guidelines address personal hygiene practices of employees (see Chapter 20).

Biofilms Aggregation in biofilms in the plant and attachment to the skin, especially feather follicles, enhances the resistance of bacteria to disinfectants, including chlorine, compared with the sensitivity of unattached suspended microbes in pure culture (Joseph et al., 2001; Kumar and Ananed, 1998). *Salmonella* and *Campylobacter* form biofilms on plastic as well as stainless steel surfaces. Although *Campylobacter* survives in biofilms, this microbe, unlike *Salmonella*, cannot replicate on poultry carcasses or on contact surfaces present in the slaughterhouse.

Additional Pathogen Reduction Strategies Significant improvement occurs when clean birds (*Campylobacter*- and *Salmonella*-free) are slaughtered before contaminated birds, as is practiced in Scandinavia. A further reduction of bacterial food-borne pathogens is achieved by freezing carcasses from known contaminated flocks (Lindqvist and Lindblad, 2008). The lower market price for frozen versus fresh poultry is a major incentive for the producer to provide *Campylobacter*-free birds in Scandinavia. Multiple hurdles may be needed. To illustrate, campylobacteriosis cases declined significantly in Iceland following consumer education, reinitiating the freezing of carcasses originating from known *Campylobacter*-contaminated flocks, heightened on-farm biosecurity and possibly climate conditions (Stern et al., 2003). In the Netherlands, Campylobacter Risk Management and Assessment (CARMA) is a multidisciplinary project to integrate information from risk assessments, epidemiology, and economics. It has provided an extensive cost–benefit analysis for reduction of *Campylobacter* from the farm through slaughter (Havelaar et al., 2007). In analyzing broiler production, CARMA summarized that although theoretically possible, attaining *Campylobacter*-free birds is unrealistic in the short term, despite aggressive on-farm practices. Thus the emphasis is on processing and consumer education. Interestingly, although chemical decontamination of carcasses is not practiced in the EU, CARMA calculates that it is less expensive than either freezing or heat treatment.

Industry-initiated HACCP strategies in place at the processing plant may be correlated with the decline in human campylobacteriosis (Stern and Robach, 2003). Pre- and post-slaughter data collected in 1995 prior to implementation of HACCP were compared with data obtained in 2001. *Campylobacter* counts on-farm in chicken feces were comparable at both sampling intervals (ca. 10^5 CFU/g). However, the levels of *Campylobacter* on broiler carcasses exiting the chiller in 2001 (3.03 $\log_{10}$ CFU/g) were lower than 1995 estimates (4.11 $\log_{10}$ CFU/g). This indicates the cost-effectiveness of bacterial pathogen reduction during processing.

Plant Sanitation HACCP guidelines address cleaning and sanitizing of the processing facilities. Proper usage of detergents and sanitizers ensures that product contact surfaces are clean. Sanitation can only be accomplished on surfaces free of organic material at the optimal concentration of sanitizers, applied at the correct temperature for the correct time interval. The modern poultry plant allocates an entire 8-h shift to cleanup at the end of the processing day.

8.3.4 Distribution and Consumption

USDA-FSIS uses advertisements and labels to educate the consumer on proper storage, transportation, cooking, and holding of meat and poultry products. To further protect consumers, the USDA requires safe-handling instructions on packages of raw or partially cooked meat and poultry product.

8.3.5 Consumer Awareness

The Partnership for Food Safety Education was formed in 1997 as a part of the National Food Safety Initiative. The Partnership—composed of industry, state, and consumer organizations and government liaisons from FDA, FSIS, Cooperative State Research, Education, and Extension Service (CSREES), CDC, and EPA—cooperatively developed the consumer-friendly FightBAC campaign (www.fightbac.org).

The messages are based on four key food safety practices:

1. *Clean*: Wash hands and surfaces often.
2. *Separate*: Don't cross-contaminate.
3. *Cook*: Cook to proper temperatures.
4. *Chill*: Refrigerate promptly.

Cross-contamination during food preparation can be averted by consumer education as well as by improved kitchen hygiene and rinsing of raw food items (Mylius et al., 2007). For example, *Campylobacter* is transmitted from raw poultry to utensils and chopping boards, which are then used to prepare to clean foods. Dining at home may actually lower the risk of campylobacteriosis. To illustrate, Hawaii has the highest infection rate of *Campylobacter* in the United States (69/100,000 population). Interestingly, a case–control study revealed that consuming ready-to-eat chicken out of the home is a significant risk factor, whereas eating chicken prepared at home is a protective factor (Effler et al., 2001). This demonstrates the need to educate food handlers on the need to cook poultry thoroughly, to keep raw and cooked food separate, and to avoid recontamination of poultry after cooking (Effler et al., 2001).

8.4 CONCLUSIONS

To minimize the risk of foodborne illness associated with poultry consumption, microbial pathogens must be properly controlled. Intervention programs at the production (day-of-hatch bird to market-weight bird), distribution, and consumer levels must be in place, monitored to determine their effectiveness and continuously improved. Future initiatives in the poultry sector will continue to yield microbiologically safe, wholesome, and high-quality poultry to the global customer.

Acknowledgments

We are indebted to the National Turkey Federation for providing us with their best management practices for the production of turkeys.

REFERENCES

Bailey JS, Stern NJ, Cox NA (2000): Commercial field trial evaluation of mucosal starter culture to reduce *Salmonella* incidence in processed broiler carcasses. *J Food Prot*. 63:867–870.

Barbut S (2001): *Poultry Products Processing: An Industry Guide*. CRC Press, Boca Raton, FL.

Berndtson E (1996): *Campylobacter* incidence on a chicken farm and the spread of *Campylobacter* during the slaughter process. *Int J Food Microbiol*. 32:35–47.

Buchanan RL, Whiting RC (1998): Risk assessment: a means for linking HACCP plans and public health. *J Food Prot*. 61:1531–1534.

CDC (Centers for Disease Control and Prevention) (2006): Preliminary FoodNet data on the incidence of infection with pathogens transmitted commonly through food—10 states, United States, 2005. *MMWR Morb Mortal Wkly Rep*. 55:392–395.

Corry JEL, Atabay HI (2001): Poultry as a source of *Campylobacter* and related organisms. *Soc Appl Microbiol Symp Ser*. 30 (90):96S–114S.

Cox NA, Berrang ME, Cason JA (2000): *Salmonella* penetration of egg shells and proliferation in broiler hatching eggs: a review. *Poult Sci*. 79:1571–1574.

Effler P, Long MC, Kimura A, et al. (2001): Sporadic *Campylobacter jejuni* infections in Hawaii: associations with prior antibiotic use and commercially prepared chicken. *J Infect Dis*. 183:1152–1155.

Genigeorgis CA, Oanca P, Dutulescu D (1990): Prevalence of *Listeria* spp. in turkey meat at the supermarket and slaughterhouse level. *J Food Prot*. 53:282–288.

Havelaar AH, Mangen MJ, de Koeijer AA, et al. (2007): Effectiveness and efficiency of controlling *Campylobacter* on broiler chicken meat. *Risk Anal*. 27:831–844.

Hinton A, Buhr RJ, Ingram KD (2000a): Physical, chemical, and microbiological changes in the ceca of broiler chickens subjected to incremental feed withdrawal. *Poult Sci*. 79:483–488.

——— (2000b): Reduction of *Salmonella* in the crop of broiler chickens subjected to feed withdrawal. *Poult Sci*. 79:1566–1570.

Hoffman S, Fischbeck P, Krupnick A, McWilliam M (2007): Using expert elicitation to link foodborne illnesses in the United States to foods. *J Food Prot*. 70:1220–1229.

Humphrey T, O'Brien S, Madsen M (2007): Campylobacters as zoonotic pathogens: a food production perspective. *Int J Food Microbiol*. 117(3):237–257.

Jacobs-Reitsma W (2000): *Campylobacter* in the food supply. In: Nachamkin I, Blaser MJ (Eds.). *Campylobacter*, 2nd ed. ASM Press, New York, pp. 467–482.

James C, James SJ, Hannay N, et al. (2007): Decontamination of poultry carcasses using steam or hot water in combination with rapid cooling, chilling, or freezing of carcass surfaces. *Int J Food Microbiol*. 114:195–203.

Joseph B, Ota WSK, Karunasagar I, Karunasagar I (2001): Biofilm formation by *Salmonella* spp. on food contact surfaces and their sensitivity to sanitizers. *Int J Food Microbiol*. 64:357–372.

Kumar C, Ananed SK (1998): Significance of microbial biofilms in food industry: a review. *Int J Food Microbiol*. 412:9–27.

Kvenberg JE, Schwalm DJ (2000): Use of microbial data for hazard analysis and critical control point verification—Food and Drug Administration perspective. *J Food Prot*. 63:810–814.

Lindqvist R, Lindblad M (2008): Quantitative risk assessment of thermophilic *Campylobacter* spp. and cross-contamination during handling of raw broiler chickens: evaluating strategies at the producer level to reduce human campylobacteriosis in Sweden. *Int J Food Microbiol*. 1221:41–52.

Line JE, Bailey JS, Stern NJ, Tompkins TA (1998): Effect of yeast-supplemented feed on *Salmonella* and *Campylobacter* populations in broilers. *Poult Sci*. 77:405–410.

Loncarevic S, Tham W, Danielsson-Tham ML (1994): Occurrence of *Listeria* species in broilers pre- and post-chilling in chlorinated water at two slaughterhouses. *Acta Vet Scand*. 35:149–154.

Mallinson ET, Myint MS, Johnson YJ, Branton SL, Gdamu N, Harter-Dennis JM (2004): Airflow at the litter/manure surface: a key HACCP consideration. In *Proc. Annual Meeting of the U.S. Animal Health Association*, Greensboro, NC, October 24–27.

McNamara AM (1997): Generic HACCP application in broiler slaughter and processing. *J Food Prot*. 60:579–604.

Meyerholz DK, Stabel TJ, Ackermann MR, Carlson SA, Jones BD, Pohlenz J (2002): Early epithelial invasion by *Salmonella enterica* serovar Typhimurium DT 104 in the swine ileum. *Vet Pathol*. 39 (6):712–720.

Miller WG, Mandrell RE (2005): Prevalence of *Campylobacter* in the food and water supply: Incidence, Outbreaks, Isolation, and Detection. In: Ketley J, Konkel ME (Eds.). Campylobacter: *Molecular and Cellular Biology*. Horizon Bioscience, Norfolk, UK, pp. 101–164.

Morningstar-Flugrad B (2006): Report of the Committee on *Salmonella:* the National Veterinary Services Laboratory Report. In *Proc. Annual Meeting of the U.S. Animal Health Association*, Mineapolis, MN, pp. 564–570.

Mylius SD, Nauta MJ, Havelaar AE (2007): Cross-contamination during food preparation: a mechanistic model applied to chicken-borne *Campylobacter*. *Risk Anal*. 27:803–813.

Newell DG, Frost JA, Duim B, et al. (2000): *Campylobacter*, 2nd ed. ASM Press, Washington, DC, pp. 27–44.

NTF (National Turkey Federation) (1999): *Food Safety: Best Management Practices for the Production of Turkeys*, 2nd ed. Hoffmann-LaRoche, Washington, DC.

Plummer RAS, Blissett SJ, Dodd CER (1995): *Salmonella* contamination of retail chicken products sold in the UK. *J Food Prot*. 58:843–846.

Rostagno MH, Wesley IV, Trampel DW, Hurd HS (2006): *Salmonella* prevalence in market-age turkeys on farm and at slaughter. *Poult Sci*. 85:1838–1842.

Sahin O, Luo N, Huang S, Zhang Q (2003): Effect of *Campylobacter*-specific maternal antibodies on *Campylobacter jejuni* colonization in young chickens. *Appl Environ Microbiol*. 69:5372–5379.

Smith DP, Berrang ME (2006): Prevalence and numbers of bacteria in broiler crop and gizzard contents. *Poult Sci*. 85:144–147.

Stern NJ, Robach MC (2003): Enumeration of *Campylobacter* spp. in broiler feces and in corresponding processed carcasses. *J Food Prot*. 66:1557–1563.

Stern NJ, Hiett KL, Alfredsson GA, et al. (2003): *Campylobacter* spp. in Icelandic poultry operations and human disease. *Epidemiol Infect*. 130:23–32.

USDA-ARS (U.S. Department of Agriculture–Agriculture Research Service) (2007): Food Availability (also known as U.S. Food Supply Data, or Disappearance Data). http://www.ers.usda.gov/data/foodconsumption/. Accessed February 2008.

USDA-FSIS (U.S. Department of Agriculture–Food Safety Inspection Service) (continuously updated-a): FSIS Recall. http://www.fsis.usda.gov/FSIS%5FRecalls/. Accessed February 2008.

——— (continuously updated-b): Baseline Data. http://www.fsis.usda.gov/Science/Baseline_Data/index.asp. Accessed March 2008.

USDHHS (U.S. Department of Health and Human Services) (continuously updated): Healthy People 2010. http://www.healthypeople.gov/Data/. Accessed February 2008.

Wenger JD, Swaminathan B, Hayes PS, et al. (1990): *Listeria monocytogenes* contamination of turkey franks: evaluation of a production facility. *J Food Prot*. 53:1015–1019.

Wesley IV, Harbaugh E, Trampel D, Rivera F, Hurd HS (2005a): The effect of perimarketing events on the prevalence of *Salmonella* in market weight turkeys. *J Food Prot*. 69:1785–1793.

Wesley IV, Hurd HS, Muraoka WT, Harbaugh E, Trampel D (2005b): The effect of transport and holding on *Salmonella* and *Campylobacter*. *World Poult*. 21:28–30

Wesley IV, Muraoka WT, Trampel DW, Hurd HS (2005c): The effect of perimarketing events on the prevalence of *Campylobacter jejuni* and *Campylobacter coli* in market-weight turkeys. *Appl Environ Microbiol*. 71:2824–2831.

Whyte P, Collins JD, McGill K, Monahan C, O'Mahony H (2001): Distribution and prevalence of airborne microorganisms in three commercial poultry processing plants. *J Food Prot*. 64:388–391.

Young KT, Davis LM, Dirita VJ (2007): *Campylobacter jejuni*: molecular biology and pathogenesis. *Nat Rev Microbiol*. 5:665–679.

CHAPTER 9

FOOD SAFETY ISSUES AND THE MICROBIOLOGY OF EGGS AND EGG PRODUCTS

JEAN-YVES D'AOUST

9.1 SHELL EGG DEVELOPMENT AND STRUCTURE

The vertically integrated poultry industry rests on grandparent (primary) breeder lineages to produce commercially valuable avian progenies (Fig. 1). The genetic cross of primary breeder birds leads to multiplier breeders whose hatchlings develop into commercial egg layer (table eggs) or broiler (meat) birds. Selection criteria for commercial egg layer hens include the number, size, and shell quality of eggs as well as feed conversion ratios and vigor of layer hen populations. The egg production period of a commercial layer hen spans from 20 to 80 weeks of age, during which time the hen produces approximately 260 eggs. The avian egg ensures the successful propagation of the species by providing a protective and highly nutritive environment during embryogenesis and contributes to the pre-hatching development of chick embryos. The dynamics of egg formation are of singular interest (Board and Fuller, 1994). During its migration from the ovary to the cloaca, the ovule is surrounded progressively by a yolk mass and then engulfed in aqueous albumen separated from the yolk by a semipermeable vitelline membrane. Two membrane structures (Fig. 2) form around the albumen as it migrates through the isthmus region of the oviduct. The innermost membrane encases the albumen, whereas the outer membrane provides the template for calcium carbonate deposition and shell formation at the level of the tubular shell gland of the oviduct. At oviposition, the formed shell egg comes into contact with the opening of the digestive tract at the level of the cloaca, where the propensity for fecal contamination of the external eggshell surface is high. The egg then undergoes several important physical changes, including the rapid maturation of the moist surface cuticle from a fragile to a more rigid and protective structure, a slow transfer of water from the albumen into the yolk, which relocates within the egg mass because

Microbiologically Safe Foods, Edited by Norma Heredia, Irene Wesley, and Santos García

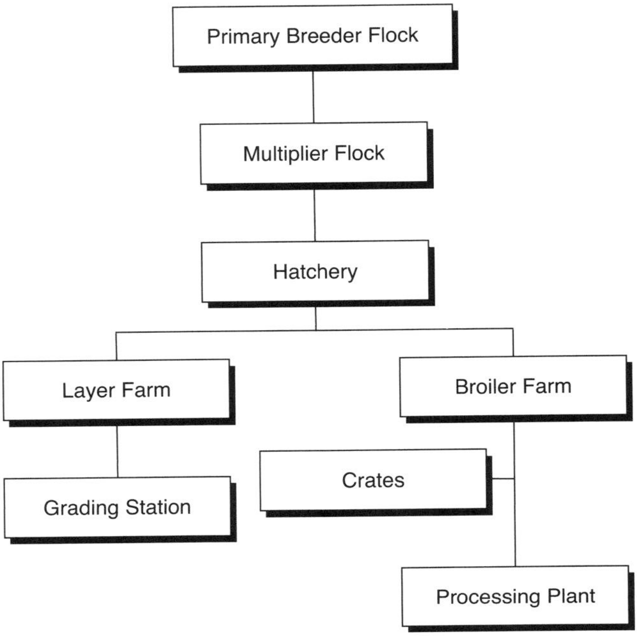

FIG. 1 Overview of the chicken industry

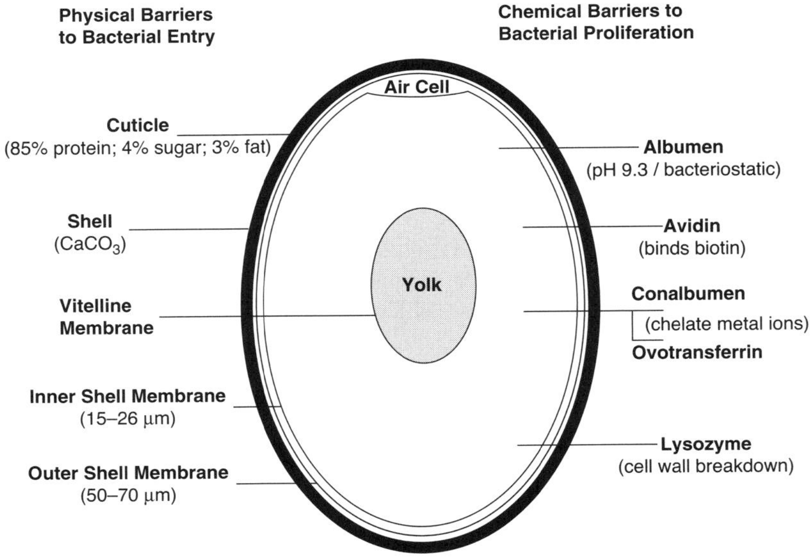

FIG. 2 Physical and chemical barriers to bacterial entry and proliferation in eggs. [Adapted from *Commun. Dis. Public Health* (1998), 1: 150–160, with permission from Health Protection Agency, London.]

of its reduced density, enlargement of the air cell located at the blunt pole of the shell egg, where significant evaporative and diffusive loss of albumen water occurs, and a significant change in the pH of albumen from approximately 7.2 in a freshly laid egg to 9.5 in stored shell eggs attributable to the loss of carbon dioxide from the egg interior.

Several structural features protect the egg against trans-shell migration of microorganisms (Board and Fuller, 1994; Mayes and Takeballi, 1983). The egg cuticle, which does not always cover the entire shell surface, is a thin, highly fissured layer of glycoprotein that provides the outermost physical line of defense against bacterial penetration and entry of water into the egg interior. The thickness and structural integrity of the cuticle decreases with increasing flock age and is adversely affected by the storage of eggs at elevated temperatures. Consequently, eggs from older layer flocks are more susceptible to internal bacterial contamination. On-farm cleaning of soiled egg surfaces with mild abrasives is generally discouraged because this practice removes the protective cuticle and potentiates the occlusion of pore canals with contaminated debris and migration of bacterial pathogens into the egg interior. The calcitic eggshell below the cuticle consists of four closely apposed structural layers, including the prominent spongiform palisade layer. The ability of egg surface contaminants such as *Pseudomonas* and *Salmonella* spp. to penetrate intact eggshells varies inversely with the thickness and the specific gravity of the shell commensurate with nutritional, genetic, and environmental determinants.

Pore canals, which facilitate gaseous exchange between the egg interior and the external environment, occur randomly in eggshells but notably in high numbers in the blunt pole of the eggshell. Water films or condensate on the surface of eggshells greatly increase the propensity for bacterial translocation through pore canals. Interestingly, the number of pore canals increases with aging of the layer flock. Hairline shell fractures favor the entry of spoilage and human pathogenic bacteria into the egg interior, thereby reducing the shelf life and safety of the product. Below the eggshell lie the closely apposed outer and inner shell membranes, which follow the contour of the shell except in the blunt region of the egg, where both membranes separate to enclose the air space (Fig. 2). The outer fibrous membrane (50 to 70 μm) is porous and closely applied to the inner surface of the eggshell, whereas the inner fibrous membrane (15 to 26 μm) intermeshed with a particulate limiting membrane (2.5 to 4.6 μm) defines the external boundary of the albumen (Liong et al., 1997). The paucity of pores and tight fiber configuration in the inner membrane confirm this layer as being the most effective surface barrier to bacterial penetration. Prolonged storage of shell eggs at temperatures favorable to bacterial growth engenders the structural deterioration of shell and vitelline membranes and the inactivation of antibacterial agents in the albumen. These conditions predispose the egg to deep bacterial penetration and growth using iron and nutrients released from the yolk through a damaged vitelline membrane.

Notwithstanding the various scenarios for trans-shell bacterial contamination of the egg interior, transovarian transmission of *Salmonella* spp. is well documented and recognized as a major contributing factor to the ongoing human pandemic of *Salmonella* Enteritidis, which was first recognized in England in 1984–1985.

The incidence of *S*. Enteritidis in egg layer flocks has ranged from 0.1 to 1.0% in multiplier and commercial egg layer flocks infected with *S*. Enteritidis phage type 4 (Humphrey, 1994). It is notable that other *Salmonella* serovars, including *S*. Gallinarum, *S*. Typhimurium, *S*. Thompson, and *S*. Menston, can also infect the ovaries of layer hens and lead to internally contaminated eggs, where salmonellae cannot be removed by current egg washing practices.

Transovarian infections with *S*. Arizonae and *S*. Enteritidis have also been reported in turkeys and ducks, respectively. Transovarian-infected eggs generally occur at a frequency of 1.0×10^{-4} eggs, are laid intermittently, and contain fewer than 10 salmonellae per egg. Extensive studies have also shown that transovarian serovars target the egg albumen and/or the external surface of the vitelline membrane. Transovarian infection could also result from the migration of infective microorganisms from the avian cloaca to the proximal shell gland in the oviduct. Early studies on the infection of ovarian tissues and internal contamination of intact shell eggs following the oral inoculation of layer hens with *S*. Enteritidis reiterate the importance of *Salmonella*-free poultry feeds and stringent control of the barn environment for the abatement of *Salmonella* within the egg industry.

In addition to its structural barriers to bacterial penetration, the intact shell egg is also endowed with several endogenous defense mechanisms (Fig. 2). The viscosity of albumen impedes bacterial translocation toward the highly nutritive yolk, whereas the high pH of albumen retards or inhibits the growth of invasive microorganisms.

Development of an alkaline pH in the albumen follows from a progressive loss of CO_2 originally acquired in the oviduct. Other deterrents to bacterial growth in the egg contents (i.e., magma) include conalbumen, which chelates albumenous cationic iron and other metal ions, whereas avidin sequesters biotin. Invasive salmonellae rely on siderophores to effectively compete with egg conalbumen for the limited amounts of essential iron in the albumen. For example, the high-affinity phenolate enterochelin (also known as enterobactin) and the lower-affinity hydroxamate aerobactin play a determinant role in the growth and survival of *Salmonella* spp. in the egg albumen (D'Aoust et al., 2001). Lysozyme in the albumen effectively disrupts the peptidoglycan layer of gram-positive bacteria, resulting in bacterial cell lysis.

Commercial egg washing is used in many but not all egg-producing countries because washing potentially facilitates permeation of eggshells by human bacterial pathogens and spoilage microflora, thereby reducing the shelf life and safety of shell eggs. Technological advances have led to the widespread use of continuous egg washers consisting of three distinct chambers. In the first chamber, eggs that had been cooled from 42°C at lay to a temperature of 10 to 14°C are sprayed with potable warm water ($\geq$ 41°C) containing alkaline detergent to clean soiled egg surfaces. The use of wash water at temperatures greater than that of shell eggs entering the washer prevents a temperature-dependent contraction of the air space and creation of a negative pressure that would draw surface contaminants through the pore canals into the egg interior. The mineral content of wash water should be low because high levels of aqueous iron could neutralize the antibacterial conalbumen and predispose eggs to accelerated spoilage. Adjustment of egg wash water to a high pH is warranted because it effectively increases the thermal susceptibility of *Salmonella* spp. and other human bacterial pathogens. Eggs are given a final aqueous rinse (pH $\geq$ 10.0) containing chlorine, calcium hypochlorite, iodine, cationic quarternary ammonium, or other high-alkaline sanitizers, such as sodium metasilicate, sodium carbonate, or trisodium phosphate. Acidic cleansers are not recommended because they adversely affect the structural integrity of the eggshell. Eggs are then dried in the third chamber using streams of warm air or heat from infrared lamps. Eggs with meat or blood spots, hairline cracks, or visible surface contamination are removed before clean sanitized eggs are packaged for commercial distribution and sale.

9.2 MICROFLORA OF SHELL EGGS

Current data on the prevalence of indigenous bacterial flora on freshly laid chicken eggs are generally lacking. Total bacterial populations on eggshells reportedly range from 10^3 to 10^5 CFU under clean environmental conditions and increase to 10^7 to 10^8 CFU under poor hygienic conditions. Cleanliness of the environment at the time of lay impact the microbial load greatly, as evidenced by higher levels of surface contamination on floor eggs than on eggs laid on clean nesting material (Mayes and Takeballi, 1983). Although clean and soiled duck eggshells can harbor 10^2 and 10^5 salmonellae, respectively, current information on the numbers of salmonellae on chicken eggshells could not be located. *Salmonella* spp. can survive for up to 26 days on the surface of shell eggs stored at 28 to 35°C. The kinetics of eggshell penetration are dependent on the temperature and relative humidity of the microenvironment and on the nature of the bacterial contaminant. Surface bacterial contaminants require 10 to 15 days to penetrate eggshells and to produce visible changes in the albumen. The microflora most commonly encountered on shell egg surfaces is not always associated with egg spoilage (Table 1). The propensity for members of the

TABLE 1 Indigenous Eggborne Microflora

Bacteria	Relative Frequency	
	Eggshell Surface	Spoiled Egg Meat
Micrococcus spp.	+++	+
Achromobacter spp.	++	+
Alcaligenes spp.	++	+++[a]
Enterobacter spp.	++	+[a]
Escherichia spp.	++	+++
Flavobacterium spp.	++	+
Pseudomonas spp.	++	+++[a,b]
Staphylococcus spp.	++	−
Proteus spp.	+	+++

Source: Adapted from Board RG and Tranter HS, *The Microbiology of Eggs*, 4th ed., Chap. 5, with permission from The Haworth Press, Binghamton, NY.
[a]Produces black rot.
[b]Produces pink or green rot.

Pseudomonas, Alcaligenes, Escherichia, and *Proteus* genera to engender spoilage and to produce characteristic rots confirms their ability to penetrate the eggshell and to metabolize components of the egg magma. The absence of egg spoilage by gram-positive organisms probably reflects their sensitivity to albumenous lysozyme.

Although *Campylobacter* spp. are frequently associated with broiler birds, the persistence of this human bacterial pathogen on the eggshell surface is distinctly short (<48 h) at room temperature. The fate of *Campylobacter* is modulated by the water activity (a_w) at the egg surface and by the low tolerance of the organism to atmospheric oxygen. Nonetheless, isolated studies have reported incidence levels of <1.6% on shell eggs, some of which were visibly contaminated with fecal material. Although campylobacters are particularly sensitive to the antibacterial agents in egg albumen, the organism can penetrate the eggshell under ideal environmental conditions. *C. jejuni* grows slowly in egg yolk and in homogenized whole egg held at 37°C but is rapidly inactivated in these foods at 20°C (Board and Fuller, 1994). Information on the ecology of *Listeria* spp. in eggs and egg products is generally lacking. However, in a study of 11 processing establishments across the United States in 1987–1988, *L. monocytogenes* was isolated from 4.8% of 42 liquid whole egg samples. In a subsequent study in the United Kingdom (Moore and Madden, 1993), *L. monocytogenes* was isolated from 27.2% in-line filters used to remove shell fragments from liquid whole eggs. The organism survives for several hours in wash water held at pH 10.5 and 42°C, and for up to 90 days on shell eggs stored at 5 to 10°C. *Listeria* spp. grow in whole liquid egg stored at refrigerator temperatures and in heat-treated (121°C, 15 min) albumen, yolk, and liquid whole egg within hours of storage at 20°C, and after 10 to 15 days storage at 5°C (Sionkowski and Shelef, 1990). The pathogen also survives spray drying during the manufacture of egg powder (Brackett and Beuchat, 1991).

Yersinia enterocolitica can penetrate and infect shell eggs. The tolerance of this organism to the high pH of egg wash water coupled with its psychrotrophy favors the survival of this human pathogen on the surface of refrigerated shell eggs and potentiates its involvement in human eggborne diseases. Authoritative reviews on egg structure and on the bacterial ecology of shell eggs by Board and Fuller (1994) and in *Microorganisms in Food* (ICMSF, 2005) are recommended as additional readings.

A nonexhaustive literature review on the prevalence of *Salmonella* spp. in chicken layer flocks and in table eggs is revealing (Table 2). The prominence of salmonellae in commercial layer flocks and their barn environment probably stems from the placement of infected replacement stocks in sanitized barns, provision of contaminated feeds and drinking water, access of infected rodents and insects into the barn environment, and human translocation of contaminated soil into barns (Board and Fuller, 1994). Propagation of salmonellae is further amplified by high bird densities maintained in barns and by avian behavioral patterns. Such conditions frequently lead to intestinal colonization of fowl, which remain asymptomatic carriers of *Salmonella* and other human bacterial pathogens. The incidence of shell eggs internally contaminated with *Salmonella* spp. occurs at a frequency of less than 3% (Table 2). It is noteworthy that salmonellae do not alter the organoleptic attributes of shell eggs, whose intact appearance conceals the presence of a potential health hazard to unsuspecting consumers. The high level of internal contamination of eggs from Germany (11.4%) was reported for eggs implicated in a major human outbreak of salmonellosis.

TABLE 2 Incidence of *Salmonella* in Chicken Layer Flocks and Table Eggs

Country	Number Tested	Percent Positive
Layer flocks		
Canada (ca. 1991)	295	52.9 (fecal/eggbelt)
Germany (1993)	2,112	13.7 (ceca/liver/spleen)
United States (1991)	406	86.5 (ceca)
United States (ca. 1995)	50	72.0 (environment)
Poland (1996–1998)	714	8.8 (environment)
Table eggs		
Canada (ca. 1995)	16,560	0.06 (content)
Canada (1996)	252[a]	0.4 (shell/content)
Denmark (1995)	14,800	0.1 (shell/content)
France (ca. 1990)	519	2.3 (shell/content)
Germany (1990)	70[b]	11.4 (content)
India (ca. 1993)	102	4.9 (shell)/0.9 (yolk)
Japan (1998)	213	3.3 (shell/content)
Northern Ireland (1996–1997)	2,090[a]	0.38 (shell)/0.05 (content)
Thailand (1991–1992)	744	13.2 (shell)/3.9 (content)
United States (1994)	647,000	0.03 (content)
The Netherlands (2005)	36[c]	13.9 (whole egg)
Duck eggs		
Thailand (1992)	564	12.4 (shell)/11.0 (content)

Source: Adapted from D'Aoust JY, *The Microbiological Safety and Quality of Food,* Vol. II, Chap. 45, with permission from Springer-Verlag GmbH.
[a]Pools of 6 shell eggs were examined.
[b]Eggs from sources associated with outbreaks of human salmonellosis.
[c]Pools of 20 shell eggs from a single producer were examined.

The similarly high incidence of internally contaminated eggs from Thailand probably resulted from the ubiquity of salmonellae in the natural environment and from animal husbandry practices in this country.

Salmonella Enteritidis can multiply rapidly in egg magma to levels of 10^9 CFU when eggs are stored for 24 h at optimal growth temperatures. Storage of shell eggs for lengthy periods of time at elevated temperatures accelerate the natural breakdown of constitutive antimicrobial barriers within shell eggs. Storage of shell eggs below 10°C retards the growth of eggborne spoilage and pathogenic bacterial contaminants and preserves the functional integrity of endogenous bacterial defense mechanisms.

9.3 SIGNIFICANCE OF THE DETECTION OF *SALMONELLA*

The prominence of *Salmonella* spp. as the principal etiologic agent associated with shell eggs and egg products predicates a need to review aspects of cultural and automated methods for the detection of foodborne salmonellae. The use of a statistically significant food sampling plan and a sensitive method for the detection of salmonellae is paramount for reliable test results. Clearly, the collection of multiple random sample units from a lot of food (i.e., 10×100 g sample units) will more accurately establish the bacteriological status of that lot than if a single 1.0-kg sample unit were withdrawn. The potential human health hazard associated with product abuse during processing and consumer handling determines the stringency of the sampling plan, which may require the collection of 5 to 60 replicate sample units per lot. Although an analytical unit of 25 g is generally specified in standard methods of analysis, the use of larger analytical units will increase method sensitivity. Standard culture methods for the detection of foodborne salmonellae typically include five distinct steps (D'Aoust, 2000).

Pre-enrichment of analytical units in a nonselective broth medium such as buffered peptone water, lactose, or nutrient broths for 18 to 24 h at 35 to 37°C ensures the resuscitation of stressed or injured salmonellae arising from abrupt temperature shifts during food processing and from prolonged storage or exposure to adverse environmental conditions, including extreme pH conditions, low water activity, and bacteriostatic agents. It is critical that all test materials, regardless of the known or suspected levels of background microflora, be pre-enriched in a nonselective broth medium. Natural antibacterial agents in foods need to be neutralized at the pre-enrichment step to ensure the successful recovery of *Salmonella* spp. For example, the use of skim milk broth for the pre-enrichment of cocoa and chocolate products is predicated on the ability of milk casein to effectively neutralize inhibitory anthocyanins in cocoa. Similarly, 0.5% K_2SO_3 (w/v) added to tryptic soy broth neutralizes endogenous propyl disulfides in onion and garlic powder. The potential impact of bactericidal and bacteriostatic compounds in cinnamon, allspice, cloves, and oregano is negated by using a food sample/pre-enrichment broth ratio of 1 : 20 and greater to dilute endogenous food toxicants (D'Aoust and Purvis, 1998; USDA, 2004).

For selective enrichment, replicate portions from individual pre-enrichment cultures are generally enriched for 18 to 24 h in two of the following broth media: tetrathionate brilliant green ($TBG_{35\text{-}43°C}$), selenite cystine ($SC_{35°C}$), or Rappaport–Vassiliadis ($RV_{41\text{-}43°C}$). The wide range of selective agents found in enrichment media and incubation of these media at elevated temperatures (41 to 43°C) synergistically repress endogenous competitive microflora to facilitate the subsequent recovery of *Salmonella* spp. on plating media. Direct suspension of test materials with high levels of background microflora in selective enrichment broth media (direct enrichment) once figured prominently in standard methods. Proponents of this analytical approach pointed to the benefits of early selective inactivation of background microorganisms to encourage a copious growth of *Salmonella* spp. through reduced bacterial competition for organic and inorganic nutrients. Cumulative reports on the low sensitivity of direct enrichment suggested that the few stressed or injured salmonellae commonly encountered in foods were rapidly inactivated by selective (toxic) agents in enrichment media, thereby leading to false-negative results. The direct enrichment approach has now fallen into disfavor.

The changing physiology of *Salmonella* spp. and the increasing ability of this pathogen to utilize lactose and/or sucrose is gradually eroding the diagnostic reliability of saccharide-dependent differential media, including brilliant green (BGA) supplemented with sulfapyridine (BGS), xylose lysine desoxycholate (XLD), xylose lysine Tergitol 4 (XLT4), and Hektoen (Hek) agar media, which are recommended by prominent regulatory agencies in the United States (Andrews and Hammack, 2004; USDA, 2004) and by the International Organization for Standardization (ISO, 2002). The high selectivity of the saccharide-independent bismuth sulfite agar coupled with its uniquely sensitive system for the detection of bacterial H_2S justifies its prominence in standard methods of analysis. The diagnostic capabilities of the novel chromogenic BD/BBL Chrom agar (BD Diagnostic, Sparks, Maryland), Rapid'Salmonella (Bio-Rad Laboratories, Inc. Marnes-la-Coquette, France), and *Salmonella* chromogenic agar (Oxoid Limited, Basingstoke, UK) are based on C8 esterase- and β-D-galactosidase-dependent breakdown of chromogenic substrates. Although the complete formulation of these novel media remains proprietary, supplementation of these media with novobiocin, amphotericin, cefsulodin, or bile salts represses the growth of *Proteus* spp., *Candida* spp., nonfermenters, and gram-positive organisms, respectively. The performance of these novel plating media has yet to be fully evaluated.

Suspect *Salmonella* isolates on differential plating media are then screened biochemically using conventional biochemical tests or commercially available identification kits and then confirmed serologically using polyvalent and single grouping somatic and flagellar antisera. Notwithstanding the diagnostic value of complete serological characterization of *Salmonella* isolates, the discriminating powers of pulsed-field gel electrophoresis (PFGE), phage-typing, and ribotyping continue to play a vital role in the timely investigation of human foodborne outbreaks by facilitating epidemiological linkages between commonly occurring *Salmonella* serovars in suspect foods and in cases of human salmonellosis.

Standard culture methods for the detection of foodborne *Salmonella* spp. generally require 4 days to obtain evidence of the absence or presumptive presence of salmonellae in a food sample. The last decade has witnessed remarkable progress in the development of novel methods for the rapid detection of salmonellae in foods and in agricultural products. Rapid methods offer different levels of sophistication and automation and are based on enzyme-linked immunosorbent assay (ELISA), nucleic acid hybridization, conductometry, immuno-immobilization, or polymerase chain reaction (PCR) technologies. Rapid methods that generally insert at the level of preenrichment or selective enrichment in standard culture methods exhibit a threshold sensitivity of 10^4 to 10^5 salmonellae per milliliter of test culture, differ widely in their sensitivity and specificity, and provide negative or presumptive-positive results 12 to 48 h earlier than with conventional culture methods (D'Aoust, 2000; D'Aoust et al., 2001). Immuno-concentration of salmonellae in pre-enrichment broth cultures is used to increase the sensitivity of several rapid methods. The diagnostic success of rapid methods rests on the affinity of antibodies for *Salmonella*-specific somatic and flagellar antigens or on the specificity of probes and primers for unique nucleic acid targets. Although antibody-dependent systems readily detect salmonellae belonging to common somatic serogroups, many systems falter in the detection of exotic *Salmonella* serovars and produce false-positive reactions with closely related members of the *Citrobacter*, *Escherichia,* and *Enterobacter* genera.

In recent years, scientific interest has focused on PCR technologies for the presumptive identification of *Salmonella* in foods and agricultural products. In PCR-dependent assays, a *Salmonella*-specific nucleic acid sequence is repeatedly amplified by means of alternate cycles of high-temperature (ca. 95°C) denaturation of double-stranded DNA into single strands, annealing (45 to 65°C) of synthetic oligonucleotide primers to a region that flanks the targeted sequence, and replication (ca. 72°C) of the targeted sequence by a heat-stable DNA polymerase. The potential inhibition of PCR reactions by components in food matrices underlines the importance of appropriate positive and negative controls for all PCR assays. Moreover, the reliability of PCR assays can be adversely affected by large populations of background microflora in test materials, and extreme care must be exercised to prevent cross-contamination of preamplification reagents and test samples with extraneous nucleic acid during PCR analyses. The performance of the commercially available colorimetric Probelia (Sanofi Diagnostics Pasteur) and the fluorometric BAX (Dupont Qualicon), TaqMan (Perkin-ElmerBiosystems), iQ-Check (Bio-Rad Laboratories Inc.), and Genevision (Warnex Inc.) PCR systems has yet to be fully evaluated.

9.4 EGGBORNE OUTBREAKS OF HUMAN SALMONELLOSIS

The consumption of raw or lightly cooked eggs figures prominently as the cause of many human *Salmonella* infections (Table 3). Concerted efforts by food service establishments and consumers to fully cook egg-containing foods and to use pasteurized eggs in foods to be lightly cooked would greatly alleviate the human epidemiological burden of eggborne outbreaks. Traditional home preparation of mayonnaise with raw eggs is a potentially hazardous practice that could lead to acute gastrointestinal and severe systemic *Salmonella* infections as well as other chronic and debilitating diseases, such as Reiter's syndrome, aseptic reactive arthritis, and ankylosing spondylitis. *Salmonella* spp. will readily survive in raw egg mayonnaise stored at physiologically permissive temperatures, particularly if the mayonnaise was acidified with a weak organic acid such as lactic or citric acid rather than acetic acid, which is more bactericidal.

The use of raw eggs in homemade ice cream is equally hazardous and is strongly discouraged, because consumers are frequently children, who are more susceptible to *Salmonella* infections. The continued prominence of human outbreaks of *S.* Enteritidis from the consumption of raw or lightly cooked shell eggs reiterates the global public health significance of avian transovarian transmission as a cryptic disease transfer mechanism. Although salmonellae figure prominently as the principal etiological agent in human eggborne outbreaks, a rare episode of campylobacteriosis was associated with the consumption of undercooked eggs (Finch and Blake, 1985). The psychrotrophy and heat resistance of *Listeria* spp. potentiate incidents of human listeriosis from the consumption of shell eggs or liquid egg products.

TABLE 3 Major Outbreaks of Eggborne Salmonellosis

Year	Country	Vehicle	Serovar	Confirmed Cases	Deaths[a]
1984	Canada	Raw egg dessert	*S.* Typhimurium PT204	249	2
1987	China	Egg drink	*S.* Typhimurium	1,113	NS
1988	England	Raw egg mayonnaise	*S.* Typhimurium PT49	120	0
	Japan	Cooked eggs	*Salmonella* spp.	10,476	NS
1991	England	Raw egg mayonnaise	*S.* Enteritidis PT4	144	0
1992	United States	Monte Cristo sandwiches	*S.* Enteritidis PT8	74	0
1993	France	Raw egg mayonnaise	*S.* Enteritidis	751	0
	United States	Homemade ice cream	*S.* Enteritidis PT13a	12	0
1994	United States	Ice cream	*S.* Enteritidis PT8	>740	0
1995	England	Raw egg marshmallow	*S.* Enteritidis PT4	26	0
1996	Ireland	Raw egg mousse	*S.* Enteritidis PT4	>233	0
	England	Raw egg mousse	*S.* Enteritidis PT4	61	3
1997	United States	Hollandaise sauce	*S.* Enteritidis PT13a	91	0
1998	Saudi Arabia	Raw egg mayonnaise	*S.* Enteritidis	159	0
1999	Canada	Homemade ice cream	*S.* Typhimurium PT1	27	0
2000	Uruguay	Egg whites in butter	*Salmonella* spp.	588	NS
2001	United States	Tuna salad with boiled eggs	*S.* Enteritidis PT2	688	0
	Latvia	Cake/raw egg sauce	*S.* Enteritidis PT4	19	0
2002	England	Bakery products	*S.* Enteritidis PT14b	>150	1
2003	Australia	Raw egg mayonnaise	*Salmonella* spp.	>106	1
	United States	Egg salad kit	*S.* Typhimurium	18	0
2005	England	Imported shell eggs	*S.* Enteritidis PT6	68	0

Source: Adapted from D'Aoust (2000), D'Aoust et al. (2001).
[a]NS, not stated.

TABLE 4 Characteristics of Liquid Egg Products

		Composition (wt %)		
Product	pH	H_2O	Protein	Lipid
Whole egg	7.3	73.6	12.8	11.8
Albumen	9.1	87.9	10.6	Trace
Yolk	6.5	48.0	16.6	32.6

Source: Adapted from Board RG, *Adv. Appl. Microbiol.*, 11:245–281 (1969), with permission from Elsevier.

9.5 THERMAL PROCESSING OF EGG PRODUCTS

The water content in whole eggs greatly exceeds that of proteins and lipids, where much of the water resides in the albumen (Table 4). Although the protein content of egg yolk and albumen is similar, the egg yolk is notable for its high lipid content. Such compositional differences strongly affect the kinetics of thermal inactivation of *Salmonella* and other bacterial pathogens in liquid whole egg, yolk, and albumen products. Bacterial heat resistance is frequently expressed in terms of decimal reduction time (D), the amount of time required at a given temperature to effect a 1.0-$\log_{10}$ reduction in the number of viable microorganisms in a heated matrix. The thermal resistance of *Salmonella* spp. increases with decreasing water activity (a_w) of the heating menstruum, decreases as pH deviates from neutrality, and can be greatly affected by dissolved solutes. For example, the D-values for *Salmonella* spp. and *L. monocytogenes* in liquid egg yolk heated at 63.3°C increase markedly when sucrose and/or NaCl are added to liquid egg yolk (Table 5). Bacterial heat resistance can also increase with increasing growth temperatures. For example, upshifts in growth temperature from 20°C to 44.0°C increased the D_{56C} of *S.* Enteritidis phage type 4 from 0.91 min to 14.4 min, respectively (D'Aoust, 2000).

TABLE 5 Bacterial Heat Resistance and Solutes in Liquid Yolk

	Salmonella[a]		*Listeria monocytogenes*[c]	
Product	$D_{63.3°C}$ (min)	$\log_{10}$ Reduction[b]	$D_{63.3°C}$ (min)	$\log_{10}$ Reduction[b]
Egg yolk	0.20	17.5	0.81	4.32
Egg yolk + 10% sucrose	0.72	4.86	1.05	3.33
Egg yolk + 10% NaCl	11.5	0.30	10.5	0.33
Egg yolk + 10% NaCl + 5% sucrose	8.13	0.43	21.3	0.16

Source: Adapted from M.S. Palumbo et al. (1995), *J. Food Prot.*, 58:960–966, with permission from the International Association for Food Protection.
[a]Cocktail of *S.* Enteritidis, *S.* Senftenberg, and *S.* Typhimurium.
[b]USDA treatment (63.3°C for 3.5 min) using glass vials submerged in a water bath.
[c]Cocktail of five strains of *L. monocytogenes*.

Pasteurization as applied in many countries targets the elimination of *Salmonella* spp. in both liquid and dried egg products. In the United States and Canada, pasteurization hinges on a 3.5-min thermal treatment of whole egg (60.0°C), albumen (54.0 to 56.7°C), yolk (61.1°C), and yolk supplemented with 5% NaCl or 5% sucrose (63.0 to 63.3°C). Since these thermal processes result in non-shelf-stable products, pasteurized egg products need to be refrigerated (4°C) or held at or below −18°C during prolonged periods of storage. Although the pasteurization of liquid whole egg and other liquid egg products originally targeted a 9.0-$\log_{10}$ reduction of salmonellae (USDA, 1969), new pasteurization guidelines for liquid egg products target a 5.0-$\log_{10}$ reduction of salmonellae (Froning et al., 2002). In Mexico, comparable margins of product safety are assured by the thermal treatment of liquid whole eggs for 2.5 min at 64.5°C, albumen for 20 min at 55.0°C, and yolk for 6.0 min at 64.0°C. Treatment of liquid whole eggs for 3.5 min at 60.0°C provides up to a 9.0-$\log_{10}$ reduction of salmonellae, but only a modest 2.0- to 3.0-$\log_{10}$ reduction of *L. monocytogenes*. In contrast, standard pasteurization of liquid egg yolk for 3.5 min at 61.1°C is considerably more bactericidal and engenders a 21.9- and 3.9-$\log_{10}$ reduction of *Salmonella* spp. and *L. monocytogenes*, respectively (Schuman and Sheldon, 1997). Such stringent processing conditions are applied because of the vulnerability of yolks in intact shell eggs to bacterial contamination and prolific growth of salmonellae in this nutritively rich environment. Interestingly, a recent study on the standard thermal processing of liquid yolk supplemented with 10% NaCl or with 10% NaCl plus 5% sucrose at 63.3°C reported a 0.43-$\log_{10}$ reduction or less in viable *Salmonella* and *L. monocytogen*es (Palumbo et al., 1995). These findings strongly suggest that current standard pasteurization conditions would not eliminate large numbers of salmonellae in liquid yolk supplemented with 10% salt or sucrose unless the liquid yolk was pasteurized separately followed by the aseptic addition of salt and/or sugar.

The thermal susceptibility of egg white proteins and the need to preserve their native rheological properties for the manufacture of bakery products precludes pasteurization of liquid albumen at or above 56.7°C. Recent data showed that the standard pasteurization (3.5 min at 56.7°C) of liquid albumen (pH 9.3) inoculated with a cocktail of *Salmonella* strains including *S.* Enteritidis phage types 4 and 13, *S.* Typhimurium, *S.* Blockey, and *S.* Heidelberg resulted in less than a 5.0-$\log_{10}$ reduction in viable salmonellae (Froning et al., 2002). Similarly, standard pasteurization of albumen (pH 8.2) inoculated with five strains of *S.* Enteritidis and *S.* Typhimurium yielded a $D_{56.7^\circ C}$ value of 2.96 min and a corresponding 1.18 $\log_{10}$ reduction in viable salmonellae (Schuman and Sheldon, 1997). Interest in methods for the effective pasteurization of albumen at low temperatures has led to several innovative processing techniques. For example, adjustment of egg albumen to pH 6.8 to 7.3 with lactic acid together with the addition of aluminum sulfate increases the heat stability of conalbumin and other sensitive albumenous proteins, thereby enabling a nondestructive pasteurization of egg albumen at 60.0 to 61.7°C for 3.5 min. Low-temperature pasteurization of albumen for 3.5 min at 51.7°C can also be achieved by the addition of 10% H_2O_2 to reduce the heat resistance of *Salmonella* spp. In this process, liquid albumen is first heated to 51.7°C for 1.5 min, after which H_2O_2 is added and allowed to react for 2.0 min. The albumen is then cooled and the excess H_2O_2 digested with catalase.

A third method for the pasteurization of egg white utilizes a high-temperature, short-time (HTST) plate pasteurization at 57°C for 3.5 min under partial vacuum.

Three methods are used commercially to prepare dry liquid egg products. Spray drying is the preferred treatment method, where contact of finely atomized liquid egg with a stream of hot air results in the rapid evaporation of water. In the less favored pan or drum drying process, liquid egg is passed over a heated surface to evaporate the aqueous phase, whereas in the freeze-drying method water is removed from frozen egg products under partial vacuum. Spray-dried and pan-dried albumen are treated with starter cultures to remove carbohydrates, which would otherwise react with egg proteins to produce off-flavors and insoluble brown reaction products (i.e., nonenzymatic Maillard reaction). In the United States and Canada, the carbohydrate-free albumen is then pasteurized at 54.0°C for 7 to10 days and at 52.0°C for 5 days, respectively. It is important to note that standard thermal pasteurization conditions for egg albumen were developed when the pH of egg albumen received belatedly at processing plants had increased from pH 7.2 at lay to pH 9.5. Major improvements in the timely on-farm collection of shell eggs provides breaking plants with egg albumen with a reduced pH of 8.2 to 8.6, which markedly enhances the heat resistance of salmonellae. A thorough assessment on the adequacy of current pasteurization regimens for liquid albumen is clearly indicated.

The pervasion of *S.* Enteritidis within the global egg industry led to numerous studies on the heat resistance of this pandemic serovar and its behavior under standard thermal processing conditions for liquid egg products. The physiological resiliency of *Salmonella* spp. in the stationary phase of growth and the acquired tolerance of salmonellae to normally injurious environmental conditions following adaptive preconditioning of cells is well documented. The early fear that eggborne *S.* Enteritidis phage types 4 and 8 were highly heat resistant proved to be unfounded. A comprehensive study (Palumbo et al., 1995) underlined the different heat responses of four strains of *S.* Enteritidis inoculated into liquid egg yolk, where $D_{60^\circ C}$ values ranged from 0.55 to 0.75 min, whereas homologous values for single strains of *S.* Senftenberg (not the 775W heat-resistant strain) and *S.* Typhimurium were 0.73 and 0.67, respectively. In a separate study, the $D_{60^\circ C}$ values for *S.* Enteritidis phage type 4 inoculated into liquid egg yolk ranged from 0.06 to 0.16 min (Humphrey, 1990). Clearly, current thermal treatments of liquid egg products provide different levels of bacterial inactivation and product safety. Risk analyses on the adequacy of home and food service cooking practices need to focus on the fate of salmonellae in egg yolk, where large populations of *S.* Enteritidis are more likely to occur.

9.6 POTENTIALLY HAZARDOUS EGG PRODUCTS IN THE HOME

Shell and transovarian contamination of shell eggs with *Salmonella* spp. potentiate serious public health consequences from the consumption of raw or lightly cooked eggs. Common cooking methods may not always eliminate *S.* Enteritidis in internally contaminated shell eggs. For example, cooking of shell eggs under nonstandardized conditions by three separate operators showed that mean endpoint temperatures of

65.0, 75.5, 83.5, and 80.0°C were measured in fried, scrambled, omelet, and hard-boiled eggs, respectively (Saeed and Koons, 1993). These endpoint temperatures were obtained after cooking for approximately 2.0 min except for hard-boiled eggs, which were cooked for 11.0 min. Fewer cooking failures were noted with eggs that had been stored at refrigerator (4°C) than those stored at ambient temperature (23°C) prior to cooking. These findings probably stem from the active growth of the internally inoculated *S.* Enteritidis phage type 8 during the greater than 5-day storage of shell eggs at room temperature and the greater heat resistance of the egg inoculum stored at room temperature than at refrigerator temperature. This report and a more recent study (De Paula et al., 2005) indicate that eggs fried "sunny-side up" in a stovetop skillet are potentially hazardous to unsuspecting consumers and should be cooked until the yolk is fully congealed.

The home preparation of mayonnaise using raw eggs is to be discouraged because of the propensity of eggborne salmonellae to survive and grow in this ready-to-eat food. Numerous studies have shown that the fate of *Salmonella* spp. in mayonnaise is temperature-, pH-, acidulant-, and vegetable oil–dependent. Several *Salmonella* strains in inoculated mayonnaise (pH 3.8 to 4.0) grew within 1 to 3 days of storage at 30°C or within 3 to 5 days of storage at 20°C; no growth was detected in mayonnaise (pH < 4.4) stored at 10°C (Ferreira and Lund, 1987). The susceptibility of *Salmonella* spp. to low pH values is acidulant-dependent. For example, the inactivation of *S.* Muenster was markedly more effective in mayonnaise acidified to pH 4.8 to 5.2 with acetic acid than with citric acid during product storage at 25°C (Collins, 1985). Similar results were reported for *S.* Enteritidis phage type 4 in mayonnaise acidified to pH 5.0 with vinegar and lemon juice (Perales and Garcia, 1990). Interestingly, storage of acidified mayonnaise at refrigerator temperatures attenuates the bactericidal action of acetic acid against *S.* Enteritidis (Kurihara et al., 1994; Lock and Board, 1995). The nature of vegetable oil used in the preparation of mayonnaise can also affect the death rate kinetics of *Salmonella* spp. Extra virgin olive oil, which is more acid and contains higher levels of phenolic compounds than do blended olive or sunflower oil, was more inhibitory to *S.* Enteritidis phage type 4 (Radford et al., 1991). The continued prominence of raw egg mayonnaise as a vehicle of human salmonellosis in Spain reiterates the need for the safe home preparation of this potentially hazardous food (Crespo et al., 2004). Isolated outbreaks of human salmonellosis from the consumption of ice cream prepared with raw eggs underline the inherent health risk associated with this traditional home-prepared food (Morgan et al., 1994).

Traditional Chinese methods of curing shell eggs are of scientific and public health interest. *Pi dan* (also known as 1000-year-old eggs) are intact chicken or duck shell eggs that have been cured for 20 to 30 days at room temperature in a highly alkaline solution of NaOH, NaCl, and black tea (Meng et al., 1990). After curing, the eggs are rinsed in water, air dried, coated with a slurry consisting of clay soil and the NaOH curing solution, and rolled in rice hulls. The pH of the albumen and yolk in *pi dan* are 11.5 and 9.4, respectively. The albumen of these eggs is coagulated and brownish, whereas the yolk is semisolid with a distinct black color from the bacterial production of H_2S. The bacterial production of NH_3 during the curing process also imparts flavor to this uncooked, ready-to-eat product. The health concern with *pi dan* stems from the slow increase in internal pH, which probably favors the adaptive survival of eggborne *Salmonella* spp. within the egg magma. *Yan dan* are intact shell eggs that have been cured for 20 to 30 days at room temperature in a 20% NaCl solution, during which time the water activity (a_w) of the albumen and yolk markedly decrease from 0.996 to 0.944 and from 0.998 to 0.963, respectively. The pH of the albumen also decreases from 9.0 to 6.7, whereas the pH of the yolk remains unchanged (Meng et al., 1990). The lowered a_w and neutral pH in salt-cured egg would increase the heat resistance of eggborne salmonellae and potentiate their survival when *yan dan* are lightly cooked in boiling water before consumption.

9.7 CONTROL

The abatement of human salmonellosis from the consumption of shell eggs and liquid egg products requires concerted and sustained efforts at all levels of the commercial egg industry to disrupt the potential transovarian and trans-shell transmission of *Salmonella* spp. (ICMSF, 1998). At the farm level, many control interventions can be applied, including the disinfection of rearing barns before the placement of new layer flocks, the use of *Salmonella*-free replacement breeder stocks and poultry feeds, construction of rearing barns with rodent- and insect-resistant materials, provision of clean litter and drinking water to bird flocks, frequent on-farm collection of shell eggs, hygienic and refrigerated storage, and shipment of shell eggs to retail outlets. The periodic bacteriological monitoring of the layer barn environment for *Salmonella* contamination is a more effective control measure than the monitoring of shell egg contents, because the incidence of shell eggs infected internally with *Salmonella* spp. is extremely low. Intervention strategies for layer barns found to be environmentally contaminated with *S.* Enteritidis have varied widely among countries. Action plans have included registration and intensive testing of multiplier breeder and layer birds, their barn environment and supply hatcheries, mandatory pasteurization of eggs from infected flocks, depopulation of infected multiplier breeder and egg layer flocks, aggressive decontamination of contaminated barns, stringent monitoring of domestic and imported animal feeds (Table 6), exclusion of animal proteins from avian feeds, and mandatory refrigeration ($\leq 8°C$) of shell eggs and coding of egg cartons by producer farms to facilitate epidemiological tracebacks. Suggestively, the weakest links in on-farm poultry husbandry practices are the provision of *Salmonella*-free replacement stocks and poultry feeds. The thermal recycling of animal offals into rendered proteins presents a formidable challenge to the feed and poultry industries because of the endogenously high levels of bacterial flora in these raw products and the multiple opportunities from bacterial cross-contamination of rendered products during bulk storage, mixing at feed mills, surface transportation to farms, and on-farm storage. Reports of *Salmonella* in up to 30% of rendered animal proteins and complete feeds are not uncommon (D'Aoust, 2000). The enduring problem of salmonellae in rendered products was addressed in recent years with the supplementation of animal feeds with formic and propionic acids and with other antimicrobial agents. Sal

TABLE 6 ***Salmonella* in Animal Feeds**

Country of Origin	Product	Number of Samples Tested	Percent Positive
Rendered animal protein			
Australia (ca. 1995)	Meat meal	72	30.6
Lebanon (ca. 1988)	Animal feed	300	19.0
The Netherlands (1990–1991)	Fish meal	130	31.0
United States (ca. 1994)	Animal protein	101	56.4
Vegetable protein			
The Netherlands (1990–1991)	Maize grits	15	27.0
United States (ca. 1994)	Vegetable protein	50	36.0
Complete feed			
Brazil (ca. 1995)	Poultry feed	200	10.0
Denmark (1995)	Swine feed	2300	0.7
	Animal feed	1669	1.2
Japan (1988–1990)	Poultry feed	115	3.5
The Netherlands (1990–1991)	Poultry feed	360	10.0
Japan (1993–1998)	Layer feed	2466	0.7

Source: Adapted from D'Aoust (2000).

Curb (Kemin Europa N.V., Belgium), available in both liquid and dry forms, exerts broad-spectrum antibacterial and antifungal activity within 24 to 48 h of application to rendered products and complete feeds. Residual levels of active ingredients also provide long-term protection against recontamination of animal feeds. Bio-Add (Trouw Nutrition, Northwich, UK) is a similar organic acid product for the control of *Salmonella* and molds in animal feeds.

On-farm control interventions can play an important role in the abatement of salmonellae in chicken breeder and commercial egg layer flocks. In its annual report (2001), the Advisory Committee on the Microbiological Safety of Food suggested that the sustained decrease in the number of human infections of *S*. Enteritidis in the United Kingdom since 1997 probably stemmed from a marked decrease in the prevalence of salmonellae in shell eggs commensurate with improved flock hygiene and a national vaccination program against *S*. Enteritidis for breeder–layer flocks.

Several vaccines are currently marketed for the protection of poultry against *S*. Enteritidis. The live Salmovac SE vaccine, consisting of a purine and histidine auxotrophic strain of *S*. Enteritidis phage type 4, is administered preferably in three separate doses before the onset of the laying period. The vaccine is strongly immunogenic, as evidenced by elevated serum levels of *S*. Enteritidis–specific IgY antibodies in vaccinated birds and reduction in the shedding and intestinal persistence of the pathogen in treated birds compared to control birds (Springer et al., 2002). It has been suggested that live vaccines should be administered to breeder flocks only and not to commercial egg layer flocks because of the concern that vaccine strains could migrate into the interior of table eggs. Salenvac (Intervet, Milton, Keynes, UK) is an inactivated iron-restricted bacterin vaccine, which when administered intramuscularly in two or three doses, reduces shedding, organ colonization, and egg contamination in layer birds challenged with *S*. Enteritidis phage type 4 (Clifton-Hadley et al., 2002).

It is clear that a significant reduction in the asymptomatic carriage and shedding of salmonellae in layer birds would greatly alleviate the potential for external and internal contamination of shell eggs. In the last two decades, the efficacy of probiotics as biological hurdles for the competitive exclusion of salmonellae in layer and broiler chickens has been investigated extensively (Stavric and D'Aoust, 1992). In this prophylactic approach, a live bacterial preparation of either an undefined or defined mixture of nonpathogenic microflora from mature *Salmonella*-free birds is administered to 1-day-old chicks. The protective mixture is administered by gavage into the crop or added to the first drinking water. Broilact (Orion Corporation, Turku, Finland) was the first commercial preparation of an undefined protective mixture to be marketed. Aviguard (Microbial Developments Ltd, Malvern, Worcestershire, England) was introduced shortly thereafter. Defined mixtures of protective strains are also available commercially. Levucell SB (Lallemand Animal Nutrition SA, Blagnac, France) is a live dry yeast vaccine of *Saccharomyces cerevisiae* type *boulardii* that has undergone field testing for the protection of poultry and other livestock against *Salmonella* and other bacterial pathogens. Preempt (MS Bioscience, Dundee, Illinois) consists of a defined mixture of 29 aerobic and anaerobic bacterial strains that is sprayed as a course mist over newly hatched chicks. The protective mixture is ingested as the chicks groom their feathers. Although the exact mechanism of bird protection has yet to be fully elucidated, it is widely held that probiotic microflora effectively compete with *Salmonella* for the limited number of binding sites on the avian intestinal wall. The production of volatile fatty acids by probiotic microflora has also been proposed as an inhibitor of commensal *Salmonella* colonization of the avian intestinal tract (Stavric and D'Aoust, 1992).

There is a growing interest in the clinical use of phage therapy to control bacterial infections with highly virulent and/or antibiotic-resistant strains in humans and in animals. The increasing incidence of bacterial pathogens that no longer respond to traditional antibiotics, combined with the increasing bacterial resistance to novel drugs such as fluoroquinolones, reinforce the potential value of bacteriophages in human and animal therapy. Lytic phage treatment of human bacterial infections is widely used in the former USSR republic of Georgia and in Poland, where prophylactic and therapeutic bacteriophage products are commercially available. In 2002, a report from the Rockefeller University (United States) confirmed the ability of a bacteriophage preparation to rapidly kill vegetative cells and germinating spores of *Bacillus anthracis*. Phages enjoy a high specificity against targeted bacterial pathogens and, in contrast to broad-spectrum antibiotics, effectively remove infectious agents without disturbing the delicate balance of endogenous microflora in the host. The potential of phage therapy to improve the microbial safety of agricultural products cannot be underestimated. In September 2005, two major biotechnology companies from the United States and India joined in a multi-million-dollar venture to develop a bacteriophage-supplemented bovine feed to inactivate verotoxigenic *E. coli*. Phage therapy could also benefit the shell egg industry by reducing the occurrence of *Salmonella* spp. on eggshell surfaces and in the egg interior. The mitigating potential of phage therapy in this era of rapid emergence of antibiotic-resistant "super bugs" cannot be minimized.

Control interventions at egg-washing and egg-grading stations generally include monitoring of chlorine levels and other disinfectants in wash water that ideally should be of low iron content, continuous inflow of fresh water to the egg washer, candling of eggs to identify and remove eggs with hairline cracks and eggs with meat or blood spots, use of chlorinated potable water for the final rinsing of shell eggs, immediate drying and refrigerated storage of sanitized eggs, and regular cleaning of egg-washing equipment. Egg centrifuges are used in some egg-processing plants, bakeries, pasta factories, and large food service kitchens to separate the egg magma from shell fragments. In this process, shell eggs are crushed when dropped into a spinning perforated basket, and liquid whole egg is separated from shell fragments by centrifugation. The use of egg centrifuges is contraindicated and even prohibited in many countries because of the likely transfer of bacterial contaminants on the eggshell surface to the liquid whole egg collected. Notwithstanding the possible creation of aerosols and contamination of the egg-processing environment, the use of this unpasteurized egg product in foods that may be subjected to light cooking clearly potentiates a human health risk. Several innovative technologies can reduce or eliminate *Salmonella* on the surface and/or within intact shell eggs without altering the physical and functional properties of egg magma. An automated process for the large-scale in-shell pasteurization of shell eggs was recently introduced by Pasteurized Eggs, L.P. (Laconia, New Hampshire). Under stringent processing conditions, flats of shell eggs are automatically weighed and transported by a conveyor belt system through a series of pasteurizing water baths. The system automatically weighs each batch of eggs and computes the processing conditions to effect a 5.0 $\log_{10}$ reduction in *Salmonella* spp. The pasteurized eggs are then cooled and the shell sealed with a food-grade wax to protect the shell from external contamination and to preserve the freshness of shell eggs. Treated shell eggs marketed as Davidson's Pasteurized Eggs are packaged and stored at 7.0°C. A similar egg pasteurization system is marketed by M.G. Waldbaum (Gaylord, Minnesota), where flats of clean graded shell eggs are placed in the pasteurizer and heat-treated at 56°C for a specified holding time. Pasteurized shell eggs are then cooled, spray rinsed, surface coated, and packaged for distribution. Another interesting technology for the in-shell pasteurization of intact eggs involves the simultaneous exposure of eggs to ultrasound and heat. The efficacy of this treatment arises in part from the ability of ultrasonication to markedly reduce the heat resistance of *S.* Enteritidis and to predispose salmonellae to inactivation at normally sublethal temperatures. Application of this treatment for approximately 7.0 min at 54°C yields a 6.0-$\log_{10}$ reduction of *S.* Enteritidis on shell egg surfaces without adversely affecting the functional properties of the egg magma. Interestingly, ultrasonication of *S.* Senftenberg ATCC 43845 under similar conditions resulted in nonpasteurizing levels of inactivation (Cabeza et al., 2005). The need for further kinetic studies on the ultrasonic inactivation of salmonellae is clearly indicated.

Current concerns for global terrorism have led to concerted research efforts in the development of methods for the prompt and reliable detection of potentially life-threatening adulterants deliberately added to national food and water supplies. Fresh shell eggs are a staple food in numerous countries and cannot be neglected as potential targets of bioterrorism. In 2004, the European Council promulgated a regulation for the mandatory stamping of shell eggs to facilitate the rapid tracking of producer farms. This approach played a key role in the rapid containment of several outbreaks of *S.* Enteritidis phage type 6 in England from shell eggs imported from a single supplier in the Netherlands. An egg-stamping identification system is also used for intact shell eggs marketed in Canada. In September 2005, Radlo Foods (Massachusetts) announced the imminent marketing of Born Free Eggs, which will be laser-etched with expiration dates and numerical codes to facilitate traceback of shell eggs to supply farms. Warnex Diagnostics Inc. (Laval, Québec) is currently considering the use of molecular bar codes to track the origin of unpackaged food products such as fresh fruits and vegetables. More specifically, a unique single-stranded DNA molecule would be incorporated in the product of a food supplier; the rapid detection of a molecular tag, using specific beacons and primers in a real-time PCR assay, would provide timely identification of the food supplier.

Shell eggs and egg products have a long history as vehicles of human bacterial diseases. It is clear that the abatement of *Salmonella* spp. and other eggborne human bacterial pathogens will require continued public health vigilance, sustained application of effective control measures by all sectors of the egg industry, and major efforts in consumer education on the safe preparation of these sensitive foods. The low human infectious dose and physiological resiliency of foodborne salmonellae (D'Aoust, 2000), the increasing food trade between developed and developing countries, and the prominence of antibiotic-resistant *Salmonella* in human medicine and in the global food supply remain major challenges to the marketing of safe shell eggs and egg products.

REFERENCES

Andrews WH, Hammack TS (2004): *Salmonella*. In: *Bacteriological Analytical Manual*, 8th ed. http://www.cfsan.fda.gov/~ebam/bam-toc.html. Accessed March 2007.

Board RG, Fuller R (1994): *Microbiology of the Avian Egg*. Chapman & Hall, London.

Brackett RE, Beuchat LE (1991): Survival of *Listeria monocytogenes* in whole egg, egg yolk powders and in liquid whole eggs. *Food Microbiol*. 8:331–337.

Cabeza MC, Garcia ML, de la Hoz L, Cambero I, Ordonez JA (2005): Destruction of *Salmonella* Senftenberg on the shells of intact eggs by thermoultrasonication. *J Food Prot*. 68: 841–844.

Clifton-Hadley FA, Dibb-Fuller MP, Sprigings KA, et al. (2002): Efficacy of Salenvac® T, an inactivated bivalent iron restricted *Salmonella enterica* serovar Enteritidis and Typhimurium dual vaccine, in reducing other *Salmonella* serogroup B infections in poultry. In *Proc. International Symposium on* Salmonella *and Salmonellosis*, St. Brieuc, France, pp. 619–620.

Collins MA (1985): Effect of pH and acidulant type on the survival of some food poisoning bacteria in mayonnaise. *Microbiol Aliments Nutr*. 3:215–221.

Crespo PS, Hernandez G, Echeita A, Torres A, Ordonez O, Aladuena A (2004): Vigilancia epidemiologica de brotes alimentarios relacionados con el consumo de huevo y derivados. España. 2002–2003. *Bol Epidemiol.* 12:233–236.

D'Aoust JY (2000): *Salmonella.* In: Lund BM, Baird-Parker TC, Gould GW (Eds.). *The Microbiological Safety and Quality of Food,* Vol. II. Aspen Publishers, Gaithersburg, MD, pp. 1233–1299.

D'Aoust JY, Purvis U (1998): Isolation and identification of *Salmonella* from foods. MFHPB-20. In: *Compendium of Analytical Methods,* Vol. 2, Health Canada, Ottawa, Ontario, Canada. http://www.hc-sc.gc.ca/fn-an/res-rech/analy-meth/microbio/volume2/mfhpb20-01_e.html. Accessed May 2008.

D'Aoust JY, Maurer J, Bailey JS (2001): Salmonella species. In: Doyle MP, Beuchat LR, Montville TJ (Eds.). *Food Microbiology: Fundamentals and Frontiers,* 2nd ed. ASM Press, Washington, DC, pp. 141–178.

De Paula CMD, Mariot RF, Tondo EC (2005): Thermal inactivation of *Salmonella enteritidis* by boiling and frying egg methods. *J Food Saf.* 25:43–57.

Ferreira MASS, Lund BM (1987): The influence of pH and temperature on initiation of growth of *Salmonella* spp. *Lett Appl Microbiol.* 5:67–70.

Finch MJ, Blake PA (1985): Foodborne outbreaks of campylobacteriosis: the United States experience, 1980–1982. *Am J Epidemiol.* 122:262–268.

Froning GW, Peters D, Muriana P, Eskridge K, Travnicek D, Sumner SS (2002): *International Egg Pasteurization Manual.* United Egg Producers, Alpharetta, GA, and American Egg Board, Park Ridge, IL.

Humphrey TJ (1990): Heat resistance in *Salmonella enteritidis* phage-type 4: the influence of storage temperatures before heating. *J Appl Bacteriol.* 69:493–497.

——— (1994): Contamination of egg shell and contents with *Salmonella enteritidis*: a review. *Int J Food Microbiol.* 21:31–40.

ICMSF (International Commission on Microbiological Specifications for Foods) (1998): *Microorganisms in Foods,* Vol. 6. Blackie Academic and Professional, London, pp. 475–520.

——— (2005): *Microorganisms in Foods,* Vol. 6, 2nd ed. Kluwer Academic/Plenum Publishers, New York, Chap. 15.

ISO (International Organization for Standardization) (2002): *Microbiology of Food and Animal Feeding Stuffs: Horizontal Method for the Detection of* Salmonella *spp.* ISO/FDIS 6579. ISO, Geneva, Switzerland.

Kurihara K, Mizutani H, Nomura H, Takeda N, Imai C (1994): Behavior of *Salmonella* Enteritidis in home-made mayonnaise and salads. *Jpn J Food Microbiol.* 11:35–41.

Liong JWW, Frank JF, Bailey S (1997): Visualization of eggshell membranes and their interaction with *Salmonella enteritidis* using confocal scanning laser microscopy. *J Food Prot.* 60:1022–1028.

Lock JL, Board RG (1995): The fate of *Salmonella enteritidis* PT4 in home-made mayonnaise prepared from artificially inoculated eggs. *Food Microbiol.* 12:181–186.

Mayes FJ, Takeballi MA (1983): Microbial contamination of the hen's egg: a review. *J Food Prot.* 46:1092–1098.

Meng YC, Dresel J, Hechelmann H, Leistner L (1990): Reproduction and survival of *Salmonella enteritidis* in eggs (Pi Dan, Yan Dan) cured using traditional Chinese methods. *Mitt Bundesanst Fleischforsch.* 107:38–44.

Moore J, Madden RH (1993): Detection and incidence of *Listeria* species in blended whole egg. *J Food Prot*. 56:652–654.

Morgan D, Mawer SL, Harman PL (1994): The role of home-made ice cream as a vehicle of *Salmonella enteritidis* phage type 4 infection from fresh shell eggs. *Epidemiol Infect*. 113:21–29.

Palumbo MS, Beers SM, Bhaduri S, Palumbo SA (1995): Thermal resistance of *Salmonella* spp. and *Listeria monocytogenes* in liquid egg yolk and egg yolk products. *J Food Prot*. 58:960–966.

Perales I, Garcia MI (1990): The influence of pH and temperature on the behaviour of *Salmonella enteritidis* phage-type 4 in home-made mayonnaise. *Lett Appl Microbiol*. 10:19–22.

Radford SA, Tassou CC, Nychas GJE, Board RG (1991): The influence of different oils on the death rate of *Salmonella enteritidis* in homemade mayonnaise. *Lett Appl Microbiol*. 12:125–128.

Saeed AM, Koons CW (1993): Growth and heat resistance of *Salmonella enteritidis* in refrigerated and abused eggs. *J Food Prot*. 56:927–931.

Schuman JD, Sheldon BW (1997): Thermal resistance of *Salmonella* spp. and *Listeria monocytogenes* in liquid egg yolk and egg white. J Food Prot. 60:634–638.

Sionkowski PJ, Shelef LA (1990): Viability of *Listeria monocytogenes* strain Brie-1 in the avian egg. *J Food Prot*. 53:15–17.

Springer S, Lehman J, Lindner T, Alder G, Selbitz HJ (2002): A new live *Salmonella* Enteritidis vaccine for chicken: experimental evidence of its safety and efficacy. In *Proc. International Symposium on* Salmonella *and Salmonellosis*, St. Brieuc, France, pp. 609–610.

Stavric S, D'Aoust JY (1992): Competitive exclusion for the control of *Salmonella* in poultry. In *Proc. International Roundtable on Animal Feed Biotechnology: Research and Scientific Regulation*, Ottawa, Ontario, Canada, pp. 75–87.

USDA (U.S. Department of Agriculture) (1969): *Egg Pasteurization Manual*. ARS 74-48. Poultry Laboratory, Agricultural Research Service. U.S. Department of Agriculture, Albany, CA.

——— (2004): *Isolation and Identification of* Salmonella *from Meat, Poultry and Egg Products. MLG* 4.03. USDA, Athens, GA.

CHAPTER 10

FOOD SAFETY ISSUES AND THE MICROBIOLOGY OF PORK

GAY Y. MILLER and JAMES S. DICKSON

10.1 INTRODUCTION

The goal of the production of pork is to provide a safe (low risk) and wholesome pork product to consumers. It is not practical or possible in most environments to eliminate all risks in pork, pork products, or any food in general. All foods have some degree of risk. Having said that, it is recognized that within the flow of animals and products that make up the pork food chain, there are many things that can be and are done to help reduce or eliminate risks at certain points in the production and processing chain. Pork food safety begins on the farm by providing for adequate hygiene (facilities and personnel), controlling rodent and other pest populations that can contribute to or transmit diseases that have food safety implications, enforcing farm biosecurity to decrease possible exposure of pigs to foodborne pathogens, controlling pig flow and pig source to provide for a healthy pig, providing good-quality feed and water that has been stored and delivered to pigs in a hygienic manner, and practicing good animal husbandry and management, which decreases pig stress and improves pig health. All are important contributors to the delivery of a high-quality pig for slaughter.

National programs for safety and quality assurance at the farm level in the pork industry include the USDA/AMS Quality Systems Certification Program, the National Pork Producers Council (NPPC) Pork Quality Assurance Program, and the NPPC *Trichinae* Program Working Group. Additionally, many farms have custom-designed programs based on their consumer base (Unnevehr et al., 1999). Some programs involve monitoring, verification, and/or certification of practices that occur on the farm. Market advantages seen with these programs include access to specific export markets or particular domestic niche markets, access to specific processor markets, and improved pork image and competitiveness.

Pork food safety continues into the transportation and lairage of pigs. Pigs' natural behavior is to investigate their environs with the snout and mouth. Thus, transported

Microbiologically Safe Foods, Edited by Norma Heredia, Irene Wesley, and Santos García

pigs will lick and chew on other pigs, their environs, and its contents. Feces are readily mouthed and eaten. On the farm, this is limited by housing, with most pigs reared on flooring where feces fall to a manure storage pit below.

Healthy, properly housed pigs appear to be fairly clean. But during transportation and lairage, such flooring is either impossible or impractical. Pigs readily become somewhat soiled and the flooring contains feces; thus, pigs can become infected with potential food pathogens during this phase of the pork chain. Indeed, *Salmonella* can be isolated from pigs previously not found to have this organism as quickly as 2 h after arriving in a slaughter plant. Slaughter plant holding pens are generally contaminated with *Salmonella*. Pigs become exposed and infected as a matter of course during shipment and lairage.

Details related to processing of the pork carcass into finished product are covered below in a separate section. Some farm practices can influence potential slaughter plant contamination. For example, feed removal prior to slaughter has been shown to decrease the incidence of visceral rupture, which will decrease the risk of pathogen contamination of carcasses (Miller et al., 1997). Needless to say, farm-to-fork pork safety is a shared responsibility by all parties, from the producer through each step in the production of finished pork products and on to the consumer. Each party must take responsibility for and control their portion of the pork chain in order for consumers of pork to continue to enjoy a high-quality, safe product.

10.2 NORMAL FLORA OF RAW PORK

The microflora that is usually found on fresh raw pork originates from both the production environment of the live animal and the microflora that may be associated with the transportation and processing equipment. This would generally consist of a mixed microflora of gram-positive and gram-negative bacteria, as well as yeasts, fungi, and possibly swine viruses. From a human perspective, the primary focus is on bacteria, which are generally thought of in terms of "spoilage" and "pathogenic" microflora. If the animals are raised with good animal husbandry practices and processed with modern hygienic standards, the populations expected on chilled pork carcasses should be quite low. In the United States, a nationwide microbiological study of chilled animal carcasses was conducted in the early 1990s, and the results for pork carcasses suggested that the mesophilic aerobic bacterial populations were less than 5000 CFU/cm^2 on the hide surface of chilled pork carcasses, and that 25% of the carcasses sampled had populations of less than 1000 CFU/cm^2 on the hide surface (USDA-FSIS, 1996a).

The bacteria that come to predominate and ultimately spoil fresh pork vary by the type of packaging method. Most of the high-value pork cuts (i.e., loins) are vacuum packaged for at least part of their shelf life. Vacuum packaging restricts the growth of microorganisms to either facultative anaerobic or strictly anaerobic bacteria. In most cases, lactic acid bacteria, such as *Lactobacillus*, *Leuconostoc*, or *Pediococcus*, become predominant in the microflora. After the vacuum package is opened, the product is frequently repackaged in a retail package, which is aerobic.

Since these bacteria are facultatively anaerobic, they continue to grow in the aerobic environment. Spoiled retail product often has a sour odor or taste as a result of the lactic acid production of these bacteria.

Potentially pathogenic bacteria which can contaminate fresh pork include, but are not limited to, both gram-negative pathogens such as *Salmonella*, the pathogenic *Escherichia coli*'s, and *Campylobacter*, as well as gram-positive bacteria such as *Bacillus cereus*, the *Clostridia*, and *Listeria*. These bacteria occur randomly on fresh pork and are commonly associated with the animal production environment and cross-contamination during processing. Generic *Escherichia coli* were found on 44% of the hide surfaces of chilled carcasses, and the mean population of the positive samples was less than 1 CFU/cm^2 (USDA-FSIS, 1998a). *Salmonella enterica* was present on 6.9% of the hide surfaces of the chilled carcasses, although the populations were not quantified. In the earlier baseline survey (USDA-FSIS, 1996a), the populations of *S. enterica* (when present) were quite low, with 55% of the positive samples testing negative by the most probable number (MPN) method (less than 0.03 MPN/cm^2).

10.3 SPOILAGE

Food spoilage can generally be described as the point at which a food becomes unacceptable to the consumer. As such, the end of shelf life is highly subjective, with people making a determination based on personal preferences. Consumers use the resources that are available to them in the determination of spoilage: namely, odor, texture, taste, purchase date, and storage (e.g., refrigerated or frozen). Because of individual preferences and variations between them, a precise scientific description of spoilage in the form of a maximum bacterial population of the results of a chemical assay is elusive.

The spoilage of food products is determined by a variety of factors, including but not limited to the initial microflora, the effects of processing, the effects of storage, and the effects of any antimicrobial process applied to the product. In the case of fresh pork, the primary factors that affect spoilage are the initial microflora and the effects of storage conditions (temperature and atmosphere). The initial microflora is contributed by the microflora in and on the live hog, the environment, and potential contamination from the processing equipment. There is a clear correlation between the initial population of bacteria on the meat and the potential shelf life. Emphasizing sanitary dressing procedures can positively affect shelf life.

Fresh pork is often vacuum packaged to extend the shelf life during storage and distribution. However, most retail presentations are repackaged into aerobic trays, because of consumer preference. The switch from the reduced oxygen vacuum package to an aerobic environment, often accompanied by increases in temperature, results in more rapid microbial growth at retail. Retail pork packages are typically labeled with a "use or freeze by" date to encourage consumers to use the meat before it spoils. These dates are very conservative and include a margin of error, simply because of the variability in temperature of home refrigerators. The predominant microflora found on fresh pork in a vacuum package is predominantly lactic acid bacteria. Upon exposure to air, some of the bacteria grow at a faster rate and are capable of producing extracellular polysaccharides, which gives the pork a slippery feel which the consumer perceives as "slime." In addition, some aerobic bacteria, such as the pseudomonads, may grow rapidly under aerobic conditions. While the lactic acid bacteria produce what the consumer perceives as "souring," the pseudomonads may produce a variety of off-odors, most characteristically one that is perceived as "fruity."

Frozen pork does not spoil as a result of microbiological action. Most frozen red meats have an estimated shelf life of 180 days at −20°C. The product ultimately becomes unacceptable due to chemical reactions, typically resulting in rancidity. The product may also become unacceptable if the packaging is not sufficient to prevent dehydration or freezer burn.

Processed meats containing pork are intended to have an extended shelf life, often measured in months. In some cases the products are shelf stable and will essentially last until chemical reactions result in a product that is deemed unsuitable. Processed meats derive this extended shelf life from a combination of processes, including a (thermal) lethality process, the addition of microbial inhibitors, and vacuum packaging. In some cases, the amount of available moisture (water activity) is also reduced. The lethality process generally results in a product with an extremely low microbial population as it exits the smokehouse.

The microflora that is on the product as it is packaged is usually derived from both the processing equipment and the environment. The result is a product with a very low initial population, which contains antimicrobial additives to slow the growth of microorganisms. When this type of product is vacuum packaged and stored at refrigeration temperatures, it may well have a shelf life of 6 months. The microorganisms that spoil processed meat products are those that can grow at low temperatures in the absence of oxygen. Typically, this includes lactic acid bacteria as well as micrococci. In most cases, lactic acid bacteria are the predominant component of the spoilage microflora (Radin et al., 2006). In rare cases, yeasts can become established and spoil the product. Typically, the yeast spores on the initial packaged product are a result of contamination from equipment. Yeast spoilage is characterized by the production of carbon dioxide in the package, resulting in swelling or ballooning of the package, and is accompanied by the characteristic yeast odor when the package is opened.

10.4 PATHOGENS OF CONCERN

Any foodborne pathogen that is transmitted by poor hygiene or poor water quality in food processing or food preparation can contaminate pork or pork products and serve as a potential foodborne hazard for people. Contamination with gut contents due to errors in slaughter and cross-contamination between carcasses can also contribute to contamination. Numerous pathogens have been associated with pork products, including *Salmonella* spp., *Staphylococcus aureus*, *Campylobacter* spp., *Clostridium botulinum*, *Yersinia enterocolitica*, *Listeria monocytogenes*, *Clostridium perfringens*, *Aeromonas hydrophila*, *Streptococcus* spp., *Escherichia coli*, *Brucella suis*, *Toxoplama gondii*, *Trichinella spiralis*, and *Taenia solium*.

Some of these could have originated directly from the pig on the farm, while others are more likely obtained from contamination that occurs during processing, or later during food preparation. These and other fecal–orally transmitted microorganisms and viruses can also occur with humans serving to contaminate pork. Additionally, temperature abuse related to either inadequate cooking time/temperatures or temperature abuse during storage can result in microbial growth and food safety risk of pork.

10.5 RISK OF CONTAMINATION DURING PROCESSING

A number of steps in processing occur to allow for consumption of high-quality pork products. Figure 1 shows the steps in going from the live animal on the farm to the consumption of pork by humans (Barber et al., 2003). Most of the steps in

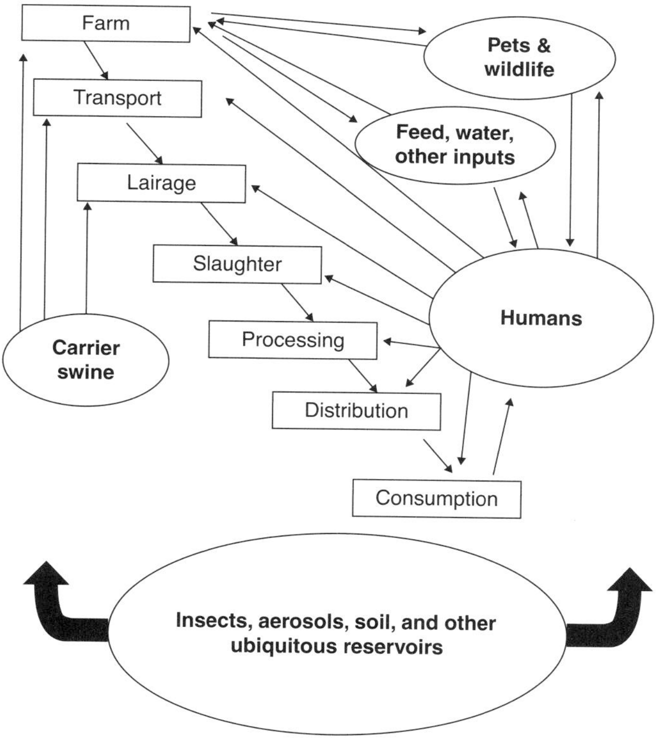

FIG. 1 Flowchart for pork microbiological contamination risks. (From Barber et al., 2003. Reprinted with permission from the *Journal of Food Protection*. Copyright © International Association for Food Protection, Des Moines, Iowa.)

slaughter and processing are designed to decrease the degree of contamination on the carcass, although there is always the possibility of introduction of contamination. There is evidence now that transportation and lairage (holding and resting of live animals between the time they arrive at the slaughter plant and the time they are killed) increases the risk of infection for the live animal and therefore increases the potential for contamination of the carcass (Hurd et al., 2001).

Scalding, singeing, and carcass washing and rinsing, steps in slaughter and processing up to the point of producing a chilled pork carcass, have all been shown to decrease the degree of exterior contamination. Evisceration and dehairing, also slaughter and processing steps, increase the risk of carcass contamination, as can final carcass inspection and carcass chilling. USDA found that there were 3.2% positive carcasses of those sampled for *Salmonella* in 2002 (Rigney et al., 2004). Although they state that this estimate cannot be construed as a true prevalence estimate, a pre-HACCP (hazard analysis of critical control points) baseline prevalence estimate of 8.7% was considerably higher. Thus, there appeared to be a declining proportion of pork carcasses found to be *Salmonella* positive during the period from 1998–2002 (post-HACCP implementation period). More is known about *Salmonella* contamination than about other organisms simply because this is the genus on which the performance standard for HACCP (discussed in more detail later) is set.

The quantitative details of the degree to which surface contamination and/or animal infection translate into product contamination are not generally known because there is so much variability found in various studies, in part due to variability seen among farms and processing plants. Some research is revealing, though. Berends et al. (1997) found that there is a strong correlation between the number of live animals entering a slaughter plant that are fecal-positive for *Salmonella* and the number of carcasses found to be *Salmonella*-positive at the end of the slaughter process. They estimated that 70% of all carcass contamination results from positive animals, while 30% of contamination occurs because of cross-contamination during slaughter from other positive carcasses. During carcass processing, inadequate cleaning of polishing machines, improper evisceration procedures, and poor hygienic practices were the most important risk factors for *Salmonella*-positive carcasses. Additionally, bacteria on equipment can generally be controlled by proper cleaning and disinfection; thus, organisms that are generally present at lower prevalence in hogs can serve as indicator organisms used to monitor the success of good management (hygiene) of processing plant practices.

In Table 1 we summarize literature documenting changes (increases or decreases) in the degree of (or log change of) product contamination for different bacteria at various steps and stages in the production of pork. The only carcass-processing steps found to increase the risk of contamination were dehairing (1 or 2 log increase) and evisceration. Other carcass preparation steps result in varying log reductions in contamination risk (see Table 1). Scalding of carcasses (used to help with dehairing as well as to clean the carcass) has been shown to decrease levels of *E. coli* significantly, while subsequent scraping increases bacteria counts (Namvar and Warriner, 2006). Bolton et al. (2002) showed that scalding, dehairing, and singeing decreased carcass bacterial numbers by approximately 4.5 log. Namvar and Warriner (2006) also suggest

TABLE 1 Production and Processing Steps and Associated Changes in Contamination Risk

Production/Processing Step	Contamination Risk	Microbe	References
On farm prevalence, market pig	6.0%	*Salmonella*	USDA-APHIS, 1997
Transportation and lairage	Prevalence increased 21× (3.4% on-farm to 71.8% after transportation and lairage)	*Salmonella*	Hurd et al., 2001
Scalding	Greater than 9 log decrease	*Salmonella*	Dickson, 2002
	2 log decrease	*Salmonella*	Berends et al., 1997
Dehairing	1 log increase	Enterobacteriaceae	Berends et al., 1997
	1 log increase	Aerobic microflora	Gill and Bryant, 1992
	2 log increase	Aerobic mesophilic bacteria	Pearce et al., 2004
Singeing	3 log decrease	*Enterobacteriaceae*	Berends et al., 1997
	no change	*Salmonella* Aerobic	Gill and Bryant, 1992
	2.5 log decrease	mesophilic bacteria	Pearce et al., 2004
Sheets of recycled hot water applied to polished, uneviscerated carcasses	At least a 2 log decrease	General carcass flora	Gill et al., 1995
Polishing and evisceration	2 log increase	Enterobacteriaceae	Berends et al., 1997
Chilled pork carcass	3.2%	*Salmonella*	USDA-FSIS, 2003b
Cumulative effects of slaughter processes	Decreased from 12% (carcass positive) to 5% (secondary cuts)	Verotoxin-producing *Escherichia coli*	Bouvet et al., 2002

that contamination of incoming pigs was of only minor importance compared with slaughterhouse environment. Although the rate of cross-contamination of carcasses is generally unknown, Vieira-Pinto et al. (2006) found that 31% of *Salmonella*-positive carcasses had a genotype of other pigs slaughtered in the same day. Warriner et al. (2002) found that cross-contamination occurs mainly during evisceration. Namvar and Warriner (2006) found that the holding and scraper areas were the most important sites of cross-contamination. This study also demonstrates the value of molecular typing of generic *E. coli* for elucidating the dynamics of contamination by enteric bacteria in the slaughter process. Pearce et al. (2006) found that air can be an important source of carcass contamination, and therefore of cross-contamination.

Eggenberger-Solorzano et al. (2002) demonstrated that hot water washing of the carcass followed by organic acid rinsing significantly decreased carcass contamination. The cumulative effects of the slaughter process result in an overall decrease in carcass contamination [this has been shown to occur for verotoxin-producing *E. coli* by Bouvet et al. (2002)].

Various treatments for microbial decontamination of pork trim have been evaluated. It has been found that water and water plus lactic acid were more favorable treatments because they reduced bacterial populations (all treatments applied reduced bacterial populations) but did not have detrimental effects on product quality (found when treatments included the use of hot air).

The quantitative contribution to contamination of packaging, transportation, and handling within production chain post-processing, including at the grocery store, in the home, and in eating establishments outside the home, is generally not known. But it is known that case-ready pork products are contaminated with bacteria (Duffy et al., 2001). Figure 1 also points to a number of important concepts related to food safety for pork; this includes the fact that cross-contamination is important at many steps in the consumption of pork by consumers, and that contamination can come from a variety of nonpig, nonpork sources.

There are additives in pork processing that prevent the growth of harmful bacteria, decrease or destroy any product contamination that exists, and preserve the pork product. Nitrate and nitrite salts and sugars are commonly used "curing" agents in the production of ham and luncheon meats that provide these functions. Additionally, acids are used and function as bacteriostatic agents.

In addition to chemical methods in processing, physical methods are used in processing to control bacteria and to enhance product shelf-life. As described previously when discussing spoilage, some pork product is smoked or cooked completely, which decreases the amount of bacteria in/on product and provides preservation. Gases (carbon dioxide and ozone) can be used to retard bacterial growth. Ionizing irradiation also destroys microorganisms in pork. Irradiated product has historically not been well received by U.S. consumers. However, a consumer acceptance study done at Kansas State University suggests that properly packaged (vacuum packaged with the right type of packaging film) irradiated pork may achieve consumer acceptance (Luchsinger et al., 1996a,b). More pronounced oxidative rancidity and less stable color were noted for samples irradiated in aerobic packaging. Optimum packaging conditions controlled color and rancidity changes in boneless chops.

10.6 SURVIVAL AND GROWTH OF PATHOGENS AND SPOILAGE ORGANISMS IN PORK PRODUCTS

Intrinsic and extrinsic factors affect the survival and growth of microorganisms in fresh and processed pork during storage. Most intrinsic parameters, such as nutrient content and biological structures, cannot be directly affected by processing. The removal of biological structures, in the form of hide removal, is arguably a source of contamination, but there are no alternatives other than sanitary dressing procedures. Water activity and pH can be adjusted to reduce the growth of microorganisms, but these adjustments are applicable only to processed pork products, not to fresh products. They are, however, very effective methods of reducing the growth of spoilage bacteria and inhibiting pathogenic bacteria.

In reality, most of the direct control of the growth of microorganisms in pork and pork products is through extrinsic factors. The primary extrinsic factors used to affect microbial growth are temperature and atmosphere. Adjustment of the external temperature to levels that are suboptimal for microbial growth is perhaps the most common method of restricting microbial growth, and the rapid cooling of freshly processed carcasses is one of the regulatory requirements. Low-temperature refrigeration (i.e., less than 5°C) radically slows the growth of most spoilage bacteria and prevents the growth of almost all of the pathogenic bacteria. The notable exception to this is *Listeria monocytogenes*, which is capable of growth at temperatures as low as 0°C (ICMSF, 1996). However, the growth rate for *Listeria* at this temperature is extremely slow.

The other aspect of temperature control is lethality (cooking) with processed meats. Many processed meats contain pork as their primary source of protein, and most of these products undergo a lethality process prior to packaging and distribution. The value of cooking in eliminating pathogenic bacteria and reducing the populations of spoilage bacteria has been documented for years. Current U.S. Department of Agriculture (USDA) regulations for fully cooked ready-to-eat meats require a lethality treatment sufficient to reduce the population of *Salmonella* by 6.5 $\log_{10}$ CFU/g of product (USDA-FSIS, 1999).

Additionally, a lethality step can be and often is applied by consumers: cooking. Even in ready-to-eat products, such a lethality step can decrease the risk of consumer exposure to most foodborne pathogens, including the risk from *L. monocytogenes*. Porto et al. (2004) showed that frankfurters that had intentionally been inoculated with 8.0-log CFU per package had a 5-log reduction if the frankfurters were reheated to a surface temperature of 70°C for about 2 min or 90°C for 0.6 min.

The other extrinsic factor that is commonly altered in pork processing is the environment. Subprimal high-value cuts (especially pork loins) are often vacuum packaged, which removes most of the oxygen from the package. Although most spoilage and many pathogenic bacteria are facultatively anaerobic, the growth rates under reduced oxygen conditions are considerably slower than those under aerobic conditions. The combination of vacuum packaging and low-temperature storage has allowed the shelf life of fresh pork products to be extended to as much as 45 days.

10.7 INDICATOR MICROORGANISMS

An ideal indicator of product quality would have the following characteristics (Jay, 2000):

- It should be present and detectable in all foods to be assessed.
- The growth and numbers should have a direct, negative correlation with quality.
- It should be easy to detect and enumerate.
- It should be enumerable in a short time period.
- The growth should not be adversely affected by food components.

When the USDA-FSIS conducted a nationwide swine baseline data collection program, they identified three groups of microorganisms that were "thought to be of value as indicators of general hygiene or process control": mesophilic aerobic bacteria, total coliforms, and *E. coli* biotype I. (USDA-FSIS, 1996a): With fresh meat products, the population of mesophilic aerobic bacteria can serve as an indicator of overall contamination. Fresh muscle tissue is considered to be essentially sterile (Ayres, 1955). However, intrinsic bacteria (bacteria that occur in the deep muscle tissue of healthy animals) have been reported for many animal species (Ingram, 1964; Ingram and Dainty, 1971). The most frequently characterized intrinsic bacteria are *Clostridium* spp. (Canada and Strong, 1964; Jensen and Hess, 1941; Narayan, 1966; Zagaevskii, 1973). However, when present, these bacteria are present in very low populations.

Mesophilic aerobic bacteria are useful indicators of contamination on animal carcasses. However, unlike beef carcasses, most hog carcasses are processed and chilled with the hide still on. The skin side of the hog carcass is not expected to be sterile, as the processes involved are not sufficient to sterilize the skin. However, scalding and dehairing can greatly reduce the initial population of bacteria that enter on live hogs. The mean population of mesophilic aerobic bacteria on hog carcasses was approximately 5000 CFU/cm^2 (USDA-FSIS, 1996a). Populations of several orders of magnitude in excess of this value may indicate a process that could be improved, or that the live animals that enter the slaughter establishment may be unusually contaminated.

The internal cavity surfaces of the carcass should have relatively low populations of bacteria, as the internal body cavity surfaces of a live hog should be essentially sterile. In this case, the presence of aerobic bacteria on the cavity surfaces may generally be attributable to the processing. Very high populations (e.g., in excess of 10,000 CFU/cm^2) may indicate a process that could be improved, since the source of these bacteria may be from ruptured viscera or from contamination deposited either by equipment or by employee's hands. The population of mesophilic aerobic bacteria enumerated by the analysis procedure is dependent on the incubation temperature of the culture medium. While the standard incubation temperature is 35°C (USDA-FSIS, 1998b), this temperature is intended to enumerate bacteria on carcasses shortly after they have been slaughtered. When fresh meat has been stored at refrigeration temperatures, a lower incubation temperature (20 to 25°C) may be more appropriate.

Bacteria that are growing actively at refrigeration temperatures may not grow on laboratory media at 35°C.

While mesophilic aerobic bacteria may also be of value as indicators of general hygiene on the surfaces of subprimal cuts derived from hog carcasses, lactic acid bacteria may be useful indicators as well. Lactic acid bacteria are often estimated by direct plating on selective agar [such as deMann, Rugosa, and Sharpe (MRS)]. These bacteria may provide an indication of potential product shelf life. However, these bacteria comprise a very small portion of the initial microflora on subprimals and do not become a predominate part of the microflora until after several days or weeks of storage.

As with product quality indicators, an ideal indicator for food safety issues should have the following characteristics (Jay, 2000):

- It is easily and rapidly detectable.
- It is easily distinguished from other microflora.
- There is a history of constant association with the pathogen of interest.
- It is always present when pathogen is present.
- The population corresponds to the pathogen population.
- The growth requirements and growth rates are comparable to those of the pathogens.
- It has a die-off rate parallel to the pathogen of concern.
- It is absent from foods free of the pathogens.

The USDA-FSIS administers meat inspection in the United States to provide a framework for slaughter and pork inspection. The FSIS instituted testing for biotype I *E. coli* as an indicator of process control for enteric pathogens in raw meat processing (USDA-FSIS, 1996b). The *E. coli* biotype I testing requirement was intended to indicate fecal contamination of carcasses. The inspection agency cited the following as justification for their actions:

> In reaching its conclusion that *E. coli* would be the most effective measure of process control for enteric pathogens, the panel considered the ideal characteristics of microbial indicators for the stated purpose. Important characteristics of *E. coli* are:
>
> There is a strong association of *E. coli* with the presence of enteric pathogens and, in the case of slaughtering, the presence of fecal contamination.
>
> *E. coli* occurs at a higher frequency than *Salmonella*, and quantitative *E. coli* testing permits more rapid and more frequent adjustment of process control.
>
> *E. coli* has survival and growth characteristics similar to enteric pathogens, such as *E. coli* O157:H7 and *Salmonella*.
>
> Analysis for *E. coli* poses fewer laboratory safety issues and testing at the establishment site is more feasible than such testing with *Salmonella*.
>
> There is wide acceptance in the international scientific community of its use as an indicator of the potential presence of enteric pathogens.

Microbiological performance standards under the hazard analysis critical control point–pathogen reduction (HACCP-PR) rule were established to monitor the food safety risk in meat using the prevalence of contamination with *Salmonella* spp. These standards monitor only the prevalence of the pathogen, not the actual population. The USDA-FSIS selected *Salmonella* as an indicator of enteric pathogens in fresh raw meat for several reasons (USDA-FSIS, 1996b):

1. It is the most common bacterial cause of foodborne illness.
2. FSIS baseline data show that *Salmonella* colonizes a variety of mammals and birds, and occurs at frequencies that permit changes to be detected and monitored.
3. Current methodologies can recover *Salmonella* from a variety of meat and poultry products.
4. Intervention strategies aimed at reducing fecal contamination and other sources of *Salmonella* on raw product should be effective against other pathogens.

The use of *Salmonella* as an indicator of potential human pathogens on fresh pork has resulted in efforts to decrease *Salmonella* during slaughter and dressing procedures. These efforts have been successful, with an observed reduction in the incidence of *Salmonella* on pork carcasses. The USDA isolated *Salmonella* spp. from 7% of carcasses tested between January 1998 and December 2000 (Rigney et al., 2004). Data from more recent monitoring suggests that the number of positive carcasses has fallen to 3.2% (USDA-FSIS, 2003b). Other bacteria have been identified as potential surrogate organisms for *Salmonella*, which would allow verification of antimicrobial processes within a slaughter establishment (Marshall et al., 2005).

There are limits to what can be done within the processing establishment, and it may be necessary to initiate *Salmonella* controls in the live animal. Berends et al. (1997) reported that carcasses produced from live animals that carried *Salmonella* were three to four times more likely to test positive for *Salmonella* than were carcasses from animals that did not harbor *Salmonella*. Recently, the USDA-FSIS has become concerned with an apparent increase in the levels of *Salmonella* in meats, especially poultry products. Although the current prevalence of *Salmonella* seen is less than the baseline levels reported in the mid-1990s, and below the levels set by the performance standards, the overall incidence (in humans) has increased. As a result, the USDA-FSIS has begun a "*Salmonella* initiative" (USDA-FSIS, 2006a), which has refocused both industry and regulatory efforts on the control of *Salmonella*.

10.8 MAINTAINING PRODUCT QUALITY AND REDUCING THE NUMBER OF MICROORGANISMS

A recent advance in improving product quality at the slaughter and processing plant is the development and implementation of the HACCP-PR system. The principles of HACCP include hazard analysis, identification of critical control points (the CCPs), followed by establishment of CCP monitoring, limits, corrective actions if limits are exceeded, verification that the HACCP system works, and documentation of all of the HACCP steps and procedures.

To augment and enhance the HACCP system, ongoing scientific advances in pathogen identification are being developed. Such methods were already in place at the time of HACCP implementation, but the usefulness of these methods is more obvious with HACCP system requirements. Rapid methods for identifying food microbiological status and verification of performance at critical control points are needed for HACCP to be effective. Improvements in analytical microbiology applications that have the potential or are finding application in pork processing include improvements in culture methods, electrical methods, ATP bioluminescence (especially for the monitoring of sanitation and cleanliness of work surfaces and processing equipment), and a variety of improved immunological and genetic techniques and assays (McMeekin, 2003).

Microbial risk assessment (MRA) is a relatively new tool for improving food quality and decreasing product contamination (Brown and Stringer, 2002). MRA involves hazard identification and characterization, exposure assessment, and risk characterization. Thus, MRA results in predictions of the likelihood of illness based on dose–response characterization, how much and how often consumers are exposed, and a synthesis of the risk chain to provide a qualitative or quantitative estimate of the risk from a particular food. A general MRA model for pork using generic *Salmonella* showed the risk of human *Salmonella* cases that are pork-associated and the associated social costs (Miller et al., 2005). Sensitivity analysis in this study demonstrated that *Salmonella* contamination during processing was more important for human health risk, and practices applied during processing to control contamination had higher benefit/cost ratios than those of on-farm strategies that controlled *Salmonella*.

10.9 MICROBIOLOGICAL METHODS FOR DETECTION AND QUANTIFICATION

Conventional bacteriological analysis of meat products may be characterized as either qualitative or quantitative. The assays for most pathogenic bacteria are qualitative, primarily because the regulatory environment is based on a presence/absence concept rather than on a population perspective. For example, the current *Salmonella* performance standards (USDA-FSIS, 1996b) are based on the percentage of samples that are positive by a presence/absence assay. Although this simplifies sample analysis and the interpretation of results, it also means that a sample with one *Salmonella* cell per 100 cm^2 is essentially equivalent to a sample that contains1000 *Salmonella* cells per square centimeter.

Most qualitative pathogen analytical methods follow the same basic format: a nonselective enrichment to recover injured bacteria, a selective enrichment to increase the population of the target bacterium, and a detection step. In some cases, the selective enrichments are combined, and in others, a confirmation step follows the detection step. Methods used presently in meat processing include traditional bacteriological methods as well as both immunological- and genetic-based detection systems. Currently, the *Microbiological Laboratory Guidebook* (MLG) (USDA-FSIS, 1998b) includes both recommended methods for detection of pathogens and performance specifications for the analytical methods (sensitivity and specificity). Any method that can be shown to meet the performance characteristics stated in MLG is considered acceptable for the detection of a specific pathogen. In practice, many commercially available analytical tests are independently verified in terms of performance characteristics so that they may be used in the microbiological analysis of food products.

Quantitative analytical methods are typically utilized for process control indicators (e.g., *E. coli* biotype I) as well as general indicators of contamination. Quantitative analytical methods are also used for the enumeration of the populations of spoilage bacteria. General methods of quantitating bacteria populations involve either direct plating on media, most probable number methods, or membrane filtration. Direct plating is by far the most common methodology, using either prepared petri dishes or Petrifilm (3M Microbiology, 2006). The most probable number technique also applies to specific pathogens, but the methodology is cumbersome, labor intensive, and lacking in precision. As with the qualitative analytical methods, the USDA-FSIS MLG describes the officially recommended analytical methods for quantitative determination of microbial populations (USDA-FSIS, 1998b).

10.10 REGULATIONS

Meat inspection in the United States is historically based on the Federal Meat Inspection Act (FIMA) of 1906. A complete history of the role of federal meat inspection may be found on the USDA-FSIS website (USDA-FSIS, 2006b). Although the FIMA has been revised continually over the years, the single greatest change in approach to inspection came with the HACCP System Final Rule of 1996 (USDA-FSIS, 1996a). This rule implemented a series of changes, including mandatory sanitation standard operating procedures, implementation of the HACCP system in meat-processing establishments, microbiological testing for *E. coli* biotype I/II, and performance standards for *Salmonella*. These changes were substantial, not only from a regulatory perspective but also from a philosophical approach, as it represented a shift in the thought processes of the agency. From a practical standpoint, implementation of HACCP was a step that had been endorsed by the scientific community for years (NRC, 1985), and the addition of microbiological testing resulted in standards for pathogens in fresh raw products for the first time in the United States.

Sanitation standard operating procedures (SSOPs) require that a meat- processing establishment have written procedures to clean and sanitize both the equipment and the processing environment. In addition, these procedures must include details on monitoring and corrective action. That is, the procedures must specifically state what is to be inspected and how it will be inspected to determine if the cleaning and sanitizing procedures have been carried out satisfactorily. In addition, corrective actions must be described to address any failures in the procedures. Although met with skepticism initially, the meat industry has generally embraced SSOPs, and they have probably been effective in improving the overall hygiene of meat-processing establishments.

Traditional inspection determines when a failure has occurred and implements procedures to address the failure. In contrast, HACCP systems focus on prevention. The development of a HACCP plan requires that a meat-processing establishment address prerequisite programs [such as sanitation and good manufacturing practices (GMPs)] as well as comprehensive risk assessment. The HACCP approach to meat processing is essentially a variant of the "modes of failure" concept in quality assurance, where possible errors in manufacturing are identified and then monitored to prevent a failure. HACCP is based on seven principles that have evolved over the years. An excellent summary of the HACCP system is that of the National Advisory Committee on Microbiological Criteria for Food (NACMCF, 1998).

The requirement for *E. coli* biotype I/II testing was based on an assumption that this group of nonpathogenic bacteria was a useful indicator of contamination in raw meat–processing systems. Although *E. coli* testing is mandatory, the results are to be used as part of statistical process control, to assure that the food-processing system is under adequate control. In contrast, the *Salmonella* performance standards are regulatory requirements to achieve a level of reduction of *Salmonella* on the product. As with any regulatory standard, there are clear actions to be taken in the event that the standard is not met. The current *Salmonella* performance standard for market hogs is 8.7%, or a maximum of 6 positive samples out of a sample set of 55.

Although there are several components of the *Salmonella* initiative (USDA-FSIS, 2006a), the most immediate is the introduction of a category system for *Salmonella* performance standards. Category 1 is considered to be plants at or below 50% of the current standard (by species); category 2 is considered to be plants between 50 and 100% of the current standard; and category 3 is considered to be plants above 100% of the standard. In other words, category 3 plants are those that fail to meet the current performance standard. In the agency's words: "The industry-wide shift to category 1 level process control for *Salmonella* is expected to be timely" (Englejohn, 2006). This, in effect, lowers the *Salmonella* performance standard for pork carcasses to 4.35% positive or less.

Listeria monocytogenes is a human pathogen of concern that may be associated with fully cooked, ready-to-eat meats. *Listeria* does not survive normal lethality processes, but does persist in the environment. Fully cooked meats may become contaminated with *Listeria* during the stabilization (cooling), slicing, or packaging processes. *Listeria* can survive and grow in vacuum packages and at low temperatures, so the possibility of multiplication exists in these products. To address this issue, the USDA-FSIS has established requirements for processors that produce fully cooked, ready-to-eat meat products (USDA-FSIS, 2003a). These regulations outline three alternatives for the control of *L. monocytogenes* in ready-to-eat products and require increased testing of establishments that rely on what the USDA-FSIS considers the lowest level (alternative 3) of control.

REFERENCES

3M Microbiology (2006): Online catalog: microbiology. http://solutions.3m.com/wps/portal/3M/en_US/Microbiology/FoodSafety/products/product-catalog/?PC_7_RJH9U523003DC023S7P92O3O87_nid=2BJ86690LFbe29BDXSBJ7Fgl. Accessed April 2008.

Ayres JC (1955): Microbial implications in the handling, slaughtering and dressing of meat animals. *Adv Food Res*. 6:109–161.

Barber DA, Miller GY, McNamara PE (2003): Modeling food safety and food-associated antimicrobial resistance risk to humans. *J Food Prot*. 66:700–709.

Berends BR, Van Knapen F, Snijders JMA, Mossel DAA (1997): Identification and quantification of risk factors regarding *Salmonella* spp. on pork carcasses. *Int J Food Microbiol*. 36:199–206.

Bolton DJ, Pearce RA, Sheridan JJ, Blair IS, McDowell DA, Harrington D (2002): Washing and chilling as critical control points in pork slaughter hazard analysis and critical control point (HACCP) systems. *J Appl Microbiol*. 92:893–902.

Bouvet J, Montet MP, Rossel R, et al. (2002): Effects of slaughter processes on pig carcass contamination by verotoxin-producing *Escherichia coli* and *E. coli* O157:H7. *Int J Food Microbiol*. 77:99–108.

Brown M, Stringer M (2002): *Microbiological Risk Assessment in Food Processing*. CRC Press, Boca Raton, FL, p. 301.

Canada JC, Strong DH (1964): *Clostridium perfringens* in bovine livers. *J Food Sci*. 29:862–864.

Dickson JS, Hurd HS, Rostagno MH (2002): *Salmonella* in the pork production chain: A review. Paper presented at the Pork Quality and Safety Summit, National Pork Producers Council, Des Moines, IA.

Duffy EA, Belk KE, Sofos JN, Bellinger GR, Pape A, Smith GC (2001): Extent of microbial contamination in United States pork retail products. *J Food Prot*. 64:172–178.

Eggenberger-Solorzano L, Niebuhr SE, Acuff GR, Dickson JS (2002): Hot water and organic acid interventions to control microbiological contamination on hog carcasses during processing. *J Food Prot*. 65:1248–1252.

Englejohn D (2006): Meeting summarization. In *Proc. Public Meeting on Advances in Post-harvest Reduction of* Salmonella *in Poultry*. http://www.fsis.usda.gov/PDF/Slides_022406_Engeljohn.pdf. Accessed April 2008.

Gill CO, Bryant J (1992): The contamination of pork with spoilage bacteria during commercial dressing, chilling and cutting of pig carcasses. *Intl J Food Microbiol*. 16 (1):51–62.

Gill CO, McGinnis DS, Bryant J, Chabot B (1995): Decontamination of commercial, polished pig carcasses with hot watter. *Food Microbiol*. 12:143–149.

Hurd SH, Mckean JD, Wesley IV, Karricker LA (2001): The effect of lairage on *Salmonella* isolation from market swine. *J Food Prot*. 64 (7):939–944.

ICMSF (International Commission on Microbiological Specifications for Foods) (1996): Listeria monocytogenes. In: Roberts TA, Baird-Parker AC, Tompkin RB (Eds.). *Microorganisms in Foods*, Vol. 5. Blackie Academic and Professional, London, pp. 141–182.

Ingram M (1964): Feeding meat animals before slaughter. *Vet Rec*. 76:1305–1315.

Ingram M, Dainty RH (1971): Changes caused by microbes in spoilage of meat. *J Appl Bacteriol*. 34:21–39.

Jay JM (2000): Indicators of food microbial quality and safety. In: Jay J (Ed.): *Modern Food Microbiology*, 6th ed. Aspen Publishers, Gaithersburg, MD, pp. 473–566.

Jensen LB, Hess WR (1941): A study of ham souring. *Food Res.* 6:272–326.

Luchsinger SE, Kropf DH, Garcia Zepeda CM, et al. (1996a): Sensory analysis and consumer acceptance of irradiated boneless pork chops. *J Food Sci.* 61:1261–1266.

Luchsinger SE, Kropf DH, Garcia Zepeda CM, et al. (1996b): Color and oxidative rancidity of gamma and electron beam-irradiated boneless pork chops. *J Food Sci.* 61:1000–1006.

Marshall KM, Niebuhr SE, Acuff GR, Lucia LM, Dickson JS (2005): The identification of *Escherichia coli* O157:H7 meat processing indicators for fresh meat through the comparison of the effects of selected anti-microbial interventions. *J Food Prot.* 68: 2580–2586.

McMeekin TA (2003): *Detecting Pathogens in Food.* CRC Press/Woodhead Publishing, Boca Raton, FL, pp. 1–365.

Miller MF, Carr MA, Bawcom DB, Ramsey CB, Thompson LD (1997): Microbiology of pork carcasses from pigs with differing origins and feed withdrawal times. *J Food Prot.* 60:242–245.

Miller GY, Liu X, McNamara PE, Barber DA (2005): The influence of *Salmonella* in pigs pre-harvest and during pork processing on *Salmonella* human health costs and risks from pork. *J Food Prot.* 68:135–145.

NACMCF (National Advisory Committee on Microbiological Criteria for Food) (1998): Hazard analysis and critical control point principles and application guidelines. *J Food Prot.* 61:1246–1259.

Namvar A, Warriner K (2006): Application of enterobacterial repetitive intergenic consensus–polymerase chain reaction to trace the fate of generic *Escherichia coli* within a high capacity pork slaughter line. *Int J Food Microbiol.* 108:155–163.

Narayan KG (1966): Studies on *Clostridia* incidence in beef cattle. *Acta Vet Acad Sci Hung.* 16:65–72.

NRC (National Research Council) (1985): *An Evaluation of the Role of Microbiological Criteria for Foods and Food Ingredients.* National Academies Press, Washington, DC.

Pearce RA, Sheridan JJ, Bolton DJ (2006): Distribution of airborne microorganisms in commercial pork slaughter processes. *Int J Food Microbiol.* 107:186–191.

Porto ACS, Call JE, Luchansky JB (2004): Effect of reheating on viability of a five-strain mixture of *Listeria monocytogenes* in vacuum-sealed packages of frankfurters following refrigerated or frozen storage. *J Food Prot.* 67:71–76.

Radin D, Niebuhr SE, Dickson JS (2006): Impact of the population of spoilage microflora on the growth of *Listeria monocytogenes* on frankfurters. *J Food Prot.* 69:679–681.

Rigney CP, Salamone BP, Anadaraman N, et al. (2004): *Salmonella* serotypes in selected classes of food animal carcasses and raw ground products of food animal carcasses and raw ground products, January 1998 through December 2000. *J Am Vet Med Assoc.* 224:524–530.

Unnevehr LJ, Miller GY, Gómez MI (1999): Ensuring food safety and quality in farm level production: emerging lessons from the pork industry. *Am J Agric Econ.* 81:1096–1101.

USDA (1997): Shedding of *Salmonella* by finisher hogs in the U.S. NAHMS Swine Survey 1995. http://www.aphis.usda.gov/vs/ceah/ncahs/nahms/swine/swine95/sw95salm.pdf. Accessed November 21, 2008.

USDA-FSIS (U.S. Department of Agriculture–Food Safety and Inspection Service) (1996a): Nationwide pork microbiological baseline data collection program: Market hogs. http://www.fsis.usda.gov/OPHS/baseline/markhog1.pdf. Accessed September 2002.

———(1996b): Pathogen reduction/hazard analysis critical control point (HACCP) systems final rule. *Fed Reg*. 61:38805–38989. http://www.fsis.usda.gov/OPPDE/rdad/FRPubs/93-016F.pdf. Accessed July 2007.

———(1998a): Nationwide sponge microbiological baseline data collection program: swine, June 1997–May 1998. http://www.fsis.usda.gov/PDF/Baseline_Data_Swine.pdf. Accessed July 2006.

———(1998b): *Microbiological Laboratory Guidebook*, 3rd ed. Current version online at http://www.fsis.usda.gov/Science/Microbiological_Lab_Guidebook/index.asp. Accessed July 2006.

———(1999): Performance standards for the production of certain meat and poultry products. *Fed. Reg*. 64:732–749. http://www.fsis.usda.gov/Frame/FrameRedirect.asp?main=http://www.fsis.usda.gov/OPPDE/rdad/FRPubs/95-033F.htm. Accessed July 27, 2006.

———(2003a): Control of *Listeria monocytogenes* in ready-to-eat meat and poultry products: final rule. *Fed reg*. 68:34207–34254. http://www.fsis.usda.gov/OPPDE/rdad/FRPubs/97-013F.htm. Accessed July 2006.

———(2003b): Progress report on *Salmonella* testing of raw meat and poultry products, 1998–2002. http://www.fsis.usda.gov/OPHS/haccp/salm5year.htm. Accessed March 2006.

———(2006a): FSIS announces initiative to reduce *Salmonella* in meat and poultry. http://www.fsis.usda.gov/news/NR_022306_01/index.asp. Accessed July 24, 2006.

———(2006b): Celebrating 100 years of FIMA (Federal Meat Inspection Act). http://www.fsis.usda.gov/About_FSIS/100_Years/index.asp. Accessed July 6, 2006.

Vieira-Pinto M, Tenreiro R, Martins C (2006): Unveiling contamination sources and dissemination routes of *Salmonella* sp. in pigs at a Portuguese slaughterhouse through macrorestriction profiling by pulsed-field gel electrophoresis. *Int J Food Microbiol*. 110:77–84.

Warriner K, Aldsworth TG, Kaur S, Dodd CER (2002): Cross-contamination of carcasses and equipment during pork processing. *J Appl Microbiol*. 93:169–177.

Zagaevskii IS (1973): Beef contamination by *Clostridium perfringens*. *Veterinariya*. 1:101–103.

CHAPTER 11

FOOD SAFETY ISSUES AND THE MICROBIOLOGY OF FISH AND SHELLFISH

LUCIO GALAVIZ-SILVA, GRACIA GOMÉZ-ANDURO,
ZINNIA J. MOLINA-GARZA, and FELIPE ASCENCIO-VALLE

11.1 INTRODUCTION

Fish and fishery products are at the forefront of food safety and quality improvement because they are among the most internationally traded food commodities. Of the products used for human consumption, fresh fish showed significant growth from 1990 to 2005 (FAO, 2007). Approximately 45% of the fish used for human consumption is sold fresh, 30% frozen, 14% canned, and 12% cured (Gram et al., 2002; Huss et al., 2003). Seafood includes cephalopods (octopus, squid), freshwater and saltwater fish (including finfish), and shellfish. Shellfish include the bivalve molluskan shellfish (oysters, cockles, clams, and mussels), gastropods (periwinkles, sea snails), and crustaceans (crab, lobster, and shrimp).

Seafood is an important part of a healthy diet. In some countries it is the main source of animal protein. Furthermore, it has become a healthy alternative to other animal protein (e.g., beef), because it contains low fat and beneficial omega-3 polyunsaturated fatty acids.

Despite its benefits, seafood consumption can cause allergic reactions, infection, or intoxication (Huss, 1997). In this chapter we focus on infection and intoxication. Infection and intoxication from seafood consumption are commonly caused by ingestion of the microorganisms that live in seafood tissue.

Foodborne illnesses from seafood are more common in countries with high seafood consumption or traditions of eating seafood raw. Twenty percent of foodborne illnesses in Australia and more than 70% in Japan were related to seafood consumption in 2003 (Butt et al., 2004). Most of the infectious outbreaks from seafood appear to be due to shellfish rather than to finfish. A study from New York attributed 64% of

Microbiologically Safe Foods, Edited by Norma Heredia, Irene Wesley, and Santos García

the seafood-related infectious outbreaks to shellfish and 31% to finfish (Butt et al., 2004). Finfish are less likely to be associated with infectious illness because they are most often eaten well cooked. Mollusks are more frequently marketed and eaten raw or only partially cooked, thereby increasing the risk of infectious illness by organisms that would otherwise be killed or inactivated by heat. In addition, mollusks are filter-feeders, which can concentrate infectious microorganisms in their tissue because they filter several liters of water a day. Oysters can concentrate fecal coliform bacteria in their tissue that is four times more concentrated than their environment (Olafsen, 2001; Olafsen et al., 1993). This selective accumulation may be seasonal and also parallel other pathogenic microorganisms or toxins (Butt et al., 2004; FAO, 2007), such as *Vibrio cholera, V. parahaemolyticus*, and biotoxins, (Flores-Luna et al., 1993; Hernández et al., 2005). Because of the public health significance of foodborne diseases associated with this commodity, in 2008 the National Advisory Committe for Microbiological Criteria for Foods drafted extensive recommended cooking parameters for fish and shellfish (NACMCF, 2008)

11.2 NORMAL FLORA OF FISH AND SHELLFISH

The total number of bacteria found on fish varies enormously. Between 10^2 and 10^7 CFU/cm^2 can be found on the skin surface and between 10^3 and 10^9 CFU/cm^2 on the intestine or gills (Liston, 1980). Fish caught in cold, clean waters tend to carry fewer microorganisms than fish caught in warm waters. Microorganism species composition in seafood can vary by temperature. *Clostridium botulinum* and *Listeria* spp. are most common in colder climates. Horse mussels (*Modiolus modiolus*) collected from 4 to 6°C in seawater 6 to 10 m below the sea surface contained bacteria in hemolymph (2.6×10^4 CFU) and soft tissues (2.9×10^4 CFU) at densities similar to those of oysters. These bacteria were primarily *Pseudomonas* (61.3%), *Vibrio* (27.0%), and *Aeromonas* spp. (11.7%) in hemolymph and *Vibrio* (38.5%), *Pseudomonas* (33.0%), and *Aeromonas* spp. (28.5%) in soft tissue (Barbieri et al., 1999; Olafsen et al., 1993).

The dominant microorganisms on, or in, temperate-water fish are psychrotrophic gram-negative rod-shaped bacteria (*Pseudomonas, Moraxella, Acinetobacter, Shewanella,* and *Flavobacterium* spp.), *Vibrio* and *Photobacterium* spp., and *Aeromonas* spp. Gram-positive bacteria (*Bacillus, Micrococcus, Clostridium, Lactobacillus*, and coryneforms) are also found on temperate fish in lower numbers.

The dominant microorganisms on warm-water fish are psychrotrophs, psychrophiles, and mesophiles. The dominant microorganisms on coastal and estuarine fish are mesophilic *V. cholerae* and *V. parahaemolyticus*, gram-positive bacteria, and enteric bacteria.

The dominant microorganisms in aquaculture are *V. anguillarum, V. salmonicida, V. vulnificus* (fish pathogens), and *V. harveyi* (shrimp pathogen, particularly in white shrimp, *Litopenaeus vannamei*, and tiger shrimp, *Penaeus monodon*). Reared fish larvae and shellfish larvae are particularly vulnerable to mortality caused by *Vibrio* spp., sometimes leading to death of the entire population (Lightner and Redman, 1998; Olafsen, 2001). In contrast, *Vibrio* spp. on plankton and particulates appear to enhance the survival and growth of reared *L. vannamei*. Healthy *L. vannamei* have approximately 10^9 CFU/g of *Vibrio* spp. and *Aeromonas* spp. in their gut tissue (up to 85% of total gut bacteria) (Moss et al., 2000) and 10^5 CFU/g and 10^4 CFU/mL *Vibrio* spp. in the hepatopancreas and hemolymph, respectively (Gomez-Gil et al., 2000).

The most abundant bacteria (1.4×10^2 to 5.6×10^2/mL) in the hemolymph and soft tissues of coldwater (1 to 8°C)-reared Pacific oysters (*Crassostrea gigas*) are *Pseudomonas* spp., *Alteromonas* spp., *Vibrio* spp., and *Aeromonas* spp.

Vibrio spp. are the most abundant microorganism across all aquatic environments combined, including aquaculture. They are very dense in and around marine organisms such as corals, fish, mollusks, sea grasses, sponges, shrimp, and zooplankton (Barbieri et al., 1999).

Many seafood species have a symbiotic relationship with the bacteria in, or on, their bodies. *Photobacterium leiognathi* and *P. phosphoreum* have symbiotic associations with fish; and *P. leiognathi*, *V. logei*, and *V. fischeri* have symbiotic associations with squid. These bacteria colonize the light-producing organs of the host and emit the light that the host uses for communication, prey attraction, and predator avoidance. In the light organs of the squid *Sepiolla* spp., the abundance of vibrios can be as high as 10^{11} cells per organ. Dense colonies of *Vibrio* (*V. anguillarum*, *V. cholerae*, *V. harveyi*, *V. parahaemolyticus*, and *V. vulnificus*) and up to 4.3×10^6/mm^2 *Photobacterium* spp. are attached to the external membrane of zooplankton in what is believed to be a symbiotic relationship (Thompson et al., 2004). *Vibrio* spp. form a biofilm on the exoskeletons of these zooplankton that may enable the plankton to cope during environmental stress (e.g., low food resources). In turn, *Vibrio* spp. trap and absorb nutrients, resist antibiotics, and establish favorable partnerships with other bacteria or hosts (Diggles et al., 2000; Zo et al., 2002).

11.3 MICROBIAL HAZARDS AND PREVENTIVE MEASURES

Seafood pathogens include pathogenic bacteria (infectious or toxin producing), biogenic amines, viruses, parasites, and aquatic biotoxins. Disease can occur without ingestion of viable bacteria. For intoxication to occur, toxin-producing bacteria need to grow to a minimum density (10^5 to 10^8 CFU/g) prior to ingestion. Lists of hazardous pathogens are available on the FDA website (USFDA, 2001) under the subcategory of Fish and Fisheries Products Hazard and Control Guidance.

11.3.1 Organisms

Seafood microorganisms can originate from the marine or freshwater environment, water pollution, or contamination. Sources of contamination include fish-processing handlers and their equipment, and the environment (Price, 2007). According to Food and Agriculture Association (FAO) specialists, seafood-borne pathogenic bacteria may conveniently be divided into three groups, depending on their ecology and origin: (1) indigenous to an aquatic environment and naturally present on fish, (2) indigenous to multiple environments and frequently found on seafood, and (3) found on the outer and inner surfaces of diseased or asymptomatic animal/human carriers (Huss et al., 2003). Group 1 includes *Clostridium botulinum* (nonproteolytic types B, E, and F); *Vibrio cholerae*, *V. parahaemolyticus*, and *V. vulnificus* (ubiquitous in salt water); *Plesiomonas shigelloides* (warm freshwater organism); and *Aeromonas*. Group 2 includes *Listeria monocytogenes*, *C. botulinum* (proteolytic types A and B), *Clostridium perfringens* (type A from soil and types B, C, and D from animals), and *Bacillus* spp. Group 3 includes *Salmonella* spp., *Shigella* spp., *Escherichia coli*, *Staphylococcus aureus*, *Campylobacter jejuni*, and other mesophilic *Campylobacter* spp. These species are initially absent on seafood, but contaminate seafood via poor hygienic and manufacturing practices (Huss et al., 2003). Some of the pathogenic bacteria in this group are also part of the natural flora on fish in their aquatic environment. Usually, these natural bacteria populations need to grow on the fish products before disease will occur in humans.

The proteolytic *C. botulinum* is frequently found in soil in the terrestrial environment and can possibly spread to the aquatic environment or fish-processing environment. *C. botulinum* contamination of seafood products can be prevented if seafood is stored continuously below 3.3°C; stored at 5 to 10°C with a shelf life of less than 5 days; heat treated at 90°C for 10 min followed by cold storage below 10°C; or the pH in the tissue set below 5.0 combined with cold storage below 10°C.

V. parahaemolyticus causes serious gastroenteritis in humans (Huss et al. 1997) (see Chapter 2). It is common in many seafood products, particularly bivalve mollusks. In its natural environment, *V. parahaemolyticus* population size is larger when temperature is higher, and probably survives colder temperatures in sediment, emerging with zooplankton when temperature rises (EC, 2001). *V. parahaemolyticus* is very heat sensitive and easily destroyed by cooking. Temperatures at 50 to 60°C for 0.3 to 0.8 min destroy these bacteria sufficiently (USFDA-CFSAN, 2001).

Human enteric viruses are the major cause of shellfish-associated disease. Over 100 enteric viruses are excreted with human feces into domestic sewage, but only a few are linked to seafood-associated illness: hepatitis A, the Norwalk virus, the Snow Mountain agent, Calicivirus spp., Astrovirus (Kilgen and Cole, 1991), and Rotavirus (USFDA-CFSAN, 2001). These viruses contaminate seafood via polluted water or infected food handlers.

Shellfish will filter-feed and concentrate waterborne viruses. Individual oysters, for example, can filter up to 1500 L/day (Gerba and Goyal, 1978), thus bioconcentrating the virus. Health officials are concerned about viruses from shellfish harvest locations because (1) many harvest locations are in areas that have natural pathogens and sewage pathogens, (2) the shellfish in these areas will filter and bioconcentrate pathogens from surrounding water; and (3) shellfish are often consumed whole and raw or partially cooked (USFDA-CFSAN, 2001).

Parasites (in the larval stage) are responsible for a substantial number of seafood-associated infections worldwide (Table 1). Consumption of raw or undercooked seafood is the factor most commonly associated with these infections. Some products that have been implicated in human infection are ceviche (fish and spices marinated in lime juice), lomi lomi (salmon marinated in lemon juice, onion, and tomato),

TABLE 1 Geographic Areas, Infective Stage, and Seafood Involved in Common Seafood-Borne Parasitic Infections

Parasite	Infective Stage	Geographic Area	Seafood (Intermediate Host)
Trematoda			
Alaria americana	Metacercaria	North America	Frogs
Centrocestus formosanus	Metacercaria	Asia	Fish
Clonorchis sinensis	Metacercaria	China, Japan, Canada	Fish
Echinoparyphium recurvatum	Metacercaria	Worldwide	Fish
Echinostoma iliocenum	Metacercaria	Asia, Kenya, Canada	Snails, clams, fish, crustaceans
Heterophyes heterophyes	Metacercaria	Asia	Fish
Nanophyetus salmincola	Metacercaria	North America	Fish
Opisthorchis viverrini	Metacercaria	Asia	Fish
Paragonimus spp.	Metacercaria	Worldwide	Freshwater crabs
Cestoda			
Diphyllobothrium latum	Plerocercoid	Japan, United States, Philippines	Fish
Nematoda			
Anisakis spp.	Larva	Worlwide	Fish
Capillaria philippinensis	Larva	Japan, United States	Fish
Dioctophyme renale	Larva	Worldwide	Fish
Echinocephalus sp.	Larva	Worldwide	Shellfish
Gnathostoma spp.	Larva	Asia and Mexico	Fish
Pseudoterranova spp.	Larva	Worldwide	Fish
Acanthocephala			
Bulbosoma spp.	Juvenile	Rusia	Fish
Corynosoma strumosum	Juvenile	Rusia	Fish

Source: Modified from Butt et al. (2004), Ferre (2001), Orlandi et al. (2002).

poisson cru (fish marinated in citrus juice, onion, tomato, and coconut milk), herring roe; sashimi (slices of raw fish), sushi (pieces of raw fish with rice and other ingredients), green herring (lightly brined herring), drunken crabs (crabs marinated in wine and pepper), cold-smoked fish, and undercooked grilled fish. Gastroenterologists confirmed that seafood-borne parasitic infections occur with sufficient frequency to make preventive controls necessary during the processing of parasite-containing species of fish that are intended for raw consumption (USFDA, 2001).

It is estimated that more than 50 million people are infected with seafood-borne trematodes (*Chlonorchis sinensis*, *Opisthorchis* spp., *Heterophyes* spp., *Metagonimus* spp., *Nanophyetus salminicola*, and *Paragonimus* spp.) worldwide (Butt et al., 2004; USFDA, 2001). The highest prevalence of these infections is in Southeast and East Asia, but increasing numbers of infections are being recognized in areas previously considered nonendemic, due largely to increased importation of seafood that may be contaminated and travel from endemic regions (Hine and Thorne, 2000). *Clonorchis sinensis* (the Chinese liver fluke) is highly prevalent in China, Korea, Taiwan, Vietnam, and Japan. More than 5 million people are thought to be infected in China alone (Dixon and Flohr, 1997) and additional cases are being diagnosed and reported in nonendemic areas. *C. sinensis* was reported to be the most common parasitic infection in Hong Kong immigrants to Canada between 1979 and 1981. In surveys in the United States in the 1990s, 1226 stool samples out of 216,275 tested were positive for the ova of *Clonorchis* or *Opisthorchis* spp., making this group the most frequently isolated trematode. Many fish species from the endemic areas harbor the parasite and have been associated with transmission of infection (Butt et al., 2004; Yu et al., 2003). *Metorchis conjunctus* (the Canadian liver fluke) caused an outbreak involving 17 of 19 persons from Quebec in 1996. They had consumed raw white sucker fish that was caught in a small river (MacLean et al., 1996).

Cestodes or tapeworms are a frequent cause of human infection in many countries. Diphyllobothriasis is an intestinal parasitosis acquired by eating raw or partially cooked fish containing *Diphyllobothrium* spp. plerocercoids. Most persons are asymptomatic, but diarrhea, abdominal pain, or discomfort may occur. Prolonged or heavy *Diphyllobothrium latum* infection may cause pernicious anemia (Beldsoe and Oria, 2001). Several species of *Diphyllobothrium* are responsible for human infection, but *D. latum* and *D. dendriticum* are the most common. These cestodes should be considered a possible hazard in all environments and cannot be ruled out from aquaculture systems. At least two known outbreaks of diphyllobothriasis associated with salmon consumption have been documented in the United States. It has been estimated that there are 13 million carriers globally, with greater prevalence in Eastern Europe (Beldsoe and Oria, 2001).

The human nematode infection most commonly associated with seafood-borne disease is the anisakiasis (see Chapter 2). The species most commonly implicated is *Anisakis simplex*, followed by *Pseudoterranova decipiens* (Herreras et al., 2000). Outbreaks of human anisakiasis have been reported from countries with a high consumption of raw or undercooked seafood (Butt et al., 2004). *Gnathostoma spinigerum* and *G. hispidus* are responsible for infections called "larva migrans" (cutaneous, ocular, visceral, or neurologic). It is endemic in Asiatic countries (Thailand, Japan, China, India, and Philippines). In Mexico, it became an important public health problem in several regions where raw or undercooked freshwater fish is consumed (Díaz-Camacho et al., 2000).

11.3.2 Biotoxins

Certain bacteria and marine algae produce potent toxins that impact human health when humans consume contaminated shellfish and finfish. Scombroid poisoning, also called histamine poisoning, is caused by the ingestion of foods that contain high levels of histamine and possibly other vasoactive amines and compounds. Histamine and other amines are formed by the growth of certain bacteria and the action of their decarboxylase enzymes on histidine and other amino acids during the spoilage of fishery products (USFDA, 1992). Symptoms include a metallic, sharp, or peppery taste, nausea, vomiting, abdominal cramps and diarrhea, oral blistering and numbness, facial swelling and flushing, headache and dizziness, palpitations, hives, rapid and weak pulse, thirst, and difficulty in swallowing (SeafoodNIC, 2007a).

Seafood products commonly implicated in scombroid poisoning include the tunas (e.g., skipjack and yellowfin), mahi mahi, bluefish, sardines, mackerel, amberjack, and abalone. Histamine production occurs rapidly at high temperatures, but slows dramatically at temperatures below 40°F (SeafoodNIC, 2007a). Distribution of the toxin within an individual fish fillet or between cans in a case lot can be uneven, with some sections of a product causing illnesses and others not. Neither cooking, canning, nor freezing reduces the toxic effect (SeafoodNIC, 2007a).

Mussels, clams, cockles, and scallops that eat toxic dinoflagellate algae (*Gambierdiscus toxicus, Alexandrium catenella*, *Dinophysis acuta*, and *Pseudonitzchia* spp.) retain a toxin for varying periods of time, depending on the shellfish type. Some clear the toxin very quickly and are toxic only during the actual bloom, while others retain the toxin for a long time, even years. Harmful aquatic algal blooms (HAB) are associated with outbreaks of ciguatera, paralytic shellfish poisoning (PSP), diarrheal shellfish poisoning (DSP), and amnesic shellfish poisoning (ASP). As little as a few micrograms of toxin can kill an adult human. Human cases of DSP have occurred in Japan, Southeast Asia, Scandinavia, Western Europe, Chile, New Zealand, and eastern Canada (USFDA-CFSAN, 2001).

Dinoflagellate toxins are very poisonous. The short history of these pathological phenomena suggests that they are increasing in frequency and expanding their geographical range (Hernández et al., 2005; Huss, 1997). In general, shrimp and fish do not carry toxins. Most of the time, contamination occurs when seafood is harvested from areas with natural toxins. Other times, however, a fish can acquire a toxin by eating toxic algae. Humans can acquire ciguatera food poisoning (CFP) if they consume fish that have eaten toxic marine algae or toxin-contaminated fish. Ciguatera and related toxins are derived from dinoflagellates (algae), which herbivorous fish consume while foraging through macro-algae.

Ciguatera is common in tropical and subtropical areas of the South Atlantic Ocean, the Caribbean Sea, the South Pacific Ocean, and the Indian Ocean. The ciguatera toxin will biomagnify in the tissue of top fish predators that feed on smaller reef fish, becoming a danger to humans who harvest the predators.

Over the past three decades, the global frequency and global distribution of harmful algal blooms and toxic algal incidents appear to have increased, and human intoxications from novel algal sources are more common, raising concerns. The increase parallels an increase in global ecologic disturbances coincidental with trends in global warming.

Some of the changes in algal bloom and toxin incidents may be due to increased awareness, aquaculture, eutrophication, and/or transport of algal cysts in ship ballast. Researchers are developing better methods for the detection of algal toxins, which accounts for some of the increases (Brett, 2003).

Marine algal toxins are responsible for an array of human illnesses associated with consumption of seafood. Approximately 20% of all foodborne disease outbreaks in the United States result from the consumption of seafood, with half of them originating from naturally occurring algal toxins (Ahmed, 1991). Worldwide, marine algal toxins are responsible for more than 60,000 intoxication incidents per year and an overall human mortality rate of 1.5% (Ahmed, 1992). Algal toxins also cause extensive die-offs of fish and shellfish and have been implicated in episodic mortalities of animals within the marine food web (e.g., birds, fish, and mammals) (Brett, 2003). Algal intoxication is generally believed to be acute, but the health effects of chronic exposure are becoming an emerging issue (Burkholder, 1998; Edmunds et al., 1999; Landsberg, 1996; Landsberg et al., 1999). Most algal toxins are tolerant of high temperatures, so cooking does not eliminate them (Van Dolah, 2000).

Worldwide, humans consume many types of mollusks, therefore, mollusks have significant commercial value. Bivalve mollusks are very important hazards because they filter-feed algae. Among the thousands of species of microscopic algae, scientists have identified a few dozen significantly toxic species. If mollusks feed on toxic algae, the toxins bioconcentrate to levels lethal to humans (Ciminiello and Fattorusso, 2006).

Pectenotoxins (PTXs) are a group of toxins isolated from dinoflagellate algae that cause diarrheal shellfish poisoning (DSP), hepatotoxic effects in humans, cytotoxic effects on human cancer cells, and are tumor promoters in animals. With advances in technology, scientists continue to identify additional new PTXs, but know little about their toxicology and potential impacts on public health, making it difficult to conduct adequate health-risk assessments (Burgess and Shaw, 2001).

Cyanobacteria (blue–green algae) produce a variety of toxins called cyanotoxins. Cyanotoxins are functionally classified as hepato-, neuro-, and cytotoxins. Cyanobacteria also produce lipopolysaccharide (LPS) irritants. Cyanotoxins are chemically classified as cyclic peptides (hepatotoxins, microcystins, and nodularin), alkaloids (anatoxin and saxitoxin neurotoxins), and LPS. Toxic cyanobacteria include *Microcystis aeruginosa*, *Planktothrix* (*Oscillatoria*) *rubescens*, *Aphanizomenon flos-aquae*, *Anabaena flos-aquae*, *Planktothrix agardhii*, and *Lyngbia* spp. (Hitzfeld et al., 2000). Rather than bioconcentrate via filter-feeding (i.e., mollusks), cyanotoxins concentrate on surface scum, where scientists have recently focused many risk assessments (Ibelings and Chorus, 2007).

Fish can accumulate cyanotoxins through predation on cyanobacteria (e.g., *Hypophthalmichthys molitrix*), uptake of dissolved cyanobacteria microcysts through gills and skin epithelium (e.g., *Jenynsia multidentata* and *Corydoras paleatus*) (Cazenave et al., 2005), or accumulation via the food web (e.g., flounder eating blue mussels that filter-fed toxic cyanobacteria).

Time is associated with toxin accumulation and depuration in animals. Cyanobacteria toxin concentrations in fish are very dependent on the length of exposure (Kankaanpaa et al., 2002). Cyanotoxins are ubiquitous and can be found in the tissue and organs of fish, mollusks, macroinvertebrates (including bivalves), and other filter-feedering aquatic organisms, some of which are consumed by humans. Saker et al. (1999) found alkaloid hepatotoxin cylindrospermopsin and microcystic cyanobacteria in *Cherax quadricarinatus* crayfish. Kankaanpaa et al. (2005) found hepatotoxins in *Penaeus monodon* tiger prawns. Chen and Xie (2005a,b) found microcystic cyanobacteria in *Palemon modestus* shrimp, *Macrobrachium nipponensis* shrimp, and *Procamburus clarkii* crayfish. Magalhaes et al. (2001) demonstrated the presence of microcystic cyanobacteria in fish (*Tilapia rendalli*). Negri et al. (2004) found microcystic cyanobacteria in *Pinctada maxima* oysters.

Cyanotoxins tend to accumulate in the less edible body parts of seafood, such as the gut or pancreas, but will still accumulate in muscle tissue. When cyanobacteria blooms disappear, toxin concentrations in animals may decrease or persist until the next season (Pires et al., 2004; Zurawell et al., 2006). The health risk from exposure to cyanotoxins is difficult to quantify, because knowledge of cyanotoxin exposure and its effects is currently inconclusive, especially for humans (Hitzfeld et al., 2000).

In health risk assessment, the goal is to apply weights to different exposure types to create allocation factors. The main source of exposure is drinking water, which has an allocation factor of 0.8, but other sources of exposure are more difficult to quantify. Scientists may currently be underestimating health risks from fish, mussels, and shellfish consumption because they often do not consider bioconcentration effects. Furthermore, exposure via consumption may vary considerably among countries and regions.

When cyanotoxin concentration in seafood reaches dangerous levels, health officials will issue consumption advisories. Responsible authorities should perform evaluations and develop action plans in conjunction with HACCP (hazard analysis of critical control points; see Chapter 22) plans for commercial seafood operations, and water safety plans that control eutrophication. In locations with significant cyanotoxin concentrations, the plan should include surveillance of seafood quality and cyanotoxin testing. Since seafood consumption rates can vary across regions, inspectors also need standardized threshold values so that they can quickly assess the need for consumption advisories (Ibelings and Chorus, 2007).

To reduce the number of seafood outbreaks, many agencies (e.g., water quality; disease surveillance; consumer education; and seafood harvesting, processing, and marketing) need to coordinate their activities. Foodborne disease surveillance data highlight where to focus prevention efforts: (1) pathogens (and their hosts) causing the largest number of seafood-associated outbreaks and illnesses: namely, shellfish-associated viral gastroenteritis and finfish-associated scombroid fish poisoning; and (2) venues where seafood illnesses were most frequently reported, such as commercial food establishments and catered events (Wallace et al., 1999).

11.4 SPOILAGE

Spoilage is currently not quantifiable, yet there are qualitative indicators (e.g., off-odor and off-flavor, slime formation, gas production, discoloration, and changes in texture) defined by a combination of microbiological, chemical, and autolytic phenomena (Gram et al., 2002; Huss, 1992; Huss et al., 2003).

Seafood is typically rich in nitrogen and protein but low in carbohydrates; therefore, postmortem pH is less than 6.0. Seafood phospholipids and lipids (mainly triglycerides) are highly unsaturated, which affects spoilage in aerobic conditions. Initially, seafood loses its quality via autolytic changes. Spoilage then occurs when microorganisms (primarily gram-negative psychrotrophic bacteria) begin to multiply.

Fish caught in tropical areas may initially carry a high load of gram-positive organisms and enteric bacteria. During storage, a characteristic flora develops in seafood, but only parts of this flora contribute to spoilage. Specific spoilage organisms (SSOs) produce metabolites that cause the undesirable odors and flavors associated with spoilage.

Shewanella putrefaciens is a typical spoilage organism in fish from temperate waters. It produces trimethylamine (TMA), hydrogen sulfide (H_2S), and other volatile sulfide metabolites that give rise to the sulfurous off-odor and off-flavor associated with spoilage. Vibrionaceae and Enterobacteriaceae spoilage organisms produce similar metabolites during spoilage at higher temperatures. Another common spoilage bacterium, the psychrophilic *Photobacterium* spp., can generate large amounts of TMA in an atypical atmosphere (i.e., more CO_2).

Pseudomonas spp. appear to be the main bacteria involved with fresh water and tropical fish spoilage during aerobic storage. It has a characteristic fruity, sulfurous odor. *Pseudomonas* spp. produce several volatile sulfides [e.g., methylmercaptan (CH_3SH) and dimethyl sulfide $(CH_3)_2S$], ketones, esters, and aldehydes.

Scientists have identified most of the SSOs as well as threshold densities for increases in spoilage rate. Spoilage proceeds very rapidly when the SSO density exceeds approximately 10^7 CFU/g (Dalgaard, 2000; Gram et al., 2002; Huss, 1997; USFDA-CFSAN, 2001). Microbiological activity will cause spoilage of preserved fish products stored at temperatures above 0°C. In most cases the specific spoilage bacteria are not known.

Preservation salts and acids influence microflora composition. The main bacteria in these products are gram-positive bacterial species (e.g., lactic acid bacteria, *Brochotrix* spp.) (Table 2) that will act as SSOs under certain conditions. Strongly preserved (salt cured and fermented) fish products usually have gram-positive halophilic or halotolerant micrococci, spore-formers, lactic acid bacteria, yeasts, and molds. *Halococcus* and *Halobacterium* spp. are extreme halophilic spoilage bacteria that cause pink discoloration of brines and salted fish during spoilage (Table 3). Some SSO halophilic molds (e.g., *Sporendonema* and *Oospora* spp.) have an undesirable appearance that depreciates the value of a product (Huss, 1995, 1997).

Seafood spoilage causes a post-harvest and post-slaughter loss of 10 to 50%. Imported fish products are most often detained at the U.S. border because they are decomposed or dirty (USFDA, 2002). At that time, if food poisoning bacteria are present (but not at detectable levels), they will probably multiply and cause illness when the seafood is later eaten (Price, 2007). Some countries (United States, Japan, and some European countries) have mandatory seafood standards that use total viable counts (TVCs) or aerobic plate counts (APCs) of microorganisms on seafood products. TVCs are unreliable because only a small fraction of microorganisms found on seafood are involved with spoilage and TVCs correlate poorly with freshness and shelf life. Specific spoilage organisms' density and metabolite concentration are much more indicative of spoilage and a better index of shelf life in seafood. Lund et al. (2000) report a high correlation between log-transformed SSO abundance

TABLE 2 Specific Spoilage Organisms of Cod

Storage Temperature (°C)	Specific Spoilage Organisms	Packing Method[a]
0	Gram-negative psychrotrophs, nonfermentative rods, *Pseudomonas* spp., *Shewanella putrefaciens, Moraxella* spp., *Acinetobacter* (*Pseudomonas*) spp.	Aerobic
	Gram-negative rods; psychrotrophs and psychrophiles (*S. putrefaciens, Photobacterium phosphoreum*)	Vacuum
	Gram-negative fermentative rods with psychrophilic character (*Photobacterium phosphoreum*), *Pseudomonas* spp., *S. putrefaciens*, gram-positive rods (lactic acid bacteria)	MAP
5	Psychotrophic gram-negative rods, Vibrionaceae (*Aeromonas* spp., *S. putrefaciens*)	Aerobic
	Psychotrophic gram-negative rods; Vibrionaceae (*Aeromonas* spp., *S. putrefaciens*)	Vacuum
	Gram-negative psychotrophic rods (*Aeromonas* spp.)	MAP
20–30	Gram-negative mesophilic fermentative rods, Vibrionaceae, Enterobacteraceae	Aerobic

Source: Modified from Huss (1997).
[a] MAP, modified atmosphere packaging.

and remaining shelf life. Seafood Spoilage and Safety Predictor (SSSP) software v. 2.0 (multilanguage version) has been developed to predict shelf life and growth of bacteria in different fresh and lightly preserved seafoods. This software can be downloaded free of charge at the SSSP page of the Danish Institute for Fisheries Research (DIFR-DTU, 2005).

Important international guidelines and regulations for FAO, the European Union, the UK, the United States, Canada, Australia, New Zealand, and Codex can be found at the Seafood Network Information Center (SeafoodNIC, 2007b).

11.5 SEAFOOD PROCESSING AND FOOD SAFETY

Seafood processing usually involves several steps. In step 1, harvesters capture the seafood from the wild or harvest it at aquaculture farms.Then they transport it and store it until distribution.

In step 2, inspectors preferably use a systematic approach to control safe distribution with the goal of providing minimal risk to human health (Huss et al., 2003).

TABLE 3 Microflora Spoilage in Light-Preserved Fish and Shellfish[a]

Seafood	Preservative	Spoilage Indicator	Specific Spoilage Organisms	Packaging
Shrimp	Benzoic acid with or without ascorbic or citric acid, pH 5.5–5.8	Slime	Lactic acid bacteria (*Leuconostoc* spp.)	Brine
		Gas production and yeast odor and flavor	Heterofermentative/lactic acid bacteria, yeast	
		Off-odor/off-flavor	*Brochotrix* spp., lactic acid bacteria	
Fish Cold smoked	Salt in water	Off-odor/off-flavor	Gram-negative rods, lactic acid bacteria	Vacuum
		Putrid appearance, sticky, sulfurous	Enterobacteriaceae, Vibrionaceae, lactic acid bacteria	
Sugar salted	Salt in water	Off-odor/off-flavor, rancidity	Occasionally gram-negative bacteria, *Brochotrix* spp., lactic acid bacteria	Vacuum
		Sour taste, putrid appearance	Enterobacteriaceae, Vibrionaceae, *S. putrefaciens*	
		Off-odor/off-flavor	Gram-positive bacteria, lactic acid bacteria	MAP[b]

Source: Modified from Huss (1997).
[a]3 to 6% saline water above 5°C and pH > 5; or another preservative.
[b]MAP, modified atmosphere packaging.

Achieving this goal meets consumer demands for safety and complies with legislative requirements (Dalgaard, 2000).

The good hygienic and manufacturing practices (GHPs/GMPs) and the HACCP programs are important for improving the safety of fish and shellfish produced for human consumption. The shellfish industry implemented the GHP/GMP program at several levels to ensure product safety. The regulations associated with the program are related to harvest area, type and size of fish, capture method, and lag time needed to decrease contamination risk.

The USFDA-CFSAN (2001) developed and implemented the HACCP program. The final regulations of this program were published in the *Federal Register* on December 18, 1995 and became effective on December 18, 1997. The program recommends seafood freshness and quality evaluations with sensory and microbiological methods, and evaluations of seafood shelf life, preferably using spoilage organism growth models that integrate time and temperature.

The goal of the HACCP program is to eliminate food safety hazards, or at a minimum, reduce them to acceptable levels. HACCP program protocol is to (1) identify the food safety hazard(s); (2) identify the processing that best controls hazards, and (3) implement a control plan (Butt et al., 2004; Huss, 1992). These steps include a risk assessment that specifies critical control points (CCPs). A control plan usually involves several steps designed to minimize or eliminate hazards. If a CCP can control a hazard completely, it is designated CCP-1, while a CCP that minimizes a hazard is designated CCP-2 (Table 4). All of these programs are species dependent (e.g., fecal coliforms).

Fecal coliforms are gram-negative bacteria associated with the waste of human beings and animals. They are often used as indicators of sanitary quality in shellfish since they provide a reasonable indication of bacterial contamination (Butt et al., 2004). Action plans that use fecal coliform counts are effective at reducing the risk of certain bacterial infections resulting from consumption of shellfish (Butt et al., 2004; Schwab et al., 1998).

Count indicators are not effective hazard indicators for all microorganisms, particularly enteric viruses. An outbreak of norovirus gastroenteritis occurred in an area where humans had consumed seafood from an estuary despite acceptable levels of fecal coliform. Polymerase chain reaction (PCR) (Butt et al., 2004; LaGuyader et al., 2006; Schwab et al., 1998) is a new molecular method that may be useful in predicting the extent of such a viral contamination. The European Commission discourages the use of *Vibrio* spp. (e.g., *V. parahaemolyticus*) counts without consideration of additional virulence factors, based on the rapid alert system for food products (EC, 2001). In 1999, the rapid alert system identified 107 hazardous seafood products from a group of 295 products (EC, 2001). Seventy-five alerts identified hazardous levels of pathogenic bacteria (*Vibrio* spp., *Salmonella* spp., *Listeria monocytogenes*, *Staphylococcus* spp., and Enterobacteriaceae "aerobic mesophiles") in, or on, chilled and frozen fish. The report also included a list of chemical (heavy metals and pesticide residues) dangers. Thirty alerts identified hazardous levels of pathogenic bacteria (*Vibrio* spp., *Salmonella* spp., and *Staphylococcus* spp.) in, or on, shrimp, crayfish, and crab. Hazardous alerts for canned, frozen, and fresh tuna, bivalve mollusks, and

TABLE 4 Hazards and Critical Control Points for Production and Processing of Fresh and Frozen Boneless Fish Fillets

Processing Step	Hazards	Preventive Measure	Control[a]
Live fish	Contamination[b] (chemicals, enteric pathogens, biotoxin)	Avoid fishing in contaminated areas with biotoxins	CCP-2
Catch handling	Growth of bacteria	Short handling time	CCP-1
	Gaping in fillets Discolorations	Avoid rough handling	CCP-2
Chilling	Growth of bacteria	Ensure low temperature	CCP-1
Arrival of raw material at factory	Substandard quality	HACCP plan or list of approved suppliers	CCP-2
		Sensory evaluation	
Chilling	Growth of bacteria (deterioration)	Ensure low temperature	CCP-1
Processing (deicing, washing, filleting, skinning, trimming, candling)	Pieces of skin, bones, and membranes left on fillet	Proper setting of machinery	CCP-2
		Adequate instructions for personnel	CCP-2
	Visible parasites left on fillet	Ensure light intensity on candling table	
		Frequent change of personnel	
Weighing	Under- and overestimated weight	Ensure accuracy of scales	CCP-1
Packaging	Deterioration during fresh/frozen storage	Ensure adequate packaging material and method (e.g., vacuum)	CCP-2
All processing steps	Growth of bacteria	Short processing time	CCP-1
	Contamination (enteric bacteria)	Factory hygiene/sanitation	CCP-2
		Good water quality	
Chilling, freezing, storage	Deterioration	Ensure correct (low) temperature	CCP-1

Source: Huss (1995).
[a]CCP, critical control point.
[b]Excess contamination with group 2 pathogenic bacteria, biotoxins, parasites, and chemicals.

other unidentified seafood often include a wide array of organisms and substances, including histamines, mercury, *Salmonella* spp., biotoxins, viruses, and fecal coliforms (Huss et al., 1995).

11.6 PRODUCT QUALITY AND MICROORGANISM REDUCTION METHODS

Currently, consumers prefer fresh over frozen seafood because they claim that fresh seafood tastes better (Goulas et al., 2005). Fresh seafood has a high water content ($a_w > 0.95$) and contains free amino acids that promote microorganism growth (Goulas et al., 2005) and could confer a contamination risk to consumers. If consumers continue to prefer fresh seafood, suppliers may need to develop methods that reduce contamination risk without freezing.

Depuration is a method in which filter-feeding bivalve mollusks are placed in tanks where they can filter clean water to remove microorganisms and toxins. Depuration significantly decreases bacterial counts but is ineffective at reducing viruses. In one study, depuration for 48 h reduced bacterial counts by 95%, but reduced norovirus concentrations by only 7% (Butt et al., 2004).

Parasitic infection is also a problem in seafood safety; visual and microscopic inspection is an alternative method for reducing the risk of seafood parasites. Inspectors remove parasites with forceps or cut off infected parts, both of which can be time consuming. The effectiveness of this inspection method is dependent on fish fillet thickness, the presence of skin, oil content, pigmentation, and the expertise of the inspector. Ultimately, heat treatment and heat smoking of seafood are the most effective methods for reducing parasite risk. Freezing seafood with dry ice is another alternative to traditional freezing methods because it freezes seafood very quickly, minimizing spoilage time. When handlers freeze Indian white shrimp (*Penaeus indicus*) with dry ice and water in the ratio 1 : 1 (w/v), store them for 24 h, and do not re-ice, the shrimp maintains flavor and quality suitable for consumption (Jeyasekarane et al., 2006). Any freezing methods must ensure that the temperature within the seafood product is low enough to minimize production of toxic biogenic amines and other pathogens. Nevertheless, using dry ice is not a practical method, due to the cost of its production.

Refrigeration combined with vacuum packaging (VP) or modified atmosphere packaging (MAP) will also increase the shelf life of seafood (Reddy et al., 1992). In MAP, handlers replace the air inside the packaging with a single gas, or a mixture of gases, that differ from normal air composition. Varying concentrations of CO_2 and N_2, coupled with refrigeration, will inhibit growth of aerobic microorganisms, proteolytic bacteria, yeasts, and fungi (Swiderski et al., 1997). Using this method, shelf life depends on species, fat content, initial microbial population, gas mixture, the ratio of gas to product, and most important, storage temperature (Sivertsvik et al., 2002). If improper storage temperature is used, toxin (such as cyanotoxin) formation can occur in VP or MAP (Eklund, 1992). Another disadvantage of MAP is that it costs twice as much as VP (Reddy et al., 1992).

Pasteurization is another alternative to traditional freezing of seafood; however, it will modify nutritional and sensory properties. High-pressure and ultraviolet (UV) techniques are other new interesting preservation techniques that avoid the use of chemical additives (Fioretto et al., 2005). Water treatment industries are interested in UV irradiation technology because it is easy to apply and maintain, requires little maintenance, reduces waterborne pathogens significantly, and has no hazardous by-products (Hijnen et al., 2006). Linden et al. (2002) found UV irradiation to have irreversible affects on *C. parvum* oocysts. Ahmed et al. (1997) tested gamma radiation on nagli fish (*Sillago sihama*) products with success.

One of the oldest methods for preserving fish is smoking, although developed countries smoke fish primarily to obtain additional flavor. Smoking methods often involve a combination of salting (brining), drying, heating, and smoking. The smoke itself usually contains an antioxidant and antimicrobial agent. To ensure product safety and storage life, the smoking process should include rapid post-smoking chilling, hygienic packaging, and well-regulated chilled storage (Cakli et al., 2006). Cold-smoking methods are risky because they cannot eliminate *C. botulinum* spores. Eklund (1992) conducted studies on the growth of *C. botulinum* and subsequent toxin formation in fish smoked inside an oxygen-impermeable film (O_2 transmission 108 cm^3/m^2 for 24 h; CO_2 transmission 526 cm^3/m^2) at 23°C for 24 h (760 mmHg; 0% relative humidity) and then packaged it inside a 1.5-mL polyethylene oxygen-permeable film (oxygen transmission 7195 cm^3/m^2; CO_2 transmission 22,858 cm^3/m^2) for 24 h. He reported that O_2-impermeable films need higher concentrations of sodium chloride than O_2-permeable films to prevent *C. botulinum* toxin formation.

11.7 MICROBIOLOGICAL METHODS FOR DETECTION AND QUANTIFICATION OF SEAFOOD PATHOGENS

Seafood freshness and quality depend on chemical, microbiological, and sensory properties. Historically, food safety personnel identified seafood microorganisms from microbes cultured on a laboratory medium. Microbiologists looked for physical and chemical changes in the medium, such as color measurement, pH, total volatile basic nitrogen (TVB-N), thiobarbituric acid, malonaldehyde per milligram, trimethylamine nitrogen (TMA-N), and sensory attributes. TVB-N and TMA-N content are the most common measurements.

TMA is a component of TVB. It is initially present in small quantities in fresh fish, but increases with storage time. TMA-N and TVB-N levels are the traditional indicators used on iced fish. Since they cause fish off-odors, they are also useful in sensory analysis. Spoilage time, as characterized by production of TMA or other volatile bases, is species-, process-, and time-dependent, partly because the composition of fish muscle and decomposition time varies by species (Ruiz-Capillas and Horner, 1999).

Seafood manufacturers and inspectors need rapid, reliable, specific, sensitive, and cost-effective methods for detecting target food pathogens; therefore, research on methods for pathogen detection has expanded (Palchetti and Mascini, 2008). New research should focus on methods that can concentrate target organisms from food, eliminate inhibitory substances, detect PCR products, simplify procedures, and reduce cost (Palchetti and Mascini, 2008). Readers are encouraged to read Chapters 2, 26, and 27 for further information on foodborne pathogens.

Vibrio parahaemolyticus causes gastroenteric infections in humans after they consume raw or undercooked contaminated seafood. Traditional methods of detection take up to 10 days (Blake et al., 1980); however, Miyamoto et al. (1990) developed a rapid and sensitive detection assay that only takes 6 h. This method cultivates cells in a specific medium and then measures intracellular trypsin-like activity of *V. parahaemolyticus*. Later, Venkateswaran et al. (1996) developed a method that uses a simple and rapid fluorogenic *V. parahaemolyticus* that does not require enrichment and isolation. More recently, Richards et al. (2005) developed a simple and rapid colony overlay procedure for peptidases for the rapid fluorogenic detection and quantification of *Vibrionaceae* from seawater, shellfish, sewage, and clinical samples. The assay detects phosphoglucose isomerase (PGI) with a lysyl aminopeptidase activity (LysAP) that is produced by Vibrionaceae family members. In this procedure the PGI-LysAP hydrolyzes the amino-terminal lysyl residue from des-Arg^{10}-kallidin, converting it to des-Arg^{9}-bradykinin (Richards, 2004). These kinin-based metabolites enhance virulence and mediate inflammatory reactions (Maeda et al., 1992).

11.8 FOOD SAFETY CHALLENGES FOR AQUACULTURE AND THE COMMERCIAL FISHING INDUSTRY

Aquaculture operations have food safety concerns at all levels, from culturing methodology to food preparation and consumption. Greater consumption of fish by humans in a world with depleted natural fish stocks puts pressure on aquaculture practices to produce more fish. Aquaculture is probably the fastest-growing food production sector in the world, with a global production growing from approximately 4 million metric tons in 1980 to 60 million metric tons in 2004, which was 43% of the global fish consumption in 2004 (FAO, 2006). Most of the growth occurred in Asia and the Pacific region; production rates in Western Europe amounted to only 2% per annum during 2000–2004 (FAO, 2006). Controversy over the safety and sustainability of farmed versus wild fish, and the impacts that fish farms may have on natural settings (e.g., the oceans) when they are located in those environments adds to the pressure placed on the aquaculture industry.

Once referred to as "extensive" systems, aquacultural systems have magnified into "semi-intensive," "intensive," and "super-intensive" systems. Similar to agricultural succession, fish farming now uses chemicals and drugs in products. In the developed world, food safety is now a major issue of concern. The world market demands healthy aquaculture practices at all levels of production. To maintain their markets, many countries now require certain safety and sustainability control measures, such as farm licensing, good farming practices, a code of conduct for sustainable aquaculture, and hazard analysis and critical control point (HACCP) programs (Chinabut and Puttinaowarat, 2005). The aquaculture industry typically controls pathogens, with preventive agents such as antibiotics, chemotherapeutics, environmentally safe vaccines, or probiotics (live microorganisms which when administered in adequate amounts confer a health benefit on the host). Managers recommend that aquaculture use good farming practices, which evaluate chemicals and antibiotics so as to establish dosage and withdrawal periods. Aquaculture has also begun to use probiotics that replace pathogenic bacteria with beneficial bacteria inside the organism. Scientists are also developing chemotherapeutants and more antibiotics that target specific bacteria. Some of these methods are new; more research is needed to determine their impacts on food and the environment.

In Europe, Japan, and the United States, vaccinations are highly effective at controlling diseases (e.g., furnunculosis, yersiniosis, and vibriosis) that arise from salmon products while reducing farmer dependence on antibiotics. In Asian countries other than Japan, vaccines are not used widely because aquaculture systems are so different and farmed fish in these areas are not valuable enough to make vaccinations cost-effective. Much effort is under way to develop vaccines against viral infections in shrimp, since it is one of the largest seafood industries; however, the efficacy of trial vaccines remains inconclusive. Research on the use of immunostimulants in the shrimp industry is promising, but also inconclusive (Chinabut and Puttinaowarat, 2005).

Many seafood farmers are now able to manage aquatic animal health at their facilities. This is possible because they have access to rapid and accurate tests and belong to strong farmer organizations that coordinate information sharing and research projects with scientists. In Asia, where farmers produce approximately 90% of the seafood worldwide, farmers are less involved with health management because they have little coordination with scientists (few farmer–science organizations), and information is difficult to disseminate because Asia has so many producers. Asia now has a better management practices program, focused largely on shrimp farming, that promotes animal health management. Asia and other countries still need to develop simple and affordable farm practices that help control aquatic animal diseases (Corsin et al., 2007).

In shellfish culture, health officials are concerned about the effects that zoonoses and drug residues have on public health. Not all diseases that affect shellfish affect humans. Most public health concerns come from the hazards associated with aquaculture methods, such as contamination by either marine algae biotoxins or by domestic sewage that contains human pathogenic bacteria and viruses. Dominant infectious bacteria are threats to aquaculture operations and expansions (Ghittino, 1985; Roberts, 2001), particularly when global trade and global warming create new bacterial colonization opportunities.

Warm-water gram-positive coccal bacteria have invaded and spread throughout Europe and are now a threat to European aquaculture. The dominant infectious bacteria, *Lactococcus garvieae* (which causes lactococcosis), reduced Italian rainbow trout production by 20% and will probably spread to cultured marine fish (Ghittino and Pedroni, 2001). The exotic pathogen *Streptococcus iniae* is currently in Europe and will probably spread to fish in many countries (including Italy), infecting trout, sea bass, and sea bream (Eldar and Ghittino, 1999). With threat of exotic invasions, fish farms should adopt preventive sanitation plans.

Responsible aquaculture practices ensure safe seafood for consumers. They promote fish health and welfare through application of vaccination programs, appropriate therapeutic cycles, and good husbandry. They preserve habitat by reducing environmental impact, and they also protect seafood industry workers from pathogens (e.g., zoonoses) by adopting programs that minimize exposure risk (Ghittino and Bozzetta, 1994).

Transmission of zoonotic agents from fish to humans occurs when humans consume uncooked contaminated seafood products (food zoonoses) or handle seafood in infected environments (professional zoonoses). Food zoonoses are most often associated with commercial fisheries, whereas professional zoonoses are most often associated with aquaculture. Professional zoonoses include *Streptococcus iniae*, *Vibrio vulnificus*, and *Mycobacterium marinum*, bacteria that infect workers when their skin is penetrated by a fish spine. Fish farmers, fish processors, and cooks are at greatest risk. Shrimp aquaculture is at high risk for pathogenic microorganism infection because it is so intensive. Most shrimp farms are located in areas where antibiotic use is not regulated (Alderman and Hastings, 1998; Holmstrom et al., 2003); thereby increasing the risk of shrimp and human pathogen resistance to antibiotics (Brown, 1989). An FDA survey of imported foods showed *Salmonella* spp. to be antibiotic resistant in aquatic food products (Zhao et al., 2006). Boinapally and Jiang (2007) found that farm-raised shrimp had significantly ($p < 0.05$) more bacteria that were resistant to ceftriaxone and tetracycline than did wild-caught shrimp. Pathogenic isolates and indicator microorganisms in imported shrimp have elevated antibiotic resistance (Alderman and Hastings, 1998). *Salmonella* and *Vibrio* spp. in shrimp are often resistant to multiple antibiotics (Boinapally and Jiang, 2007). All present a biosafety hazard to shrimp handlers and consumers.

Fish bioengineering is a new and controversial method of preventing fish disease. Growth-enhanced transgenic salmon may become the first bioengineered animal product approved for use as food in the United States. Bioengineered (transgenic) fish may boost future salmon harvests, increase aquaculture productivity, and lower consumer prices for fish. The public often opposes the practice, investors are reluctant, and scientists are skeptical, primarily due to environmental concerns. In the United States, opposition may be sufficient to prevent the use and development of transgenic technology despite an elaborate regulatory framework. Analogous to genetically modified food crops, the consumer market will probably determine the future of transgenic fish (Aerni, 2004).

11.9 EFFECTS OF CLIMATE ON WATERBORNE AND FOODBORNE SEAFOOD PATHOGENS

Humans are exposed to waterborne and foodborne pathogens when they drink water contaminated with feces, eat produce that was irrigated or processed with contaminated water, or eat seafood contaminated with hazardous microbes, toxins, or wastewater. Weather affects the transport and dissemination of these microbial agents during rainfall and runoff events and the survival and/or growth of the agents as temperatures change. Federal and state laws and regulatory programs protect much of the U.S. population from waterborne disease, but if climate becomes more variable and/or extreme, watershed protection, infrastructure, and storm drainage systems may be compromised in ways that increase contamination. At least in the marine environment, few studies address the potential health effects of climate variability in combination with other stresses, such as overfishing, introduced species, and a rise in sea level (Rose et al., 2001).

Three environmentally overlapping health-related areas are affected by weather and climate: (1) waterborne disease from drinking and recreational waters, (2) foodborne disease from water contamination, and (3) harmful algal blooms in marine and coastal environments and ecologic disruption. Drinking water disease outbreaks occur when a number of events happen simultaneously: contamination of source water, contamination of water intake systems, and insufficient treatment (Rose et al., 2001).

Seasonal warming of sea-surface temperatures enhances plankton blooms of copepods (Colwell, 1996), hosts for *V. cholera*. In the wake of an El Niño event affecting the Bay of Bengal, a copepod bloom preceded an increase in cholera cases (Lobitz et al., 2000). Pascal et al. (2000) found occurrences of this same relationship in Bangladesh over an 18-year period, and Speelmon et al. (2000) found a similar link between elevated temperature and *V. cholerae* presence in Peru.

Changing weather parameters are sometimes correlated with contamination of coastal waters and shellfish-related disease. *Vibrio* spp. and associated disease is strongly correlated (r^2 of 0.60) with weather factors, particularly temperature (Motes et al., 1998), which dictates *Vibrio* spp. seasonality and geographic distribution (Lipp and Rose, 1997). *V. vulnificus* is rarely found in temperate estuaries during winter months, but is found year-round in subtropical regions when water temperature is about 17°C (Lipp et al., 2001).

Changes in weather, ocean temperature, and ocean upwelling can affect the prevalence of algal blooms (NRC, 1999). Harmful algal blooms are globally more common (Hallegraff, 1993; Sournia, 1995). Of the approximate 5000 identified marine microalgae, the number known to be toxic or harmful has increased to around 86 species (Burkholder and Glasgow, 1997). Some of the increase may be due to expanded identification efforts and improved methodology for identifying toxic species.

11.10 CONCLUSIONS

Many factors influence seafood safety, including environment type (e.g., marine vs. freshwater, natural vs. aquaculture), native microorganism composition, water pollution, microbe contamination, and product handling (transportation, storage, distribution, and marketing). Thus, food safety strategies that include effective international guidelines and regulations for safe seafood have to be conducted by food industry and food safety officers to identify and measure infection risk and to eliminate or reduce hazards.

REFERENCES

Aerni P (2004): Risk, regulation and innovation: The case of aquaculture and transgenic fish. *Aquat Sci.* 66:327–341.

Ahmed FE (Ed.) (1991): *Seafood Safety*. National Academies Press, Washington, DC, p. 432.

Ahmed FE (1992): Review: assessing and managing risk due to consumption of seafood contaminated with micro-organisms, parasites, and natural toxins in the United States. *Int J Food Sci Technol.* 27:243–260.

Ahmed IO, Alur MD, Kamat AS, Bandekar JR, Thomas P (1997): Influence of proccesing on the extension of shelf life of nagli fish (*Sillago sihama*) by gamma radiation. *Int J Food Sci Technol.* 32:325–332.

Alderman DJ, Hastings TS (1998): Antibiotic use in aquaculture: development of antibiotic resistance—potential for consumer health risks. *Int J Food Sci Technol.* 33:139–155.

Barbieri E, Falzano L, Fiorentini C, et al. (1999): Occurrence, diversity, and pathogenicity of halophilic *Vibrio* spp. and non-O1 *Vibrio cholerae* from estuarine waters along the Italian Adriatic coast. *Appl Environ Microbiol.* 65:2748–2753.

Beldsoe GE, Oria MP (2001): Potential hazards in cold-smoked fish: parasites. *J Food Sci.* 66:S1058–S1133.

Blake PA, Weaver RE, Hollis DG (1980): Diseases of humans (other than cholera) caused by vibrios. *Annu Rev Microbiol.* 34:341–367.

Boinapally K, Jiang X (2007): Comparing antibiotic resistance in commensal and pathogenic bacteria isolated from wild-caught South Carolina shrimps vs. farm-raised imported shrimps. *Can J Microbiol.* 53:919–924.

Brett MM (2003): Food poisoning associated with biotoxins in fish and shellfish. *Curr Opin Infect Dis.* 16:461–465.

Broadbent JR, Chou YC, Gillies K, Kondo JK (1989): Nisin inhibits several gram-positive, mastitis-causing pathogens. *J Dairy Sci.* 72:3342–3345.

Brown JH (1989): Antibiotics: their use and abuse in aquaculture. *World Aquacult.* 20: 34–43.

Burgess V, Shaw G (2001): Pectenotoxins—an issue for public health: a review of their comparative toxicology and metabolism. *Environ Int.* 27:275–283.

Burkholder JM (1998): Implications of harmful microalgae and heterotrophic dinoflagellates in management of sutainable fisheries. *Ecol Appl.* 8:S37-S62.

Burkholder JM, Glasgow HBJ (1997): *Pfiesteria piscicida* and other pfiesteria-like dinoflagellates: behavior, impacts and environmental controls. Part 2. *Limnol Oceanogr.* 42:1052–1075.

Butt AA, Aldridge KE, Sanders CV (2004): Infections related to the ingestion of seafood. II: parasitic infections and food safety. *Lancet Infect Dis.* 4:294–300.

Cahu C, Salen P, de Lorgeril M (2004): Farmed and wild fish in the prevention of cardiovascular diseases: assessing possible differences in lipid nutritional values. *Nutr Metab Cardiovasc.* 14:34–41.

Cakli S, Kilinc B, Dincer T, Tolasa S (2006): Comparison of the shelf lifes of map and vacuum packaged hot smoked rainbow trout (*Onchoryncus mykiss*). *Eur Food Res Technol.* 224:19–26.

Calo-Mata P, Arlindo S, Boehme K, Miguel T, Pascoal A, Barros-Velazquez J (2008): Current applications and future trends of lactic acid bacteria and their bacteriocins for the biopreservation of aquatic food products. *Food Bioprocess Technol.* 1:43–63.

Cazenave J, Wunderlin DA, Bistoni MA, et al. (2005): Uptake, tissue distribution and accumulation of microcystin-RR in *Corydoras paleatus*, *Jenynsia multidentata* and *Odontesthes bonariensis*: a field and laboratory study. *Aquat Toxicol.* 75:178–190.

Chen J, Xie P (2005a): Tissue distributions and seasonal dynamics of the hepatotoxic microcystins-LR and -RR in two freshwater shrimps, *Palaemon modestus* and *Macrobrachium nipponensis*, from a large shallow, eutrophic lake of subtropical China. *Toxicon.* 45:615–625.

——— (2005b): Seasonal dynamics of the hepatotoxic microcystins in various organs of four freshwater bivalves from the large eutrophic lake Taihu of subtropical China and the risk for human consumption. *Environ Toxicol.* 20:572–584.

Chinabut S, Puttinaowarat S (2005): The choice of disease control strategies to secure international market access for aquaculture products. Dev Biol (Basel). 121:255–261.

Chinabut S, Somsiri T, Limsuwan C, Lewis S (2006): Problems associated with shellfish farming. *Rev Sci Tech.* 25:627–635.

Christian B, Luckas B (2007): Determination of marine biotoxins relevant for regulations: from the mouse bioassay to coupled LC-MS methods. *Anal Bioanal Chem.* 391:117–134.

Ciminiello P, Fattorusso E (2006): Bivalve molluscs as vectors of marine biotoxins involved in seafood poisoning. *Prog Mol Subcell Biol.* 43:53–82.

Colwell RR (1996): Global climate and infectious disease: the cholera paradigm. *Science.* 274:2025–2031.

Corsin F, Giorgetti G, Mohan CV (2007): Contribution of science to farm-level aquatic animal health management. *Dev Biol (Basel).* 129:35–40.

Dalgaard P (2000): *Freshness, Quality and Safety in Seafoods.* Flair-Flow Europe Technical Manual. F-FE 380A/00. National Food Center. Lyngby, Denmark.

Dalgaard P, Vancanneyt M, Euras Vilalta N, Swings J, Fruekilde P, Leisner JJ (2003): Identification of lactic acid bacteria from spoilage associations of cooked and brined shrimps stored under modified atmosphere between 0°C and 25°C. *J Appl Microbiol.* 94:80–89.

Díaz-Camacho SP, Cruz-Otero MC, Manning KW (2000): Gnathostomiasis. *Rev Fac Med UNAM.* 43:192–201.

DIFR-DTU (Danish Institute for Fisheries Research–Technical University of Denmark) (2005): Seafood Spoilage and Safety Predictor (SSSP) software v. 2.0 (multilanguage version). http://www.dfu.min.dk/micro/sssp/Home/Home.aspx. Accessed June 2008.

Diggles BK, Carson J, Hine PM, Hickman RW, Tait MJ (2000): *Vibrio* species associated with mortalities in hatchery-reared turbot (*Colistiumnudipinnis*) and brill (*C. guntheri*) in New Zealand. *Aquaculture.* 183:1–12.

Dixon BR, Flohr RB (1997): Fish- and shellfish-borne trematode infections in Canada. *Southeast Asian J Trop Med Public Health.* 28:58–64.

EC (European Commission) (2001): Opinion of the Scientific Committee on veterinary measures relating to public health on *Vibrio vulnificus* and *Vibrio parahaemolyticus* (in raw and undercooked seafood). Report adopted September 20, 2001. Health and Consumer Protection Directorate General.

Edmunds JSG, McCarthy RA, Ramsdell JS (1999): Ciguatoxin reduces larval survivability in finfish. *Toxicon.* 37:1827–1832.

Eklund MW (1992): Control in fishery products. In: Hauschild AHW, Dodds KL (Eds.). Clostridium Botulinum*: Ecology and Control in Foods*. Marcel Dekker, New York, pp. 209–232.

Eldar A, Ghittino C (1999): *Lactococcus garvieae* and *Streptococcus iniae* infections in rainbow trout *Oncorhynchus mykiss*: similar, but different diseases. *Dis Aquat Org*. 36: 227–231.

FAO (Food and Agriculture Organization) (2006): *State of World Aquaculture: 2006 Advance Copy*. FAO Fisheries Technical Paper 500. FAO Fisheries Department, Rome.

——— (2007): *El Estado Mundial de la Pesca y la Acuicultura 2006*. Organización de las Naciones Unidas para la Agricultura y la Alimentación, Rome, pp. 1–198.

Ferre I (2002): Anisakiosis y otras zoonosis parasitarias transmitidas por consumo de pescado. Revista AquaTIC 14. Updated June 2002. http://www.revistaaquatic.com/aquatic/art.asp?t=&c=122. Accessed June 2008.

Fioretto F, Cruz C, Largeteau A, Sarli TA, Demazeau G, Moueffak AE (2005): Inactivation of *Staphylococcus aureus* and *Salmonella enteritidis* in tryptic soy broth and caviar samples by high pressure processing. *Braz J Med Biol Res*. 38:1259–1265.

Flores-Luna JL, Martínez-Fuentes JC, Casillas-Gómez FJ (1993): *Manual de Buenas Prácticas de Higiene y Sanidad*. Subsecretaría de Regulación y Fomento Sanitario, Secretaría de Salud, México.

Gerba CP, Goyal SM (1978): Detection and occurrence of enteric viruses in shellfish: a review. *J Food Prot*. 41:742–750.

Ghittino P (1985): *Technology and Pathology in Aquaculture*, Vol. 2. Bono, Turin, Italy.

Ghittino C, Bozzetta E (1994): Prophylaxis of zoonoses of fish origin. *Prev Vet Med*. 7:5–6.

Ghittino C, Pedroni A (2001): Main bacterial pathologies in salmonid fish: diagnosis, therapy and prevention. In: Baruchelli G (Ed.): *Modern Trout Farming, Trento, Italy. ESAT News*. 17(4 Suppl):41–56.

Gomez-Gil BA, Roque A, Turnbull JF (2000): The use and selection of probiotic bacteria for use in the culture of larval aquatic organisms. *Aquaculture*. 191:259–270.

Goulas AE, Chouliara I, Nessi E, Kontominas MG, Savvaidis IN (2005): Microbiological, biochemical and sensory assessment of mussels (*Mytilus galloprovincialis*) stored under modified atmosphere packaging. *J Appl Microbiol*. 98:752–760.

Gram L, Ravn L, Rasch M, Bruhn JB, Christensen AB, Givskov M (2002): Food spoilage: interactions between food spoilage bacteria. *Int J Food Microbiol*. 78:79–97.

Guillotreau P (2004): How does the European seafood industry stand after the revolution of salmon farming: an economic analysis of fish prices. *Mar Policy*. 28:227–233.

Hallegraeff GM (1993): A review of harmful algal blooms and their apparent global increase. *Phycologia*. 32:79–99.

Hernández GC, Ulloa PJ, Vergara OJA, Romilio ET, Cabello CF (2005): *Vibrio parahaemolyticus* infections and algal intoxications as emergent public health problems in Chile. *Rev Med Chile*. 133:1081–1088.

Herreras MV, Aznar FJ, Balbuena JA, Raga JA (2000): Anisakid larvae in the musculature of the Argentinean hake, *Merluccius hubbsi*. *J Food Prot*. 63:1141–43.

Hijnen WA, Beerendonk EF, Medema GJ (2006): Inactivation credit of UV radiation for viruses, bacteria and protozoan (oo)cysts in water: a review. *Water Res*. 40:3–22.

Hine PM, Thorne T (2000): A survey of some parasites and diseases of several species of bivalve mollusc in northern Western Australia. *Dis Aquat Organ*. 40:67–78.

Hitzfeld BC, Höger SJ, Dietrich DR (2000): Cyanobacterial toxins: removal during drinking water treatment, and human risk assessment. *EHP Suppl.* 108; 113–122.

Holmstrom K, Graslund S, Wahlstrom A, Poungshompoo S, Bengtsson BE, Kautsky N (2003): Antibiotic use in shrimp farming and implications for environmental impacts and human health. *Int J Food Sci Technol.* 38:255–266.

Huang CH, Huang SL (2004): Effect of dietary vitamin E on growth, tissue lipid peroxidation, and liver glutathione level of juvenile hybrid tilapia, *Oreochromis niloticus* × *O. aureus*, fed oxidized oil. *Aquaculture.* 237:381–389.

Huss HH (1992): Development and use of the HACCP concept in fish processing. *Int J Food Microbiol.* 15:33–44.

——— (1995): *Quality and Quality Changes in Fresh Fish.* FAO Fisheries Technical Paper. 348. FAO, Rome.

——— (1997): *Aseguramiento de la Calidad de los Productos Pesqueros.* FAO Documento Técnico de Pesca 334. FAO, Rome.

Huss HH, Ababouch L, Gram L (2003): *Assessment and Management of Seafood Safety and Quality.* FAO Fisheries Technical Paper 444. FAO, Rome.

Ibelings BW, Chorus I (2007): Accumulation of cyanobacterial toxins in freshwater "seafood" and its consequences for public health: a review. *Environ Pollut.* 150:177–192.

Jeyasekaran G, Ganesan P, Anandaraj R, Jeya Shakila R, Sukumar D (2006): Quantitative and qualitative studies on the bacteriological quality of Indian white shrimp (*Penaeus indicus*) stored in dry ice. *Food Microbiol.* 23:526–533.

Kankaanpaa H, Vuorinen PJ, Sipia V, Keinanen M (2002): Acute effects and bioaccumulation of nodularin in sea trout (*Salmo trutta* m. *trutta L.*) exposed orally to *Nodularia spumigena* under laboratory conditions. *Aquat Toxicol.* 61:155–168.

Kankaanpaa HT, Holliday J, Schroder H, Goddard TJ, von Fister R, Carmichael WW (2005): Cyanobacteria and prawn farming in northern New South Wales, Australia case study on cyanobacteria diversity and hepatotoxin bioaccumulation. *Toxicol Appl Pharmacol.* 203:243–256.

Kilgen MB, Cole MT (1991): Viruses in seafood. In: Ward DR, Hackney C (Eds.). *Microbiology of Marine Food Products.* Van Nostrand Reinhold, New York, pp 197–209.

LaGuyader FS, Bon F, DeMedici D, et al. (2006): Detection of muiltiple noroviruses associated with an international gastroenteritis outbreak linked to oyster consumption. *J Clin Microbiol.* 44:3878–3782.

Landsberg JH (1996): Neoplasia and biotoxins in bivalves: Is there a connection? *J Shellfish Res.* 15:203–230.

Landsberg JH, Balazs GH, Steidinger KA, Baden DG, Work TM, Russel DJ (1999): The potential role of natural tumor promotors in marine turtle fibropapillomatosis. *J Aquat Anim Health.* 11:199–210.

Lightner DV, Redman RM (1998): Shrimp diseases and current diagnostic methods. *Aquaculture.* 164:201–220.

Linden KG, Shin G, Faubert G, Cairns W, Sobsey MD (2002): UV disinfection of *Giardia lamblia* cysts in water. *Environ Sci Technol.* 36:2519–2522.

Lipp EK, Rose JB (1997): The role of seafood in foodborne diseases in the United States of America. *Rev Sci Tech.* 16:620–640.

Lipp EK, Rodriguez-Palacios C, Rose JB (2001): Occurrence and distribution of the human pathogen *Vibrio vulnificus* in a subtropical Gulf of Mexico estuary. *Hydrobiologia.* 460:165–173.

Liston J (1980): Microbiology in fishery science. In: Connell JJ (Ed.): *Advances in Fishery Science and Technology*. Fishing News Books, Farnham, UK, pp. 138–157.

Lobitz B, Beck L, Huq A, et al. (2000): Climate and infectious disease: use of remote sensing for detection of *Vibrio cholerae* by indirect measurement. *Proc Natl Acad Sci USA*. 97:1438–1443.

Lund BM, Baird-Parker AC, Gould GW (2000): *The Microbiological Safety and Quality of Foods*. Aspen Publishers, Gaithersburg, MD.

MacLean JD, Arthur JR, Ward BJ, Gyorkos TW, Curtis MA, Kokoskin E (1996): Common-source outbreak of acute infection due to the North American liver fluke *Metorchis conjunctus*. *Lancet*. 347:154–158.

Maeda H, Mauro K, Akaike T, Kaminishi H, Hagiwara Y (1992): Microbial proteinases as an universal trigger of kinin generation in microbial infections. *Agents Actions Suppl*. 38:362–369.

Magalhaes VF, Soares RM, Azevedo S (2001): Microcystin contamination in fish from the Jacarepagua Lagoon (Rio de Janeiro, Brazil): ecological implication and human health risk. *Toxicon*. 39:1077–1085.

Manerio E, Rodas VL, Costas E, Hernandez JM (2008): Shellfish consumption: a major risk factor for colorectal cancer. *Med Hypotheses*. 70:409–412.

Miyamoto T, Miwa H, Hatano S (1990): Improved fluorogenic assay for rapid detection of *Vibrio parahaemolyticus* in foods. *Appl Environ Microbiol*. 56:1480–1484.

Moss SM, LeaMaster BR, Sweeney, JN (2000): Relative abundance and species composition of gram-negative, aerobic bacteria associated with the gut of juvenile white shrimp *Litopenaeus vannamei* reared in oligotrophic well water and euritrophic pond water. *J World Aquacult Soc*. 31:255–263.

Motes ML, DePaola A, Cook DW, et al. (1998): Influence of water temperature and salinity on *Vibrio vulnificus* in northern gulf and atlantic coast oysters (*Crassostrea virginica*). *Appl Environ Microbiol*. 64:1459–1465.

NACMCF (National Advisory Committee on Microbiological Criteria for Foods) (2008): Response to the questions posed by the Food and Drug Administration and the National Marine Fisheries Service regarding determination of cooking parameters for safe seafood for consumers. *J Food Prot*. 71:1287–1308.

Nawa Y, Hatz C, Blum J (2005): Sushi delights and parasites: the risk of fishborne and foodborne parasitic zoonoses in Asia. *Clin Infect Dis*. 41:297–1303

Negri AP, Bunter O, Jones B, Llewellyn L (2004): Effects of the bloom forming alga *Trichodesmium erythraeum* on the pearl oyster *Pinctada maxima*. *Aquaculture*. 232: 91–102.

Nes IF, Diep DB, Holo H (2007): Bacteriocin diversity in *Streptococcus* and *Enterococcus*. *J Bacteriol*. 189:1189–1198.

NRC (National Research Council) (1999): *From Monsoons to Microbes: Understanding the Ocean's Role in Human Health*. National Academies Press, Washington, DC.

Olafsen JA (2001): Interactions between fish larvae and bacteria in marine aquaculture. *Aquaculture*. 200:223–247.

Olafsen JA, Mikkelsen HV, Giæver HM, Hansen GH (1993): Indigenous bacteria in hemolymph and tissues of marine bivalves at low temperatures. *Appl Environ Microbiol*. 59:1848–1854.

Orlandi PA, Chu DM, Bier JW, Jackson GJ (2002): Parasites and the food supply. *Food Technol*. 56:72–81.

Palchetti I, Mascini M (2008): Electroanalytical biosensors and their potential for food pathogen and toxin detection. *Anal Bioanal Chem*. E-pub ahead of print.

Pascal M, Rodo X, Ellner SP, Colwell R, Bouma MJ (2000): Cholera dynamics and El Niño–Southern Oscillation. *Science*. 289:1766–1769.

Pires LMD, Karlsson KM, Meriluoto JAO, et al. (2004): Assimilation and depuration of microcystin-LR by the zebra mussel, *Dreissena polymorpha*. *Aquat Toxicol*. 69:385–396.

Price RJ (2006): Cross-contamination. *Seafood Today*. April–May 2006.

——— (2007): Why seafood spoils. Department of Food Science and Technology, University of California, Davis, CA., http://seafood.ucdavis.edu/pubs/spoils.htm. Accessed March 2008.

Reddy NR, Amstrong DJ, Rhodehamel EJ, Kauter DA (1992): Shelf life extension and safety concerns about fresh fishery products packaged under modified atmospheres: a review. *J Food Saf*. 12:87–118.

Reilly A, Káferstein F (1997): Food safety hazards and the application of the principles of the hazard analysis and critical control point (HACCP) system for their control in aquaculture production. *Aquaculture Res*. 28:735–752.

Richards GP (2004): Structural and functional analyses of phosphoglucose isomerase from *Vibrio vulnificus* and its lysyl aminopeptidase activity. *Biochem Biophys Acta*. 1702: 89–102.

Richards GP, Watson MA, Parveen S (2005): Development of a simple and rapid fluorogenic procedure for identification of *Vibrionaceae* family members. *Appl Environ Microbiol*. 71:3524–3527.

Roberts RJ (2001): *Fish Pathology*, 3rd ed. Baillière Tindall, London.

Rose JB, Epstein PR, Lipp EK, Sherman BH, Bernard SM, Patz JA (2001): Climate variability and change in the United States: potential impacts on water- and foodborne diseases caused by microbiologic agents. *Environ Health Perspect*. 109 (S2): 211–221.

Ruiz-Capillas C, Horner WFA (1999): Determination of trimethylamine nitrogen and total volatile basic nitrogen in fresh fish by flow injection analisis. *J Sci Food Agric*. 79: 1982–1986.

Ruxton CH, Reed SC, Simpson MJ, Millington KJ (2004): The health benefits of omega-3 polyunsaturated fatty acids: a review of the evidence. *J Hum Nutr Diet*. 17:449–459.

Ryan MP, Meaney WJ, Ross RP, Hill C (1998): Evaluation of lacticin 3147 and a teat seal containing this bacteriocin for inhibition of mastitis pathogens. *Appl Environ Microbiol*. 64:2287–2290.

Saker ML, Neilan BA, Griffiths DJ (1999): Two morphological forms of *Cylindrospermopsis raciborskii* (Cyanobacterta) isolated from Solomon Dam, Palm Island, Queensland. *J Phycol*. 35:599–606.

Schwab KJ, Neill FH, Estes MK, Metcalf TG, Atmar RL (1998): Distribution of Norwalk virus within shellfish following bioaccumulation and subsequent depuration by detection using RT-PCR. *J Food Prot*. 61:1674–1680.

SeafoodNIC–UCDavis (Seafood National Information Center–University of California at Davis) (2007a): Recommendations for on board handling of albacore tuna. http://seafood.ucdavis.edu/Pubs/albacore.htm. Accessed June 2008.

——— (2007b): Guidelines and regulations. http://seafood.ucdavis.edu/guidelines.html. Accessed June, 2008.

Sidhu KS (2003): Health benefits and potential risks related to consumption of fish or fish oil. *Regul Toxicol Pharmacol*. 38:336–344.

Sivertsvik M, Jeksrud WK, Rosnes JT (2002): A review of modified atmosphere packaging of fish and fishery products: significance of microbial growth activities and safety. *Int J Food Sci Technol*. 37:107–127.

Sournia A (1995): Red tide and toxic marine phytoplankton of the world ocean: an inquiry into biodiversity. In: Lassus P, Arzal G, Erard-Le-Den E, Gentien P, Marcaillou-Le-Baut C (Eds.). *Harmful Marine Algal Blooms*. Lavoisier, Paris, pp. 103–112.

Speelmon EC, Checkley W, Gilman RH, Patz J, Calderon M, Manga S (2000): Cholera incidence and El Niño–related higher ambient temperature [Letter]. *JAMA*. 283:3072–3074.

Srionnual S, Yanagida F, Lin LH, Hsiao KN, Chen YS (2007): Weissellicin 110, a newly discovered bacteriocin from *Weissella cibaria* 110, isolated from plaa-som, a fermented fish product from Thailand. *Appl Environ Microbiol*. 73:2247–2250.

Swiderski F, Russel S, Waszkiewicz-Robak B, Cholewinska E (1997): Evaluation of vacuum-packaged poultry meat and its products. *Rocz Panstw Zakl Hig*. 48:193–200.

Thompson FL, Iida T, Swings J (2004): Biodiversity of vibrios. *Microbiol Mol Biol Rev*. 68:403- 431.

Uchiyama H, Ehira S (1974): Relation between freshness and acid-soluble nucleotides in aseptic cod and yellowtail muscles during ice storage. *Bull Tokai Reg Fish Lab*. 78: 23–31.

USFDA (U.S. Food and Drug Administration) (1992): Scombrotoxin. Updated 2007 http://www.cfsan.fda.gov/~mow/chap38.html. Accessed June 2008.

——— (2001): Fish and fisheries products hazards and control guidance. Updated February 2008. http://www.cfsan.fda.gov/~comm/haccp4.html. Accessed June 2008.

——— (2002): Import refusal reports for OASIS. http://www.fda.gov/ora/oasis/ora_oasis_ref.html. Accessed March 2008.

USFDA-CFSAN (U.S. Food and Drug Administration–Center for Food Safety and Applied Nutrition) (2001): Fish and fisheries products hazards and controls guidance. http://www.cfsan.fda.gov/~comm/haccp4.html. Accessed March 2008.

Van Dolah FM (2000): Marine algal toxins: origins, health effects, and their increased occurrence. *Environ Health Perspect*. 108 (S1): 133–141.

Venkateswaran K, Kurusu T, Satake M, Shinoda S (1996): Comparison of a fluorogenic assay with a conventional method for rapid detection of *Vibrio parahaemolyticus* in seafoods. *Appl Environ Microbiol*. 62:3516–3520.

Verbeke W, Sioen I, Brunsø K, De Henauw S, Van Camp J (2007): Consumer perception versus scientific evidence of farmed and wild fish: exploratory insights from Belgium. *Aquacult Int*. 15:121–136.

Viviani R (1992): Eutrophication, marine biotoxins, human health. *Sci Total Environ*. Suppl:631–662.

Walker E, Pritchard C, Forsythe S (2003): Hazard analysis critical control point and prerequisite programme implementation in small and medium size food businesses. *Food Control*. 14:169–174.

Wallace BJ, Guzewich JJ, Cambridge M, Altekruse S, Morse DL (1999): Seafood-associated disease outbreaks in New York, 1980–1994. *Am J Prev Med*. 17:48–54.

Watanabe F, Goto M, Abe K, Nakano Y (1996): Glutathione peroxidase activity during storage of fish muscle. *J Food Sci.* 61:734–735.

Yaron S, Matthews KR (2002): A reverse transcriptase–polymerase chain reaction assay for detection of viable *Escherichia coli* O157:H7: investigation of specific target genes. *J Appl Microbiol.* 92:633–640.

Yu SH, Kawanaka M, Li XM, Xu LQ, Lan CG, Rui L (2003): Epidemiological investigation on *Clonorchis sinensis* in human population in an area of South China. *Jpn Infect Dis.* 56:168–171.

Zhao S, McDermott PF, Friedman S, Qaiyumi S, Abbott J, Kiessling C, Ayers S, Singh R, Hubert S, Sofos J, White DG (2006): Characterization of antimicrobial-resistant *Salmonella* isolated from important foods. *J Food Prot.* 69 (3):500–507.

Zo YG, Rivera IN, Russek-Cohen E, et al. (2002): Genomic profiles of clinical and environmental isolates of *Vibrio cholerae* O1 in cholera endemic areas of Bangladesh. *Proc Natl Acad Sci.* 99:12409–12414.

Zorrilla I, Chabrillón M, Arijo S, et al. (2003): Bacteria recovered from diseased cultured gilthead sea bream (*Sparus aurata* L.) in southwestern Spain. *Aquaculture.* 218:11–20.

Zurawell RW, Chen H, Burke JM, Prepas EE (2006): Hepatotoxic cyanobacteria: a review of the biological importance of microcystins in freshwater environments. *J Toxicol Environ Health Pt B Crit Rev.* 8:1–37.

CHAPTER 12

FOOD SAFETY ISSUES AND THE MICROBIOLOGY OF FRUITS AND VEGETABLES

JUAN S. LEÓN, LEE-ANN JAYKUS, and CHRISTINE L. MOE

12.1 INTRODUCTION

Production and consumption of fresh produce, including fruits and vegetables, increases worldwide every year (Fig. 1). Increased demand for fresh produce is related to their numerous health benefits, which include improving nutrition and reducing disease risk (Ness and Powles, 1997). For example, in the United States the American Dietetic Association currently recommends the consumption of at least five servings of produce per day as part of a healthy diet. The lowering of trade restrictions (e.g., the formation of the European Union) and the ease of transport worldwide have contributed to variety and year-round availability of produce items. As a consequence, increased demand has resulted in an increase in production, and much of our produce now comes from many different countries around the world.

This increase in produce consumption has been accompanied by a rise in the number of produce-associated foodborne disease outbreaks worldwide. Based on data analyzed from the U.S. Foodborne Outbreak Surveillance System from 1973 through 1997, the median number of reported produce-associated outbreaks in the United States increased from two outbreaks per year in the 1970s, to seven per year in the 1980s, to 16 per year in the 1990s. The proportion of foodborne disease outbreaks linked to produce contamination over the past two decades has increased almost 10-fold (from 0.7% in the mid-1970s to 6% in the mid-1990s), even after adjusting for improved surveillance and reporting (De Waal et al., 2006; Sivapalasingam et al., 2004). From 1990 to 2004, produce items were linked to 19.3% of foodborne disease outbreaks and 33.8% of cases (De Waal et al., 2006). The increase in the number of

Microbiologically Safe Foods, Edited by Norma Heredia, Irene Wesley, and Santos García

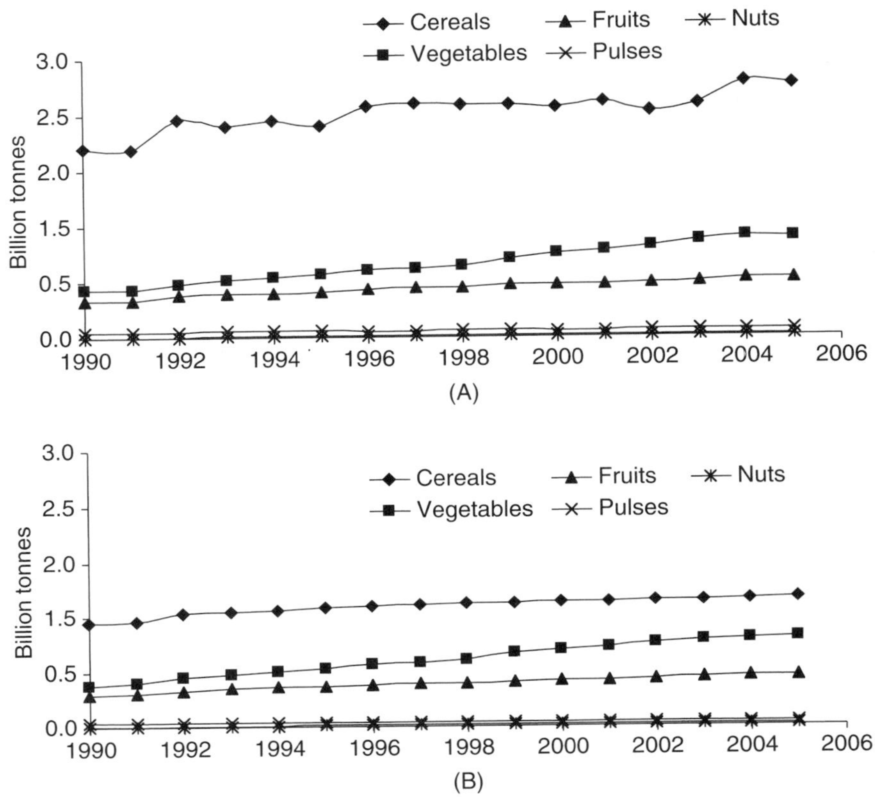

FIG. 1 Worldwide consumption (A) and production (B) of fruits and vegetables. (Data to create these graphs were obtained from the consumption and production online databases of FAOSTAT, faostat.fao.org/. Commodities under each category are specified in faostat.fao.org/site/370/default.aspx. Data accessed: April 30, 2007, FAOSTAT, Statistics Division, Food and Agriculture Organization of the United Nations.)

outbreaks has also been associated with an increase in the number of ill persons per outbreak (Sivapalasingam et al., 2004).

The purpose of this review is to discuss our current state of knowledge about the microbial safety of fresh produce by identifying pathways and factors affecting contamination and discussing candidate interventions to reduce the risk of contamination. Because the topic is global in scope, we draw on examples from around the world. The reader is also encouraged to review four recent books on the general topic of produce safety (James, 2006b; Matthews, 2005a; Sapers et al., 2006; Sumner, 2003)and other reviews more focused on the safety of organically grown produce (Bourn and Prescott, 2002; Fonseca, 2005; Matthews, 2005b). One book, two additional book chapters, and one review focus exclusively on the microbiology of fresh-cut produce

(Bhagwat, 2005; Gil and Selma, 2006; Lamikanra, 2002; Nguyen-the and Carlin, 1994).

12.2 NORMAL MICROFLORA OF FRESH PRODUCE

The types and levels of microbes on fresh fruits and vegetables vary with commodity and level of post-harvest processing. In general, *Pseudomonas fluorescens*, *Erwinia herbicola*, and *Enterobacter agglomerans* are major components of the epiphytic microflora of many vegetables (reviewed in Nguyen-the and Carlin, 1994). *Leuconostoc* spp., *Lactobacillus* spp., *Enterobacter agglomerans*, molds, and yeasts can also be found on various fruits and vegetables (Zagory, 1999). Pectinolytic *P. fluorescens*, *Xanthomonas* spp., *Cytophaga* spp., and *Flavobacterium* spp. have also been isolated. These bacteria are normally present and not considered harmful to humans.

The type of produce has a significant influence on microbial populations. Seed sprouts (e.g., mung bean, alfalfa, clover, radish, broccoli) in particular frequently have higher microbial levels, including fecal coliforms, than other produce items (Fett et al., 2005). This occurs because of the unique features of seed sprout production, including limited sources of seed lots and the elevated temperatures and relative humidity using during production, which simultaneously promote the growth of bacterial contaminants (Matos et al., 2002). The types and levels of commensal microbes may also vary depending on the stage of plant growth, environmental conditions (temperature, moisture), harvesting and packing practices (washing and decontamination), and packaging (Nguyen-the and Carlin, 1994). The interaction of normal produce-associated microflora with foodborne pathogens on fruits and vegetables has not been well studied, but it is likely that normal flora may inhibit, or perhaps even promote, the growth of certain foodborne pathogens (Nguyen-the and Carlin, 1994).

12.3 SPOILAGE OF FRESH PRODUCE

Spoilage of produce has been characterized as a brown discoloration, necrosis of tissue, loss of texture, and exudation and production of off-flavors and off-odors (Nguyen-the and Carlin, 1994). The causes of produce spoilage are frequently commodity-specific and may be due either to microbial agents or to senescence. Microbiological spoilage is caused by yeasts, molds, and sometimes bacteria (reviewed in Filtenborg et al., 1996; Tournas, 2005), and prevention of spoilage is approached by implementation of decontamination procedures, temperature control, and/or modified atmosphere packaging. In some instances, total bacterial numbers bear little relationship to spoilage, produce quality, or shelf life (reviewed in Nguyen-the and Carlin, 1994; Zagory, 1999). In this case, spoilage is not associated with any particular microorganism(s) but instead, is caused by senescence (ripening) of produce tissue, which occurs as a result of intrinsic enzymatic processes, including respiration (Nguyen-the and Carlin, 1994). When this occurs, it can promote microbial growth and further damage to tissues. Operations that reduce injury and preserve the integrity of fresh produce can slow this process, while conditions that damage or abuse the tissues can result in higher microbial populations (Zagory, 1999).

12.4 HUMAN PATHOGENS ASSOCIATED WITH PRODUCE

Produce-associated foodborne disease outbreaks are usually caused by bacteria, viruses, and parasites, and only rarely by chemical toxins. With a few exceptions, human pathogens should not be present on fresh produce and certainly not at levels that can cause disease. Except for instances in which small amounts of the contaminant may be present on produce as a result of normal environmental contacts with water and soil (e.g., *Listeria monocytogenes*, *Clostridium botulinum*, *and Bacillus cereus*), most produce items become contaminated with pathogens by contact with human or animal feces. The bacterial pathogens *Salmonella* spp. and *E. coli* O157:H7 (and other pathogenic *E. coli*) tend to be transmitted predominantly by animal fecal wastes, either directly or indirectly through fecal-contaminated water or soil. The source of contamination with human enteric viruses (hepatitis A virus and the noroviruses) and *Shigella* spp. is contact with human fecal matter via contaminated human hands, contact with human sewage, or indirectly through sewage-contaminated water or soil. *Cryptosporidium*, a protozoan parasite, can be found in both human and animal feces. Both viruses and parasites require a human and/or animal host to replicate and do not increase in number during subsequent product storage. On the other hand, many bacteria, including pathogens, are free-living and not dependent on cells to replicate. Their levels may increase during storage, although the degree of that increase depends on produce type (one important factor being product pH) and storage conditions (e.g., temperature, humidity).

Salads and produce "dishes" are the most commonly recognized vehicles of produce-associated outbreaks. For example, in the United States, an analysis conducted by the Center for Science in the Public Interest (CSPI) found that between 1990 and 2004, salads were associated with 28% of all produce-associated outbreaks, while produce dishes caused 15% of all produce-associated outbreaks (De Waal et al., 2006). These data suggest that contamination occurred just prior to consumption in these cases, probably during food preparation and serving of produce (e.g., raw, cooked). In the United States, the individual crops most often associated with produce outbreaks were lettuce (8%), potatoes (6%), melons (5%), sprouts (5%), and berries (3%). The viral, bacterial, and parasitic protozoan pathogens most commonly implicated among *all* produce-associated outbreaks between 1990 and 2004 ($n = 639$) were noroviruses (39%), *Salmonella* (19%), and *Cyclospora* (3%) (Table 1). Table 2 lists the pathogens involved in produce-associated outbreaks, their clinical symptoms, representative outbreaks, and relevant vehicles. This list is representative but not meant to be all-inclusive. Other produce pathogen lists describe pathogens detected on produce regardless of whether they have been associated with outbreaks (Beuchat, 1998).

TABLE 1 Contribution of Pathogens to Produce-Associated Outbreaks in the United States, 1990–2004

	Outbreaks		Cases	
Cause	Number	Percent	Number	Percent
Viral				
Norovirus	251	39	9746	31
Hepatitis	25	4	1832	6
Other virus	20	3	1115	4
Bacterial				
Salmonella	120	19	7628	24
Shigella	25	4	2829	9
Escherichia	48	8	2103	7
Clostridium	42	7	1519	5
Campylobacter	17	3	795	3
Bacillus	21	3	193	1
Staphylococcus	20	3	160	1
Pseudomonas	1	<1	7	<1
Vibrio	1	<1	2	<1
Parasitic				
Cyclospora	16	3	3233	10
Cryptosporidium	1	<1	54	<1
Giardia	2	<1	47	<1
Other parasites	1	<1	8	<1
Other chemicals/toxins	28	4	225	1
Total	639		31,496	

Source: Data from CSPI (2006). For additional details on these data, including collection, refer to De Waal et al. (2006).

12.5 FACTORS THAT INFLUENCE SURVIVAL AND GROWTH OF ORGANISMS

Multiple factors affect the survival and growth of pathogens and spoilage organisms on produce, and these are usually commodity-specific. For example, the physical characteristics of individual produce items, such as the rough irregular surfaces of leafy greens (Badawy et al., 1985) or the ridges of cantaloupe, may sequester microorganisms and protect them from removal or inactivation. A larger number of crevices and ridges is proportional to a greater overall surface area and provide increased opportunities for pathogen attachment. These crevices and the hydrophobic nature of the waxy cuticle on fruits and vegetables may prevent sanitizing solutions and treatments from reaching hidden microorganisms (Annous et al., 2001; Beuchat, 1998). Fruit and vegetable tissue components can also neutralize chlorine, rendering it inactive against microorganisms (Beuchat, 1998; Gonzalez et al., 2004). Certain produce items may also exhibit potent antibacterial and antiviral properties. For example, carrots and fennel inhibited the survival of hepatitis A virus (Croci et al.,

TABLE 2 Pathogens Linked to Produce-Associated Outbreaks[a]

Pathogen	Source[b]	Main Clinical Characteristics[c] Associated with Foodborne Outbreaks	References	Vehicles
Bacteria				
Bacillus cereus	E	Gastroenteritis	Portnoy et al., 1976	Sprouts
Campylobacter	E, H	Gastroenteritis, Guillain–Barré syndrome, reactive arthritis (Reiter's syndrome), septic arthritis, osteomyelitis	CDC, 2005	Melon, strawberries, tomato, green salad
Clostridium botulinum	E	Nerve impairment, descending weakness or paralysis	Reviewed in Sobel et al., 2004	Canned asparagus, squash, peppers
Enterohemorhagic *Escherichia coli*	E, H	Gastroenteritis, possibly hemolytic uremic syndrome (HUS) or thrombotic thrombocytopenia purpura (TTP)	Doorduyn et al., 2006; Anonymous, 2006; Ferguson et al., 2005	Lettuce, spinach, sprouts
Listeria monocytogenes	E	Meningoencephalitis and/or septicemia, pregnant women may exhibit fever and abortion, normal host may exhibit only mild febrile illness	Aureli et al., 2000; Farber et al., 1990; Junttila and Brander, 1989; Schlech et al., 1983	Corn, alfalfa tablets, salted mushrooms, coleslaw
Salmonella spp.	H	Gastroenteritis, enterocolitis, septicemia	Anonymous, 2005; CDC, 2002, 2004a, 2004b; Takkinen et al., 2005; Sivapalasingam et al., 2003	Lettuce, mangoes, tomatoes, cantaloupes, almonds
Shigella	H	Gastroenteritis, perhaps toxemia, dysentery, convulsions, HUS, Reiters syndrome, toxic megacolon	Reller et al., 2006; CDC, 1999	Tomatoes, parsley

Staphylococcus aureus	H	Varied symptoms from skin lesions, to pneumonia, sepsis, and sometimes death	Martin et al., 2004	Vegetables
Pseudomonas aeruginosa	E	Mostly affects immunocompromised persons; causes systemic infections (e.g., pneumonia, gastrointestinal, bone infections)	Correa et al., 1991	Lettuce, onion
Vibrio cholera	E, H	Severe gastroenteritis	Mujica et al., 1994; CDC, 2004c	Fruits and vegetables
Yersinia enterocolitica, Y. pseudotuberculosis	E	Enterocolitis, bloody diarrhea, mesenteric lymphadenitis complicated by erythema nodosum	Jalava et al., 2006, discussed in Cover and Aber, 1989	Sprouts, carrots
Parasites				
Cryptosporidium parvum	E, H	Gastroenteritis, may also involve other organs: gallbladder, lungs, eyes, vagina	Blackburn et al., 2006; CDC, 1998	Apple cider, green onions
Cyclospora cayetanensis	H	Gastroenteritis	Herwaldt and Beach, 1999; Ho et al., 2002; Doller et al., 2002; Lopez et al., 2001	Basil, raspberries, snow peas
Fasciola hepatica	E	Liver function abnormalities, eosinophilia, biliary colic, jaundice	Marcos et al., 2005; Bjorland et al., 1995; Mailles et al., 2006	Aquatic plant, watercress, salads
Giardia lamblia	E, H	Gastroenteritis, steatorrhea	CDC, 2005; Mintz et al., 1993	Raw vegetables, fresh fruit

(Continued)

TABLE 2 ***(Continued)***

Pathogen	Source[b]	Main Clinical Characteristics Associated with Foodborne Outbreaks[c]	References	Vehicles
Viruses				
Hepatitis A	H	Jaundice, fever, nausea, abdominal discomfort	Calder et al., 2003; Hutin et al., 1999; Wheeler et al., 2005	Blueberries, green onions, strawberries
Noroviruses		Gastroenteritis	Hjertqvist et al., 2006, Cotterelle et al., 2005; Falkenhorst et al., 2005; Holtby et al., 2001; Le Guyader et al., 2004	Raspberries, salad
Rotavirus	E, H	Gastroenteritis	Gallimore et al., 2005	Salad

[a]Outbreaks searched on Pubmed, various reviews, and the U.S. Centers for Disease Control and Prevention's foodborne outbreak database until 2006 (CDC, 2004).
[b]Source information obtained from Johnston et al. (2006b) and Heymann (2004). E, environmental (including animal): H, human.
[c]Clinical characteristics obtained from Heymann (2004).

2002), although the presence of antimicrobial agents on produce may not always inhibit growth of a microorganism (Kurdziel et al., 2001). Wounding of produce by cutting, peeling, or shredding may bring internal antibacterial and antiviral agents in contact with microorganisms. For example, in carrots, cutting had an inhibitory effect on the survival of *L. monocytogenes* (Beuchat and Brackett, 1990; Nguyen-the and Lund, 1991). The pH of the produce has an enormous influence on pathogen (and commensal) growth. As an example, *L. monocytogenes* is inhibited on sliced tomatoes but grows well on whole tomatoes, an effect probably due to the acidic juice released by slicing (Beuchat and Brackett, 1991). The oxidation–reduction potential on the surfaces of fruits and vegetables can also affect pathogen growth (IFT, 2001). Finally, vegetables with moist surfaces, such as lettuce and celery, may facilitate prolonged bacterial and virus survival (Badawy et al., 1985; Konowalchuk and Speirs, 1975; Kurdziel et al., 2001), while pathogens are inactivated more quickly under dry conditions.

12.6 MICROBIOLOGICAL METHODS FOR DETECTION AND QUANTIFICATION

Conventional, rapid, and cutting-edge approaches to microbial detection and quantification in foods are discussed in Chapters 26 and 27. These techniques and methods are applicable to produce, and the reader is encouraged to read those chapters. In this section we supplement some of these topics and provide a discussion of viral detection strategies. Sampling fresh produce is complicated because in many cases, only a small proportion of an entire harvest may be contaminated, called *focal contamination*. Consequently, detection of pathogens in contaminated produce is a relatively rare event (USFDA-CFSAN, 2001a, 2003). Even in the case of a produce-associated outbreak investigation, the contaminant may be detected only sporadically in the food item implicated (Calder et al., 2003; Nuorti et al., 2004). Sampling strategies are not discussed in this section but must be considered when designing microbiological detection and surveillance programs.

Conventional methods for the detection of bacterial foodborne pathogens involve three main steps: cultural enrichment, selective plating, and confirmation (reviewed in Jaykus, 2003). "Rapid" first-generation detection methods such as nucleic acid hybridization and immunoassays allow for decreased time to detection by providing a substitute for the selective plating step. Rapid second-generation detection methods such as PCR (polymerase chain reaction)-based methods, should, in theory, replace these three steps with just one step. In practice, the cultural enrichment and confirmation steps (usually by conventional cultural methods) are still necessary.

Viruses and certain parasites present additional detection challenges (reviewed in D'Souza et al., 2006; Jaykus, 2001; Koopmans and Duizer, 2004; Leggitt and Jaykus, 2000; Richards, 1999; Sair Al et al., 2002). Because produce samples usually have low levels of contamination and the organisms cannot be "enriched" by culture methods, scientists must process produce items before detection to (1) concentrate the pathogen, (2) purify it from the sample matrix, and (3) amplify its numbers, usually though nucleic acid amplification [e.g., PCR or real time (RT)-PCR]. Unfortunately, these technologies cannot distinguish between infectious and noninfectious viruses or parasitic protozoa. Infectivity assays have not yet been developed for norovirus or wild-type hepatitis A virus, the main viruses responsible for produce-associated outbreaks (Table 1). In the case of norovirus detection, an additional challenge is that because of the vast genetic diversity of norovirus strains, no single set of primers has proven effective for universal norovirus detection (Vinje et al., 2003).

12.7 INDICATOR MICROORGANISMS

Detection of pathogens in produce is difficult for many reasons, not the least of which is the extended time to detection, complicated methodology, and high cost. For this reason, the detection and enumeration of microbiological indicator organisms is often used in place of pathogen detection. The presence of these organisms often results from direct or indirect fecal contamination of foods, and hence serves as a "marker" that fecal contamination has occurred, and hence the potential for pathogen presence. Product quality indicators are available as well, but this discussion will be limited to those used for safety purposes (Bhagwat, 2005).

Numerous criteria have been identified as essential for an "ideal" microbiological indicator. Some examples of these are as follows: easy and rapid detection and enumeration; readily distinguishable from commensal microflora; consistent association (presence, concentration, and absence) with the pathogen whose presence it is intended to indicate; growth rate similar to that of the pathogen; and inactivation rate similar to, but slightly slower than, the pathogen of concern (reviewed in Jay, 2005; Pierson and Smoot, 2007; USFDA-CFSAN, 2001b). No currently identified indicator meets all these criteria. Some of the indicator organisms that are most commonly used to ensure food safety include coliform bacteria, fecal coliform bacteria, *E. coli*, total *Enterococcus* spp., and aerobic plate count (APC) (reviewed in Jay, 2005; Pierson and Smoot, 2007). Coliphage have been proposed as an alternative indicator of contamination with viral pathogens, but they are still not widely used. APC is used to estimate the total number of viable aerobic bacteria in a sample, while coliforms are indicators of general environmental contamination (filth). Total coliforms may not be the best organism to use as an indicator of fecal contamination on produce because they may be present in high numbers in soil. Fecal coliforms are associated with the intestinal tracts of warm-blooded animals (including humans). *E. coli*, which is a member of the fecal coliform group, is found exclusively in the intestinal tracts of animals and humans and is one of the most commonly used indicator organisms. It is well accepted that the presence of *E. coli* in produce may indicate the potential presence of many other enteric pathogens. Some species of the *Enterococcus* genus are found almost exclusively in the intestinal tracts of humans and animals, while others are general environmental contaminants present in soil, water, and vegetation. They are more resistant to refrigeration, freezing, drying, low pH, and NaCl, and hence more persistent, than are the gram-negative coliform indicators.

12.8 SOURCES OF PRODUCE CONTAMINATION

Multiple sources in the farm-to-fork pathway can cause produce contamination. The continuum can be divided into the following stages: pre-harvest, harvest, post-harvest, and retail–consumer. Produce may become contaminated with a human pathogen at any stage in the continuum. If no additional control measures are used to ameliorate contamination, the pathogen may persist and perhaps even grow. Depending on host factors, pathogen virulence, and dose, consumption of contaminated produce may result in illness and, occasionally, death. Several reviews (D'Souza et al., 2006; Guzewich and Ross, 1999; Leon and Moe, 2006; Richards, 2001; Seymour and Appleton, 2001; Tran et al., 2006; USFDA-CFSAN, 2001c) have addressed the mechanism of produce contamination at these various stages, and the descriptions below have been synthesized from these reviews.

12.8.1 Pre-harvest

There are some documented instances (such as for sprouts) in which seeds are contaminated with pathogens. Nonetheless, pre-harvest is considered the earliest phase of the farm-to-fork continuum, and includes planting, growing, irrigating, and other activities and treatments associated with the production of the mature plant. The significance of contamination of produce during growing and harvesting is not well characterized because once an outbreak occurs, it is often difficult to determine the specific pre-harvest source of contamination (reviewed in Richards, 2001; Seymour and Appleton, 2001). Although for most products contamination occurs on the surface of produce, there is some evidence that pathogens may be taken up by capillary action into spaces or crevices (e.g., carrots) and/or damaged plant tissues during production (Petterson et al., 2001).

The pre-harvest stage has several risk factors for produce contamination. In 1998, the U.S. Food and Drug Administration (FDA) developed guidance documents related to good agricultural practices (GAPs) entitled A *Guide to Minimize Microbial Food Safety Hazards for Fresh Fruits and Vegetables* (USFDA-CFSAN, 1998). This document identifies risk factors and areas for which control of microbial contamination of produce may be implemented at the pre-harvest stage. This includes such issues as the microbial quality of water, manure use and composting, animal and pest management, traceback, cleaning and sanitation, and worker health and hygiene. GAPs are similar to good manufacturing practices (GMPs) used in the food-processing industry, but they address agricultural practices rather than processing activities.

Contamination of produce at the pre-harvest phase frequently occurs as a consequence of exposure to contaminated water or soil. The guide states: "Wherever water comes into contact with fresh produce, its quality dictates the potential for pathogen contamination." The source of irrigation water, how it is distributed, and the type of irrigation process used are important factors that influence the potential for produce contamination (USFDA-CFSAN, 1998). In general, groundwater may be less likely to be contaminated than surface waters. Surface water quality may be affected by land-use patterns in the watershed. These patterns can affect the presence of human and animal feces in water, such as in point-source (sewage) and non-point-source (runoff) as well as by topography and fluctuations in rainfall. The type of irrigation used for produce may also affect produce contamination, especially if the irrigation source is questionable and/or irrigation occurs close to harvest time. Irrigation practices that maximize exposure to the edible portion of produce (e.g., wetting the entire plant) may also increase the likelihood of produce contamination. Drip, trickle, or subirrigation can minimize wetting the edible portion of the plant. Unfortunately, there is widespread use of untreated wastewater for irrigation, especially in developing countries. Untreated wastewater may also increase the risk of produce contamination.

Contaminants can be introduced into soil if the land was previously used for animal production or industrial dumping, or if biosolids or sludge, manure, or animal waste were applied as fertilizer or for waste disposal. Manure use may be particularly risky, as animal feces may contain pathogens which then make their way to produce items grown in the field. Close proximity of manure to produce, inappropriate containment of manure, recontamination of manure from pests, and improper composting (e.g., temperature of piles below the minimum heat and time requirements) all increase the risk of produce contamination. Banning the use of manure as fertilizer may reduce the risk of product contamination, but would also eliminate the positive benefits of manure in terms of growth enhancement, not to mention providing a useful role for animal waste and a means of disposal. Because it is not possible to remove bacteria, parasites, and viruses completely from manure, growers can instead focus on strategies to minimize the levels of microbial contaminants. One such strategy is through active (e.g., proper composting, pasteurization, among others) or passive (e.g., passage of time) treatments. A particularly contentious issue is the time between manure application and harvest. The National Organic Standards recommend a 90- to 120-day interval between application of raw manure and harvest, depending on whether the edible portion of the crop contacts the soil, without distinction for type of crop. Some produce buyers request that manure not be applied for 5 years prior to planting, or in extreme cases, that manure never be applied to land for crops (Bihn and Gravani, 2005).

Proximity to wildlife (e.g., birds, mammals, reptiles) has gained interest as a potential source of produce contamination. By way of example, in our work, we observed that several farms had no barriers to prevent domestic animals or wildlife from entering the fields, and most farms reported animals near their water sources (Clayton, 2006). Other factors, such as cleaning and sanitation and worker health and hygiene, may play a somewhat minor role on contamination at this stage. These factors are discussed in the next section.

12.8.2 Harvest

Harvest is the stage where produce is collected by human or mechanical means. The sources of contamination at this phase differ somewhat from those occurring during pre-harvest. In addition, the type of contaminants occurring during and after harvest are affected by whether the produce items are field packed (i.e., packed in the field ready for immediate distribution) or the product is subjected to washing and subsequent packing at a processing plant (packing shed).

Microbiological contamination of produce may occur through contact with contaminated equipment. Unfortunately, it is difficult to ascertain the degree to which equipment surfaces serve as the source of contamination to produce, or vice versa. Equipment surfaces in contact with produce should always be washed and sanitized. A survey performed in 1999 of farm and packing shed practices suggested that washing of equipment surfaces did not occur in 0 to 18% of packing sheds, and sanitizing of food contact surfaces did not occur in 13 to 47% of packing sheds (USDA, 2001). The percentage range was based on the equipment and tool washing frequency for various equipment and tools used for fruits and vegetables. These data are based on 2868 reports from packing sheds across the United States. Packing shed personnel were asked to fill out surveys on packing shed practices, including washing and sanitizing of equipment surfaces, for a maximum of two produce commodities.

Contamination may also occur during handling of produce by workers during harvesting (Hernandez et al., 1997). A survey of farm and packing shed practices across several U.S. states suggested that 94% of all fruit acres and 87% of all vegetable acres surveyed were harvested by hand (USDA, 2001). In addition, certain produce items, such as green onions, are handled extensively during harvest. The practices of the food handlers picking and packing produce items can have a significant influence in the type and magnitude of the hazards that follow the food into processing and consumption. Some significant worker hygiene issues may include contaminated hands, lack of hygiene, dirty clothes and hair, and open cuts, sores, and infections on hands. Workers may also be ill (e.g., gastroenteritis or hepatitis) or may be asymptomatic carriers of enteric pathogens. Some outbreaks have been linked to infected field workers (Ramsay and Upton, 1989; Reid and Robinson, 1987). The presence of children in fields during picking may provide an additional contamination risk. Poor or inconsistent hand-washing practices, limited access to latrines, and defecation in fields can also serve as sources of contamination on produce. In our work, we identified high levels of fecal coliforms and *E. coli* on farmworkers' hands, suggesting the presence of fecal contamination and the potential for enteric pathogens (Clayton, 2006).

Farm practices related to worker hygiene may also influence produce contamination. For example, in our work we found that some farms had no worker training programs on issues such as personal hygiene, nor did they have protective measures in place for workers with cuts and sores on their hands. The majority of farms responding to interview questions did not require workers to wash their hands prior to harvesting crops. Few farm personnel were familiar with relatively common quality control terms mentioned in the FDA guide, such as good manufacturing practices (GMPs), good agricultural practices (GAPs), or hazard analysis of critical control points (HACCP) (Clayton, 2006).

12.8.3 Post-harvest

Post-harvest covers what happens to a food product (in this case, fresh produce) after harvest, up through shipment to distribution and/or retail establishments. The term *processing* is often used for this phase and is appropriate for instances in which a raw material is converted to a value-added product, such as would be the case for potatoes being converted into a boxed instant mashed product or oranges into juice. Raw produce receives less extensive post-harvest treatment; some produce items are packed and shipped without further handling, while others are washed or sanitized and packed prior to shipment. Fresh items that receive the most extensive treatment are fresh-cut produce, which is washed in multiple steps, cut, repackaged in sealed plastic bags (which may or may not be modified atmosphere packages), and is ready for immediate use by the consumer.

Many produce items pass through specialized facilities called packing sheds. The role of the packing shed is to prepare produce that comes directly from the field for subsequent distribution. Packing sheds may also repackage crops that come from other countries to meet buyers' and distributors' specifications. Packing sheds frequently specialize in specific crops because handling and packaging requirements differ by produce commodity. Crops may undergo washing steps, where they are immersed in water wash tanks, sprayed, or rinsed, after which they are frequently transported by conveyor belts and/or are handled manually prior to being placed in the final distribution container (e.g., box). These may sometimes be topped with ice to maintain low temperatures. Our work and that of other investigators has indicated that certain crops, such as cantaloupe, cilantro, and parsley, have significantly higher microbial loads when they leave the packing shed than when they enter directly from the field (Castillo et al., 2004; Johnston et al., 2005, 2006a). This suggests that certain processes that occur in packing sheds may result in cross-contamination and/or microbial proliferation.

We have identified several areas of concern with regards to cross-contamination in packing sheds. For example, the microbial load on conveyor belts appears to be highly correlated with microbial levels on produce (Etienne, 2006). Second, similar to the findings of others, we have observed instances where there were high levels of fecal coliforms and *E. coli* on shed workers' hands, suggesting that food handlers may be a source of contamination on produce (Blanding, 2006). Third, produce collected from certain end-stage locations in the shed (e.g., conveyor belt, merry-go-round, and box) was at an increased risk of *E. coli* contamination compared to identical products collected at earlier stage locations (e.g., bin, wash tank) (Ailes et al., 2008), also suggesting that contaminated food contact surfaces may contaminate produce. Finally, we found that certain packing shed practices (e.g., cleanliness, presence of rodents, absence of training) may contribute to produce contamination (Blanding, 2006). On the other hand, we observed little relationship between the levels of indicator organisms in water used for packing and the microbial quality of produce items. The packing shed waters screened in our study were generally clean (absence of or low levels of microbial indicators), probably because they came from a chlorinated municipal source (Hall, 2005). In the United States, between 50 and 60% of packing facilities treated their produce wash waters with sanitizer (USDA, 2001). This may not always be the case for water used in packing sheds in other countries.

Even though fresh-cut produce may be considered "cleaner" than produce items that receive less post-harvest processing, there are unique opportunities for contamination in this product. Because it undergoes multiple washing steps, fresh-cut produce items may have more wounding of the plant tissue, predisposing it to microbial contamination (Bhagwat, 2005). Microbes tend to attach more easily to cut or bruised surfaces than to intact produce. The injured tissue and liquids may also interfere with sanitizing treatments, such as chlorine. Considerations for control of microbial contamination of fresh-cut produce are similar to those for less highly processed products. Accordingly, strict maintenance of equipment sanitation, attention to worker health and hygiene, and the quality of the water used in processing are all critical. Because washes are the only steps in which pathogens can be removed, processors should be particularly cognizant of the potential for cross-contamination and the need to assure the use of high-quality water and appropriate concentrations of disinfectants in washing steps. This is particularly important when using re-circulating water, which is common in the fresh-cut industry (Bhagwat, 2005).

Contamination may also occur at various transportation steps as produce items move from the farm to the packing shed (e.g., unclean truck) or from the packing shed to the warehouse for eventual distribution. Contamination may be kept at a minimum during transportation by ensuring hygienic conditions and adherence to safe temperature ranges. For example, if produce is contaminated in the field, keeping transportation and storage temperatures below 4°C can prevent growth of bacteria in those products having intrinsic parameters that might support pathogen growth.

12.8.4 Retail and Consumer Handling

Food handlers can do much to influence the microbial load on fresh produce. Although it is generally recognized that simple water washing at the retail or home level cannot completely eliminate pathogens present on fresh produce, it may be able to reduce the numbers. Food handlers may themselves contaminate produce by inattention to recommended hygiene practices, such as washing hands before preparing foods or preventing cross-contamination between raw meat products and salad items. Certainly, inclusion of a single contaminated produce item in a salad mix will result in commingling and may increase the number of people exposed to a contaminated product. The reader is referred to two reviews that specifically address the role of consumer behavior in contamination of produce (Bruhn, 2005, 2006).

12.9 MAINTAINING PRODUCE QUALITY AND REDUCING THE NUMBER OF MICROORGANISMS

As discussed previously, produce contamination may take place anywhere along the farm-to-fork continuum. Produce that becomes contaminated during pre-harvest, harvest, or post-harvest phases tend to cause more widespread outbreaks because one lot may be distributed across state or even country borders. However, these outbreaks may also be focal in nature, as would occur when a single lot is contaminated inconsistently or sporadically. Traceback investigations rarely identify the source of contamination because of the time lapse between identification and investigation of the outbreak and sometimes poor consumer recall about food consumption. Produce that is contaminated at the food preparation stage tends to cause isolated outbreaks. In the vast majority of cases, when this type of produce-associated outbreak is identified, an infected food handler is usually the source of contamination. Unfortunately, it is often difficult to confirm this causal relationship.

In general, most pathogen contamination of food occurs as a consequence of some sort of fecal–oral contamination. Interventions intended to prevent contamination can be divided into two categories: primary and secondary barriers (reviewed in Leon and Moe, 2006). Primary barriers are those interventions that prevent pathogens from getting into the environment. Examples of these primary barriers would be safe containment and disposal of feces (e.g., encouraging workers to use toilets). Secondary barriers are those interventions that prevent pathogens from infecting a host once the contaminants are in the environment. Examples of these secondary barriers may include destruction of pathogens (e.g., cooking produce or disinfecting equipment surfaces in contact with produce) or avoiding unsafe foods (e.g., avoiding raw produce or salads when traveling abroad). In addition, two reviews on the effects of water and sanitation on enteric illness morbidity list several interventions (e.g., good water quality, hand washing, safe excreta disposal) that could interrupt the fecal–oral transmission pathway, especially in developing countries (Esrey et al., 1991; Fewtrell and Colford, 2004).

12.9.1 Controlling Contamination During Growing, Harvesting, and Post-harvest

General recommendations to minimize contamination during growing, harvesting, and post-harvest have been published by the U.S. Food and Drug Administration [good agricultural practices (GAPs)] and detailed in several reviews (D'Souza et al., 2006; Guzewich and Ross, 1999; Leon and Moe, 2006; Richards, 2001; Seymour and Appleton, 2001; Tran et al., 2006; USDA-CFSAN, 1999, 2001c, 2004, 2007). These recommendations are somewhat general (i.e., not produce commodity–specific) and at the time of writing are recommended but not mandatory. In the United States, packing sheds are encouraged but not required by law, to follow current good manufacturing practices (cGMPs; see Chapter 20). These provide guidance on the safe handling of product in buildings used for food processing (Food cGMP Modernization Working Group, 2005). Four important recommendations on washing, sanitizing, hand cleansing, and temperature are detailed below.

Washing Washing can decrease contamination but cannot be relied upon to eliminate foodborne pathogens. Several reviews have focused on various washing materials and protocols (D'Souza et al., 2006; Richards, 2001; Sapers, 2006; Seymour and Appleton, 2001). In general, disinfectants approved for food applications (such as chlorine, chlorine dioxide, and ozone) are effective at reducing levels of bacteria, parasites, and viruses on produce (D'Souza et al., 2006; Leon and Moe, 2006; Sapers, 2006; USFDA-CFSAN, 2001d). One disadvantage of ozone is that it is unstable and therefore must be generated on-site, but industry suppliers are working on appropriate ozone systems for washing fresh produce. It is also important to note that some European Union countries have outlawed the use of chlorine as an additive to wash water. The efficacy of disinfectants varies with different fruits and vegetables based on surface characteristics, temperature, and type of pathogen. The efficacy of a disinfectant such as chlorine may be reduced by organic material in the water or on the surface of the produce; if not replenished appropriately, the disinfectant has minimal effect (Parnell et al., 2005). Therefore, leaving fruits and vegetables in the sanitizing or washing water for an extended period of time may consume the disinfectant residual and possibly lead to cross-contamination, thus counteracting the beneficial effect of the disinfectant (Beuchat, 1998; Rajkowski and Rice, 2004). A balance must be established between effective disinfection of produce and the effect of disinfectants on taste and shape (organoleptic properties) of produce. Finally, there has been concern about the possible migration of pathogens into the core tissue of fruits and vegetables during washing. A negative temperature differential between the water and produce, together with unique produce surface characteristics of produce items, can result in the uptake of bacterial cells (and perhaps other microbes). This has been demonstrated in both cantaloupe, tomatoes, and apples (Buchanan et al., 1999; Ibarra-Sanchez et al., 2004; Richards and Beuchat, 2004).

Sanitizing Equipment Surfaces The same agents used for produce surface decontamination (chlorine and chlorine dioxide) can also be used to disinfect equipment surfaces (reviewed in D'Souza et al., 2006; Fonseca, 2005; Richards, 2001; Sapers, 2006; Seymour and Appleton, 2001). Quaternary ammonium–based sanitizers are also effective. Some of these sanitizers, such as sodium hypochlorite, are not very effective against hepatitis A virus and human rotaviruses (reviewed in Koopmans and Duizer, 2004). As mentioned previously, our research indicated a significant correlation between the level of microbiological indicator organisms on produce items and on the equipment surfaces with which they came in contact (Etienne, 2006). Although not yet tested in controlled studies, one could speculate that improved sanitation of equipment surfaces may decrease the microbial load of produce.

Hand Cleansing As mentioned previously, many produce items are manipulated by hand during picking and washing, so the cleanliness of the hands of field and shed workers is important. Indeed, our work has shown that both farm and shed workers can have high levels of fecal indicator organisms on their hands (Blanding, 2006; Clayton, 2006). Hand contamination may be controlled by promoting regular and proper hand-washing practices, including ready access to soap and water and educational programs aimed at training employees about appropriate hand hygiene practices. Even with these policies, compliance will remain an issue. The routine use of hand disinfectants may also help. Several studies have examined the effects of hand disinfectants on the inactivation of foodborne pathogen and recommended hygiene practices for agricultural workers (reviewed in Barry and Todd, 2006; D'Souza et al., 2006; Guzewich and Ross, 1999; Michaels and Todd, 2006; Richards, 2001). In general, chlorhexidine gluconate and alcohol-based hand disinfectants, although effective at reducing bacterial levels, are not effective at reducing levels of foodborne viruses and parasitic protozoa (Mbithi et al., 1993; Weir et al., 2002). Hand washing with soap reduces levels of bacteria and viruses but does not always eliminate viruses.

A survey of several soaps found that those containing Triclosan, a chlorophenol, were effective at reducing hepatitis A levels on hands (Mbithi et al., 1993). Additional work to identify hand sanitizers that are effective against nonenveloped enteric viruses such as hepatitis A and noroviruses is a critical need for the produce industry.

Temperature In general, lower temperatures will maintain better produce quality and ensure longer shelf life, although a number of produce items are sensitive to refrigeration (e.g., bananas) (Elmé, 2006). For products that can support bacterial growth, lowering the storage and transport temperature may also help maintain food safety because it prevents the growth of pathogenic bacteria. However, enteric viruses and parasites are likely to survive longer at cooler temperatures. Packing sheds use a variety of methods for rapid cooling: forced-air cooling, hydrocooling, vacuum cooling, and icing. Forced-air cooling is probably the least likely to result in cross-contamination, as there is no contact between produce and water. If water is used in the cooling process, it must be potable and adequately disinfected (USFDA-CFSAN, 1998). Storage of produce is also an important step, and both hygienic conditions and safe temperature ranges will prevent the occurrence or exacerbation of contamination.

12.9.2 Controlling Contamination During Processing (Fresh-Cut Produce)

Unlike most food processors, the fresh-cut produce industry has the difficult challenge of ensuring microbiological safety without implementing a thermal inactivation step and/or manipulating intrinsic and extrinsic parameters to prevent microbial growth. Certainly, implementation of a hazard analysis of critical control point (HACCP) program can supply some degree of protection for the product. HACCP is a preventive approach that focuses on controlling pathogen contamination at the source (see Chapter 22). Although not mandatory for the fresh-cut industry, the International Fresh-Cut Produce Association (IFPA) has been encouraging its members to implement HACCP programs in their plants voluntarily. IFPA also has been proactive in offering educational and training programs to its members. Although HACCP addresses an important point in the farm-to-fork continuum, the need for adequate controls at the pre-harvest phase cannot be overlooked simply because a post-harvest HACCP program is in place. Indeed, comprehensive programs that include HACCP together with GAPs (recommended), cGMPs (required by U.S. law for the fresh-cut industry), and sanitation standard operating procedures (SSOPs) help ensure the safety of fresh-cut fruits and vegetables. These programs all require adequate and clear documentation and auditing to assure that they are functioning as intended. For more detail about specific food safety recommendations for the fresh-cut industry (e.g., pre-washing/sorting, peeling, packaging), the reader is encouraged to consult various reviews and books (Bhawat, 2005; Gil and Selma, 2006; Nguyen-the and Carlin, 1994).

12.9.3 Controlling Contamination During Retail and Home Preparation

At the retail level, the single most important intervention is assuring appropriate hygiene practices and sanitary conditions when working with produce (e.g., frequent hand washing, use of gloves, hair nets). Poor personal hygiene and, to a lesser degree, unsafe food sources, are the most commonly identified factors associated with foodborne disease outbreaks (Bean et al., 1996; Olsen et al., 2000). Although any ready-to-eat food that has received extensive human handling may become contaminated with pathogens, certain ready-to-eat foods have repeatedly been associated with outbreaks, including salads and raw fruits and vegetables (reviewed in De Waal et al., 2006; Guzewich and Ross, 1999; Richards, 2001). Cross-contamination of processed products by contaminated surfaces (especially raw foods) and utensils is another important risk factor for outbreaks, and appropriate cleaning and sanitation practices must be maintained to prevent cross-contamination (reviewed in Rooney et al., 2004).

In recent years, there has been increased focus on the need to furlough food handlers who are symptomatic for enteric illness for a predetermined period of time (usually, 2 to 3 days) to prevent contamination that might occur due to poor personal hygiene. For hepatitis A virus and the noroviruses in particular (and some bacterial pathogens), it is known that people may shed the agents in feces many days before symptom onset or after symptoms have resolved (Graham et al., 1994; Irwin and Millership, 1999; Latham and Schable, 1982; Patterson et al., 1993; Rockx et al., 2002). Unfortunately, mandatory exclusion of ill food workers is complicated by a number of factors, including the fact that exclusion usually occurs without pay, and hence there is no incentive for ill workers to report their health status. Further, asymptomatic shedding means that even with this type of restriction policy, some persons shedding pathogens will remain in the employment pool. Finally, mandatory vaccination of all food handlers against hepatitis A virus has been proposed but has not been advocated universally, due to cost and inconvenience (Fiore et al., 2006; Franco et al., 2003; Meltzer et al., 2001).

As stated previously, washing of produce cannot be relied upon to eliminate bacterial, parasitic, or viral pathogens, and simple practices such as peeling and cooking may be a more effective means for reducing the risk from pathogens (Bruhn et al., 2004; USFDA, 2000). However, this is not practical for many produce items. As at the retail level, washing of hands prior to food preparation and attention to surface sanitation, including the prevention of cross-contamination, is important (Bruhn et al., 2004; USFDA, 2000). There is an ongoing debate as to whether commercially available produce "disinfectant" solutions are effective against pathogens. To date, there is no convincing evidence that using these products is superior to water rinsing (Crowe et al., 2004; Kilonzo-Nthenge et al., 2006; Michaels et al., 2003; Parnell and Harris, 2003; Parnell et al., 2005; Simmone, 2006). Consumer educational programs have had some impact on modifying food-handling behavior, and these are reviewed elsewhere (Bruhn, 2005).

12.9.4 Risk Assessment: HACCP

Multiple reviews and several regulatory representatives (USFDA-CFSAN, 2007) have encouraged the produce industry in the United States to adopt a HACCP approach to food safety, similar to other food industries, such as red meat and poultry. Some challenges in implementing HACCP in the U.S. produce industry include the following: (1) lack of coordination between the many diverse organizations in the produce industry (packing shed industry, retailers, farmers, and transport industry work separately), (2) limited research identifying appropriate critical control points and appropriate critical limits at these points, and (3) lack of governmental regulations. This may be changing in the wake of several high-profile produce-associated outbreaks that occurred in the United States during the fall of 2006. Interestingly, Europe has implemented legislation to encourage a HACCP approach to produce safety [Regulation (EC) No. 852/2004 of the European Parliament].

One tool to assist the development of food safety regulations is microbial risk assessment. For additional information on risk assessment, see Chapter 19. Particularly relevant to produce is the product pathway approach to risk assessment, which examines the factors that influence risk associated with food–hazard pairs along a specific product production, processing, distribution, and point-of-consumption pathway. These types of risk assessments can be used to identify critical factors that affect exposure to the pathogen of interest. They can also be used to identify points in the farm-to-fork pathway that increase or decrease the risk of microbial contamination and estimate the impact of specific mitigation strategies on overall exposure and disease risk (Jaykus et al., 2006).

As is the case for some of the other foodborne pathogen–commodity combinations, risk modeling for produce safety is complicated. Certainly, there are pathogen-specific differences in prevalence in the population, environmental occurrence and survival, and amplification, as well as produce-specific differences in production, packing, and handling practices. The wide range of product–pathogen combinations makes this a daunting task. By way of example, the single-input "pathogen levels" will differ by produce type (e.g., leafy greens vs. carrots) and pathogen type (bacteria, virus, or parasitic protozoa).

A comprehensive risk model for produce contamination and subsequent human disease has yet to be designed. By way of illustration, we attempted to create a very basic exposure model that estimates pathogen levels through the farm-to-fork pathway (Fig. 2). While contamination can occur at any point in the farm-to-fork pathway, for simplicity we assumed that contamination occurs exclusively at the pre-harvest step. An additional assumption was that bacterial levels will increase; however, it is recognized that some vegetative bacteria will not grow on certain produce items. Based on existing data, we propose three major factors that influence the presence and concentrations of pathogens on produce:

- The first of these factors is the packing shed, as multiple studies have demonstrated that microbial levels on certain produce (e.g., cantaloupe, cilantro, parsley) increase during the packing process (Castillo et al., 2004; Johnston et al., 2005, 2006a).

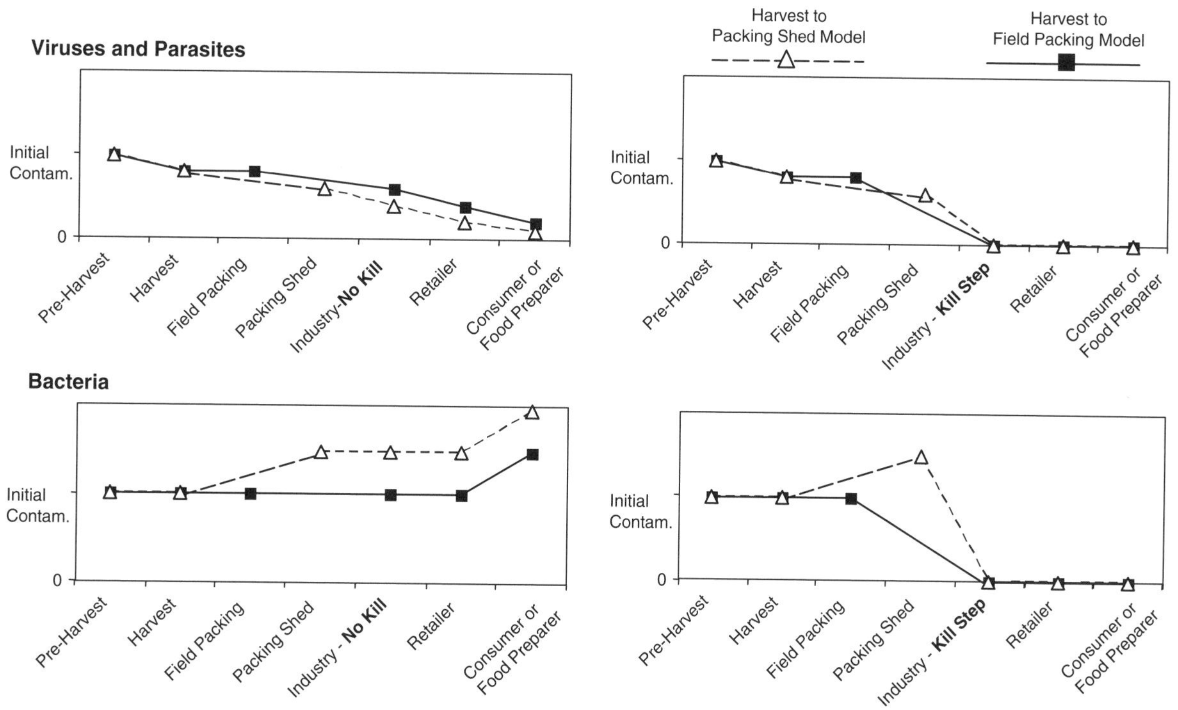

FIG. 2 Models of pathogen levels through produce farm-to-fork pathway. The model assumes that only one contamination event occurs at pre-harvest (Initial Contam.). Produce may be field packed or sent to a packing shed. The left panels assume that the pathway has no kill step (e.g., preparing bagged spinach). The right panels assume that the pathway includes a kill step (e.g., processed commercially sterile tomato sauce). Both models assume that bacteria grow during the pathway, although there are some vegetative bacteria that do not grow or there may be some environmental conditions that do not favor growth. Horizontal lines indicate no change in microbial levels.

- The second factor is whether the pathway includes a "kill" step (such as cooking or other thermal processing), which should result in pathogen elimination.
- The third factor is food handler practices, which vary by produce item as discussed previously.

The final assumption was that pathogen levels on all produce are affected by these factors, although in reality, pre-harvest pathogen levels may not be affected by sanitary packing shed or food handler practices. We also limited the number of farm-to-fork pathways in this model to four. The scenarios differed as to whether or not the produce was field-packed (therefore bypassing the packing shed) and whether or not the produce item was subjected to a kill step. Given these assumptions and restrictions, the model demonstrated that the levels of viruses and parasitic protozoa on produce decreased through the pathway and were eliminated if the industry or consumer implemented a kill step. In contrast, bacterial levels on produce increased if the product was processed through a packing shed and was not subjected to a kill step. Bacterial levels increased further on arrival at the consumer or food preparer. These types of models provide initial conceptualization of the process and can be thought of as a preliminary step to more thorough quantitative risk assessment efforts.

12.10 REGULATIONS

12.10.1 Regulatory Agencies with Oversight Over Produce

Individual countries and regions have their own organizations (e.g., ministries of health) charged with protecting the public health of their citizens, which often includes disease and outbreak surveillance activities. Two very different examples of oversight over the safety of fresh produce will be discussed in this section: the approaches used in the United States and in the European Union (EU).

The primary agencies in the United States that play a major role in the identification and investigation of foodborne illness outbreaks are the Centers for Disease Control and Prevention (CDC), state and local health departments, public health laboratories, and the Council of State and Territorial Epidemiologists (CSTE). The primary agencies that have regulatory authority over foods are state departments of agriculture, the U.S. Food and Drug Administration (FDA), and the U.S. Department of Agriculture (USDA). There are a number of other federal agencies that also have jurisdiction over some aspect of food safety. Consistent communication and collaboration both within and between agencies is essential to preventing foodborne disease. Currently, the FDA is responsible for the safety of produce, both domestic and imported, and because of recent interest in this problem, it is possible that more stringent regulations for this commodity will soon be implemented.

In the EU, the Directorate General for Health and Consumer Protection is in charge of keeping food safety laws up to date and making sure that member countries are enforcing these regulations properly. It is the responsibility of individual national governments to apply the EU food safety regulations. In 2002, the EU adopted general principles of food safety in a regulation called the General Food Law, Regulation (EC) No. 178/2002. This law contains stringent regulations on release, marketing, labeling, and traceability of crops and foodstuffs. In 2006, the EU also adopted Regulation (EC) No. 852/2004, which addresses food hygiene among other issues. The Directorate General for Health and Consumer Protection depends on the European Food Safety Authority (EFSA), headquartered in Parma, Italy, to provide scientific data on food safety. In 2005, the European Centre for Disease Control and Prevention was formed to fulfill a similar role as the U.S. CDC, including the detection, surveillance, and investigation of foodborne illness. Currently, food safety organizations in Europe have more legal authority over produce than do their counterparts in the United States, although this may change in the coming years.

12.10.2 Surveillance Systems and Produce Safety

There are few commodity-specific monitoring programs worldwide that systematically or routinely test for pathogens or indicator organisms on samples of produce. Instead, individual countries may perform epidemiologic surveillance for outbreaks and/or diseases associated with certain foodborne pathogens. However, many of these organisms can be transmitted through multiple routes, and contaminated foods are only a single vehicle. The degree to which foods in general are the cause of these diseases (called attributable risk) is not well characterized. Certainly, produce items are implicated in outbreaks of foodborne disease, and hopefully, those outbreaks and cases will be reported to a surveillance system. However, it is likely that there are many more produce-associated foodborne disease outbreaks and cases that are not recognized and/or reported in routine epidemiological surveillance activities.

In the United States, two limited "snapshot" surveillance studies have lead to the establishment of a permanent produce-monitoring system. In 1999 and 2000, the FDA performed two national surveys of imported and domestic crops at high risk for foodborne pathogen contamination (USFDA-CFSAN, 2001a, 2003). They sampled 1003 imported samples and 1028 domestic samples of various commodities and found the highest foodborne pathogen isolation rates on cantaloupe (7.3% imported, 3.0% domestic), cilantro (9.0% imported, 1.2% domestic), and parsley (2.4% imported, 1.1% domestic). Although imported crops had a higher prevalence of pathogens, the survey was not specifically designed to compare domestic and imported crops. In 2002, the U.S. Department of Agriculture (USDA) began the Microbiological Data Program (MDP) (www.ams.usda.gov/science/MPO/Mdp.htm) to assess trends in certain produce commodities over time. The goal of the program is to provide statistically reliable information regarding targeted foodborne pathogens (currently, pathogenic *E. coli* and *Salmonella*) on selected produce (to date, five to eight commodities, including cantaloupe, celery, cilantro, green onion, leaf and romaine lettuce, parsley, and tomato). This is a voluntary data-gathering program, not a regulatory enforcement effort, and encompasses 11 states in the United States. From 2002 to 2006, the MDP collected between 7000 and 11,000 produce samples each year from both terminal markets and wholesale locations. The origin of produce samples collected through the MDP differs by year but ranges from 61 to 86% domestic origin, 11 to 34% imported samples, and 3 to 5% samples of unknown origin. To date, no significant difference in the frequency of pathogen detection from imported produce versus domestic produce has been identified for any of the sampling years, 2002 through 2006.

The U.S. government has also instituted two systems to monitor and track the incidence of diseases that are commonly transmitted by contaminated foods. FoodNet (www.cdc.gov/foodnet) is a collaborative project of the CDC, 10 emerging infections program sites (10 states), the USDA, and the FDA. This is an active surveillance system set up to (1) determine the burden of foodborne illness in the United States, (2) monitor trends in the burden of specific foodborne illness over time, and (3) attribute the burden of foodborne illness to specific foods and settings. The second system is PulseNet (www.cdc.gov/pulsenet), which is a national network of public health and food regulatory agency laboratories coordinated by the CDC. The network consists of state and local health departments and federal agencies (CDC, USDA-FSIS, FDA). PulseNet participants perform standardized molecular subtyping (or "fingerprinting") of foodborne pathogenic bacteria using pulsed-field gel electrophoresis (PFGE). Fingerprinting allows the identification of bacteria associated with separate outbreaks to facilitate linking apparently unrelated cases and/or sources in space and time. This system is limited to bacteria and the samples received by the reference laboratory. Often, an average of 15 days elapses between the recognition of an outbreak and the posting of a fingerprint pattern on PulseNet. These two systems strengthen the capacity of U.S. federal health and food safety agencies to detect and contain produce-associated outbreaks.

The European equivalents of these networks are Enter-Net and Salm-gene for detection of outbreaks associated with pathogenic *E. coli* and *Salmonella* (Fisher and Threlfall, 2005), respectively; PulseNet Europe (www.pulsenet-europe.org) for fingerprinting of pathogenic bacteria isolated from sporadic cases and outbreaks; and the European Foodborne Viruses Network (www.eufoodborneviruses.co.uk/) for detection of foodborne viral disease outbreaks (Koopmans, 2004). The PulseNet system has also expanded globally to include Canada and countries in Latin America and the Asia Pacific (links under www.cdc.gov/pulsenet/participants.htm). All PulseNet sites share the same protocols and databases for standardized and rapid identification of common outbreak strains. As mentioned previously, other countries may also have instituted their own surveillance systems, such as OzFoodNet for Australia (www.ozfoodnet.org.au/).

12.10.3 Standards and Guidelines

Each country or region may or may not have specific standards related to produce safety. For example, Canada and Australia are among the few countries that have irrigation water quality guidelines (ANZECC/ARMCANZ, 2000; CCME, 2005). The United States, on the other hand, has no strict irrigation or processing water guidelines (reviewed in Bihn and Gravani, 2005). The closest type of guidance on irrigation water quality for the United States are two recommendations published by the Center for Food Safety and Applied Nutrition (CFSAN) of the FDA for all produce (USFDA-CFSAN, 1998) and sprouts (USFDA-CFSAN, 1999), which include general recommendations on testing of irrigation water for pathogens and indicators and types or water used for irrigation, among other recommendations. The World Health Organization has water quality guidelines for produce production, including recommendations on maximum bacterial load and specific types of water used for irrigation (Carr et al., 2004). It is clear that guidelines and standards, based on scientifically valid research, are important for decreasing the risk of produce-associated disease.

At the international level, the United Nations' Food and Agricultural Organization (FAO) and World Health Organization (WHO) have created the *Codex Alimentarius* Commission to enhance food safety by promoting the use of best practices for food production, processing, and handling, and by setting uniform standards. The *Codex* has developed two codes related to produce safety; one focuses on primary production, the other focuses on precut, ready-to-eat fruits and vegetables. There are also several food assurance systems, programs, and standards. Examples of global standards include EurepGAP Fruit and Vegetable Standard and Safe Quality Food 1000 Code. National or regional standards include Assured Produce Scheme (UK), SwissGAP (Switzerland), and US-GAP (United States), among others (reviewed in Elmé, 2006).

EurepGAP is a private-sector quality assurance system that sets voluntary good agricultural practices (GAPs) standards for the certification of agricultural products around the globe. Safe Quality Food (SQF) 1000 is designed specifically for agricultural producers and is a food safety audit and certification program based on *Codex Alimentarius* and HACCP guidelines. British standards, such as assured produce schemes, combine ISO, HACCP, and GAP standards. Both SwissGAP and US-GAP are country-specific GAP standards.

In the United States, in addition to the guide that introduced the concept of GAPs (USFDA-CFSAN, 1998), the FDA later implemented a regulation referred to as the Recording and Reporting Rule of the Bioterrorism Act (2002) (Cupp et al., 2004). Under this rule, food companies must provide the FDA with data on the source of all ingredients used in food production and processing. For produce, this includes information on the shipper, date harvested, field, and picker. This has facilitated the identification of produce items associated with foodborne disease outbreaks. In 2004, the FDA launched the Action Plan to Minimize Foodborne Illness Associated with Fresh Produce Consumption, which was intended to provide a framework to reduce the number of illnesses per produce-associated outbreak (USFDA-CFSAN, 2004). Finally, in 2007, FDA-CFSAN published the *Guide to Minimize Microbial Food Safety Hazards of Fresh-Cut Fruits and Vegetables*, which focuses more specifically on worker hygiene, layout, and practices in the processing of this product (USFDA-CFSAN, 2007).

Despite significant efforts in the development of guidelines to assure the safety of fresh produce, they remain quite general and provide little guidance for prioritizing specific practices in the production of specific commodities. This means that at present, the U.S. agricultural community does not have a clear understanding of the relative importance of specific risk factors for produce contamination. If such risk factors were better identified and prioritized, they could be incorporated into GAPs (as preferred by the U.S. produce industry) (Elmé, 2006) or in a HACCP model (as advocated by the FDA) (USFDA-CFSAN, 2007). Produce organizations are beginning to work with researchers and public health officials to identify high-risk practices and to develop and enforce more specific guidelines to prevent produce contamination and subsequent human disease.

In most instances, the U.S. food service industry is regulated by the *Food Code*; the most recent edition appeared in 2005. The code is produced as a collaborative effort between FDA, USDA, and CDC and is a reference manual for regulatory agencies to ensure the maintenance of safe food produced in food service establishments, retail food stores, and institutional settings such as nursing homes and child care centers. The code provides practical evidence-based recommendations for addressing risk factors associated with foodborne illness, such as specific food storage temperatures and handling conditions. These differ by commodity, of course, but include produce items of all sorts.

12.10.4 Third-Party Auditing

In countries that lack national regulations and standards on produce safety, such as the United States, the produce industry has used third-party auditors to help assure consumers that due diligence programs are in place. Countries or regions that have strict regulations and standards on produce safety, such as the European Union, may also use these third-party audit companies to assure consumers that appropriate food safety laws are enforced. In the United States, large retailers are also beginning to use these third-party audit companies to ensure that individual suppliers (farms and packing sheds) enforce appropriate practices to assure produce safety, including GAPs, GMPs, and HACCP. These auditing companies have no regulatory or legal authority to enforce produce safety standards. However, because large purchasers of produce may require farms and packing sheds to show evidence of routine audit and good practices, these companies may have substantial economic clout. In countries like the such as the United States, produce growers and packers have several concerns about routine third-party auditing, including the lack of government regulation of the auditors, the high cost associated with auditing, the lack of industry standards for routine auditing, and inappropriate application of protocols designed for the nonagricultural food sector to agricultural fields, farms, and packing sheds (James, 2006a). Nonetheless, such auditing practices are likely to continue as the seeks an appropriate manner by which to ensure the safety of produce produced within and imported into the United States.

In response to several U.S. produce-associated outbreaks in 2007, various trade groups serving the conventional produce industry and supervised by the California Department of Food and Agriculture formed a Leafy Green Product Handler Marketing Agreement, which would require those handlers who sign on to agree to adhere to best practices and to buy or handle leafy green products only from growers who have grown the produce in accordance with the best practices (www.caleafygreens.ca.gov).

Those who advocate use of the best practices approach cite advantages such as more specific guidelines (e.g., maximum bacterial counts in irrigation or manure samples) and easy-to-use decision trees. Several groups have criticized this approach and stated that (1) these recommendations are not based on produce-specific research, (2) that the board may be composed solely of industry representatives and may be biased, (3) that the guidelines proposed are established by industry without public input, and (4) that since participation is voluntary, the marketing agreement does not cover all leafy green growers and processors (Odabashian, 2007). The debate surrounding the use of best practices illustrates the need to implement control measures in a transparent manner that engages all stakeholders and is structured to accommodate change that may occur as a result of the continuous input of new research.

12.11 CONCLUSIONS

Produce production and consumption will continue to increase worldwide in the coming years, and this trend will probably lead to increased numbers of produce-associated disease outbreaks. We need to move toward a global multitiered approach to produce safety that will provide assurances for both consumers and the industry. Several recent initiatives indicate progress in this direction: multinational regulations, foodborne disease surveillance, research on produce production and safety, and efforts in creating regional or global standards. Continued and effective dialogue between scientists, policymakers, business groups, and regulators is needed if we are to continue to improve global produce safety. Multidisciplinary (e.g., agronomy, microbiology, epidemiology, policy, engineering, behavioral sciences) and applied research that is sensitive to the needs of governments, industry, and consumers will become increasingly important. Together, these efforts will reduce the risk of produce-associated disease and provide safer produce to support the sustenance and health of consumers worldwide.

Acknowledgments

The authors are grateful to Farida Bhuiya and the staff at the Center for Science in the Public Interest for providing produce specific data on outbreaks (Table 1). We also thank Peter Teunis, RIVM (National Institute for Public Health and Environment), the Netherlands, for thoughtful insights in produce risk assessment modeling and revisions to the manuscript, and Erin Floyd and Marisol Lopez for assistance on this chapter. We appreciate Barry Palevitz's (University of Georgia, Athens) guidance in the botanical classification of fruits and vegetables for Fig. 1. Thank you to Albert DiChiara and the staff at FAOSTAT for checking and verifying Fig. 1. The authors gratefully acknowledge USDA CSREES, National Research Initiative, Epidemiological Approaches to Food Safety Program, award numbers 99-35212-8564 and 2002-35212-12386, for support of this work. Juan Leon was funded by a fellowship from the Dana-Irvington Institute for Immunological Research.

REFERENCES

Ailes EC, Leon JS, Jaykus L, Johnston LM, Clayton HA, Blanding S, Kleinbaum DG, Backer LC, Moe CL (2008): Microbial concentrations on fresh produce are affected by post-harvest processing, importation, and season. *J Food Prot.* 71(12):2389–2397.

Annous BA, Sapers GM, Mattrazzo AM, Riordan DC (2001): Efficacy of washing with a commercial flatbed brush washer, using conventional and experimental washing agents, in reducing populations of *Escherichia coli* on artificially inoculated apples. *J Food Prot.* 64:159–163.

Anonymous (2005): Outbreaks of *Salmonella* infections associated with eating Roma tomatoes—United States and Canada, 2004. *MMWR Morb Mortal Wkly Rep.* 54: 325–328.

——— (2006): Ongoing multistate outbreak of *Escherichia coli* serotype O157:H7 infections associated with consumption of fresh spinach—United States, September 2006. *MMWR Morb Mortal Wkly Rep.* 55:1045–1046.

ANZECC/ARMCANZ (Australian and New Zealand Environment and Conservation Council/Agriculture and Resource Management Council of Australia and New Zealand) (2000): Water quality for irrigation and general use. In: *Australian and New Zealand Guidelines for Fresh and Marine Water Quality*. pp. 9.2-1 to 9.2-104.

Aureli P, Fiorucci GC, Caroli D, et al. (2000): An outbreak of febrile gastroenteritis associated with corn contaminated by *Listeria monocytogenes*. *N Engl J Med.* 342:1236–1241.

Badawy AS, Gerba C, Kelley LM (1985): Survival of rotavirus SA-11 on vegetables. *Food Microbiol.* 2:199–205.

Barry M, Todd E (2006): Food worker personal hygiene requirements during harvesting, processing and packaging of plant products. In: James JL (Ed.): *Microbial Hazard Identification of Fresh Fruit and Vegetables*. Wiley, Hoboken, NJ, pp. 115–153.

Bean NH, Goulding JS, Frederick CL, Angulo FJ (1996): Surveillance for foodborne-disease outbreaks—United States, 1988–1992. *MMWR Morb Mortal Wkly Rep.* 45:1–55.

Beuchat L (1998): Surface decontamination of fruits and vegetables eaten raw: a review. http://www.who.int//fsf/Documents/Surface_decon.pdf. Accessed March 2007.

Beuchat LR, Brackett RE (1990): Inhibitory effects of raw carrots on *Listeria monocytogenes*. *Appl Environ Microbiol.* 56:1734–1742.

——— (1991): Behavior of *Listeria monocytogenes* inoculated into raw tomatoes and processed tomato products. *Appl Environ Microbiol.* 57:1367–1371.

Bhagwat A (2005): Microbiological safety of fresh cut produce: Where are we now? In: Matthews KR (Ed.). *Microbiology of Fresh Produce: Emerging Issues in Food Safety*. ASM Press, Washington, DC, pp. 121–165.

Bihn EA, Gravani RB (2005): Good agricultural practices in produce safety. In: Matthews KR (Ed.): *Microbiology of Fresh Produce: Emerging Issues in Food Safety*. ASM Press, Washington, DC, pp. 21–53.

Bjorland J, Bryan RT, Strauss W, Hillyer GV, McAuley JB (1995): An outbreak of acute fascioliasis among Aymara Indians in the Bolivian Altiplano. *Clin Infect Dis.* 21: 1228–1233.

Blackburn BG, Mazurek JM, Hlavsa M, et al. (2006): Cryptosporidiosis associated with ozonated apple cider. *Emerg Infect Dis.* 12:684–686.

Blanding S (2006): An analysis of the relationship between packing shed processes and microbial contamination of produce in packing sheds in the southern United States. M.P.H. thesis, Emory University.

Bourn D, Prescott J (2002): A comparison of the nutritional value, sensory qualities, and food safety of organically and conventionally produced foods. *Crit Rev Food Sci Nutr.* 42: 1–34.

Bruhn CM (2005): Consumer handling of fresh produce. In: Matthews KR (Ed.). *Microbiology of Fresh Produce: Emerging Issues in Food Safety.* ASM Press, Washington, DC, pp. 167–219.

——— (2006): Consumer handling of fresh produce from supermarket to table. In: James JL (Ed.). *Microbial Hazard Identification of Fresh Fruit and Vegetables.* Wiley, Hoboken, NJ, pp. 261–278.

Bruhn CM, Cohen AL, Harris LJ, Spitler-Kashuba A (2004): Safe handling of fruits and vegetables. http://anrcatalog.ucdavis.edu/pdf/8121.pdf. Accessed March 2007.

Buchanan RL, Edelson SG, Miller RL, Sapers GM (1999): Contamination of intact apples after immersion in an aqueous environment containing *Escherichia coli* O157:H7. *J Food Prot.* 62:444–450.

Calder L, Simmons G, Thornley C, et al. (2003): An outbreak of hepatitis A associated with consumption of raw blueberries. *Epidemiol Infect.* 131:745–751.

Carr RM, Blumenthal UJ, Mara DD (2004): Guidelines for the safe use of wastewater in agriculture: revisiting WHO guidelines. *Water Sci Technol.* 50:31–38.

Castillo A, Mercado I, Lucia LM, et al. (2004): *Salmonella* contamination during production of cantaloupe: a binational study. *J Food Prot.* 67:713–720.

CCME (Canadian Council of Ministers of the Environment) (2005): Canadian water quality guidelines for the protection of agricultural water uses. *Updated October 2005.* http://www.ccme.ca/assets/pdf/wqg_ag_summary_table.pdf.

CDC (Centers for Disease Control and Prevention) (1998): Foodborne outbreak of cryptosporidiosis—Spokane, Washington, 1997. *MMWR Morb Mortal Wkly Rep.* 47:565–567.

——— (1999): Outbreaks of *Shigella sonnei* infection associated with eating fresh parsley—United States and Canada, July–August 1998. *MMWR Morb Mortal Wkly Rep.* 48:285–289.

——— (2002): Multistate outbreaks of *Salmonella* serotype Poona infections associated with eating cantaloupe from Mexico, United States and Canada, 2000–2002. *MMWR Morb Mortal Wkly Rep.* 51:1044–1047.

——— (2004a): Outbreak of *Salmonella* serotype Enteritidis infections associated with raw almonds, United States and Canada, 2003–2004. *MMWR Morb Mortal Wkly Rep.* 53:484–487.

——— (2004b): Foodborne Outbreak Response and Surveillance Unit. Foodborne and Diarrheal Diseases Branch. http://www.cdc.gov/foodborneoutbreaks/us_outb.htm. Accessed November 2004.

——— (2004c): Cholera epidemic associated with raw vegetables—Lusaka, Zambia, 2003–2004. *MMWR Morb Mortal Wkly Rep.* 53:783–786.

CDC (2005): Foodborne Outbreak Response and Surveillance Unit. http://www2.cdc.gov/ncidod/foodborne/fbsearch.asp, http://www.cdc.gov/foodborneoutbreaks/outbreak_data.htm. Accessed March 2007.

Clayton H (2006): An epidemiologic study to describe the relationship between farming practices and microbial indicator concentrations on produce from farms in the southern United States. M.P.H. thesis, Emory University.

Correa CM, Tibana A, Gontijo Filho PP (1991): Vegetables as a source of infection with *Pseudomonas aeruginosa* in a university and oncology hospital of Rio de Janeiro. *J Hosp Infect.* 18:301–306.

Cotterelle B, Drougard C, Rolland J, et al. (2005): Outbreak of norovirus infection associated with the consumption of frozen raspberries, France, March 2005. *Eur Surveill.* 10: E050428–E050421.

Cover TL, Aber RC (1989): *Yersinia enterocolitica. N Engl J Med.* 321:16–24.

Croci L, De Medici D, Scalfaro C, Fiore A, Toti L (2002): The survival of hepatitis A virus in fresh produce. *Int J Food Microbiol.* 73:29–34.

Crowe K, Bushway A, El-Begearmi M (2004): Best ways to wash fruits and vegetables. *Food Safety Facts.* http://www.umext.maine.edu/onlinepubs/htmpubs/4336.htm. Accessed March 2007.

CSPI (Center for Science in the Public Interest) (2006): Outbreak Alert! database. Revised and updated 2006. http://www.cspinet.org/new/pdf/outbreakalertlinelisting2006.pdf. Accessed March 2007.

Cupp OS, Walker DE, Hillison J (2004): Agroterrorism in the U.S.: key security challenge for the 21st century. Biosecurity and bioterrorism: biodefense strategy. *Pract Sci.* 2:97–105.

De Waal CS, Johnson K, Bhuiya F (2006): Outbreak alert! Closing the gaps in our food-safety net. Center for Science in the Public Interest, Review. http://www.cspinet.org/foodsafety/outbreak_alert.pdf. Accessed March 2007.

Doller PC, Dietrich K, Filipp N, et al. (2002): Cyclosporiasis outbreak in Germany associated with the consumption of salad. *Emerg Infect Dis.* 8:992–994.

Doorduyn Y, de Jager CM, Van Der Zwaluw WK, et al. (2006): Shiga toxin–producing *Escherichia coli* (STEC) O157 outbreak, The Netherlands, September–October 2005. *Eur Surveill.* 11.

D'Souza DH, Moe C, Jaykus LA (2006): Foodborne viral pathogens. In: Doyle MP, Beuchat LR, Montville TJ (Eds.). *Food Microbiology: Fundamentals and Frontiers*, 2nd ed. ASM Press, Washington, DC, pp. 581–610.

Elmé C (2006): Microbiological risk in produce from the field to packing. In: James JL (Ed.). *Microbial Hazard Identification of Fresh Fruit and Vegetables.* Wiley, Hoboken, NJ, pp. 73–94.

Esrey SA, Potash JB, Roberts L, Shiff C (1991): Effects of improved water supply and sanitation on ascariasis, diarrhoea, dracunculiasis, hookworm infection, schistosomiasis, and trachoma. *Bull World Health Organ.* 69 (5):609–621.

Etienne K (2006): An epidemiologic study to describe the relationship between microbial indicator concentrations on produce, workers' hands, and equipment surfaces in farms and packing sheds in the southern United States. M.P.H. thesis, Emory University.

Falkenhorst G, Krusell L, Lisby M, Madsen SB, Bottiger B, Molbak K (2005): Imported frozen raspberries cause a series of norovirus outbreaks in Denmark, 2005. *Eur Surveill.* 10:E050922.

Farber JM, Carter AO, Varughese PV, Ashton FE, Ewan EP (1990): Listeriosis traced to the consumption of alfalfa tablets and soft cheese. *N Engl J Med.* 322:338.

Ferguson DD, Scheftel J, Cronquist A, et al. (2005): Temporally distinct *Escherichia coli* 0157 outbreaks associated with alfalfa sprouts linked to a common seed source, Colorado and Minnesota, 2003. *Epidemiol Infect.* 133:439–447.

Fett WF, Fu TJ, Tortorello ML (2005): Seed sprouts: the state of microbiological safety. In: Matthews KR (Ed.). *Microbiology of Fresh Produce: Emerging Issues in Food Safety.* ASM Press, Washington, DC, pp. 167–219.

Fewtrell L, Colford JM (2004): *Water, Sanitation and Hygiene: Interventions and Diarrhoea—A Systematic Review and Meta-analysis.* World Bank, Washington, DC, pp. 47–53.

Filtenborg O, Frisvad JC, Thrane U (1996): Moulds in food spoilage. *Int J Food Microbiol.* 33:85–102.

Fiore AE, Wasley A, Bell BP (2006): Prevention of hepatitis A through active or passive immunization: recommendations of the Advisory Committee on Immunization Practices (ACIP). *MMWR Recomm Rep.* 55:1–23.

Fisher IS, Threlfall EJ (2005): The Enter-net and Salm-gene databases of foodborne bacterial pathogens that cause human infections in Europe and beyond: an international collaboration in surveillance and the development of intervention strategies. *Epidemiol Infect.* 133:1–7.

Fonseca J (2005): Postharvest handling and processing. In: Matthews KR (Ed.). *Microbiology of Fresh Produce: Emerging Issues in Food Safety.* ASM Press, Washington, DC, pp. 85–120.

Food cGMP Modernization Working Group (2005): Current good manufacturing practices (cGMPs). http://www.cfsan.fda.gov/~dms/cgmps.html. Accessed March 2007.

Franco E, Giambi C, Ialacci R, Coppola RC, Zanetti AR (2003): Risk groups for hepatitis A virus infection. *Vaccine.* 21:2224–2233.

Gallimore CI, Pipkin C, Shrimpton H, et al. (2005): Detection of multiple enteric virus strains within a foodborne outbreak of gastroenteritis: an indication of the source of contamination. *Epidemiol Infect.* 133:41–47.

Gil MI, Selma MV (2006): Overview of hazards in fresh-cut produce production: control and management of food safety hazards. In: James JL (Ed.). *Microbial Hazard Identification of Fresh Fruit and Vegetables.* Wiley, Hoboken, NJ, pp. 155–219.

Gonzalez RJ, Luo Y, Ruiz-Cruz S, McEvoy JL (2004): Efficacy of sanitizers to inactivate *Escherichia coli* O157:H7 on fresh-cut carrot shreds under simulated process water conditions. *J Food Prot.* 67:2375–2380.

Graham DY, Jiang X, Tanaka T, Opekun AR, Madore HP, Estes MK (1994): Norwalk virus infection of volunteers: new insights based on improved assays. *J Infect Dis.* 170:34–43.

Guzewich J, Ross MP (1999): Evaluation of risks related to microbiological contamination of ready-to-eat food by food preparation workers and the effectiveness of interventions to minimize those risks. http://www.cfsan.fda.gov/~ear/rterisk.html Accessed Feburary 2007.

Hall R (2005): An epidemiologic study to describe the relationship between concentrations of microbial indicators on produce samples with those in corresponding irrigation and processing water samples collected from farms and packing sheds in the southern United States. M.P.H. thesis, Emory University.

Hernandez F, Monge R, Jimenez C, Taylor L (1997): Rotavirus and hepatitis A virus in market lettuce (*Latuca sativa*) in Costa Rica. *Int J Food Microbiol.* 37:221–223.

Herwaldt BL, Beach MJ (1999): The return of *Cyclospora* in 1997: another outbreak of cyclosporiasis in North America associated with imported raspberries. *Cyclospora* Working Group. *Ann Intern Med.* 130:210–220.

Heymann DL (Ed.) (2004): *Control of Communicable Diseases Manual.* American Public Health Association, Washington, DC.

Hjertqvist M, Johansson A, Svensson N, Abom PE, Magnusson C, Olsson M, Hedlund KO, Andersson Y (2006): Four outbreaks of norovirus gastroenteritis after consuming raspberries, Sweden, June–August 2006. *Eur Surveill.* 11 (36):pii=3038. http://www. eurosurveillance.org/ViewArticle.aspx?ArticleId=3038.

Ho AY, Lopez AS, Eberhart MG, et al. (2002): Outbreak of cyclosporiasis associated with imported raspberries, Philadelphia, Pennsylvania, 2000. *Emerg Infect Dis.* 8:783–788.

Holtby I, Tebbutt GM, Green J, Hedgeley J, Weeks G, Ashton V (2001): Outbreak of Norwalk-like virus infection associated with salad provided in a restaurant. *Commun Dis Public Health.* 4:305–310.

Hutin YJ, Pool V, Cramer EH, et al. (1999): A multistate, foodborne outbreak of hepatitis A: National Hepatitis A Investigation Team. *N Engl J Med.* 340:595–602.

Ibarra-Sanchez LS, Alvarado-Casillas S, Rodriguez-Garcia MO, Martinez-Gonzales NE, Castillo A (2004): Internalization of bacterial pathogens in tomatoes and their control by selected chemicals. *J Food Prot.* 67:1353–1358.

IFT (Institute of Food Technologists) (2001): Factors that influence microbial growth. In: *IFT Evaluation and Definitions of Potentially Hazardous Foods*, Chap. 3. http://www.foodprotect.org/pdf/hazard_foods/chapter3.pdf. Accessed May 2007.

Irwin DJ, Millership S (1999): Control of a community hepatitis A outbreak using hepatitis A vaccine. *Commun Dis Public Health.* 2:184–187.

Jalava K, Hakkinen M, Valkonen M, et al. (2006): An outbreak of gastrointestinal illness and erythema nodosum from grated carrots contaminated with *Yersinia pseudotuberculosis*. *J Infect Dis.* 194:1209–1216.

James JL (2006a): Overview of microbial hazards in fresh fruits and vegetables operations. In: James JL (Ed.). *Microbial Hazard Identification of Fresh Fruit and Vegetables.* Wiley, Hoboken, NJ, pp. 2–36.

——— (Ed.) (2006b): *Microbial Hazard Identification of Fresh Fruit and Vegetables.* Wiley, Hoboken, NJ.

Jay JM (2005): Indicators of food microbial quality and safety. In: Jay JM, Loessner MJ, Golden DA (Eds.). *Modern Food Microbiology*, 7th ed. Springer Science + Business Media, New York, pp. 473–496.

Jaykus LA (2001): Detection of human enteric viruses in foods. In: Hui YH, Sattar SA, Murrell KD, Nip W, Stanfield PS (Eds.). *Foodborne Diseases Handbook, Vol. 2, Viruses, Parasites, Pathogens and HACCP*, 2nd ed. Marcel Dekker, New York, pp. 137–163.

——— (2003): Challenges to developing real-time methods to detect pathogens in foods. *ASM News.* 69:341–343.

Jaykus L, Dennis S, Bernard D, et al. (2006): Issue paper: using risk analysis to inform microbial food safety decisions. Council for Agricultural Science and Technology, Ames, IA.

Johnston LM, Jaykus LA, Moll D, et al. (2005): A field study of the microbiological quality of fresh produce. *J Food Prot.* 68:1840–1847.

Johnston LM, Jaykus LA, Moll D, Anciso J, Mora B, Moe CL (2006a): A field study of the microbiological quality of fresh produce of domestic and Mexican origin. *Int J Food Microbiol.* 112:83–95.

Johnston LM, Moe C, Moll D, Jaykus LA (2006b): The epidemiology of produce-associated outbreaks for foodborne disease. In: James JL (Ed.). *Microbial Hazard Identification of Fresh Fruit and Vegetables*. Wiley, Hoboken, NJ, pp. 37–72.

Junttila J, Brander M (1989): *Listeria monocytogenes* septicemia associated with consumption of salted mushrooms. *Scand J Infect Dis*. 21:339–342.

Kilonzo-Nthenge A, Chen FC, Godwin SL (2006): Efficacy of home washing methods in controlling surface microbial contamination on fresh produce. *J Food Prot*. 69:330–334.

Konowalchuk J, Speirs JI (1975): Survival of enteric viruses on fresh vegetables. *J Milk Food Technol*. 38:469–472.

Koopmans M (Ed.) (2004): *Food-borne Viruses in Europe Final Report, June 2004*. European Commission, Bilthoven, The Netherlands.

Koopmans M, Duizer E (2004): Foodborne viruses: an emerging problem. *Int J Food Microbiol*. 90:23–41.

Kurdziel AS, Wilkinson N, Langton S, Cook N (2001): Survival of poliovirus on soft fruit and salad vegetables. *J Food Prot*. 64:706–709.

Lamikanra O (2002): *Fresh-Cut Fruits and Vegetables: Science, Technology and Market*. CRC Press, Boca Raton, FL.

Latham RH, Schable CA (1982): Foodborne hepatitis A at a family reunion use of IgM-specific hepatitis a serologic testing. *Am J Epidemiol*. 115:640–645.

Leggitt PR, Jaykus LA (2000): Detection methods for human enteric viruses in representative foods. *J Food Prot*. 63:1738–1744.

Le Guyader FS, Mittelholzer C, Haugarreau L, et al. (2004): Detection of noroviruses in raspberries associated with a gastroenteritis outbreak. *Int J Food Microbiol*. 97:179–186.

Leon JS, Moe C (2006): Role of viruses in foodborne disease. In Morris P (Ed.). *Food Consumption and Disease Risk: Consumer–Pathogen Interactions*. Woodhead Publishing, Cambridge, UK, pp. 309–342.

Lopez AS, Dodson DR, Arrowood MJ, et al. (2001): Outbreak of cyclosporiasis associated with basil in Missouri in 1999. *Clin Infect Dis*. 32:1010–1017.

Mailles A, Capek I, Ajana F, Schepens C, Ilef D, Vaillant V (2006): Commercial watercress as an emerging source of fascioliasis in northern France in 2002: results from an outbreak investigation. *Epidemiol Infect*. 134:942–945.

Marcos L, Maco V, Terashima A, Samalvides F, Espinoza JR, Gotuzzo E (2005): Fascioliasis in relatives of patients with *Fasciola hepatica* infection in Peru. *Rev Inst Med Trop Sao Paulo*. 47:219–222.

Martin MC, Fueyo JM, Gonzalez-Hevia MA, Mendoza MC (2004): Genetic procedures for identification of enterotoxigenic strains of *Staphylococcus aureus* from three food poisoning outbreaks. *Int J Food Microbiol*. 94:279–286.

Matos A, Garland JL, Fett WF (2002): Composition and physiological profiling of sprout-associated microbial communities. *J Food Prot*. 65:1903–1908.

Matthews KR (Ed.) (2005a): *Microbiology of Fresh Produce: Emerging Issues in Food Safety*. ASM Press, Washington, DC.

Matthews KR (2005b): Microorganisms associated with fruits and vegetables. In: Matthews KR (Ed.). *Microbiology of Fresh Produce: Emerging Issues in Food Safety*. ASM Press, Washington, DC, pp. 1–19.

Mbithi JN, Springthorpe VS, Sattar SA (1993): Comparative in vivo efficiencies of hand-washing agents against hepatitis A virus (HM-175) and poliovirus type 1 (Sabin). *Appl Environ Microbiol.* 59:3463–3469.

Meltzer MI, Shapiro CN, Mast EE, Arcari C (2001): The economics of vaccinating restaurant workers against hepatitis A. *Vaccine.* 19:2138–2145.

Michaels B, Todd E (2006): Food worker personal hygiene requirements during harvsting, processing and packaging of plant products. In: James JL (Ed.). *Microbial Hazard Identification of Fresh Fruit and Vegetables.* Wiley, Hoboken, NJ, pp. 115–153.

Michaels B, Gangar V, Schattenberg H, Blevins M, Ayers T (2003): Effectiveness of cleaning methodologies used for removal of physical, chemical and microbiological residues from produce. *Food Service Technol.* 3:9.

Mintz ED, Hudson-Wragg M, Mshar P, Cartter ML, Hadler JL (1993): Foodborne giardiasis in a corporate office setting. *J Infect Dis.* 167:250–253.

Mujica OJ, Quick RE, Palacios AM, et al. (1994): Epidemic cholera in the Amazon: the role of produce in disease risk and prevention. *J Infect Dis.* 169:1381–1384.

Ness, AR, Powles JW (1997): Fruit and vegetables, and cardiovascular disease: a review. *Int J Epidemiol.* 26:1–13.

Nguyen-the C, Carlin F (1994): The microbiology of minimally processed fresh fruits and vegetables. *Crit Rev Food Sci Nutr.* 34:371–401.

Nguyen-the C, Lund BM (1991): The lethal effect of carrot on *Listeria* species. *J Appl Bacteriol.* 70:479–488.

Nuorti JP, Niskanen T, Hallanvuo S, et al. (2004): A widespread outbreak of *Yersinia pseudotuberculosis* O:3 infection from iceberg lettuce. *J Infect Dis.* 189:766–774.

Odabashian E (2007): Comments of Elisa Odabashian, Director, West Coast Office Consumers Union At California Department of Food and Agriculture Public Hearing to Consider the Implementation of the Proposed California Leafy Green Products Handler Marketing Agreement. http://www.consumersunion.org/pub/core_food_safety/004152.html. Accessed May 2007

Olsen SJ, MacKinnon LC, Goulding JS, Bean NH, Slutsker L (2000): Surveillance for foodborne-disease outbreaks—United States, 1993–1997. *MMWR Morb Mortal Wkly Rep.* 49:1–62.

Parnell TL, Harris LJ (2003): Reducing *Salmonella* on apples with wash practices commonly used by consumers. *J Food Prot.* 66:741–747.

Parnell TL, Harris LJ, Suslow TV (2005): Reducing *Salmonella* on cantaloupes and honeydew melons using wash practices applicable to postharvest handling, foodservice, and consumer preparation. *Int J Food Microbiol.* 99:59–70.

Patterson T, Hutchings P, Palmer S (1993): Outbreak of SRSV gastroenteritis at an international conference traced to food handled by a post-symptomatic caterer. *Epidemiol Infect.* 111:157–162.

Petterson SR, Teunis PF, Ashbolt NJ (2001): Modeling virus inactivation on salad crops using microbial count data. *Risk Anal.* 21:1097–1108.

Pierson M, Smoot L (2007): Indicator microorganisms and microbiological criteria. In: Doyle MP, Beuchat LR, Montville TJ (Eds.). *Food Microbiology: Fundamentals and Frontiers*, 2nd ed. ASM Press, Washington, DC, pp. 78–81.

Portnoy BL, Goepfert JM, Harmon SM (1976): An outbreak of *Bacillus cereus* food poisoning resulting from contaminated vegetable sprouts. *Am J Epidemiol.* 103:589–594.

Rajkowski KT, Rice EW (2004): Effect of alfalfa seed washing on the organic carbon concentration in chlorinated and ozonated water. *J Food Prot.* 67:813–817.

Ramsay CN, Upton PA (1989): Hepatitis A and frozen raspberries. *Lancet.* 1:43–44.

Reid TM, Robinson HG (1987): Frozen raspberries and hepatitis A. *Epidemiol Infect.* 98:109–112.

Reller ME, Nelson JM, Molbak K, et al. (2006): A large, multiple-restaurant outbreak of infection with *Shigella flexneri* serotype 2a traced to tomatoes. *Clin Infect Dis.* 42:163–169.

Richards GP (1999): Limitations of molecular biological techniques for assessing the virological safety of foods. *J Food Prot.* 62:691–697.

——— (2001): Enteric virus contamination of foods through industrial practices: a primer on intervention strategies. *J Ind Microbiol Biotechnol.* 27:117–125.

Richards GM, Beuchat LR (2004): Attachment of *Salmonella* Poona to cantaloupe rind and stem scar tissues as affected by temperature of fruit and inoculum. *J Food Prot.* 67:1359–1364.

Rockx B, De Wit M, Vennema H, et al. (2002): Natural history of human calicivirus infection: a prospective cohort study. *Clin Infect Dis.* 35:246–253.

Rooney RM, Cramer EH, Mantha S, et al. (2004): A review of outbreaks of foodborne disease associated with passenger ships: evidence for risk management. *Public Health Rep.* 119:427–434.

Sair AI, D'Souza DH, Jaykus LA (2002): Human enteric viruses as causes of foodborne disease. *Compr Rev Food Sci Food Saf.* 1:73–89.

Sapers GM (2006): Washing and sanitizing treatments for fruits and vegetables. In: Sapers GM, Gorny JR, Yousef AE (Eds.). *Microbiology of Fruits and Vegetables.* CRC Taylor & Francis, Boca Raton, FL, pp. 375–400.

Sapers GM, Gorny JR, Yousef AE (Eds.) (2006): *Microbiology of Fruits and Vegetables.* CRC Taylor & Francis, Boca Raton, FL.

Schlech WF III, Lavigne PM, Bortolussi RA, et al. (1983): Epidemic listeriosis: evidence for transmission by food. *N Engl J Med.* 308:203–205.

Seymour IJ, Appleton H (2001): Foodborne viruses and fresh produce. *J Appl Microbiol.* 91:759–773.

Simmone A (2006): To wash or not to wash: a tale of two products—raw meats versus raw produce. *Research news you can use.* http://fycs.ifas.ufl.edu/newsletters/rnycu06/2006/07/to-wash-or-not-to-wash-tale-of-two.html. Accessed March 2007.

Sivapalasingam S, Barrett E, Kimura A, et al. (2003): A multistate outbreak of *Salmonella enterica* serotype Newport infection linked to mango consumption: impact of water-dip disinfestation technology. *Clin Infect Dis.* 37:1585–1590.

Sivapalasingam S, Fiedman CR, Cohen L, Tauxe RV (2004): Fresh produce: a growing cause of outbreaks of foodborne illness in the United States, 1973 through 1997. *J Food Prot.* 67:2342–2353.

Sobel J, Tucker N, Sulka A, McLaughlin J, Maslanka S (2004): Foodborne botulism in the United States, 1990–2000. *Emerg Infect Dis.* 10:1606–1611.

Sumner SS (2003): *Microbiology of Fruits and Vegetables*, CRC Press, Boca Raton, FL.

Takkinen J, Nakari UM, Johansson T, Niskanen T, Siitonen A, Kuusi M (2005): A nationwide outbreak of multiresistant *Salmonella* Typhimurium in Finland due to contaminated lettuce from Spain, May 2005. *Eur Surveill.* 10:E050630–050631.

Tournas VH (2005): Spoilage of vegetable crops by bacteria and fungi and related health hazards. *Crit Rev Microbiol.* 31:33–44.

Tran N, Miller AJ, Rachman N (2006): Exposure assessment for foodborne pathogens. In: Morris P (Ed.). *Food Consumption and Disease Risk: Consumer–Pathogen Interactions.* Woodhead Publishing, Cambridge, UK, pp. 113–139.

USDA (U.S. Department of Agriculture) (2001): Agricultural chemical usage: fruit and vegetable agricultural practices. http://usda.mannlib.cornell.edu/MannUsda/viewDocumentInfo.do?documentID=1568. Accessed March 2007.

USFDA (U.S. Food and Drug Administration) (2000): FDA advises consumers about fresh produce safety. http://www.cfsan.fda.gov/~lrd/tpproduc.html. Accessed March 2007.

USFDA-CFSAN (U.S. Food and Drug Administration–Center for Food Safety and Applied Nutrition) (1998): Guide to Minimize Microbial Food Safety Hazards for Fresh Fruits and Vegetables. http://www.cfsan.fda.gov/~dms/prodguid.html. Accessed March 2007.

——— (1999): Sampling and microbial testing of spent irrigation water during sprout production. http://www.cfsan.fda.gov/~dms/sprougd2.html. Accessed March 2007.

——— (2001a): FDA survey of imported fresh produce. http://www.cfsan.fda.gov/~dms/prodsur6.html. Accessed February 2007.

——— (2001b): The use of indicators and surrogate microorganisms for the evaluation of pathogens in fresh and fresh-cut produce. Analysis and Evaluation of Preventive Control Measures for the Control and Reduction/Elimination of Microbial Hazards on Fresh and Fresh-Cut Produce. http://www.cfsan.fda.gov/~comm/ift3-7.html. Accessed Februrary 2007.

——— (2001c): Production practices as risk factors in microbial food safety of fresh and fresh-cut produce. http://www.cfsan.fda.gov/~comm/ift3-2a.html. Accessed Februrary 2007.

——— (2001d): Methods to reduce/eliminate pathogens from fresh and fresh-cut produce. Analysis and Evaluation of Preventive Control Measures for the Control and Reduction/Elimination of Microbial Hazards on Fresh and Fresh-Cut Produce. http://www.cfsan.fda.gov/~comm/ift3-5.html. Accessed Februrary 2006.

——— (2003): FDA survey of domestic fresh produce. http://www.cfsan.fda.gov/~dms/prodsu10.html. Accessed February 2007.

——— (2004). Produce safety from production to consumption: 2004 action plan to minimize foodborne illness associated with fresh produce consumption. http://www.cfsan.fda.gov/~dms/prodpla2.html. Accessed March 2007.

——— (2007): Guide to minimize microbial food safety hazards of fresh-cut fruits and vegetables. http://www.cfsan.fda.gov/~dms/prodgui3.html. Accessed March 2007.

Vinje J, Vennema H, Maunula L, et al. (2003): International collaborative study to compare reverse transcriptase PCR assays for detection and genotyping of noroviruses. *J Clin Microbiol.* 41:1423–1433.

Weir SC, Pokorny NJ, Carreno RA, Trevors JT, Lee H (2002): Efficacy of common laboratory disinfectants on the infectivity of *Cryptosporidium parvum* oocysts in cell culture. *Appl Environ Microbiol.* 68:2576–2579.

Wheeler C, Vogt TM, Armstrong GL, et al. (2005): An outbreak of hepatitis A associated with green onions. *N Engl J Med.* 353:890–897.

Zagory D (1999): Effects of post-procesing handling and packaging on microbial populations. *Postharvest Biol Technol.* 15:313–321.

CHAPTER 13

FOOD SAFETY ISSUES AND THE MICROBIOLOGY OF FRUIT BEVERAGES AND BOTTLED WATER

MICKEY E. PARISH

13.1 INTRODUCTION

A variety of fruit juices, beverages, and bottled waters, with or without added flavors, are currently available on the world market and are increasing in popularity with consumers. Despite their low pH, fruit juices and beverages may have significant problems related to microbial spoilage and safety. Most safety issues involve pathogenic bacteria such as *Salmonella* spp. or *E. coli* O157:H7 in "fresh" unpasteurized juices; however, outbreaks from other bacteria, viruses, and protozoans in a variety of juice products have occurred. Although growth is unlikely at low pH, it is well documented that pathogenic microorganisms may survive in fruit juices and beverages for extended periods and can cause outbreaks of foodborne illnesses. Serious disease outbreaks from low-acid fruit and vegetable juices have also occurred. Similarly, pathogens may survive in water for extended periods, although disease outbreaks from bottled water have been less frequent.

Non-safety-related spoilage of fruit juices and beverages is due to growth of fermentative yeasts, aciduric/acidophilic bacteria, and/or filamentous fungi. Such growth usually results in deleterious effects on the sensory quality of the beverage. Microbiological standards, antimicrobial treatments, and regulatory oversight contribute to the safety of these products.

13.2 NORMAL MICROFLORA

Beverage manufacturers monitor the microbial populations in their products as an indicator of possible safety and spoilage issues. Since microorganisms are widespread in nature, it should not be surprising that beverages such as juices, juice drinks, and

Microbiologically Safe Foods, Edited by Norma Heredia, Irene Wesley, and Santos García

TABLE 1 Genera of Microorganisms Isolated from Raw Citrus Juices

Alicyclobacillus	Enterobacter	Leuconostoc	Salmonella
Alternaria	Erwinia	Metschnikowia	Schwanniomyces
Aspergillus	Escherichia	Monilia	Serratia
Aureobasidium	Fusarium	Mrakia	Sporobolomyces
Bacillus	Geotrichum	Mucor	Streptococcus
Brettanomyces	Gluconobacter	Penicillium	Torulaspora
Byssochlamys	Hanseniaspora	Pichia	Torulopsis
Candida	Hansenula	Proteus	Trichoderma
Citrobacter	Klebsiella	Rhizopus	Trichosporon
Cladosporium	Kloekera	Rhodotorula	Xanthomonas
Cryptococcus	Lactobacillus	Saccharomyces	Zygosaccharomyces

water contain a large variety of microorganisms prior to processing and packaging. Juice may become contaminated by using fruit that is on the ground in contact with soil, water, sewage, or manure that harbor pathogens (Beuchat et al., 2006). For example, Table 1 shows representative genera of microorganisms isolated from raw citrus juices. It would be expected that unpasteurized juices from other fruits would also contain a large and diverse microflora. Many of the microorganisms in raw juices are benign and represent no spoilage or public health problems; however, other genera are known vectors of safety and spoilage concerns. Sources of these organisms can include the raw fruits used for juice production, contaminated processing equipment, untreated water, and human and animal contact, among others. A similar situation exists for water prior to bottling. Bottled water may contain microorganisms, although the population size and diversity will probably be considerably smaller than for fruit juices and juice-based beverages. Table 2 shows genera of microorganisms isolated from bottled water by other researchers.

TABLE 2 Genera of Microorganisms Isolated from Bottled Water

Achromobacter	Cytophaga	Ochrobactrum
Acinetobacter	Enterobacter	Pasteurella
Actinomyces	Enterococcus	Providencia
Aeromonas	Flavobacterium	Pseudomonas
Alcaligenes	Flexibacter	Serratia
Arthrobacter	Gluconacetobacter	Sphaerotilus
Bacillus	Klebsiella	Staphylococcus
Bordetella	Leptothrix	Stenotrophomonas
Caulobacter	Micrococcus	Streptococcus
Chromobacterium	Moraxella	Vibrio
Corynebacterium	Mycobacterium	Xanthomonas
Citrobacter	Nocardia	Yersinia

Source: Edberg et al. (1997), Moore et al. (2002), Venieri et al. (2006), Warburton (1993).

After being properly processed and bottled under sanitary conditions, few microorganisms should exist in the finished juice or water product. If a kill step such as pasteurization is employed, all vegetative microbial cells should be eliminated from the juice, beverage, or water. Spores of heat-resistant bacteria might remain viable in these products, although the vast majority of these will not outgrow under low-pH conditions. If a kill step is not employed, sanitation along with good manufacturing practices should reduce the microbial populations to very low levels. In low-acid pasteurized juices, refrigeration is critical to prevent germination and outgrowth of bacterial spores.

The normal microflora of bottled water varies depending on the water source, type of water treatment, handling protocols, and sanitation practices. Numerous species of microorganisms have been isolated from bottled water (Edbrg et al., 1997; Venieri et al., 2006; Warburton, 1993). Concerns about pathogens in bottled water have been expressed, although documented outbreaks have been few in number (Kramer et al., 1996; Tamagnini and Gonzalez, 1997; Warburton, 2000).

13.3 SPOILAGE

Fruit juices generally contain large concentrations of nutrients, making them microbiologically unstable. Spoilage occurs in juices when microorganisms utilize these nutrients to produce metabolic end products at concentrations that cause detrimental sensory characteristics.

Due to antimicrobial activity associated with the low-pH conditions of most fruit juices, spoilage is caused only by acid-tolerant microorganisms such as fermentative yeasts or lactic acid bacteria. These organisms are generally ubiquitous and will quickly cause spoilage in a nonpasteurized product or in pasteurized juice contaminated after heat treatment. In addition to inherent low pH, factors such as heat pasteurization and low-temperature storage have traditionally been used to extend juice shelf life, making fruit juice marketing commercially feasible. Despite advances in processing technologies, certain yeasts, molds, and bacteria may survive low-pH, processing, and storage conditions to cause spoilage problems in fruit juice products. The onset of spoilage depends on fruit quality, holding and handling conditions, grading, processing conditions, cleaning/sanitation efficiency, and temperature of product storage.

Fungi are naturally occurring contaminants of raw fruit and cause important microbiological spoilage problems in fruit juices. Yeast spoilage of fruit juice products is caused by many species, which may include *Brettanomyces, Kloeckera, Saccharomyces, Schizosaccharomyces, Torulopsis,* and *Zygosaccharomyces* as well as others (Murdock, 1977; Patrick and Hill, 1959; Splittstoesser, 1982). Perhaps the most common yeast spoilage is due to alcoholic fermentation by species of *Saccharomyces*. This spoilage is characterized by production of CO_2, various alcohols, and fermented aroma in conjunction with a decrease in sugar content. Other fermentative and nonfermentative yeasts may occasionally cause biodeterioration of fruit juices; however, changes in juice constituents due to growth of these yeasts are not as well characterized as for *S. cerevisiae*.

Yeasts are common spoilage agents in processed citrus juice products. Total microflora in concentrated citrus juice varies widely from one processor to another and can range from less than 100 to 10,000 or more CFU/mL (in reconstituted juice), of which up to 50% may be yeasts. Yeasts are not resistant to typical thermal processing regimes used by juice processors and when found in the finished product, are probably post-pasteurization contaminants. Molds have only infrequently been associated with juice spoilage, due to their aerobic nature and slow growth rates relative to yeasts and bacteria; however, certain types of juice packaging that extend the refrigerated shelf life have resulted in more favorable conditions for growth of filamentous fungi (Narciso and Parish, 1997, 2000). Molds that occasionally cause spoilage of fruit juice products include species of *Acremonium, Alternaria, Aspergillus, Aureobasidium, Botrytis, Byssochlamys, Cladosporium, Eupenicillium, Fonseceae, Fusarium, Geotrichum, Humicola, Monilia, Mucor, Neosartorya, Penicillium, Rhizopus*, and *Talaromyces*. Mold spoilage is poorly characterized but can include visual observation of fungal mycelia, off-flavors, and discoloration. Cloud destruction in citrus juice due to production of extracellular pectic enzymes by molds may also occur.

The mode of entry by which a mold becomes established in a juice is either post-pasteurization contamination or survival of the heat treatment. Molds that produce structures resistant to thermal time/temperature relationships in fruit juice processing are of particular concern from a spoilage standpoint and include: *Byssochlamys fulva, B. nivea, Eupenicillium brefeldianum, Neosartoya fischeri*, and *Talaromyces flavus*.

Juices packaged in cartons containing paperboard are at risk of contamination and spoilage by filamentous fungi harbored in the paper fibers. Many species of molds have been isolated from the paperboard fibers in gable-top carton material and have been linked to spoilage of fruit juices and juice beverages (Narciso and Parish, 1977, 2000).

Growth of filamentous fungi in fruit juice may also result in production of mycotoxins, chemical compounds that cause toxic symptoms when ingested by people or animals. Patulin, a widespread mycotoxin produced by species of *Penicillium, Aspergillus*, and *Byssochlamys*, has been reported in juices of apple, grape, blueberry, red raspberry, and boysenberry. A maximum limit of 50 ppb patulin in apple juice has been set in the United States and other countries.

Lactic acid bacteria (LAB) is a group of microorganisms composed mainly of the genera *Lactobacillus, Lactococcus, Leuconostoc, Pediococcus, Sporolactobacillus*, and *Weisella*; however, individual species of *Bacillus, Bifidobacterium, Brochothrix, Microbacterium, Micrococcus, Propionibacterium*, and *Ruminococcus* may also produce lactic acid as a major metabolic end product. Major spoilage products formed during growth of LAB include carbon dioxide, diacetyl, ethanol, and lactic acid. Although easily controlled by proper sanitation and pasteurization, lactic acid bacteria of the genera *Lactobacillus, Leuconostoc*, and *Weisella* sometimes spoil citrus juices, especially during warm weather (Murdock, 1977; Patrick and Hill, 1959). Biodeterioration of citrus juices by these bacteria is denoted primarily by production of organoleptically detectable quantities of diacetyl, which imparts a "buttery" or "buttermilk-like" flavor to juice. Occasionally fruit juices may undergo spoilage by acetic acid bacteria, including species of *Acetobacter* or *Gluconobacter*, both of which produce a "vinegary" acetic aroma.

Most spore-forming bacteria, such as species of *Bacillus*, are not capable of growth at pH levels common to fruit juices (<4.3) and will not cause spoilage. In recent years, spore-forming thermoacidophilic rod-shaped bacteria of the genus *Alicyclobacillus* have been implicated in several spoilage outbreaks of shelf-stable fruit juices stored at room temperature. These organisms require warm temperatures for growth (at least room temperature) and prefer growth at low pH. They can be controlled by product refrigeration; however, juices for markets where refrigeration is not common may be susceptible to this organism. Research indicates that alicyclobacilli strains are widespread in nature and may be associated with condensate water usage in citrus-processing plants (Parish, 2005; Wisse and Parish, 1998).

Bottled water typically has few spoilage problems, although microbial growth from residual nutrients in bottled water has been shown to occur. When fruit flavors, juice, sugar, or other ingredients are added, spoilage may result (Moore et al., 2002).

13.4 PATHOGENS

Until recent years, it was widely accepted that most low-pH, high-acid fruit juices were of minimal concern for food poisoning outbreaks, due to the presence of organic acids such as citric or malic acid. However, juice-related outbreaks from *Salmonella, E. coli* O157:H7, and *Cryptosporidium parvum* increased in frequency during the 1990s and were often traced to unpasteurized juices (Parish, 1997; Vojdani et al., 2008). When coupled with previous reports of outbreaks, these events provide a significant challenge to juice processors, government regulators, and the consuming public.

Table 3 lists documented disease outbreaks from consumption of various juices. Paquet (1923) described an outbreak of typhoid fever from consumption of unpasteurized apple juice. This indicates that the connection of fruit juices with foodborne disease has been known at least since the early twentieth century. The 1944 outbreak from orange juice produced 18 cases of typhoid fever and one death (Duncan et al., 1946). An asymptomatic restaurant worker who prepared orange juice at the hotel was implicated in the outbreak, as was the case in the 1989 typhoid fever outbreak from reconstituted orange juice (Birkhead et al., 1993). The 1974 salmonellosis outbreak from apple cider (fresh-pressed, nonpasteurized apple juice) is of interest since the use of animal manure as fertilizer was indicated as a possible source of the pathogen (CDC, 1975). Manure is suspected to be the primary source of contamination in at least two other outbreaks (Mazzotta, 2001; Millard et al., 1994).

Although *E. coli* O157:H7 was not described as a human pathogen until 1982, it is probable that the 1980 outbreak of diarrhea and hemolytic uremic syndrome (HUS) from apple cider was caused by this organism (Steele et al., 1982). A report of the 1991 HUS outbreak indicated that *E. coli* O157:H7 survived 20 days at refrigerated temperature when inoculated into apple cider (Besser et al., 1993). These

TABLE 3 Documented Disease Outbreaks from Consumption of Fruit Juices

Year	Disease Vehicle	Causative Microorganism	Reference
1922	Apple juice	*Salmonella* Typhimurium	Paquet, 1923
1944	Orange juice	*S.* Typhimurium	Duncan et al., 1946
1962	Orange juice	Hepatitis	Eisenstein et al., 1963
1974	Apple juice	*S.* Typhimurium	CDC, 1975
1980	Apple juice	Enterotoxigenic *E. coli*	Steele et al., 1982
1989	Orange juice	*S.* Typhimurium	Birkhead et al., 1993
1991	Coconut milk	*Vibrio cholerae*	CDC, 1991
	Apple juice	*E. coli* O157:H7	Besser et al., 1993
1992	Orange juice	Enterotoxigenic *E. coli*	Singh et al., 1996
1993	Apple juice	*Cryptosporidium*	Millard et al., 1994
	Orange juice	Unknown agent, yeast fermentation suspected	Millard et al., 1994
	Watermelon juice	*Salmonella* spp.	USFDA, 1999
1994	Orange juice	Unknown agent, yeast fermentation suspected	USFDA, 1999
1995	Orange juice	*Salmonella* Hartford, Gaminara, and Rubislaw	Cook et al., 1998
1996	Apple juice	*E. coli* O157:H7	CDC, 1996
	Apple juice	*E. coli* O157:H7	CDC, 1997
	Apple juice	*E. coli* O157:H7	USFDA, 1998
	Apple juice	*Cryptosporidium parvum*	CDC, 1997
	Orange juice	Unknown agent	USFDA, 1998
1999	Orange juice	*Salmonella* Typhimurium phage type 135A	ANZFA, 1999
	Orange juice	*Salmonella* Muenchen	CDC, 1999
	Orange juice	*Salmonella* Anatum	Krause et al., 2001
	Apple juice	*E. coli* O157:H7	Winslow, 1999
	Mamey puree	*Salmonella* Typhimurium	USFDA, 1999
2000	Orange juice	*Salmonella* Enteritidis	Keville, 2000
2002	Apple juice	Unknown agent	Vojdani et al., 2008
2003	Apple juice	*Cryptosporidium parvum*	Vojdani et al., 2008
	Apple juice	Unknown agent	Vojdani et al., 2008
2004	Apple cider	*Cryptosporidium parvum*, *E. coli* O111	Coronado et al., 2005
2005	Orange juice	*Salmonella* Saintpaul and Typhimurium	Vojdani et al., 2008
	Mixed fruit juice	Unknown agent	Vojdani et al., 2008
2006	Carrot juice	*Clostridium botulinum*	CDC, 2006

data confirmed previous observations that pathogens can survive in acidic products long enough to transmit disease (Mossel and de Bruin, 1960). In addition to bacterial diseases, viruses and yeast may also be transmitted via fruit juices. Hepatitis A virus was transmitted through consumption of contaminated orange juice in the 1960s (Eisenstein et al., 1963). A 2005 outbreak in an Illinois middle school resulted in

TABLE 4 Microbial Populations in Bottled Nonpasteurized Orange Juice from the Citrus-Processing Plant Implicated in the 1995 Salmonellosis Outbreak in Florida

Juice-Processing Date[a]	Aciduric Count (CFU/mL)	*E. coli* (MPN/mL)	*Salmonella* Detection
July 13	100,000,000	15	None
July 15	42,000,000	>110	*S.* Gaminara
July 27	2,400,000	>110	*S.* Rubislaw
July 31	380,000	>110	None
August 3	2,200,000	>110	None
September 12	16,000	None	None

[a]Samples in July and August represent commercially bottled juice. September 12 was a test run preceded by thorough cleaning and sanitation.

21 cases from an unknown agent and incriminated a mixed fruit juice. A high level of yeast was cultured from the multifruit juice and fruit cups involved in a later outbreak (Vojdani et al., 2008). Yeast fermentation of juices was also implicated in causing emetic responses of schoolchildren in Ohio (1993) and Alabama (1994).

The 1995 salmonellosis outbreak from unpasteurized Florida orange juice represents the first documented outbreak in which a citrus-processing facility was implicated (Parish, 1998a). Salmonellae were isolated from various samples, including unopened bottles of orange juice, unwashed fruit surfaces, and amphibians found in close proximity to the processing facility. The concurrent isolation of *Salmonella* serovars from the patients, the juice, and the processing environment, along with epidemiological data, established a probable link between the processing facility and the outbreak. Data in Table 4 show results of microbiological testing of orange juice processed before commercial production ceased in August 1995 and during a September test run in which the plant was thoroughly cleaned and sanitized. These data clearly indicate the important role of proper cleaning and sanitation in controlling the potential for juice contamination at a processing facility.

Other *Salmonella* outbreaks from unpasteurized orange juice occurred in 1999, 2000, and 2005. One outbreak was traced to unpasteurized juice transported by tanker truck from Mexico to Arizona (CDC, 1999). This outbreak caused one death. In 2005, unpasteurized orange juice was the vehicle of transmission in an outbreak in 23 states reporting 152 cases of salmonellosis. The juice was traced back to the producer, which was found in noncompliance with the plant's HACCP plan (Jain et al., 2006).

Cases of diarrhea and HUS from *E. coli* O157:H7 in apple cider were reported in the western United States and Canada during the fall of 1996 (CDC, 1996, 1997). The majority of those cases involved production of nonpasteurized apple juice and juice blends at a large processing facility in California. The death of a 16-month-old Colorado child due to HUS was reported. Apples implicated in the disease were mostly from a juice production date late in the harvest season and were of minimal quality by company standards. Extensive grading was necessary to remove unacceptable fruit before milling and pressing. *E. coli* O111– and *Cryptosporidium parvum*–contaminated apple juice was involved in an outbreak in New York in which 213 cases were reported. Contamination was traced to fresh-pressed untreated apple cider (Coronado et al., 2005).

In 2006, *Clostridium botulinum* toxin type A was involved in a four-case disease outbreak from carrot juice. Since carrot juice is not a high-acid product, the juice probably received thermal abuse by remaining nonrefrigerated for an extended period of time, allowing growth of the pathogen and toxin production.

Microbiological surveys of bottled water have detected bacterial endotoxins, *Alkaligenes fecalis*, *Corynebacterium*, *E. coli*, *Pseudomonas* spp., *Streptococcus fecalis*, *Staphylococcus*, and a host of fungi (Raj, 2005; Reyes et al., 2008; Ribeiro et al., 2006; Zamberlan et al., 2008). Bottled water has occasionally been involved in disease outbreaks, including cholera, typhoid fever, and "travelers' diarrhea" (Warburton, 1993); however, there have been fewer outbreaks from bottled water than from fruit juices. Outbreaks involving bottled water have been traced to *Salmonella* in infants in Spain and to *Pseudomonas aeruginosa* in an intensive care unit in Germany (Eckmanns et al., 2008; Palmera-Suárez et al., 2007) as well as non-01 *Vibrio cholerae* from commercially bottled water in the Northern Mariana Islands, a U.S. territory, in 1994.

13.5 MAINTAINING PRODUCT QUALITY AND REDUCING MICROBIAL NUMBERS

Pasteurization procedures as currently practiced for acid foods adequately control pathogens and most spoilage microorganisms in fruit juices. Temperatures used for thermal processing of juices range from 65°C for lemon and lime to as high as 99°C for orange or grapefruit juices. It should be noted that primary pasteurization conditions for orange and grapefruit juices are designed to inactivate the enzyme pectinmethylesterase and are much higher than necessary to destroy all common safety and spoilage organisms except *Alicyclobacillus*. The thermal sensitivity of important spoilage microbes in fruit juices varies depending on the type of cell (vegetative, bacterial spore, conidia, ascospore), pH, solids content, and water activity of the suspension medium.

Nonthermal and minimal processing methods for inactivating microorganisms in fruit juices have been an active area of research since the late 1980s when reports that juices could be stabilized by high-pressure treatment were published (Buzrul et al., 2008; Ogawa et al., 1989). Since then, high-pressure treatment has been shown to produce juices of superior flavor quality to thermally pasteurized juices (Parish, 1998b; Zook et al., 1999). Other "nonthermal" research areas for fruit juices include high pressure plus CO_2, pulsed electric field, and irradiation. Another nonthermal technique is the use of ultraviolet (UV) light to treat fresh-pressed apple juice. This technology is widely accepted in the United States and was approved for use by the U.S. FDA under 21 CFR 179.39 (Worobo, 1998). This technology provides the desired 5-log reduction in pathogens and is sufficiently portable and inexpensive for use by small apple processors.

Some processors use a minimal thermal pasteurization regime to give a theoretical 99.999% reduction of any possible pathogens in juice so that they can comply with the FDA juice HACCP (hazard analysis of critical control points) regulation. The time–temperature relationship for flash pasteurization will change depending on the type of juice, pH, and target microorganism; however, published research indicates that 71.1°C for 3 s will produce at least a 5-log reduction of *Salmonella* and *E. coli* O157:H7 in certain fruit juices (Mazzotta, 2001). FDA suggests that 6 s is needed at this temperature to provide a 5-log reduction in *Cryptosporidium*.

Antimicrobial activities related to organic acids are well known; however, effects of acids on microbial viability vary with acid concentration, buffering capacity of the food system, type and physiological state of the microorganism, and time of exposure. These acids are commonly found in fruit juices and fermented foods, or they may be added to low-acid foods as preservatives. Organic acids are generally microbiostatic in nature but may, on occasion, exhibit microbicidal characteristics. Yeasts and molds are less affected by organic acids than the bacteria.

Although organic acids exhibit bacteriostatic or bacteriocidal activity, some species of *Enterococcus, Escherichia, Listeria*, *Salmonella*, and *Streptococcus* can adapt to acid conditions for survival. This acid tolerance response is activated under sublethal pH conditions and may account for long-term survival of these organisms at pH levels common to fruit juices. If contamination of the juice occurs, certain pathogens, such as *E. coli* O157:H7 and *Salmonella*, may survive long enough to cause disease outbreaks upon consumption of the juice.

Bottled water may be treated in various manners to reduce the risk of disease outbreaks. In the United States, treatment by distillation, ion exchange, filtration, ultraviolet light, reverse osmosis, carbonation, pasteurization, or other procedures are allowed and must be conducted in a manner that effectively eliminates pathogens from the water.

13.6 U.S. REGULATIONS

As of January 2002, the U.S. Food and Drug Administration (FDA) implemented a rule to regulate all juices produced or consumed in the United States. The Juice HACCP Rule (21 CFR 120) requires all juice-processing facilities in the United States to employ an HACCP plan and to ensure that juices are processed in a manner that results in a theoretical 5-log (99.999%) reduction in the population of certain pathogenic microorganisms (USFDA-CFSAN, 2003a). In addition to the 5-log performance standard, FDA has indicated that processors of apple juice should consider setting a maximum standard of 50 ppb for the mycotoxin, patulin.

According to the juice HACCP rule, juice manufacturers must also fully employ current good manufacturing practices (cGMPs) as described in 21 CFR 110 (USFDA-CFSAN, 2003c) and must follow written procedures for eight specific sanitation standard operating procedures (SSOPs), including water safety, food contact surfaces, cross-contamination, hand washing and toilet facilities, protection from contamination, toxic compounds, employee health, and pest control. The HACCP rule is currently effective for most juice processors in the United States. The regulation also applies to juice imported into the United States Imported juices, whether imported in bulk or in the finished package, must be produced using HACCP or an equivalent system recognized by the FDA as yielding products that are safe for consumption.

Subpart B of the juice HACCP regulation sets the 5-log performance standard for all juices. Manufacturers of unpasteurized citrus juices may apply the 5-log performance standard to fruit surface treatments since the juice extraction process allows only minimal contact between the fruit surface and extracted juice. Manufacturers of fresh squeezed, unpasteurized citrus juices must conduct regular microbiological testing on 20-mL Juice samples to demonstrate that the juice is free of biotype I *E. coli*. If *E. coli* is detected in two of seven sequential samples, the HACCP plan is considered inadequate and must be reviewed and reverified. In the state of Florida, retail juice operations that are not covered by the federal FDA rule are covered by a state regulation, FDOC 20-49. This mandates HACCP and requires end-product testing similar to the federal rule.

In 1998 the FDA implemented a labeling rule [21 CFR 101.17(g)] for juices that do not receive a treatment that will reduce pathogens by 99.999%, specifically unpasteurized, freshly extracted juices such as apple cider and fresh-squeezed orange juice (USFDA-CFSAN, 2002). This rule requires that the following warning label appear on juices that are subject to the regulation:

> WARNING: This product has not been pasteurized and therefore may contain harmful bacteria that can cause serious illness in children, the elderly, and persons with weakened immune systems.

Very small juice processors not covered by 21 CFR 120 must use the warning label if they do not meet the 5-log performance standard. The decline in the number of reported juice-associated outbreaks prior to and after implementation of HACCP has been documented (Vojdani et al., 2008), although it should be noted that correlation does not necessarily reflect causality and that outbreaks from facilities with HACCP plans have occurred.

The International Bottled Water Association estimates that 5 billion gallons of bottled water were consumed in North America in 2001 (Reyes et al., 2008). Bottled water is regulated in the United States by the FDA under 21 CFR 129 and 21 CFR 165 (USFDA-CFSAN, 2003b,d). Part 129 describes sanitation and process controls and requires weekly microbiological testing on the product. Part 165 sets standards for microbiological testing by most probable number (MPN) and membrane filter methods. For most probable number tests, no more than one analytical unit in a 10-unit sample can have 2.2 or more coliform organisms per 100 mL, and no analytical unit can have an MPN of 9.2 or more coliform organisms per 100 mL. For the membrane filter test, not more than one of the analytical units in the sample can have 4.0 or more coliform organisms per 100 mL, and the arithmetic mean of the coliform density of the sample cannot exceed one coliform organism per 100 mL.

13.6.1 Acknowledgments

Production of this manuscript was supported by the University of Maryland, College of Agriculture and Natural Resources, Department of Nutrition and Food Science and by the Florida Agricultural Experiment Station.

REFERENCES

ANZFA (Australia New Zealand Food Authority) (1999): Media release: Foodborne illness in Australia—How bad is it? What are the solutions? Tuesday, May 25.

Besser R, Lett S, Weber J, et al. (1993): An outbreak of diarrhea and hemolytic uremic syndrome from *Escherichia coli* O157:H7 in fresh-pressed apple cider. *JAMA*. 269:2217–2220.

Beuchat LR (2006): Vectors and conditions for preharvest contamination of fruits and vegetables with pathogens capable of causing enteric diseases. *Br Food J*. 108:38–53.

Birkhead GS, Morse D, Levine W, et al. (1993): Typhoid fever at a resort hotel in New York: a large outbreak with an unusual vehicle. *J Infect Dis*. 167:1228–1232.

Buzrul S, Alpas H, Largeteau A, Demazeau G (2008): Inactivation of *Escherichia coli* and *Listeria innocua* in kiwifruit and pineapple juices by high hydrostatic pressure. *Int J Food Microbiol*. April 1. E-pub ahead of print.

CDC (Centers for Disease Control and Prevention) (1975): *Salmonella typhimurium* outbreak traced to a commercial apple cider—New Jersey. *MMWR Morb Mortal Wkly Rep*. 24:87.

——— (1991): Cholera associated with imported frozen coconut milk—Maryland. *MMWR Morb Mortal Wkly Rep*. 40:844–843.

——— (1996): Outbreak of *Escherichia coli* O157:H7 infections associated with drinking unpasteurized commercial apple juice—British Columbia, California, Colorado, and Washington, October 1996. *MMWR Morb Mortal Wkly Rep*. 45:975.

——— (1997): Outbreaks of *Escherichia coli* O157:H7 infection and cryptosporidiosis associated with drinking unpasteurized apple juice—Connecticut and New York, October 1996. *MMWR Morb Mortal Wkly Rep*. 46:4–8.

——— (1999): Outbreak of *Salmonella* serotype Muenchen infections associated with unpasteurized orange juice—United States and Canada, June 1999. *MMWR Morb Mortal Wkly Rep*. 48:582–585.

——— (2006): Botulism associated with commercial carrot juice—Georgia and Florida, September 2006. *MMWR Morb Mortal Wkly Rep* 55 (Dispatch):1–2.

Cook K, Dobbs T, Hlady W, et al. (1998): Outbreak of *Salmonella* serotype Hartford infections associated with unpasteurized orange juice. *JAMA*. 280:1504–1509.

Coronado F, Johnson G, Kacica M, et al. (2005): A large outbreak of cryptosporidiosis and *Escherichia coli* O111 infections associated with consumption of unpasteurized apple cider—New York, 2004. In *Abstracts of the 54th Annual Epidemic Intelligence Service Conference*, Atlanta, GA, p. 37.

Duncan TG, Coull J, Miller E, Bancroft H (1946): Outbreak of typhoid fever with orange juice as the vehicle illustrating the value of immunization. *Am J Public Health*. 36:34–36.

Eckmanns T, Oppert M, Martin M, et al. (2008): An outbreak of hospital-acquired *Pseudomonas aeruginosa* infection caused by contaminated bottled water in intensive care units. *Clin Microbiol Infect*. 114:454–458.

Edberg S, Kops S, Kontnick C, Escarzaga M (1997): Analysis of cytotoxicity and invasiveness of heterotrophic plate count bacteria (HPC) isolated from drinking water on blood media. *J Appl Microbiol*. 82:455–461.

Eisenstein AB, Aach R, Jacobsohn W, Goldman A (1963): An epidemic of infectious hepatitis in a general hospital. *JAMA*. 185:171–174.

Jain S, Bidol S, Lockett J, et al. (2006): Final trip report: multistate outbreak of *Salmonella* Typhimurium infections associated with inadequately treated orange juice—United States, 2005. In *Abstracts of the 55th Epidemic Intelligence Service Conference*, Atlanta, GA, p. 38.

Keville E (2000): FDA letter. http://www.fda.gov/foi/warning_letters/archive/m4161n.pdf. Accessed May 2008.

Kramer MH, Herwaldt BL, Craun GF, Calderon RL, Juranek DD (1996): Surveillance for waterborne-disease outbreaks—United States, 1993–1994. *MMWR Morb Mortal Wkly Rep*. 45 (SS-1):1–31.

Krause G, Terzagian R, Hammond R (2001): Outbreak of *Salmonella* serotype Anatum infection associated with unpasteurized orange juice. *South Med J*. 94:1168–1172.

Mazzotta A (2001): Thermal inactivation of stationary-phase and acid-adapted *Escherichia coli* O157:H7, *Salmonella* and *Listeria monocytogenes* in fruit juices. *J Food Prot*. 64:315–320.

Millard PS, Gensheimer K, Addiss D (1994): An outbreak of cryptosporidiosis from fresh-pressed apple cider. *JAMA*. 272:1592.

Moore J, Xu J, Heaney N, Millar B (2002): Spoilage of fruit-flavoured bottled water by *Gluconacetobacter sacchari*. *Food Microbiol*. 19:399–401.

Mossel DAA, de Bruin AS (1960): The survival of Enterobacteriaceae in acid liquid foods stored at different temperatures. *Ann Inst Pasteur Lille*. 11:65–72.

Murdock DI (1977): Microbiology of citrus products. In: Nagy S, Shaw PE, Veldhuis MK (Eds.). *Citrus Science and Technology*, Vol. 2. AVI Publishing, Westport CT, pp. 445–481.

Narciso JA, Parish M (1997): Endogenous mycoflora of gable-top carton paperboard. *J Food Sci*. 62:1223–1239.

——— (2000): Relationship of molds in paperboard packaging to food spoilage. *Dairy Food Environ San*. 20:944–951.

Ogawa H, Fukuhisa K, Fukumoto H, Hori K, Hayashi R (1989): Effect of hydrostatic pressure on sterilization and preservation of freshly-squeezed, non-pasteurized citrus juice. *Nippon Nōgeikagaku Kaishi*. 63:1109–1114.

Palmera-Suárez R, Garcia P, Garcia A, Barrasa A, Herrera D (2007): *Salmonella* Kottbus outbreak in infants in Gran Canaria (Spain), caused by bottled water, August–November 2006. *Eur Surveill*.12:3235.

Paquet P (1923): Épidémie de fièvre typhoïde: déterminé par la consommation de petit cidre. *Rev Hyg*. 45:165–169.

Parish ME (1997): Public health and non-pasteurized fruit juices. *Crit Rev Microbiol*. 23:109–119.

——— (1998a): Coliforms, *E. coli* and *Salmonella* associated with a citrus processing facility implicated in a salmonellosis outbreak. *J Food Prot*. 61:280–284.

——— (1998b): Orange juice quality after treatment by thermal pasteurization or isostatic high pressure. *Lebens Wissen Technol*. 31:439–442.

———(2005): Spoilage of juices and beverages by *Alicyclobacillus* species. In: Sapers G, Yousef A, Gorny J (Eds.). *Microbiology of Fruits and Vegetables*. CRC Press, Boca Raton FL, pp. 159–186.

Patrick R, Hill E (1959): Microbiology of citrus fruit processing. *Agric Exp Sta Bull.* 618:62.

Raj SD (2005): Bottled water: How safe is it? *Water Environ Res*. 77:3013–3018.

Reyes MI, Perez CM, Negron EL (2008): Microbiological assessment of house and imported bottled water by comparison of bacterial endotoxin concentration, heterotrophic plate count, and fecal coliform count. *Puerto Rico Health Sci J*. 27:21–26.

Ribeiro A, Machado AP, Kozakiewicz Z, et al. (2006): Fungi in bottled water: a case study of a production plant. *Rev Iberoam Micol*. 23:139–144.

Singh B, Kulshreshtha S, Kapoor K (1996): An orange juice–borne outbreak due to enterotoxigenic *Escherichia coli*. *J Food Sci Technol India*. 32:504–506.

Splittstoesser DF (1982): Microorganisms involved in the spoilage of fermented fruit juices. *J Food Prot*. 45:874–877.

Steele BT, Murphy N, Rance C (1982): An outbreak of hemolytic uremic syndrome associated with ingestion of fresh apple juice. *J Pediatr*. 101:963–966.

Tamagnini L, Gonzalez R (1997): Bacteriological stability and growth kinetics of *Pseudomonas aeruginosa* in bottled water. *J Appl Microbiol*. 83:91–94.

USFDA (U.S. Food and Drug Administration) (1998): Hazard Analysis and Critical Control Point (HACCP), Procedures for the Safe and Sanitary Processing and Importing of Juice; Food Labeling: Warning Notice Statements; Labeling of Juice Products; Proposed Rules. *Fed Reg*. 63:20450–20451.

———(1999): Enforcement Report, April 21. http://www.fda.gov/bbs/topics/ENFORCE/ENF00586.html. Accessed May 2008.

USFDA-CFSAN (U.S. Food and Drug Administration–Center for Food Safety and Applied Nutrition) (2002): Exemptions from the Warning Label Requirement for Juice—Recommendations for Effectively Achieving a 5-Log Pathogen Reduction. http://www.cfsan.fda.gov/~dms/juicgui6.html. Accessed May 2008.

———(2003a): 21 CFR 120, Hazard analysis and critical control point (HACCP) systems. http://www.cfsan.fda.gov/~lrd/fcf120.html. Accessed May 2008.

———(2003b): 21 CFR 129. Processing and bottling of bottled drinking water. http://www.cfsan.fda.gov/~lrd/FCF129.html.

———(2003c): 21 CFR 110, Current good manufacturing practice in manufacturing, packing or holding human food. http://www.cfsan.fda.gov/~lrd/cfr110.html. Accessed May 2008.

———(2003d): 21 CFR 165, Beverages. http://vm.cfsan.fda.gov/~lrd/fcf165.html. Accessed May 2008.

Venieri D, Vantarakis A, Komninou G, Papapetropoulou M (2006): Microbiological evaluation of bottled non-carbonated ("still") water from domestic brands in Greece. *Int J Food Microbiol*. 107 (1):68–72.

Vojdani JD, Beuchat LR, Tauxe RV (2008): Juice-associated outbreaks of human illness in the United States, 1995 through 2005. *J Food Prot*. 71:356–364.

Warburton D (1993):A review of the microbiological quality of bottled water sold in Canada. 2: The need for more stringent standards and regulations. *Can J Microbiol*. 39:158–168.

——— (2000): Methodology for screening bottled water for the presence of indicator and pathogenic bacteria. *Food Microbiol.* 17:3–12.

Winslow L (1999): *E. coli* sickens two more. Tulsa World, October 21.

Wisse CA, Parish M (1998): Isolation and enumeration of thermoacidophilic bacterial spore-formers from citrus processing environments. *Dairy Food Environ San.* 18:504–509.

Worobo R (1998): Apple cider safety, regulations and processing alternatives. *NY Fruit Q.* 6:13–16.

Zamberlan Da Silva ME, Santana RG, Guilhermetti M, et al. (2008): Comparison of the bacteriological quality of tap water and bottled mineral water. *Int J Hyg Environ Health.* January 16. E-pub ahead of print.

Zook CD, Parish M, Braddock R, Balaban M (1999): Isostatic high pressure inactivation kinetics of *Saccharomyces cerevisiae* ascospores in fruit juice and a model juice buffer. *J Food Sci.* 64:533–535.

CHAPTER 14

FOOD SAFETY ISSUES AND THE MICROBIOLOGY OF CANNED AND FROZEN FOODS

NINA G. PARKINSON

14.1 INTRODUCTION

In this chapter we review the history of canned and frozen foods, as well as the principles involved in preserving them. Microbiological safety and spoilage issues are discussed along with the U.S. regulations involved with each type of product.

14.2 HISTORY OF CANNED FOODS

In various parts of the world, there is an abundance of food, and to make it available to everyone throughout the year, we have developed ways to preserve it. In ancient times this involved drying, salting, and fermenting foods. In the past 150 years, we have developed canning procedures, and more recently, freezing procedures to preserve foods. It is vital that the methods used prevent the growth of spoilage and, more important, pathogenic microorganisms. The preservation process also needs to assure that the food retains a palatable appearance, flavor, and texture and its nutritional value.

Typically, preservation accomplishes one or more of the following objectives: killing the microorganisms; inhibiting microbial growth; removing microorganisms; destroying enzymes, and retarding chemical changes.

Our ancestors used procedures that were available to them to accomplish these objectives. Among the most common were drying or salting, which was commonly used to preserve meats or adding sugar to fruits. In both of these, the technical explanation was that they were reducing the water activity. In some cultures, acid was added to vegetables, or foods were treated in a way where acid was produced

Microbiologically Safe Foods, Edited by Norma Heredia, Irene Wesley, and Santos García

and the food subsequently preserved. These techniques are the basics of pickling or fermentation processes, which were used to make sauerkraut, yogurt, and pickled meats. Finally, true fermentations of wine and beer were ways of preserving grapes and grains.

Canning is a science that resulted from the French military offering a reward for anyone who came up with a way that could be used to feed hungry soldiers during the French Revolution and the Napoleonic wars. In 1809, Nicolas Appert, a French confectioner, developed a process for canning foods. After 17 years of studying different approaches, he finally came up with the idea of heating foods in a container and sealing the container. Appert really did not have the scientific explanation for why heat and a good seal were important; he just determined that food did not spoil if he did those two things.

In 1806, the French military used some "canned" foods. However, these were originally produced in glass jars, and there were problems with weight and glass breakage. So in 1820, Peter Durand introduced tin-plated wrought-iron cans. The tin plate kept the iron from rusting. This design was basically a cylinder with both ends soldered onto it, and the top had a small hole through which the food could be added. The hole was then soldered closed. The solder contained about 10% tin and 90% lead. The production of these cans was extremely slow and labor intensive. Later, lead was found to have health consequences, so it has been minimized or eliminated. This was an extremely time-consuming process.

In 1849, Henry Evans developed a machine that made can ends in a single operation, making the manufacture of containers slightly more efficient. During this time there was much concern with the container itself, but nobody was thinking about the difficulties that were being encountered in trying to get the food out of the can for consumption. In 1858 the can opener was finally patented. Until that time, cans were opened with various tools and great difficulty.

During the 1860s, Louis Pasteur did extensive laboratory work to determine why the canning process worked. He determined that microorganisms caused foods to spoil, that heating destroys enzymes and microorganisms found in foods, and that a hermetic seal ensures that no microorganisms or oxygen enter, thereby preserving the food.

Late in the nineteenth century the first automatic can-making machines were introduced, and in 1898 the sanitary can was developed. The sanitary can is the prototype of the modern can. During the first part of the twentieth century there was more emphasis on studying the thermal processes than improving the can and opening mechanisms. In 1906, the National Canners Association [later, the National Food Processors Association (NFPA)] was founded to study canned food processes.

In 1964 the two-piece can, which used more lightweight metal in the containers and no side seam, was introduced. In 1965, tin-free steel cans were developed and became very popular. In the 1990s, lead solder was considered to be a contributing factor to lead in the U.S. diet. Much information was available that lead causes problems to the human brain, and it is believed that lead is leached out of the lead solder in the side seams of cans. Lead was banned for use in the side seam of cans in the United States. However, other countries may still use it.

14.3 CATEGORIES OF CANNED FOODS

Canned foods fall into two categories. The first is *low-acid canned foods* (LACFs), which have a pH above 4.6. These foods must receive a severe thermal process designed to destroy *Clostridium botulinum* spores. The cans are thermally processed at temperatures of 240 to 250°F (116 to 121°C). The type of food and the size of the container determine the exact time and conditions necessary to achieve commercial sterility in the United States. All processes must be approved by the U.S. Food and Drug Administration (FDA). It has been determined that *C. botulinum* spores will not germinate or grow in foods with a pH below pH 4.6, which is considered the dividing line between low-acid and acidified foods. The regulation that covers the production and controls of low-acid canned foods is found in the U.S. *Code of Federal Regulations* (CFR), Title 21, part 113. This is frequently termed "21 CFR 113" (USFDA-CFSAN, 2002a).

The second category of canned foods includes those that have a pH of 4.6 or lower. These are referred to as *acid or acidified foods*. Since we are not concerned with the outgrowth of *C. botulinum* in these foods, they can receive a milder heat treatment, typically referred to as pasteurization. A common practice used in the canning to accomplish this in the food industry is referred to as *hot-fill-hold*. In this practice, acidified foods are filled at an elevated temperature into a can or bottle and the container is sealed. The temperature is maintained for a specific period of time and the container is then cooled. These heat treatments are designed to destroy vegetative cells of spoilage and pathogenic microorganisms. The regulation that covers the production and controls of acidified foods is 21 CFR 114 (USFDA-CFSAN, 2002b).

14.4 SAFETY OF CANNED FOODS

While *C. botulinum* is by far the most dangerous pathogen of concern in low-acid canned foods, strict regulations and controls have minimized these incidents in the United States in the past 50 years. There was an incident of *Staphylococcus* enterotoxin in canned mushrooms from China in 1989 (Anonymous, 1989). In this outbreak, approximately 100 people became ill with typical *Staphylococcus* poisoning symptoms in various parts of the United States after consuming a variety of foods, all containing canned mushrooms. The common food was determined to be cans of mushrooms from China. Several investigations were done and visits made to the cannery in China where the mushrooms were made. They found that the working conditions were extremely poor and that good manufacturing practices (GMPs) were minimal. Personnel practices were also deficient. The employees apparently contaminated the mushrooms with *Staphylococcus aureus*, and the mushrooms were handled in such a way that they were allowed to sit for extended periods of time prior to receiving the thermal process, allowing production of the toxin. When the mushrooms were processed, the *S. aureus* bacteria were destroyed, but since the enterotoxin is very heat stable, it survived the thermal process. The cans and product appeared normal, but the toxin was present, causing the illnesses. Although this was an unusual event, it has made us aware of the importance of GMPs and the heat resistance of this toxin.

Acid or acidified foods have the advantage that pathogens cannot grow at low pHs, but in the past few years we have learned that they can survive under acidic conditions. In the 1990s there were several outbreaks of *Salmonella* spp. in unpasteurized orange juice products and a tragic outbreak of *E. coli* 0157:H7 in unpasteurized apple juice in which several people were sickened and one child died (Bean et al., 1996; Olsen et al., 2000).

14.5 MICROBIAL SPOILAGE OF CANNED FOODS

Although not usually a safety concern, spoilage of canned foods is frequently an economic concern for the canned food industry. Microbial spoilage is usually due to one of the following causes: incipient spoilage, post-process contamination, underprocessing, or thermophilic spoilage. There are nonmicrobial factors that can cause a canned food to deteriorate: product container interaction, enzymatic spoilage/deterioration and rancidity, or color changes from the presence of oxygen (Denny and Parkinson, 2001). Below we discuss the microbiological causes of spoilage of canned foods.

14.5.1 Incipient Spoilage

Incipient spoilage is attributed to microbial growth that occurs if a product is held for an extended period of time between container closing and retorting. The microorganisms reproduce in the can, which may result in adulterated product. These microorganisms may produce acid or gas, which typically results in lack of vacuum and/or a slight off-flavor or off-odor. The microorganisms are usually killed during the thermal process, so there is no additional evidence of spoilage and no viable microorganisms are recovered when the product is subcultured (Denny and Parkinson, 2001).

14.5.2 Post-Process Contamination (Leaker Spoilage)

Leaker spoilage typically occurs during the cooling step after the retort process. It is generally caused by inadequately formed seams, container damage and/or abuse, or contaminated cooling water. This is by far the most common type of spoilage in canned foods (Denny and Parkinson, 2001; USFDA-CFSAN, 2003e).

14.5.3 Underprocessing

Low-acid canned foods must have a specific process that is delivered in a specific manner. If this is not attained, the food may not get adequate heat and microorganisms could survive, including *C. botulinum*. Frequently, this type of spoilage results from (but is not limited to) a heat process not established properly, or the heat process is not applied properly because of mechanical or personnel failure. This type of spoilage is also seen in acid or acidified foods, resulting in the growth of lactic acid bacteria, yeast, and/or mold (Denny and Parkinson, 2001).

14.5.4 Thermophilic Spoilage

Thermophilic spores are very heat resistant, and thermal processes are not designed to destroy them. If present in canned food and under the proper conditions, thermophiles will grow and spoil the food. The recommendations are to take precautions to minimize their presence and opportunities to multiply, including using good-quality ingredients, making sure that hot product is not allowed to stagnate in kettles or in pipes, and that finished product is cooled to below 105°F (41°C) and stored below 95°F (35°C).

Although canned foods have the potential of spoilage, they also have some great advantages, including the fact that canned foods and vegetables have been found to be nutritionally equal to, and sometimes higher than, their fresh and frozen counterparts. The reason for this is that fruits and vegetables are canned within hours of harvest, when nutrient content is at its peak. Canned foods are very convenient, and consumers still appreciate their ease of preparation; they are shelf-stable for extended periods of time (more than 2 years) as long as the container is not damaged; and the fact that preservatives are not used is considered an advantage.

14.6 HISTORY OF FROZEN FOODS

Frozen foods are another group of preserved foods that are gaining popularity in the United States. This method of food preservation started early in the twentieth century when Clarence Birdseye worked near the Arctic and observed fish being frozen after being caught. When thawed and eaten, these fish still had their fresh characteristics. Birdseye organized his own company in 1922 (Birdseye Seafoods, Inc.) and began freezing and selling fish fillets in New York. In 1934 he developed low-temperature display cases for supermarkets. By this time he was freezing meats, fish, oysters, vegetables, and fruit. In 1944, he developed the idea of insulated railroad cars to transport his products around the United States, and the frozen food industry gained in popularity.

In the 1940s new types of frozen products were introduced, including puff pastries, hors d'oeuvres, soups, entrees, French fries, Mexican cuisine, whipped topping, meat pies, seafood, and pizza. In the 1950s the first TV dinner was introduced and the Frozen Food Handling Code was adopted to provide guidelines on the production and handling of frozen foods (FAO/WHO, 1976).

In the 1960s frozen mixed vegetable and main courses became popular, and the microwave oven was introduced, which had a significant effect on the frozen food industry. But it took several years for the ovens to gain acceptance, increasing in popularity only in the 1980s.

In the 1990s the FDA declared that frozen fruit and vegetables have equivalent or superior nutrient profiles to their fresh counterparts. Changes in family structures in the United States, including the emergence of single-parent households and both parents working outside the home, increased the popularity of frozen home meal replacements. The next segment in which frozen foods gained popularity is the food service area.

14.7 PRINCIPLES OF FROZEN FOOD PRESERVATION

When water is frozen (ice), it is no longer available for microorganisms to use; thus, they cannot grow and spoil or decompose the food. The technology of freezing foods quickly has gained in popularity because of the high-quality finished product that is obtained. Plant cells remain virtually intact when quick frozen, whereas slow freezing can cause deterioration of the plant cell and consequently a mushier, deteriorated product. When a food is thawed, the bacteria become active again and begin to grow, and in some cases they grow more rapidly than prior to freezing.

The types of microbiological concerns with frozen foods are that they must be manufactured in a clean environment with strict adherence to good manufacturing practices (FAO/WHO, 1976; USFDA-CFSAN, 2003e). The second concern is of the potential for temperature abuse during manufacture, storage, and more important, when out of the control of the manufacturer during transport, at the retail level, and by the consumer.

14.8 SAFETY AND SPOILAGE OF FROZEN FOODS

With frozen foods, temperature abuse can result in loss of product quality as well as outgrowth of microorganisms. There have been a few incidents of foodborne illnesses attributed to commercially prepared frozen foods in recent years. The following represent typical examples of these incidents.

The first example is a case of *Salmonella* Enteritidis in commercially produced ice cream which occurred during the summer and fall of 1994 (Olsen et al., 2000). Approximately 593 cases were confirmed; an estimated 224,000 cases and no deaths were reported across United States. In this incident, ice cream mixes were prepared with pasteurized milk at one facility and transported to a second facility using tanker trucks. At the second facility the mixes were passed through a receiving system and then transferred to holding tanks. Investigators suspect that the tankers were contaminated with *Salmonella* since they had been used to transport unpasteurized whole eggs prior to transporting the ice cream mix. The condition of the inside of the tankers showed some cracks where the bacteria could have remained after the trucks were cleaned and sanitized.

In 1997, frozen strawberries were contaminated with the hepatitis A virus (Anonymous, 1997). The strawberries were grown and harvested in Mexico and processed in California and sold frozen in individual serving cups to the school lunch program. Approximately 150 cases of children with hepatitis A were reported in Michigan. Poor-quality water and sanitary conditions probably resulted in the contamination, and since the berries did not receive thermal processing, the virus was able to survive in the frozen product.

These incidents emphasize the need to minimize the presence of microorganisms in food preparation. This can be achieved by employing various methods, including using good agricultural practices (GAPs), using clean ingredients (using microbiological specifications, letters of guarantee, etc.), assuring an excellent cleaning and sanitation program in the processing environment, assuring that employee practices are adequate for the operation (including continuing training and education programs), and minimizing environmental contaminants. In plants with HACCP (hazard analysis of critical control points) programs, these are sometimes considered prerequisite (USDA-FSIS, 1996).

14.9 U.S. REGULATIONS

In the United States the Code of Federal Regulations (CFR) lists requirements that must be followed for the various types of foods produced and exported to the United States. One of these regulations, which has gained international acceptance, is 21 CFR 110 (USFDA-CFSAN, 2003), also known as current good manufacturing practices (cGMPs or GMPs). This regulation addresses employee practices, building and equipment, cleaning and sanitation, and temperature control measures, with the objective of preventing adulteration of foods. The Food, Drug and Cosmetic Act of 1936 (Chapter 4) (USFDA-CFSAN, 2003e) defines the term *adulterated* (in part) as follows:

- 402(a)(1)—if it bears or contains poisonous or deleterious substance which may render it injurious to health . . . .
- 402(a)(3)—if it consists in whole or in part of any filthy, putrid, or decomposed substance or if it is otherwise unfit for food.
- 402(a)(4)—if it has been prepared, packed or held under insanitary conditions whereby it may be contaminated with filth, or whereby it may have been rendered injurious to health . . . .

Currently, the HACCP concept has also gained international acceptance in the production of safe foods. This concept is based on the prevention of problems before they occur through having a clear understanding of potential hazards that may threaten a particular food and by applying stringent control measures to prevent them from occurring. The LACF and acidified foods regulations (21 CFR 113 and 21 CFR 114) (USFDA-CFSAN, 2002a,b) employ many of these concepts. In the United States, three segments of the food industry are currently required to have HACCP systems in place (NACMCF, 1977): meat and poultry production facilities (9 CFR 304) (USDA-FSIS, 1996); fish and fishery products (21 CFR 123) (USFDA-CFSAN, 2003b), and the juice industry (21 CFR 120) (USFDA-CFSAN, 2003a). All other products usually employ HACCP programs because it has been found to be an efficient system in controlling food safety hazards.

There are several regulations and guidelines for the production of frozen foods in the United States and internationally, including 21 CFR 135 and 158 (USFDA-CFSAN, 2003c,d) and the International Code of Practice for the Processing and Handling of Quick Frozen Foods (FAO/WHO, 1976).

REFERENCES

Anonymous (1989): Multiple outbreaks of staphylococcal food poisoning caused by canned mushrooms. *MMWR Morb Mortal Wkly Rep*. 38:417–419.

———(1997): Hepatitis A associated with consumption of frozen strawberries—Michigan. *MMWR Morb Mortal Wkly Rep*. 46:288–295.

Bean NH, Goulding JS, Frederick CL, Angulo J (1996): Surveillance for foodborne-disease outbreaks—United States, 1988–1992. *MMWR Morb Mortal Wkly Rep*. 45:1–55.

Denny CB, Parkinson NG (2001): Canned foods: tests for cause of spoilage. In: Downes FP, Ito K (Eds.). *Compendium of Methods for the Microbiological Examination of Foods*, 4th ed. American Public Health Association, Washington, DC, Chap. 61.

FAO/WHO (Food and Agriculture Organization/World Health Organization) (1976): Recommended international code of practice for the processing and handling of quick frozen foods. CAC/RCP 8. http://www.codexalimentarius.net/download/standards/285/CXP_008e.pdf. Accessed May 2008.

NACMCF (National Advisory Committee on Microbiological Criteria for Foods) (1977): Hazard analysis and critical control points: principles and application guidelines. Adopted August 14, 1997. http://www.cfsan.fda.gov/~comm/nacmcfp.html. Accessed May 2008.

Olsen SJ, MacKinon LC, Goulding JS, Bean NH, Slutsker L (2000): Surveillance for foodborne disease outbreaks—United States, 1993–1997. *MMWR Morb Mortal Wkly Rep*. 49:1–51.

USDA-FSIS (U.S. Department of Agriculture–Food Safety and Inspection Service) (1996): 9 CFR 304 (et al.) Pathogen reduction; hazard analysis and critical control point (HACCO) systems; final rule. http://www.fsis.usda.gov/OPPDE/rdad/FRPubs/93-016F.pdf. Accessed May 2008.

USFDA (U.S. Food and Drug Administration) (2003): Federal Food, Drug, and Cosmetic Act, Chapter IV. http://www.fda.gov/opacom/laws/fdcact/fdcact4.htm. Accessed May 2008.

USFDA-CFSAN (U.S. Food and Drug Administration–Center for Food Safety and Applied Nutrition) (2002a): 21 CFR 113 Thermally processed low-acid foods packaged in hermetically sealed containers. http://www.cfsan.fda.gov/~lrd/cfr113.html. Accessed May 2008.

———(2002b): 21 CFR 114 Acidified foods regulation. http://www.cfsan.fda.gov/~lrd/cfr114.html. Accessed May 2008.

———(2003a): 21 CFR 120 Juice and juice products. http://www.cfsan.fda.gov/~lrd/FCF120.html. Accessed May 2008.

———(2003b): 21 CFR 123 Fish and fishery products. http://www.cfsan.fda.gov/~lrd/FCF123.html. Accessed May 2008.

———(2003c): 21 CFR 135 Frozen desserts. http://www.cfsan.fda.gov/~lrd/FCF135.html. Accessed May, 2008.

———(2003d): 21 CFR 158 Frozen vegetables. http://www.cfsan.fda.gov/~lrd/FCF158.html. Accessed May 2008.

———(2003e): 21 CFR 110 Current good manufacturing practices in manufacturing, packing, or holding human food (GMPs). http://www.cfsan.fda.gov/~lrd/cfr110.html. Accessed May 2008.

CHAPTER 15

FOOD SAFETY ISSUES AND THE MICROBIOLOGY OF CEREALS AND CEREAL PRODUCTS

LLOYD B. BULLERMAN and ANDREIA BIANCHINI

15.1 INTRODUCTION

Cereals and cereal products are significant and important human food resources and livestock feeds worldwide. Cereal grains and legumes are food staples in many, if not most, countries and cultures and are the raw materials of many of our foods and certain beverages. The main cereal grains used for foods include corn (maize), wheat, barley, rice, oats, rye, millet, and sorghum. Soybeans are not a cereal product, but rather, are legumes or a pulse, but are often considered with cereals because of their importance as a food source.

Examples of cereal products that are derived from cereal grains include wheat, rye, and oat flours and semolina, cornmeal, corn grits, doughs, breads, breakfast cereals, pasta, snack foods, dry mixes, cakes, pastries, and tortillas. In addition, cereal products are used as ingredients in numerous products, such as batters and coatings, thickeners and sweeteners, processed meats, infant foods, confectionary products, and beverages such as beer. Because of their extensive use as human foods and livestock feeds, the microbiology and safety of cereal grains and cereal products is a very important area.

The sources of microbial contamination of cereals are many, but all are traceable to the environment in which grains are grown, handled, and processed. Microorganisms that contaminate cereal grains may come from air, dust, soil, water, insects, rodents, birds, animals, humans, storage and shipping containers, and handling and processing equipment. Many factors that are a part of the environment influence microbial contamination of cereals, including rainfall, drought, humidity, temperature, sunlight, frost, soil conditions, wind, insect, bird and rodent activity, harvesting equipment, use of chemicals in production vs. organic production, storage and handling, and moisture control.

Microbiologically Safe Foods, Edited by Norma Heredia, Irene Wesley, and Santos García

The microflora of cereals and cereal products is varied and includes molds, yeasts, bacteria (psychrotrophic, mesophilic, and thermophilic/thermoduric), lactic acid bacteria, rope-forming bacteria (*Bacillus* spp.), bacterial pathogens, coliforms, and Enterococci. Bacterial pathogens that contaminate cereal grains and cereal products and cause problems include, *Bacillus cereus, Clostridium botulinum, Clostridium perfringens, Escherichia coli*, *Salmonella,* and *Staphylococcus aureus.* Coliforms and enterococci also occur as indicators of unsanitary handling and processing conditions and possible fecal contamination (Richter et al., 1993; Sauer et al., 1992).

Bacteria are frequent surface contaminants of cereal grains. For bacteria to grow in cereal grains, they require high moisture or water activity (a_w) in equilibrium, with high relative humidity. Generally, bacteria are not significantly involved in the spoilage of dry grain and become a spoilage factor only after extensive deterioration of the grain has occurred and high moisture conditions exist. However, bacterial pathogens and spoilage bacteria, such as spore-forming bacteria that cause ropiness in bread, may survive and carry through to processed products and become problems. Lactic acid bacteria may also be present in the raw grain and carry over into flour and cornmeal and spoil doughs prepared with them. Yeasts present on cereal grains may also carry through into processed products. The main spoilage organisms in cereal grains however, are molds (Hesseltine et al., 1969; Richter et al., 1993; Sauer et al., 1992; Thompson et al., 1993).

There are more than 150 species of filamentous fungi and yeasts on cereal grains. But again, the most important of these are the filamentous fungi or molds. The filamentous fungi that occur on cereal grains are divided into two groups, depending on when they predominate in grain in relation to available moisture in the grain. These groups have been referred to as field fungi and storage fungi. Field fungi invade grain in the field when the grain is high in moisture (18 to 30%) (i.e., at high a_w) and at high relative humidities (90 to 100%). Field fungi include species of *Alternaria, Cladosporium, Fusarium*, and *Helminthosporium*. Storage fungi invade grain in storage at lower moisture contents (14 to 16%), lower a_w and lower relative humidities (65 to 90%). These main storage fungi are species of *Eurotium, Aspergillus*, and *Penicillium*. To prevent spoilage by storage fungi, the moisture content of starchy cereal grains should be below 14.0%, soybeans 12.0%, and other oilseeds, such as peanuts, and sunflower seeds, 8.5%. Certain molds, such as *Eurotium glaucus*, may initiate growth at low a_w and moisture contents (i.e., 15 to 16% moisture) and through their respiration increase a_w and raise the moisture content, facilitating molds to grow, thus ultimately leading to spoilage (Christensen and Meronuck, 1986; Reed, 2006; Sauer et al., 1992). More information on storage fungi and moisture contents in various commodities is given in Table 1.

The major effects of fungal deterioration of grains include decreased germination, discoloration, development of visible mold growth, musty or sour odors, dry matter loss and nutritional heating, caking, and the potential for production of mycotoxins in the grain (Christensen and Meronuck, 1986). Decreased germination of the grain occurs when storage fungi invade the germs or embryos of the grain kernel. The embryos are weakened and die as the storage fungi attack and parasitize the embryo to utilize its oils and other nutrients. Decreased germination caused by storage fungi

TABLE 1 Major Storage Fungi and the Moisture Contents of Commodities at Which Mold Invasion May Occur

Major Storage Fungi	Commodity	Moisture (%)
Aspergillus restrictus (blue eye)	Starchy cereals	14.0–14.5
	Soybeans	12.0–12.5
	Sunflower, safflower, peanuts	8.5–9.0
Eurotium glaucus (blue eye)	Starchy cereals	14.5–15.0
	Soybeans	12.5–13.0
	Sunflower, safflower, peanuts	9.0–9.5
A. candidus	Starchy cereals	15.5–16.0
	Soybeans	14.5–15.0
	Sunflower	9.0–9.5
A. ochraceus	Starchy cereals	15.5–16.0
	Soybeans	14.5–15.0
	Sunflower	9.0–9.5
A. flavus	Starchy cereals	17.0–18.0
	Soybeans	17.0–17.5
Penicillium (blue eye in corn)	Starch grains	16.5–20.0
	Soybeans	17.0–20.0
	Sunflower	10.0–15.0

Source: Christensen and Meronuck (1986).

usually precedes discoloration. However, discoloration can be caused by both field and storage fungi and can result in brown to black germs in wheat and corn and "blue eye" in corn, due to the presence of blue *Aspergillus* and *Penicillium* species. Musty odors may become apparent before mold growth becomes visible and is an early warning of mold activity, as is heating. Heating often starts in the fine materials or dust associated with the grain and is due to the growth of storage fungi. If sufficient heating occurs, the grain becomes dark and blackened. Further growth of storage fungi may result in surface growth and binding of the grain kernels together by mold hyphae, which is manifested as caking of the grain (i.e., large masses of the kernels bound together). By the time caking occurs, mold growth has become extensive and the grain is in advanced stages of decay. At this point the moisture content of the grain is increasing due to the respiration of the molds, and growth of yeasts and bacteria may also occur (Christensen and Meronuck, 1986; Reed, 2006).

15.2 HEALTH IMPLICATIONS OF FUNGAL DETERIORATION OF GRAINS

Both human and animal health may be affected by fungal deterioration of grain. Some molds, such as *Aspergillus fumigatus*, are pathogens and can cause respiratory and systemic infections in humans and animals. Other molds, which are not normally pathogens, may also cause infections of immunocompromised person such as AIDS patients, those undergoing radiation or chemotherapy, and the elderly. Aspergillosis is a serious lung infection in humans and animals that may originate in grain. Storage molds are also capable of causing allergic responses, such as "hay fever" or nasal allergies due to the presence of large numbers of spores in grain dusts (Cross, 1997; Denning, 1998; Latge, 1999).

15.3 MYCOTOXINS

The word *mycotoxin* is derived from the Greek word *mykes*, meaning fungus or mold, and the Latin word *toxicum*, poison or toxin. Thus, mycotoxin is a general term meaning fungus poison or mold toxin. Mycotoxins are toxic secondary metabolites produced by filamentous microfungi or molds. These secondary metabolites are distinguished from primary metabolites because they are not required for the growth of the fungus and have no apparent purpose in the metabolism of the organism. It has been speculated that mycotoxins are waste products or defense mechanisms. Mycotoxins are toxic and harmful in varying degrees to humans and animals, and may contaminate cereal grains in the field and in storage (Bennett et al., 1996; Bennett and Klich, 2003). Mycotoxins are stable compounds that resist destruction by food-processing methods and which may carry through and contaminate finished processed foods.

There are numerous specific mycotoxins that may contaminate cereal grains, such as aflatoxins, ochratoxin, fumonisins, moniliformin, deoxynivalenol, T-2 toxin, and zearalenone. Mycotoxin research began in 1960 with the outbreak of Turkey "X" disease in England, where thousands of turkey poults and other young farm animals were lost due to poisoning by a fungal metabolite produced by *Aspergillus flavus* in peanut meal. The toxic substance was called *aflatoxin* (*A. flavus* toxin) (Blount, 1961). Since 1960, many other toxic mold metabolites have been described. Those mycotoxins currently thought to be most important in cereal grains are listed in Table 2 along with the molds that produce them.

TABLE 2 Mycotoxins of Greatest Concern in Grain and the Molds That Produce Them

Mycotoxins	Molds
Aflatoxins	*Aspergillus flavus, A. parasiticus, A. nomius*
Ochratoxin	*Aspergillus ochraceus, A. niger, Penicillium verrucosum*
Fumonisins	*Fusarium verticillioides (moniliforme) F. proliferatum, F. subglutinans*
Moniliformin	*F. proliferatum, F. subglutinans*
Deoxynivalenol (DON, vomitoxin)	*Fusarium graminearum, F. culmorum, F. crookwellense*
Zearalenone	*Fusarium graminearum, F. culmorum, F. crookwellense*

Mycotoxins exhibit a range of toxicological properties, including acute toxicity or poisoning, which often results in death, and subacute or chronic toxicity, which may not result in death directly but which gradually weakens and lowers the general health of an animal or human due to effects on the immune system (Chen et al., 2008; Girish et al., 2008; Orciuolo et al., 2007). Chronic toxicity may result in greater susceptibility to secondary bacterial infections. Some mycotoxins are carcinogenic and may cause cancers; some are mutagenic and are capable of causing mutations; they may also be teratogenic and embryo toxic, causing deformities and death in developing embryos (Bennett and Klich, 2003).

15.3.1 Aflatoxins

Aflatoxins are produced by *A. flavus* and *A. parasiticus* (Bennett and Klich, 2003). Aflatoxins are most commonly found contaminating commodities and foods in the tropical regions of Africa, Southeast Asia, and South America (Egal et al., 2005; Park et al., 2004; Pineiro et al., 1996). In North America aflatoxins may occasionally occur in the southern and southeastern United States in peanuts, corn, and pecans and in the southwest in cottonseed (Wood, 1989). Aflatoxin may also occur in the midwestern U.S. corn belt in times of extreme drought stress and insect activity (Russell et al., 1991; Wood, 1992). The molds that produce aflatoxins may be found both as field and storage fungi. *Aspergillus flavus* may invade corn and cottonseed in the field when there is drought stress, insect or hail damage, and excess moisture. *Aspergillus parasiticus* may invade peanuts in the field and during harvest if there is excess moisture such as heavy rains when the peanuts are drying. Aflatoxin-producing fungi may also invade during storage if moisture conditions become favorable for growth (Bennett and Klich, 2003).

Aflatoxins are a group of structurally related compounds, the most important of which are aflatoxins B_1, B_2, G_1, G_2, M_1, and M_2 (Fig. 1). Aflatoxins B_1 and B_2 are produced by strains of *A. flavus* and are most common in corn. These strains of *A. flavus* do not normally produce the G toxins. *Aspergillus parasiticus* produces aflatoxins B_1, B_2, G_1, and G_2. Thus, corn is most commonly contaminated with aflatoxins B_1 and B_2 and peanuts with aflatoxins B_1, B_2, G_1, and G_2 (Cvetnic and Pepeljnjak, 1995; Horn et al., 1995). Aflatoxins M_1 and M_2 are hydroxylated forms of aflatoxins B_1 and B_2 and are found in milk and other body fluids, since the animal body adds the hydroxyl groups in an effort to make the toxins more soluble in aqueous solutions in order to increase excretion of the substances (Van Egmond, 1989). Besides being acutely toxic, aflatoxins may cause chronic toxicity and are potent carcinogens, affecting mainly the liver (hepatocarcinogens). Aflatoxins are considered to be involved in liver cancer worldwide. Liver cancer is most prevalent in the tropical regions of the world, such as sub-Saharan Africa, Southeast Asia, and to a lesser extent, India (Williams et al., 2004; Wogan, 1975). Aflatoxins may also cause immunotoxicity (Bondy and Pestka, 2000).

Aflatoxins are considered to be stable in most food processes. High temperatures, as are reached in flaking, roasting, and extrusion, may reduce the level of aflatoxins but do not eliminate them (Castelo, 1999; Hameed, 1993). High temperatures combined

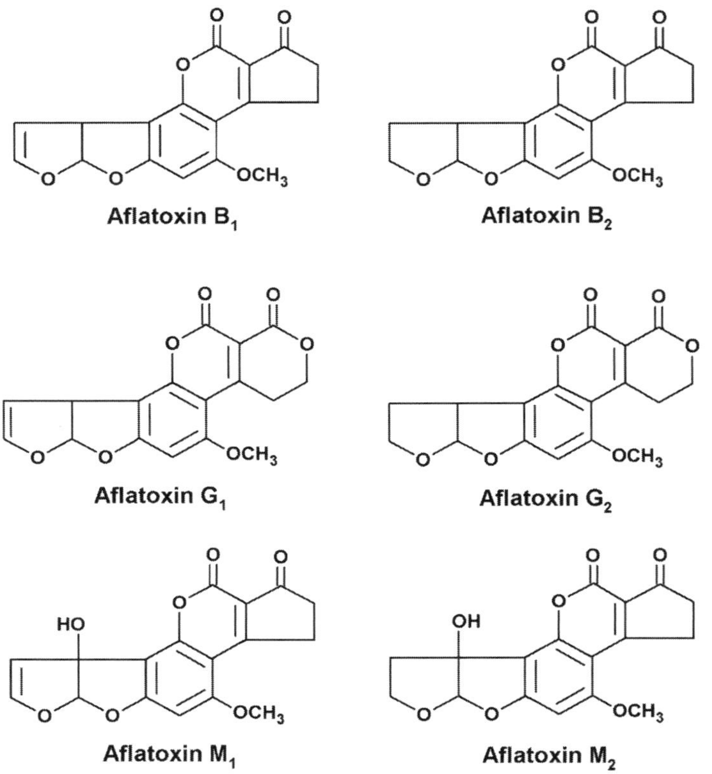

FIG. 1 Chemical structures of the principal aflatoxins.

with alkaline pH, such as with ammoniation, destroy aflatoxin in corn, but the process lowers the quality of the grain, making treated grain suitable only for animal feed (Park, 2002). The process of ammoniation has not been approved by the U.S. Food and Drug Administration (FDA) for treating human foods. The high pH of the tortilla process (nixtamalization) appears to destroy aflatoxin by opening the bifuran rings of the molecule. However, there is evidence that the rings may re-form in acidic conditions, such as may occur in the stomach, and become toxic again (Torres et al., 2001). The FDA action levels for aflatoxin in cereal products are given in Table 3. The action levels vary depending on the use of the commodity. The action level in the United States for most human food is 20 ppb (μg/kg), but for milk and certain dairy products is 0.5 ppb (μg/kg). Other countries may have different action or tolerance levels.

15.3.2 Ochratoxin

Ochratoxin A is produced by *Aspergillus ochraceus, A. carbonarius*, and *Penicillium verrucosum* (Abarca et al., 1994; Bayman et al., 2002; Frisvad and Lund, 1993;

TABLE 3 U.S. FDA Action Levels for Aflatoxin Cereal Products

Commodity	Action Level [ppb (μg/kg)]
Human food and feed for dairy cattle and immature livestock	20
Milk and dairy products	0.5
Feed for breeding, cattle, swine, and mature poultry	100
Feed for finishing swine (100 lb+)	200
Feed for finishing beef cattle	300

Source: USFDA (2000).

Pitt, 1987). Ochratoxin is a dihydroisocoumarin linked to L-β-phenylalanine (Fig. 2). Ochratoxin A is the most common form of the toxin, but two other forms, ochratoxins B and C, also exist. Ochratoxin A is also the most toxic of the group. *Aspergillus ochraceus* and *A. carbonarius* are the main sources of ochratoxin in warmer climates, with *A. ochraceus* found in green coffee beans and *A. carbonarius* found on grapes and in vineyards. *P. verrucosum* is the main source of ochratoxin in cooler climates and is found in barley (Pitt, 2000). Ochratoxin is toxic to kidneys (nephrotoxin) and also is considered to be a carcinogen (Gekle and Silbernagl, 1993; Pfohl-Leszkowicz and Manderville, 2007). Ochratoxin has been implicated as the causative agent of porcine nephropathy, a common disease of swine in Denmark caused by feeding moldy barley. There is a comparable human disease known as Balkan endemic nephropathy, which is found in Balkan countries of Central Europe and may involve human exposure to ochratoxin (Pfohl-Leszkowicz and Manderville, 2007).

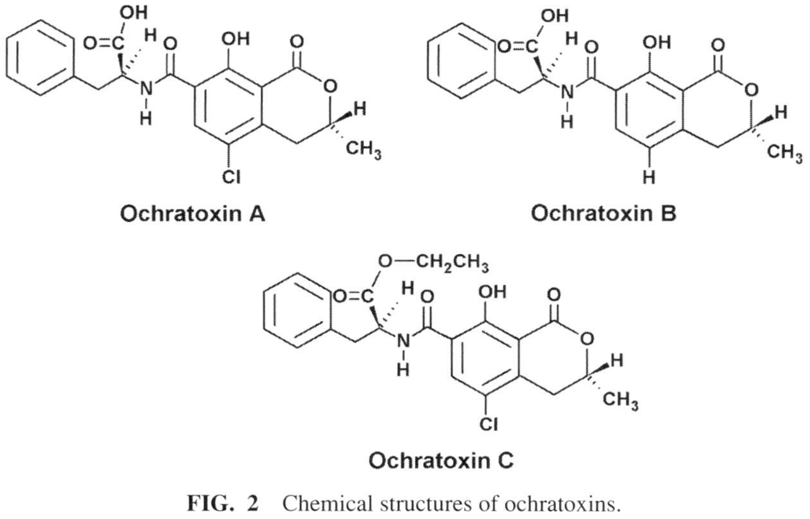

FIG. 2 Chemical structures of ochratoxins.

In addition to nephrotoxicity, ochratoxin is embryo toxic, capable of causing fetal death, and teratogenic, capable of causing deformities in developing embryos (Kittane et al., 1984).

In terms of cereals, ochratoxin occurs primarily in small grains such as wheat and barley. Ochratoxin is fairly stable in food-processing systems. It is stable during milling and divides into various milled fractions (Scudamore et al., 2003). Ochratoxin also is stable during baking, flaking, and cooking of mash for beer (Chu et al., 1975; Scudamore et al., 2003). It has been found in beer and in human blood samples in Canada and Europe (Anselme et al., 2006; Sangare-Tigori et al., 2006). Ochratoxin appears to be destroyed during roasting of coffee but has also been found in wine (Battilani et al., 2006; Chiodini et al., 2006; Pérez de Obanos, 2005).

15.3.3 *Fusarium* Mycotoxins

Fusarium molds are frequent contaminants of cereal grains in the field, including corn (maize), wheat, barley, and sorghum. They also are found in oilseeds and beans. The toxic *Fusarium* species most commonly associated with corn in all corn-growing regions are *F. verticillioides* (former *moniliforme*), *F. proliferatum*, and *F. graminearum* (Pitt, 2000). These organisms produce symptomless infections of corn plants and infect both food- and feed-grade corn. Some lots of corn may have 100% kernel infections with no outward signs of moldiness. *Fusarium verticillioides* may also cause a type of ear rot in which there is extensive visible growth of the mold (Bacon et al., 1992; Davis et al., 1989; Logrieco et al., 2002). *Fusarium graminearum* and *F. culmorum* are two closely related species that also occur in corn, wheat, and barley. In corn they cause ear rots and in wheat and barley they cause fusarium head blight, also known as scab (Logrieco et al., 2002; Parry et al., 1995). *Fusarium verticillioides* and *F. proliferatum* both produce a mycotoxin known as fumonisin, and *F. proliferatum* and *F. subglutinans* (also found in corn) produce a toxin called moniliformin. *F. graminearum* produces the mycotoxins deoxynivalenol and zearalenone (Pitt and Hocking, 1999).

Fumonisins These toxins consist of several related compounds, of which the most common are fumonisin B_1 (FB_1), fumonisin B_2 (FB_2), and fumonisin B_3 (FB_3). The structure of FB_1 (Fig. 3) consists of a long carbon chain with two tricarballylic acid side chains and an amino group. The toxin resembles sphingosine, a component of membranes and nerve cells (Merrill et al., 1993). Fumonisins disrupt sphingosine metabolism and cause different disease manifestations in different animal species. In horses and other equines fumonisins cause equine leukoencephalomalacia (ELEM), a fatal brain-destroying syndrome, where the brain tissue is liquefied and destroyed (Marasas et al., 1988). In swine, fumonisins cause porcine pulmonary edema (PPE), in which fluid accumulates in the lungs, causing death by suffocation (Haschek et al., 2001). Fumonisins have also been shown in experiments to cause liver cancer in rats and atherosclerosis in monkeys (Fincham et al., 1992; Howard et al., 2001). Human diseases associated with fumonisins are esophageal cancer, common in areas where corn is a dietary stable, such as the Transkei region of South Africa, northeastern

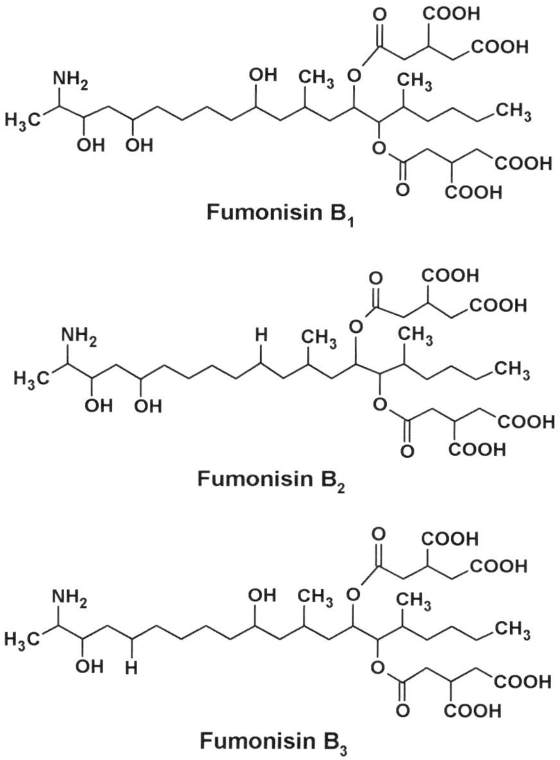

FIG. 3 Chemical structures of fumonisins.

Italy, and northern China, and a condition known as neural tube defects in developing embryos (Chu and Li, 1994; Marasas et al., 2004; Rheeder et al., 1992). In 1990 and 1991, in Cameron County, Texas, along the U.S.–Mexican border, a higher than normal number of anencephalic births (two to three times the normal rate) occurred among Hispanic women. A drought in 1988 and 1989 caused high levels of fumonisin in corn grown in the region. It has been suggested that the Hispanic women living along the Texas–Mexico border had consumed large amounts of corn in the form of tortillas and other corn products that were contaminated by high levels of fumonisin (Missmer et al., 2006).

The highest levels of fumonisins are found in corn products that receive just a physical process, such as the milled products cornmeal and corn flour. However, the fumonisin content is divided among the different fractions that come out of the process, and the concentrations are higher in the germ and bran fractions (Brera et al., 2004; Katta et al., 1997). *Fusarium verticillioides* invades corn kernels through the silks into the tip of the kernel (Munkvold et al., 1997). The hyphae grow under the seed coat and remain near the tip end of the kernel, where they may produce fumonisins. Since the hyphae do not normally spread into the endosperm, the grit

TABLE 4 U.S. FDA Guidance Levels for Fumonisins in Cereal Products

Commodity	Guidance Level [ppm (μg/kg)]
Degermed dry-milled corn	2
Whole or partially degermed dry-milled corn products	4
Dry-milled corn bran	4
Cleaned corn intended for masa production	4
Cleaned corn intended for popcorn	3

Source: USFDA (2001).

fractions of the corn tend to remain free of fumonisins or have very low concentrations (Brera et al., 2004; Katta et al., 1997). This helps in part to explain why more highly processed corn-based foods, made from various grit fractions, such as cornflakes, corn breakfast cereals, tortillas, and tortilla chips, have the lowest levels of fumonisins. Fresh and canned sweet corn and popcorn may also be contaminated with low levels of fumonisins (Machinski and Soares, 2000). Fumonisins are stable in food processes such as baking, ordinary cooking, canning, and flaking, while some losses occur in higher-temperature processes such as roasting and extrusion (Castelo et al., 1998a,b). At temperatures above 150°C and in alkaline treatment of the tortilla process fumonisins appear to be destroyed, or at least lowered in concentration. However, these processes are thought to produce hydrolyzed FB_1, which may remain toxic (Dombrink-Kurtzman et al., 2000; Hendrich et al., 1993). Heating in the presence of glucose results in the formation of *N*-(1-deoxy-D-fructos-1-yl)FB_1 (NDF-B_1) and *N*-(carboxymethyl)FB_1 (NCM-FB_1), which appear to be less toxic than FB_1 (Howard et al., 1998; Polling et al., 2002). So processing corn at temperatures above 150°C in the presence of glucose by processes such as extrusion appears to lower toxicity due to FB_1 (Castelo et al., 1998a). The U.S. FDA has issued advisory levels for fumonisins in corn products. These are given in Table 4.

Moniliformin This is a mycotoxin produced by *F. proliferatum* and *F. subglutinans* (Fig. 4) (Pitt and Hocking, 1999). Moniliformin is a cardiotoxin and is very toxic to chickens, but its toxicity to humans is unknown (Engelhardt et al., 1989; Vesonder and Wu, 1998). Since moniliformin is produced by *Fusarium* species that occur frequently in corn, there is the possibility for it to co-occur with fumonisins, and in fact it has been reported co-occurring with fumonisins in corn and commercial

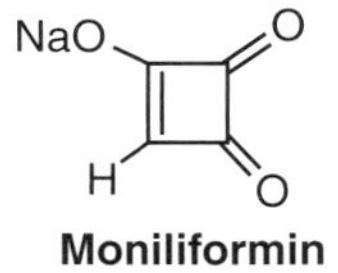

FIG. 4 Chemical structure of moniliformin.

corn-based food products (Gutema et al., 2000). Moniliformin may have synergistic effects with fumonisins, and it appears to be stable in many food processes, including baking, cooking, and canning. Some losses have been observed in processes that employ high temperatures, such as roasting and extrusion (Castells et al., 2005; Pineda-Valdes et al., 2003). Losses of moniliformin were also observed with the tortilla process (Pineda-Valdes et al., 2002).

Deoxynivalenol Another group of *Fusarium* species, *F. graminearum, F. culmorum*, and *F. crookwellense*, are widely distributed in the soil and cause diseases of cereal grains, including *Gibberella* ear rots of corn and *Fusarium* head blight of wheat and barley (Logrieco et al, 2002; Parry et al., 1995). These organisms infect grain in temperate climates, and the species that predominates is temperature dependent. *Fusarium graminearum* is found more in the warmer-temperature regions, such as North America, whereas *F. culmorum* is found in the cooler-temperature regions of northern Europe and has been suggested as the causative agent of *Fusarium* head blight in Denmark, Romania, Bulgaria, the Netherlands, and Belgium (Doohan et al., 2003; Tóth et al., 2004). The mycotoxin profiles of these species are also slightly different; *F. graminearum* isolates from North America tend to produce deoxynivalenol, whereas *F. graminearum* isolates from Europe, Africa, and Asia tend to produce nivalenol (Lee et al., 2001). *Fusarium crookwellense* produces nivalenol and/or zearalenone (Vesonder et al., 1991).

Deoxynivalenol (Fig. 5) is one of a group of mycotoxins known as trichothecenes and is, in fact, the most commonly occurring trichothecene in cereal grains. Its

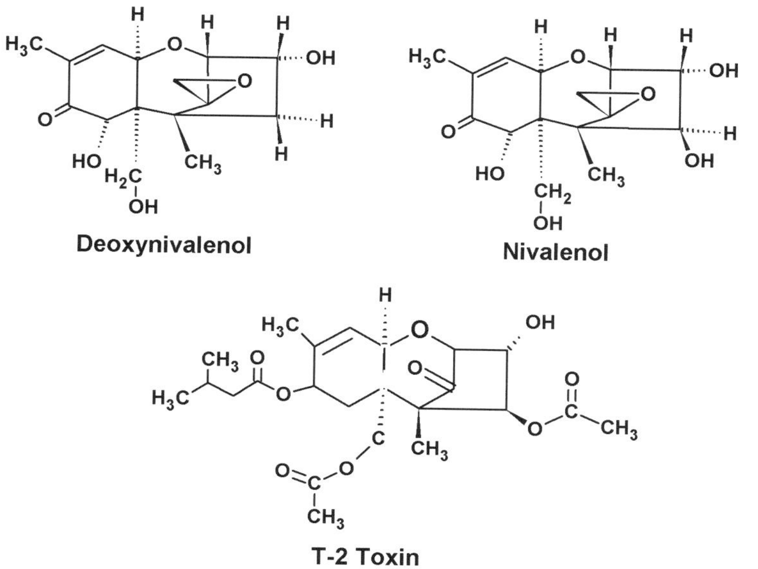

FIG. 5 Chemical structures of deoxynivalenol, nivalenol, and T-2 toxin.

chemical structure is characteristic of this group of mycotoxins. Derivatives of deoxynivalenol, which is also called DON and vomitoxin, also occur. The two most common are 3-acetyldeoxynivalenol (3-ADON) and 15-acetyldeoxynivalenol (15-ADON) (Lee et al., 2001). The 3-ADON is more commonly found in Europe, Asia, Australia, and New Zealand, while 15-ADON is more common in North America (Goswami and Kistler, 2004; Mirocha et al., 1989). Nivalenol (Fig. 5) is very similar to deoxynivalenol in structure but is more toxic (Coulombe, 1993; Ueno, 1984).

Deoxynivalenol causes vomiting or emesis in swine, dogs, cats, and humans (Bhat et al., 1989; Forsyth et al., 1977; Pestka and Smolinski, 2005). Human illnesses that have been associated with *F. graminearum* and deoxynivalenol have been called by different names in different regions of the world and include drunken bread, akakabi-byo, or scabby grain intoxication or red mold disease, and foodborne illness or gastroenteritis. The diseases appear to be the same or slightly different manifestations of the same disease. Foodborne gastroenteritis associated with *F. graminearum* and DON has been reported in several countries, including Japan, Korea, China, India, eastern Russia, and Siberia. The outbreaks have been associated with foods made from wheat and barley, most commonly breads, where the grain was infected with *Fusarium* molds (Beardall and Miller, 1994; Bhat et al., 1989; Li et al., 1999; Pestka and Smolinski, 2005). The incubation or onset times of the illnesses are characteristically short, ranging from 5 to 30 min up to 15 to 60 min, suggesting the presence of a preformed toxin. Symptoms of the illnesses include nausea, facial rash (reddening), headache, throat irritation, fever, chills, vomiting, abdominal pain, flatulence, and diarrhea. Deoxynivalenol has also been reported to affect immune systems, with both immunosuppression and immunostimulation observed in animals. Immunosuppression affects β- and T-cell responses in lymphocytes, resulting in suppressed immune activity and increased susceptibility to infectious diseases. Immunostimulation can lead to autoimmune disorders (Pestka et al., 2004). Deoxynivalenol has been shown to cause elevated immunoglobulin A (IgA) levels in mice, leading to kidney damage known as IgA nephropathy (Greene et al., 1994). There is a similar human kidney condition known as glomerulonephritis, which is an IgA nephropathy and which has been associated with grain-based diets.

Deoxynivalenol is the most common trichothecene found in cereal grains, and there is a potential for DON to contaminate finished, processed grain-based foods (Abbas et al., 1985). Many foods, such as breads, pastas, breakfast cereals, and beer, may contain at least trace amounts of DON (Anselme et al., 2006; Martins and Martins, 2001). However, unlike fumonisins, where the background contamination tends to be constant, DON contamination is more sporadic and varies from year to year depending on weather conditions, field conditions, hail damage, and incidence levels of *Gibberella* ear rot in corn and *Fusarium* head blight in wheat and barley. Deoxynivalenol is stable in most food processes, but some incomplete loss may occur at very high temperatures in processes such as roasting and extrusion and under alkaline conditions and high temperatures, as those that occur in the tortilla process (Cazzaniga et al., 2001). The FDA advisory levels for deoxynivalenol (vomitoxin) in cereal products are given in Table 5.

TABLE 5 U.S. FDA Advisory Levels for Deoxynivalenol (Vomitoxin) in Cereal Products

Commodity	Advisory Level [ppm (μg/kg)]
Human foods (finished products)	1
Grains or grain by-product destined for swine (all grains, <20% of diet)	5 (1 ppm in final diet)
Grains or grain by-product destined for cattle and chickens (all grains, <50% of diet)	10 (5 ppm in final diet)
Grains or grain by-product destined for all other animals (all grains, <40% of diet)	5 (2 ppm in final diet)

Source: USFDA (1993).

T-2 Toxin T-2 toxin and HT-2 toxin are structurally very similar to DON (Fig. 5); however, they are much more toxic but less common (Coulombe, 1993). These toxins are produced by *Fusarium poae, F. sporotrichioides*, and *F. tricinctum* (Burmeister, 1971; Pitt and Hocking, 1999). These species grow well at low temperatures, near freezing. They have low optimum growth temperatures and have optimum temperatures for production of the toxin of around 6 to 12°C (Pitt and Hocking, 1999). Maximum toxin production occurs under conditions of alternating freeze–thaw cycles. T-2 toxin inhibits protein synthesis and disrupts DNA and RNA (Khachatourians, 1990). It is a severe dermal toxin and is immunotoxic and suppresses immune systems (Pang et al., 1987; Ueno, 1984). Chickens and turkeys are quite sensitive to T-2 toxin, in which it causes severe oral lesions and necrosis of oral tissue, severe edema of the body cavity, hemorrhage of the large intestines, neurotoxic effects, and death (Chi et al., 1977). In dairy cattle it has been described to induce inappetence, abortion, visceral hemorrhage, and death (Hsu et al., 1972). T-2 toxin also causes dermal toxicity in humans and animals, with severe burning and reddening of the skin and hemorrhaging from mucous membranes. A human disease attributed to consumption of grain contaminated with T-2 toxin is alimentary toxic aleukia (ATA), a disease that destroys the bone marrow and blood-forming capacity of the body, resulting in severe anemia and susceptibility to secondary bacterial infections. The mortality rate may be as high as 60%. Severe outbreaks of ATA occurred in Russia and Siberia during World War II and caused thousands of human deaths (Bamburg et al., 1969; Yagen and Joffe, 1976).

Zearalenone Another metabolite of *F. graminearum, F. culmorum*, and *F. crookwellense* that can affect animal health, and possibly humans is zearalenone (Fig. 6). This substance is included with mycotoxins but has very low acute toxicity. However, zearalenone is biologically active as an estrogenic compound and is considered to be an endocrine disrupter. It causes estrogenic responses in swine, where it causes swollen vulva in sows and gilts, spontaneous abortions in pregnant sows and feminization of young male pigs.

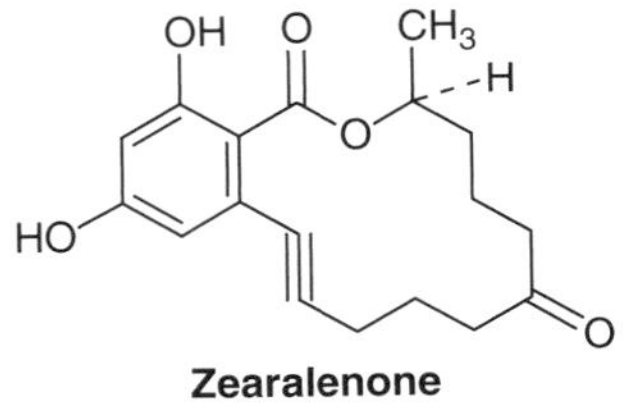

FIG. 6 Chemical structure of zearalenone.

Exposure occurs through feed for pigs and through sow milk for nursing piglets, and for swine 1 to 5 ppm (μg/g) in the diet is estrogenic. Zearalenone production most commonly occurs in high-moisture corn subjected to an early killing frost. It can also contaminate wheat, barley, and processed foods in low amounts (Zinedine et al., 2007). The effects of zearalenone in humans are unknown; however, it was suspected as the potential cause of an outbreak of precocious pubertal development in children in Puerto Rico, but never proven (Schoental, 1983). There is also speculation that zearalenone could be a contributing factor in some cases of human breast and cervical cancer because of its status as an endocrine disrupter. This is speculation only, however Zearalenone is quite stable in food processes but is partially destroyed at temperatures above 150°C (Ryu et al., 1999).

15.4 MEDIA AND METHODS FOR MOLDS AND MYCOTOXINS

The media and methods for detection and enumeration of molds in cereal products are summarized in Table 6. The media presented are all recommended by the International Commission on Food Mycology (ICFM) as well as given in the *Compendium of Methods for the Microbiological Examination of Foods* (Downes and Ito, 2001). Dichloran rose bengal chloramphenicol (DRBC) agar is recommended as a general-purpose medium for direct plating of grain kernels and for plate counts of flours, meals, and processed products for total counts (Hocking et al., 2006). Dichloran with 18% glycerol (DG18) is also recommended for these uses, especially for direct plating kernels for xerophilic molds, which prefer low a_w and dry conditions. For plating dry

TABLE 6 Media and Methods for Detection and Enumeration of Molds

Medium[a]	Method/Use
DRBC	General purpose, direct plating of kernels, and plate counts of flours, meals, and processed products for total counts
DG-18	Direct plating of kernels for xerophilic molds
AFPA	Direct plating of kernels and plate counts of *A. flavus* and *A. parasiticus*
CZID	Direct plating of kernels and plate counts of *Fusarium* species

[a]DRBC, dichloran rose bengal chloramphenicol agar; DG-18, dichloran 18% glycerol agar; AFPA, *Aspergillus flavus–parasiticus* agar; CZID, Czapek's agar plus iprodione and dichloran.

grains and cereal products, DG18 may actually be better than DRBC and the medium of choice (Hocking and Pitt, 1980). Two differential media may also be used for detection and enumeration of specific molds in cereals. *Aspergillus flavus–parasiticus* agar (AFPA) can be used as a differential medium for direct plating of kernels and plate counts of *A. flavus* and *A. parasiticus* (Pitt et al., 1983). Czapek agar with iprodione and dichloran added (CZID) is widely used as a differential medium for detecting and enumerating *Fusarium* species from cereals (Thrane, 1996).

The simplest way to evaluate the internal microflora of seeds and kernels is the direct plating method, which involves surface sanitizing seeds or kernels in full strength or 50% household bleach for 1 min to kill surface microflora. The kernels or seeds are then rinsed in sterile distilled water and dried on sterile paper towels. The seeds or kernels are then placed directly on an agar surface in a petri dish and incubated at 25 to 30°C to allow molds located in the interior of the seed or kernel to grow out. The number of kernels with internal mold is counted and the results are expressed as a percentage of infected kernels. The amount of internal infection of the grain is an indicator of quality and storability of the grain. The technique can also give some information about the safety of the grain if AFPA or CZID have been used, indicating whether or not potentially toxic *A. flavus*, *A. parasiticus*, or *Fusarium* species are present.

Methods for detecting mycotoxins are summarized in Table 7. Chromatographic methods have been used from the beginning of mycotoxin research and are still used for detecting, quantifying, and confirming the presence of mycotoxins. These methods have evolved, been improved, and have become more sophisticated. Chromatographic methods in use include thin-layer chromatography (TLC), high-performance liquid chromatography (HPLC), liquid chromatography combined with mass spectrometry (LC-MS), gas chromatography (GC), and gas chromatography combined with mass spectrometry (GC-MS). Various detection methods, such as fluorescence, ultraviolet absorption, and others, have been combined with chromatographic methods. New methods based on the production of antibodies specific for individual mycotoxins have also been developed and include enzyme-linked immunosorbent assays (ELISA) and immunoaffinity columns (IAC). These methods allow for specific and precise detection and quantification of specific mycotoxins. This has lead to test kits for mycotoxins which are rapid and simple to use and can be used in the field, country elevators, grain-buying stations, feed mills, and processing plants.

TABLE 7 Methods for Detection of Mycotoxins

Mycotoxin	Method
Aflatoxins	TLC, HPLC, ELISA, immunoaffinity column
Ochratoxins	TLC, HPLC, ELISA, immunoaffinity column
Fumonisins	HPLC, ELISA, immunoaffinity column
Moniliformin	HPLC
Deoxynivalenol	GC, HPLC, ELISA, immunoaffinity column
Zearalenone	TLC, HPLC, ELISA, immunoaffinity column

REFERENCES

Abarca ML, Bragulat MR, Sastella G, Cabanes FJ (1994): Ochratoxin A production by strains of *Aspergillus niger* var. *niger*. *Appl Environ Microbiol*. 60:2650–2652.

Abbas HK, Mirocha CJ, Pawlosky RJ, Pusch DJ (1985): Effect of cleaning, milling, and baking on deoxynivalenol in wheat. *Appl Environ Microbiol*. 50:482–485.

Anselme M, Tangni EK, Pussemier L, et al. (2006): Comparison of ochratoxin A and deoxynivalenol in organically and conventionally produced beers sold on the Belgian market. *Food Addit Contam*. 23:910–918.

Bacon CW, Bennett RM, Hinton DM, Voss KA (1992): Scanning electron microscopy of *Fusarium moniliforme* within asymptomatic corn kernels and kernels associated with equine leukoencephalomalacia. *Plant Dis*. 76:144–148.

Bamburg JR, Strong FM, Smalley EB (1969): Toxins from moldy cereals. *J Agric Food Chem*. 17:443–450.

Battilani P, Magan N, Logrieco A (2006): European research on ochratoxin A in grapes and wine. *Int J Food Microbiol*. 111:S2–S4.

Bayman P, Baker JL, Doster MA, Michailides TJ, Mahoney NE (2002): Ochratoxin production by the *Aspergillus ochraceus* group and *Aspergillus alliaceus*. *Appl Environ Microbiol*. 68:2326–2329.

Beardall JM, Miller JD (1994): Diseases in humans with mycotoxins as possible causes. In: Miller JD, Trenholm HL (Eds.). *Mycotoxins in Grain: Compounds Other Than Aflatoxin*. Eagan Press, St. Paul, MN, pp. 487–539.

Bennett JW, Klich M (2003): Mycotoxins. *Clin Microbiol Rev*. 16:497–516.

Bennett GA, Richard JL, Eckhoff SR (1996): Distribution of fumonisins in food and feed products prepared from contaminated corn. In: Jackson LS, DeVries JW, Bullerman LB (Eds.). *Fumonisin in Food*. Plenum Press, New York, pp. 317–332.

Bhat RV, Beedu SR, Ramakrishna Y, Munshi KL (1989): Outbreak of trichothecenes mycotoxicosis associated with consumption of mould-damaged wheat production in Kashmir Valley, India. *Lancet*. 1:35–37.

Blount WP (1961): Turkey "X" disease. *Turkeys*. 9:55–58, 61, 77.

Bondy GS, Pestka JJ (2000): Immunomodulation by fungal toxins. *J Toxicol Environ Health Pt B Crit Rev*. 3:109–143.

Brera C, Debegnach F, Grossi S, Miraglia M (2004): Effect of industrial processing on the distribution of fumonisin B_1 in dry milling corn fractions. *J Food Prot*. 67:1261–1266.

Burmeister HR (1971): T-2 toxin production by *Fusarium tricinctum* on solid substrate. *Appl Microbiol*. 21:739–742.

Castells M, Marín S, Sanchis V, Ramos AJ (2005): Fate of mycotoxins in cereals during extrusion cooking: a review. *Food Addit Contam*. 22:150–157.

Castelo MM (1999): Stability of mycotoxins in thermally processed corn products. Ph.D. dissertation. University of Nebraska, Lincoln. Available at UNL Libraries, LD3656.5 1999. C378.

Castelo MM, Katta SK, Sumner SS, Hanna MA, Bullerman LB (1998a): Extrusion cooking reduces recoverability of fumonisin B_1 from extruded corn grits. *J Food Sci*. 63:696–689.

Castelo MM, Sumner SS, Bullerman LB (1998b): Stability of fumonisins in thermally processed corn products. *J Food Prot*. 61:1030–1033.

Cazzaniga D, Basílico JC, González RJ, Torres RL, Greef DM (2001): Mycotoxins inactivation by extrusion cooking of corn flour. *Lett Appl Microbiol.* 33:144–147.

Chen DC, Lee YY, Yeh PY, Lin JC, Chen YL, Hung SL (2008): Eugenol inhibited the antimicrobial functions of neuthrophils. *J Endod.* 34:176–180.

Chi MS, Mirocha CJ, Kurtz HF, Weaver G, Bates F, Shimoda W (1977): Effects of T-2 toxin on reproductive performance and health of laying hens. *Poult Sci.* 56:628–637.

Chiodini AM, Scherpenisse P, Bergwerff AA (2006): Ochratoxin A contents in wine: comparison of organically and conventionally produced products. *J Agric Food Chem.* 54:7399–7404.

Christensen CM, Meronuck RA (1986): *Quality Maintenance in Stored Grains and Seeds.* University of Minessota Press, Minneapolis, MN.

Chu FS, Li GY (1994): Simultaneous occurrence of fumonisin B_1 and other mycotoxins in moldy corn collected from the People's Republic of China in regions with high incidences of esophageal cancer. *Appl Environ Microbiol.* 60:847–852.

Chu FS, Chang CC, Ashoor SH, Prentice N (1975): Stability of aflatoxin B_1 and ochratoxin A in brewing. *Appl Microbiol.* 29:313–316.

Coulombe RA Jr (1993): Symposium: biological action of mycotoxins. *J Dairy Sci.* 76:880–891.

Cross S (1997): Mould spores: the unusual suspects in hay fever. *Community Nurse.* 3:25–26.

Cvetnic Z, Pepeljnjak S (1995): Aflatoxin-producing potential of *Aspergillus flavus* and *Aspergillus parasiticus* isolated from samples of smoked-dried meat. *Nahrung.* 39:302–307.

Davis RM, Kegel FR, Sills WM, Farrar JJ (1989): *Fusarium* ear rot of corn. *Calif Agric.* 43:4–5.

Denning DW (1998): State-of-the-art clinical article: Invasive aspergillosis. *Clin Infect Dis.* 26:781–805.

Dombrink-Kurtzman MA, Dvorak TJ, Barron ME, Rooney LW (2000): Effect of nixtamalization (alkaline cooking) on fumonisin-contaminated corn for production of masa and tortillas. *J Agric Food Chem.* 48:5781–5786.

Doohan FM, Brennan J, Cooke BM (2003): Influence of climatic factors on *Fusarium* species pathogenic to cereals. *Eur J Plant Pathol.* 109:755–768.

Downes FP, Ito K (Eds.) (2001): *Compendium of Methods for the Microbiological Examination of Foods.* American Public Health Association. Washingtom, DC.

Egal S, Hounsa A, Gong YY, et al. (2005): Dietary exposure to aflatoxin from maize and groundnut in young children from Benin and Togo, West Africa. *Int J Food Microbiol.* 104:215–224.

Engelhardt JA, Carlton WW, Tuite JF (1989): Toxicity of *Fusarium moniliforme* var. *subglutinans* for chicks, ducklings, and turkey poults. *Avian Dis.* 33:357–360.

Fincham JE, Marasas WFO, Taljaard JJF, et al. (1992): Atherogenic effects in a non-human primate of *Fusarium moniliforme* cultures added to a carbohydrate diet. *Atherosclerosis.* 94:13–25.

Forsyth DM, Yoshizawa T, Morooka N, Tuite J (1977): Emetic and refusal activity of deoxynivalenol to swine. *Appl Environ Microbiol.* 34:547–552.

Frisvad JC, Lund F (1993): Toxin and secondary metabolite production by *Penicillium* species growing in stored cereals. In: Scudamore KA (Ed.). *Proc. United Kingdom Workshop on*

Occurrence and Significance of Mycotoxins. Central Science Laboratory, Slough, UK, April 21–23, pp. 146–171.

Gekle M, Silbernagl S (1993): Mechanism of ochratoxin A–induced reduction of glomerular filtration rate in rats. *J Pharmacol Exp Ther*. 267:316–321.

Girish CK, Smith TK, Boermans HJ, Karrow NA (2008): Effects of feeding blends of grains naturally contaminated with *Fusarium* mycotoxins on performance, hematology, metabolism, and immunocompetence of turkeys. *Poult Sci*. 87:421–432.

Goswami RS, Kistler HC (2004): Heading for disaster: *Fusarium graminearum* on cereal crops. *Mol Plant Pathol*. 5:515–525.

Greene DM, Azcona-Olivera JI, Pestka JJ (1994): Vomitoxin (deoxynivaleno)-induced IgA nephropathy in the B6C3F1 mouse: dose response and male predilection. *Toxicology*. 92:245–260.

Gutema T, Munimbazi C, Bullerman LB (2000): Occurrence of fumonisins and moniliformin in corn and corn-based food products of U.S. origin. *J Food Prot*. 63:1732–1737.

Hameed HG (1993): Extrusion and chemical treatments for destruction of aflatoxin in naturally-contaminated corn. M.Sc. thesis. University of Arizona, Tucson, AZ.

Haschek WM, Gumprecht LA, Smith G, Tumbleson ME, Constable PD (2001): Fumonisin toxicosis in swine: an overview of porcine pulmonary edema and current perspectives. *Environ Health Perspect*. 109:251–257.

Hendrich S, Miller KA, Wilson TM, Murphy PA (1993): Toxicity of *Fusarium proliferatum*-fermented nixtamalized corn-based diets fed to rats: effect of nutritional status. *J Agric Food Chem*. 41 (10):1649–1654.

Hesseltine CW, Graves RR, Rogers R, Burmeister HR (1969): Aerobic and facultative microflora of fresh and spoiled refrigerated dough products. *Appl Microbiol*. 18:848–853.

Hocking AD, Pitt JI (1980): Dichloran-glycerol medium for enumeration of xerophilic fungi from low-moisture foods. *Appl. Environ Microbiol*. 39 (3):488–492.

Hocking AD, Pitt JI, Samson RA, Thrane U (Eds.) (2006): *Advances in Food Mycology: Recommended Methods for Food Mycology*, Vol. 571 of Advances in Experimental Medicine and Biology. Springer Science and Business Media, New York, pp. 343–357.

Horn BW, Greene RL, Dorner JW (1995): Effect of corn and peanut cultivation on soil populations of *Aspergillus flavus* and *A. parasiticus* in southwestern Georgia. *Appl Environ Microbiol*. 61:2472–2475.

Howard PC, Churchwell MI, Couch LH, Marques MM, Doerge DR (1998): Formation of *N*-(carboxymethyl)fumonisin B_1, following the reaction of fumonisin B_1 with reducing sugars. *J Agric Food Chem*. 46:3546–3557.

Howard PC, Eppley RM, Stack ME, et al. (2001): Fumonisin B_1 carcinogenicity in a two-year feeding study using F344 rats and $B6C3F_1$ mice. *Environ Health Perspect*. 109:277–282.

Hsu I-C, Smalley EB, Strong FM, Ribelin WE (1972): Identification of T-2 toxin in moldy corn associated with a lethal toxicosis in dairy cattle. *Appl Microbiol*. 24:684–690.

Katta SK, Cagampang AE, Jackson LS, Bullerman LB (1997): Distribution of *Fusarium* molds and fumonisins in dry-milled corn fractions. *Cereal Chem*. 74:858–863.

Khachatourians GG (1990): Metabolic effects of trichothecene T-2 toxin. *Can J Physiol Pharmacol*. 68:1004–1008.

Kittane M, Stein AO, Berndt WO, Phillips TD (1984): Teratogenic effects of ochratoxin A in rats with impaired renal function. *Toxicology*. 32:277–285.

Latge JP (1999): *Aspergillus fumigatus* and aspergillosis. *Clin Microbiol Rev.* 12:310–350.

Lee T, Oh D-W, Kim H-S, et al. (2001): Identification of deoxynivalenol- and nivalenol-producing chemotypes of *Gibberella zeae* by using PCR. *Appl Environ Microbiol.* 67:2966–2972.

Li F-Q, Luo X-Y, Yoshizawa T (1999): Mycotoxins (trichothecenes, zearalenone, and fumonisins) in cereals associated with human red-mold intoxications stored since 1989 and 1991 in China. *Nat Toxins.* 7:93–97.

Logrieco A, Mulè G, Moretti A, Bottalico A (2002): Toxigenic *Fusarium* species and mycotoxins associated with maize ear rot in europe. *Eur J Plant Pathol.* 108:597–609.

Machinski M Jr, Soares LMV (2000): Fumonisin B_1 and B_2 in Brazilian corn-based food products. *Food Addit Contam.* 17:875–879.

Marasas WFO, Kellerman TS, Gelderblom WCA, Coetzer JAW, Thiel PG, Van Der Lugt JJ (1988): Leukoencephalomalacia in horse induced by fumonisin B_1 isolated from *Fusarium moniliforme. Onderstepoort J Vet Res.* 55:197–203.

Marasas WFO, Riley RT, Hendricks KA, et al. (2004): Fumonisins disrupt sphingolipid metabolism, folate transport, and neural tube development in embryo culture and in vivo: a potential risk factor for human neural tube defects among populations consuming fumonisin-contaminated corn. *J Nutr.* 134:711–716.

Martins ML, Martins HM (2001): Determination of deoxynivalenol in wheat-based breakfast cereals marketed in Portugal. *J Food Prot.* 64:1848–1850.

Merrill Jr AH, van Echten G, Wnag E, Sandhoff K (1993): Fumonisin B1 inhibits sphingosine (sphinganine) *N*-acyltransferase and de novo sphingolipid biosynthesis in cultured neurons in situ. *J Biol Chem.* 268:27299–27306.

Mirocha CJ, Abbas HK, Windels CE, Xie W (1989): Variation in deoxynivalenol, 15-acetyldeoxynivalenol, 3-acetyldeoxynivalenol, and zearalenone production by *Fusarium graminearum* isolates. *Appl Environ Microbiol.* 55:1315–1316.

Missmer SA, Suarez L, Felkner M, et al. (2006): Exposure to fumonisins and the occurrence of neural tube defect along the Texas–Mexico border. *Environ Health Perspect.* 114: 237–241.

Munkvold GP, McGee DC, Carlton WM (1997): Importance of different pathways for maize kernel infection by *Fusarium moniliforme. Ecol Epidemiol.* 87:209–217.

Orciuolo E, Stanzani M, Canestraro M, et al. (2007): Effects of *Aspergillus fumigatus* gliotoxin and methylprenisolone on human neutrophils: implications for the pathogenesis of invasive aspergillosis. *J Leukoc Biol.* 82:839-848.

Pang VF, Felsburg PJ, Beasley VR, Buck WB, Haschek WM (1987): The toxicity of T-2 toxin in swine following topical application. II: Effects of hematology, serum biochemistry, and immune response. *Fundam Appl Toxicol.* 9:50–59.

Park DL (2002): Effect of processing on aflatoxin. *Adv Exp Med Biol.* 504:173–179.

Park JW, Kim EK, Kim YB (2004): Estimation of the daily exposure of Koreans to aflatoxin B1 through food consumption. *Food Addit Contam.* 21:70–75.

Parry DW, Jenkinson P, McLeod L (1995): *Fusarium* ear blight (scab) in small grain cereals: a review. *Plant Pathol.* 44:207–238.

Pérez de Obanos A, González-Peñas E, López de Cerain A (2005): Influence of roasting and brew preparation on the ochratoxin A content in coffee infusion. *Food Addit Contam.* 22:463–471.

Pestka JJ, Smolinski AT (2005): Deoxynivalenol: toxicology and potential effects on humans. *J Toxicol Environ Health Pt B Crit Rev*. 8:39–69.

Pestka JJ, Zhou H-R, Moon Y, Chung YJ (2004): Cellular and molecular mechanisms for immune modulation by deoxynivalenol and other trichothecenes: unraveling a paradox. *Toxicol Lett*. 153:61–73.

Pfohl-Leszkowicz A, Manderville RA (2007): Ochratoxin A: an overview on toxicity and carcinogenicity in animals and humans. *Mol Nutr Food Res*. 51:61–99.

Pineda-Valdes G, Ryu D, Jackson DS, Bullerman LB (2002): Reduction of moniliformin during alkaline cooking of corn. *Cereal Chem*. 79:779–782.

Pineda-Valdes G, Ryu D, Hanna MA, Bullerman LB (2003): Reduction of moniliformin in corn by heat processing. *J Food Sci*. 68:1031–1035.

Pineiro M, Dawson R, Costarrica ML (1996): Monitoring program for mycotoxin contamination in Uruguayan food and feeds. *Nat Toxins*. 4:242–245.

Pitt JI (1987): *Penicillium viridicatum, Penicillium verrucosum,* and production of ochratoxin A. *Appl Environ Microbiol*. 53:266–269.

——— (2000): Toxigenic fungi: Which are important? *Med Mycol*. 38:17–22.

Pitt JI, Hocking AD (1999): *Fungi and Food Spoilage*, 2nd ed. Aspen Publishers, Gaithersburg, MD.

Pitt JI, Hocking AD, Glenn DR (1983): An improved medium for the detection of *Aspergillus flavus* and *A. parasiticus*. *J Appl Bacteriol*. 54:109–114.

Polling SM, Plattner RD, Weisleder D (2002): *N*-(1-Deoxy-D-fructos-1-yl)fumonisin B1, the initial reaction product of fumonisin B1 and D-glucose. *J Agric Food Chem*. 50:1318–1324.

Reed CR (2006): *Managing Stored Grain to Preserve Quality and Value*. AACC International, St. Paul, MN.

Rheeder JP, Marasas WFO, Thiel PG, Sydenham EW, Shephard GS, van Schalkwyk DJ (1992): *Fusarium moniliforme* and fumonisins in corn in relation to human esophageal cancer in Transkei. *Phytopathology*. 82:353–357.

Richter KS, Dorneanu E, Eskridge KM, Rao CS (1993): Microbiological quality of flours. *Cereal Foods World*. 38:367–369.

Russell L, Cox DF, Larsen G, Bodwell K, Nelson CE (1991): Incidence of molds and mycotoxins in commercial animal feed mills in seven midwestern states 1988–1989. *J Anim Sci*. 65:5–12.

Ryu D, Hanna MA, Bullerman LB (1999): Stability of zearalenone during extrusion of corn grits. *J Food Prot*. 62:1482–1484.

Sangare-Tigori B, Moukha S, Kouadio JH, et al. (2006): Ochratoxin A in human blood in Abidjan, Côte d'Ivoire. *Toxicon*. 47:894–900.

Sauer DB, Meronuck A, Christensen CM (1992): Microflora. In: Sauer DB (Ed.). *Storage of Cereal Grains and Their Products*, 4th ed. AACC International, St. Paul, MN, pp. 313–339.

Schoental R (1983): Precocious sexual development in Puerto Rico and oestrogenic mycotoxins (zearalenone). *Lancet*. 1:537.

Scudamore KA, Banks J, MacDonald SJ (2003): Fate of ochratoxin A in the processing of whole wheat grains during milling and bread production. *Food Addit Contam*. 20:1153–1163.

Thompson JM, Dodd CER, Waites WM (1993): Spoilage of bread by *Bacillus*. *Int Biodeterior Biodegrad*. 32:55–66.

Thrane U (1996): Comparison of three selective media for detecting *Fusarium* species in foods: a collaborative study. *Int J Food Microbiol*. 29:149–156.

Torres P, Guzmán-Ortiz M, Ramírez-Wong B (2001): Revising the role of pH and thermal treatments in aflatoxin content reduction during the tortilla and deep frying processes. *J Agric Food Chem*. 49:2825–2829.

Tóth B, Mesterházy A, Nicholson P, Téren J, Varga J (2004): Mycotoxin production and molecular variability of European and American isolates of *Fusarium culmorum*. *Eur J Plant Pathol*. 110:587–599.

Ueno Y (1984): Toxicological features of T-2 toxin and related thrichothecenes. *Fundam Appl Toxicol*. 4:S124–S132.

USFDA (U.S. Food and Drug Administration) (1993): Guidance for industry and FDA: letter to state agricultural directors, state feed control officials, and food, feed, and grain trade organizations. http://www.cfsan.fda.gov/~dms/graingui.html. Accessed May 2008.

——— (2000): Action levels for poisonous or deleterious substances in human food and animal feed. http://www.cfsan.fda.gov/~lrd/fdaact.html#afla. Accessed May 2008.

——— (2001): Guidance for industry: fumonisin levels in human foods and animal feeds. http://www.cfsan.fda.gov/~dms/fumongu2.html. Accessed May 2008.

Van Egmond HP (1989): Aflatoxin M1: occurrence, toxicity, regulation. In: van Egmond HP (Ed.). *Mycotoxins in Dairy Products*. Elsevier Applied Science, London, pp. 11–55.

Vesonder RF, Wu W (1998): Correlation of moniliformin, but not fumonisin B1 levels, in culture materials of *Fusarium* isolates to acute death in ducklings. *Poult Sci*. 77:67–72.

Vesonder RF, Golinski P, Plattner R, Zietkiewicz DL (1991): Mycotoxin formation by different geographic isolates of *Fusarium crookwellense*. *Mycopathologia*. 113:11–14.

Williams JH, Phillips TD, Jolly PE, Stiles JK, Jolly CM, Aggarwal D (2004): Human aflatoxicosis in developing countries: a review of toxicology, exposure, potential health consequences, and interventions. *Am J Clin Nutr*. 80:1106–1122.

Wogan GN (1975): Dietary factors and special epidemiological situations of liver cancer in Thailand and Africa. *Cancer Res*. 35:3499–3502.

Wood GE (1989): Aflatoxins in domestic and imported foods and feeds. *J AOAC*. 72:543–548.

Wood GE (1992): Mycotoxins in foods and feeds in the United States. *J. Anim Sci*. 70(12):3941–3949.

Yagen B, Joffe AZ (1976): Screening of toxic isolates of *Fusarium poae* and *Fusarium sporotrichioides* involved in causing alimentary toxic aleukia. *Appl Environ Microbiol*. 32:423–427.

Zinedine A, Soriano JM, Moltó JC, Mañes J (2007): Review on the toxicity, occurrence, metabolism, detoxification, regulations and intake of zearalenone: an oestrogenic mycotoxin. *Food Chem Toxicol*. 45:1–18.

CHAPTER 16

FOOD SAFETY ISSUES AND THE MICROBIOLOGY OF SPICES AND HERBS

KEITH A. ITO

16.1 INTRODUCTION

Spices have played an important role in the lives of people since ancient times. At one time spices were so valued that they were literally worth their weight in gold. They were of such value that only royalty or those who were very rich could afford them. They were valued for their antiseptic and preservative capabilities. The ancient Egyptians utilized cinnamon, cassia, and other spices for embalming purposes. Aromatic woods such as frankincense were burned as incense to purge unpleasant odors and fumigate homes. The ancient Chinese used cassia for medicinal purposes. A variety of herbs and spices were also much sought for their ability to add flavor and aroma to foods and beverages. Many of these were used to offset the flavors and aromas of spoilage and oxidation.

Today we find that spices and herbs come from many places in the world. Even though distances from area of production to area of use can still be far, the time required to bring the product from one area of the world to another is much shorter today than in ancient times. It is also far safer to transport than in ancient times.

Immigrants to the United States brought with them their culture, eating habits, and ethnic dishes. They brought spices and condiments to flavor their foods. As the populations of various immigrant groups have grown, the food and associated spices and flavorings have become more mainstream and readily available. In addition, with air travel, increases in leisure travel, and the worldwide nature of business, people are savoring the foods in their places of origin. We seem to enjoy these cultural experiences, and when we return we want to have similar authenticity when we go out to eat. This has added to the popularity of ethnic foods. Ethnicity has led not

Microbiologically Safe Foods, Edited by Norma Heredia, Irene Wesley, and Santos García

only to the generalization, but also to specific regionalizing of foods, such as not only Chinese food but, more specifically, Szechwan Chinese food.

People have become more health conscious in their eating habits. This can mean less salt, sugar, and fats in their foods. To help enhance the flavor and taste of foods while reducing or eliminating the salt, sugar, or fat, spices and herbs are added.

In addition to the flavor and aroma, which spices and herbs impart to food, there is also a perceived health benefit, as illustrated by garlic. Thus, instead of using one clove for the flavor and aroma, three, four, or more cloves may be used because of the perceived health benefits, such as its cardiovascular effects or potential for cancer reduction (Banerjee et al., 2006; Kris-Etherton et al., 2002).

What are herbs, spices, and condiments? There appear to be differences of opinion on the definition. *Webster's Dictionary* (1961) defines *spice* as any of various aromatic vegetable products used in cooking to season foods and to flavor foods. An *herb* is a seed-producing annual, biennial, or herbaceous perennial that does not develop persistent woody tissue but dies down at the end of the growing season; a plant or plant part valued for its medicinal, savory, or aromatic qualities. *Condiment* is an ingredient added to or served with food to enhance its flavor or to give it added flavor.

The U.S. Food and Drug Administration (USFDA, 2008) [21 CFR 101.22 (a)(2)] defines spice as any aromatic vegetable substance in the whole, broken, or ground form, except for those substances that have traditionally been regarded as foods, such as celery, onion, and garlic; whose significant function in foods is seasoning rather than nutritional. They also include a list of spices in this section and in 21 CFR 182.10 (USFDA, 2002b).

The International Commission on Microbiological Specifications for Foods (ICMSF, 1998) has broadly defined spices herbs and condiments as follows:

- *Spices*: any of various aromatic plant products used primarily to season, flavor, or impart aroma to foods
- *Herbs*: leafy parts of soft-stemmed plants
- *Condiments*: spices alone or blends of spices that have been formulated with other flavor adjuvants to enhance the flavor of foods

This broad definition seems to fit the current usage pattern of spices and herbs in the U.S. market. However, from a regulatory compliance standpoint, it is necessary to comply with the regulatory requirements.

16.2 USE OF SPICES AND HERBS IN FOODS

People are looking more and more to alternative health care to help them to prevent and relieve various ailments. As part of this trend, herbs have been found to be able to complement the more conventional modern approach to medicine. The conventional pharmaceutical companies as well as food processors have noticed this trend. The dietary supplement industry has grown rapidly to encompass some of these products. Dietary supplements used to be thought of as vitamin pills but now encompass a vast array of health and energy supplements. The food industry has provided new products in the "nutraceutical" and/or functional food category. Some of these have been foods supplemented with a variety of herbs and/or spices, purporting to have health and other benefits. However, because this is a subject in itself, we will not spend additional time on it but will concentrate on the use of spices and herbs as ingredients in foods for flavor and taste enhancement.

In the last five or more years, the use of fresh herbs has increased. Chefs are finding that the use of herbs enhances their dishes. It also enables them to produce new and different dishes so that they are able to expand their menus. The advent of popular cooking shows on television has exposed many consumers to the use of herbs and spices. It shows them how they can be used and the types of foods in which they can be used. The popularity of the home spice garden is fueled by these shows and by home gardening shows, which provide information on the ease with which such cultivation can be undertaken.

The commercial food processor has found that it is profitable to use spices and herbs. They have been able to provide more ethnically oriented specialties, they are getting greater acceptance from consumers for variously seasoned foods, processors have found that it can be a point of difference for their products, and there is pressure from consumers who want good-tasting foods that are low in salt, fat, and calories.

U.S. spice consumption has grown steadily over the last 20 years (ASTA, 2001). The current consumption is over a billion pounds a year, more than a 30% increase from 10 years ago. The current per capita consumption is about 4 pounds per year, which is a 50% increase in consumption from 20 years ago and about a 25% increase from 10 years ago. Table 1, which lists the 12 major spices by volume, shows that garlic and onion are the largest, nearly double the volume of the second product, mustard seed. The list also indicates that peppers in total have the highest volume of any spice, except for the combination of garlic and onion. Seven countries provide 84% of the spices consumed by volume (ASTA, 2001). Of this amount, the United States provides 39%, and the other countries, lesser amounts. Countries provide a number of different products; for example, India has 19 different products and Mexico, 10. The value of imported spices is considerable and in general has increased over the last 4 years (USDA-FAS, 2002). Garlic imports are valued at about $250 million and the value has increased about 100% in the last 4 years. On the other hand, cinnamon is valued at $31 million and has decreased in value about 50% in the last 4 years. Cloves have the most increase on the list, but it started with a smaller base and the total value of the import is only $6.6 million.

16.3 ANTIMICROBIAL EFFECTS

Spices and herbs are of interest to microbiologists for several reasons, including the fact that they exhibit antimicrobial activity (Shan et al., 2007). They normally

TABLE 1 Top 12 Spices by Volume, 2000

Spice	Thousands of Pounds[a]	Major Suppliers[b]
Dehydrated onion/garlic	321,171	United States, China
Mustard seed	172,494	Canada, United States
Red pepper	109,416	United States, India, Mexico, China
Sesame seed	108,133	Guatemala, India, Mexico, Venezuela
Black pepper	102,495	Indonesia, India, Brazil
Paprika	52,771	United States, Spain, Chile
Cinnamon	37,022	Indonesia, Sri Lanka, Vietnam
Cumin seed	17,234	Syria, Turkey, India
White pepper	16,113	Indonesia, Malaysia, China
Oregano	14,522	Turkey, Mexico, Greece
Poppy seed	11,682	Australia, the Netherlands, Turkey
Ginger	10,894	China, India, Nigeria
Total	973,947	

Source: ASTA (2001).
[a] Includes domestic production as well as imports.
[b] In order of volume supplied.

contain large numbers of microorganisms, they can spoil the spice or herb or products to which they are added, and they have been associated with food-poisoning incidents.

Normally, spices are not added to foods because of their antimicrobial properties; they are added primarily for the flavor and aroma they impart to the food. The use of spices and herbs as antimicrobials is challenging due to the complexity of the interaction with the food, the various factors that influence preservation, and the various chemical and sensory effects associated with specific spices and herbs and their mixtures.

As noted earlier, spices are regulated, by the FDA as a food. If the intent of the addition of the spice or herb is to act as an antimicrobial, it may need to be regulated under a different section of the FDA regulation, the section dealing with preservatives. There is then a need to prove effectiveness, toxicity, use concentrations, and so on.

The scientific literature describes the antimicrobial properties of spices. The amount of microbial inhibition depends on a variety of factors, including the type of food in which the testing occurred, the concentration of the spice in the media, and the manner in which the spice was added to the medium and the type of organism against which the spice was tested. Thus, it is very difficult to compare the results of various studies to reach a conclusion on the specific concentration needed to act effectively as a microbial inhibitor.

Based on published studies, there is general consensus that most herbs and spices do not possess sufficient antimicrobial activity to exert any effect at concentrations used in foods. The antimicrobial effect of spices and herbs is due in part to the presence of essential oils (Burt, 2004). The nature of essential oils varies from spice to spice as well as within the same spice. The amount present is dependent on a number of factors, including how the spice is grown, where it is grown, and the conditions under

TABLE 2 Allspice[a]

Antimicrobial Concentrate			
Spice (%)	Essential Oil (ppm)	Organism	Reference
		S. cerevisiae	Conner and Beuchat, 1984
		S. Typhimurium	Karapinar and Aktuğ, 1987
		V. parahaemolyticus	Karapinar and Aktuğ, 1987
2		*P. citrinum*	Azzouz and Bullerman, 1982
	2	*C. botulinum*	Huhtanen, 1980
0.5		Various gram-negative and gram-positive vegetative cells	

[a]The essential oil in whole spice is 3 to 5% and the antimicrobial compound is eugenol (80%).

which it is grown. Some of the antimicrobial essential oils of spices are well known and have been utilized in studies to determine their antimicrobial effect.

Based on a review of a number of studies, Zaika (1988) classified a number of spices into strong, moderate, and weak microbial inhibitors. Cinnamon, clove, mustard, and garlic are considered to be strong inhibitors, while pepper and ginger are weak inhibitors. A number of other spices are considered moderate inhibitors, and some of this is dependent on the concentration of the essential oil in the spice tested. Conner and Beuchat (1984) screened 32 essential oils against various yeasts and also found that cinnamon, allspice, and cloves were among the most inhibitory materials tested.

We have summarized some of the studies involving three of these strong inhibitors and three of the moderate inhibitors. In general, the results are variable, depending on the organism tested and the method used for the test.

In allspice (Table 2), Conner and Beuchat (1984) used a standard zone of inhibition test in yeast–malt extract–peptone–glucose agar with 95% ethanol solutions of the essential oil placed on a sensi-disk on a spread plate of yeast cells. They found that 100 ppm inhibited *S. cerevisiae* and *R. rubra*, but not several other yeast species. Karapinar and Aktuğ (1987) added ethanol solutions of the essential oil to nutrient agar for *S. typhimurium* growth and tryptic soy agar with 3% salt for the determination of *V. parahaemolyticus* growth. They found 100 ppm to inhibit the growth of *S. typhimurium* and 50 ppm to inhibit the growth of *S. aureus*. Shelef et al. (1980) tested dried spices added to the growth medium, nutrient agar, or tryticase soy agar with 3% salt. Various gram-positive and gram-negative vegetative cells were tested. About 0.5% of the dried spice was required for inhibition. Azzouz and Bullerman (1982) used ground spices added to potato dextrose agar to determine the effect upon various molds. *P. citrinum* was inhibited at 2%, whereas a number of other molds were not inhibited at that amount. Huhtanen (1980) used an alcoholic extract of dried spices in an assay medium to determine inhibition against *C. botulinum*, and he found that 2000 ppm was needed for the inhibition.

TABLE 3 Clove[a]

Antimicrobial Concentrate			
Spice (%)	Essential Oil (ppm)	Organism	Reference
	100	*R. rubra*	Conner and Beuchat, 1984
2		*Aspergillus, Penicillium*	Azzouz and Bullerman, 1982
	250	*A. parasiticus*	Bullerman et al., 1977
	500	*Aspergillus*	Hitokoto et al., 1980
	100	S. Typhimurium	Karapinar and Aktuğ, 1987
	50	*V. parahaemolyticus*	Karapinar and Aktuğ, 1987
	500	*C. botulinum*	Huhtanen, 1980
	150	*C. botulinum* B	Ismaiel and Pierson, 1990
0.5	500	*C. botulinum* A	Ueda et al., 1982
1.0	1000	*B. cereus, B. subtilis*	Ueda et al., 1982

[a]The essential oil in whole spice is 17% and the antimicrobial compound is eugenol (93%).

In cloves (Table 3), Conner and Beuchat (1984) showed inhibition of *R. rubra* with 100 ppm of essential oil. Azzouz and Bullerman (1982) attained inhibition of *Penicillium* and *Aspergillus* species with 2% ground spice. Bullerman et al. (1977) added essential oil to yeast extract with sucrose and found that 200 to 250 ppm inhibited *Aspergillus parasiticus*. Hitokoto et al. (1980) obtained essential oil by steam distillation from powdered spices. These were suspended in ethanol for testing on potato dextrose agar. They found 500 ppm to be inhibitory to several *Aspergillus* species. Karapinar and Aktuğ (1987) found 100 ppm inhibitory to *S. typhimurium,* and 50 ppm inhibitory to *V. parahaemolyticus*. Huhtanen (1980) found 500 ppm of spice extract to inhibit *C. botulinum*. Ismaiel and Pierson (1990) used essential oils in ethanol in thiotone yeast extract glucose medium and found 150 ppm to be inhibitory to *C. botulinum* type B. Ueda et al. (1982) used powdered spice as well as essential oils in ethanol for their tests in trypticase soy broth for *B. cereus* and trypticase–peptone–glucose–yeast extract broth for *C. botulinum*. With essential oils, they found that 500 ppm inhibited *C. botulinum* type A, and 1000 ppm inhibited *B. cereus*. With the powdered spices, 0.5% was needed to inhibit *C. botulinum* type A, and 1% was needed to inhibit *B. cereus*.

In cinnamon (Table 4), Conner and Beuchat (1984) showed inhibition of *R. rubra* at 100 ppm. Azzouz and Bullerman (1982) had inhibition of *Penicillium* at 2% ground spices. Bullerman et al. (1977) had inhibition of *A. parasiticus* at 200 ppm of essential oil. Huhtanen (1980) had inhibition of *C. botulinum* at 2000 ppm using a spice extract, while Ismaiel and Pierson (1990) using essential oil had inhibition of *C. botulinum* type B at 100 ppm, and Ueda et al. (1982) using powdered spices had inhibition at 1%, while with essential oil they had inhibition of *C. botulinum* type A at 130 ppm. They also had inhibition of *B. cereus* at at 4% using spice powders and at 500 ppm using essential oil.

In garlic (Table 5), Conner and Beuchat (1984) found *R. rubra* and *S. cerevisiae* to be inhibited by 25 ppm. Kyung et al. (1996) placed crushed garlic into tryptic soy

TABLE 4 Cinnamon Bark[a]

Antimicrobial Concentrate			
Spice (%)	Essential Oil (ppm)	Organism	Reference
	100	*R. rubra*	Conner and Beuchat, 1984
2		*Penicillium*	Azzouz and Bullerman, 1982
	200	*A. parasiticus*	Bullerman et al., 1977
	2000	*C. botulinum*	Huhtanen, 1980
	100	*C. botulinum* B	Ismaiel and Pierson, 1990
0.5–1.0	130	*C. botulinum* A	Ueda et al., 1982
4	500	*B. cereus, B. subtilis*	Ueda et al., 1982

[a]The essential oil in whole spice is 0.9 to 2.3% and the antimicrobial compound is cinnamic aldehyde (65 to 75%).

broth or yeast extract–malt extract–peptone–glucose broth. They also used a water solution of methyl methanethiosulfonate (MMTSO), a thiol inhibitor, which acts like allicin in the media. *S. cerevisiae* was inhibited by 40 ppm MMTSO. Inhibition was also achieved with 1% garlic extract. With *L. mesenteroides* and *L. plantarum*, inhibition was achieved with 100 ppm and 20 ppm of MMTSO, respectively. It took 10% garlic extract to inhibit *L. mesenteroides*. Karaioannoglou et al. (1977) prepared a water extract of garlic and placed it into brain heart infusion broth. They found that a 1% extract inhibited *L. plantarum*. Kyung et al. (1996) found *S. aureus* to be inhibited by 40 ppm MMTSO and 1% garlic extract. Mantis et al. (1978), using a water extract of garlic placed into brain heart infusion broth, found *S. aureus* to be inhibited by 5% garlic extract. Dababneh and Al-Delaimy (1984), using garlic extract

TABLE 5 Garlic[a]

Antimicrobial Concentrate			
Spice (%)	Essential Oil (ppm)	Organism	Reference
	25	*R. rubra, S. cerevisiae*	Conner and Beuchat, 1984
	40	*S. cerevisiae*	Kyung et al., 1996
10	100	*L. mesenteroides*	Kyung et al., 1996
	20	*L. plantarum*	Kyung et al., 1996
1		*L. plantarum*	Karaioannoglou et al., 1977
1	40	*S. aureus*	Kyung et al., 1996
5		*S. aureus*	Mantis et al., 1978
1		*S. aureus*	Dababneh and Al-Delaimy, 1984
5		*S.* Typhimurium	Juven et al., 1994
5		*B. cereus*	Saleem and Al-Delaimy, 1982
	>2000	*C. botulinum*	Huhtanen, 1980
	100	*C. botulinum* B	Ismaiel and Pierson, 1990
	1500	*C. botulinum* A	DeWit et al., 1979

[a]The essential oil in whole spice is 0.2% and the antimicrobial compounds are diallyl trisulfide (20%) and diallyl disulfide (60%).

TABLE 6 Oregano[a]

Antimicrobial Concentrate			
Spice (%)	Essential Oil (ppm)	Organism	Reference
	100	*R. rubra*	Conner and Beuchat, 1984
1		*B. cereus, B. subtilis*	Ueda et al., 1982
	15–20	*B. cereus*	Ultee et al., 1999
0.5		*C. botulinum* A	Ueda et al., 1982
	500	*C. botulinum*	Huhtanen, 1980
	100	*C. botulinum* B	Ismaiel and Pierson, 1990

[a]The essential oil in whole spice is 0.2 to 0.8% and the antimicrobial compounds are thymol and carvacrol (60 to 85%).

and mannitol salt agar plates, found *S. aureus* to be inhibited at 1% garlic extract. Johnson and Vaughn (1969) used powdered garlic in saline solution and found that 5% caused inhibition of *S.* Typhimurium. Saleem and Al-Delaimy (1982) used a water extract of garlic in nutrient agar to determine that *B. cereus* was inhibited at a concentration of 5%. Huhtanen (1980) found that more than 2000 ppm was required to inhibit *C. botulinum,* while Ismaiel and Pierson (1990) found that 100 ppm inhibited *C. botulinum* type B. DeWit et al. (1979) placed garlic oil in a meat slurry and found that 1500 ppm inhibited *C. botulinum* types A, but not types B and E.

For oregano (Table 6), Conner and Beuchat (1984) found 100 ppm inhibitory to *R. rubra*. Ueda et al. (1982) found that 1% spice extract was inhibitory to *B. cereus* and *B. subtilis*. Ultee et al. (1999) used an ethanol solution of oil in buffer solution with plating on brain heart infusion to determine the inhibition. They found that 15 to 20 ppm inhibited *B. cereus*. Ueda et al. (1982) found 0.5% spice extract to inhibit *C. botulinum* type A, while Huhtanen (1980) found that 500 ppm was needed, and Ismaiel and Pierson (1990) found *C. botulinum* type B to be inhibited by 100 ppm.

With thyme (Table 7), Hitokoto et al. (1980) found that 400 ppm inhibited *A. flavus*. Conner and Beuchat (1984) found that 100 ppm inhibited *S. cerevisiae* and *R. rubra*. Karapinar and Aktuğ (1987) found that 25 ppm inhibited *S. aureus* and that 75 ppm inhibited *V. parahaemolyticus*. Juven et al. (1994) used a water solution of the essential oil in nutrient agar plates and found that *S.* Typhimurium inhibited by 175 ppm. Kim et al. (1995) found 250 ppm to inhibit *S.* Typhimurium. Ueda et al (1982) found that 2% inhibited *B. cereus* and *B. subtilis*, while Ultee et al. (1999) found that 15 to 20 ppm of essential oil inhibited *B. cereus*. Ueda et al. (1982) also found that 0.5% of spice was needed to inhibit *C. botulinum* type A, while Huhtanen (1980) found that 500 ppm of spice extract inhibited *C. botulinum*, and Ismaiel and Pierson (1990) found that 100 ppm of the oil inhibited *C. botulinum* type B.

Thus, one can see that there is quite a bit of variability in the antimicrobial quality of spices. There is variation depending on species and within species and by test procedures. Because of this variability, a considerable amount of additional work will need to be done if the antimicrobial characteristic of the spice is to be used as a specific inhibitor for microorganisms in food.

TABLE 7 Thyme[a]

Antimicrobial Concentrate			
Spice (%)	Essential Oil (ppm)	Organism	Reference
	400	*Aspergillis*	Huhtanen, 1980
	100	*R. rubra, S. cerevisiae*	Conner and Beuchat, 1984
	25	*S. aureus*	Karapinar and Aktuğ, 1987
	75	*V. parahaemolyticus*	Karapinar and Aktuğ, 1987
	175	*S. typhimurium*	Juven et al., 1994
	250	*S. typhimurium*	Kim et al., 1995
2		*B. cereus, B subtilus*	Ueda et al., 1982
	15–20	*B. cereus*	Ultee et al., 1999
0.5		*C. botulinum* A	Ueda et al., 1982
	500	*C. botulinum*	Huhtanen, 1980
	100	*C. botulinum* B	Ismaiel and Pierson, 1990

[a]The essential oil in whole spice is 2.5% and the antimicrobial compounds are thymol and carvacrol (40 to 45%).

16.4 CONTAMINATION OF SPICES AND HERBS

Spices and herbs are agricultural products that are grown and harvested similar to other agricultural products. They can become contaminated with the microorganisms, which are normally present in the environment. In addition, they can become contaminated with other environmental contaminants, such as insects, feces, and other material from rodents and birds, dust and other extraneous material. Water, which is used for irrigation and/or washing, can also be a source of contamination. Spices and herbs are often grown in areas that are conducive to the growth of microorganism. They are most often found in tropical or subtropical areas of the world. In addition, the many steps involved in the harvesting, handling, and transportation of spices and herbs provide ample opportunities for contamination (De Boer et al., 1985; McKee, 1995).

Studies in different countries on the microbiology of herbs and spices have demonstrated the presence in these products of important and potential foodborne bacteria and toxigenic molds, including *Salmonella*, *Escherichia coli*, *Clostridium perfringens*, *Bacillus cereus*, and aflatoxigenic *Aspergillus* (for example, USFDA, 2002a). Furthermore, herbs and spices may introduce potential food spoilage organisms to a range of food types (Aguilera et al., 2005; García et al., 2001). Fungi are the predominant contaminants of spices, but such microbial populations are probably regarded as commensal residents on the plant that survived drying and storage.

Spices are often contaminated with mycotoxins. Of the different mycotoxins, aflatoxin is the most common contaminant in spices. Aflatoxin contamination of ground red pepper has been reported in several countries such as Ethiopia, Italy, Korea, Turkey, and Portugal, where 5 to 43% of the samples had concentrations ranging from 0.8 to 525 μg/kg (Cho et al., 2008; Fazekas et al., 2005; Romagnoli et al., 2007).

TABLE 8 Microbial Contamination of Spices

Spice	Untreated[a] APC (CFU/g)	Australia[b] APC (CFU/g)	Austria[c] APC (CFU/g)	Mexico[d] APC (CFU/g)
Allspice	10^3–10^7		10^6	
Bay	<10–10^7			<10^2–10^7
Cinnamon	<10–10^7	<10–10^6	10^3–10^5	
Cloves	<10–10^6	<10–10^3	10^4	
Garlic	10^3–10^7	10^3–10^6	10^4	10^3–10^8
Oregano	<10–10^7	10^2–10^6	10^6	<10^2–10^7
Pepper				
Black	10^3–>10^7	10^6–>10^8	10^7	10^4–10^8
White	10^3–>10^7	10^4–10^7	10^2–10^5	
Thyme	10^3–10^7		10^6	

From [a]ICMSF (1998).
From [b]Pafumi (1986).
From [c]Kneifel and Berger (1994).
From [d]Garcia et al. (2001).

Microbial counts can vary over a wide range, depending on the spice, where it is harvested, and how it is handled during harvesting, processing, and transportation. At time of use, the microbial load is dependent on the original load, the ability to control the growth during the handling, and any die-off or killing that has occurred during processing. Thus, for any one type of spice or herb, the microbial count can vary widely.

Some examples of aerobic plate counts (APC) obtained are shown in Table 8. The untreated numbers are for spices not treated with any agents or procedures designed to reduce the viable number of microorganisms and represent a composite of numbers from various regions of the world. The numbers from the specific areas of the world represent samples from retail taken in the country noted. The numbers of organisms represent a broad range and appear similar despite the sampling in different parts of the world.

Burnett and Beuchat (2001) compared sample preparation methods in recovering *Salmonella* from raw fruits, vegetables, and herbs. They found that preparation procedure did not influence the number of *salmonellae* recovered. Regardless of the preparation procedure used, the recovery from herbs was always less than from fruits and vegetables. They attributed this in part to the antimicrobials released from the herbs during the preparation procedure.

The U.S. Food and Drug Administration (USFDA-CFSAN, 2001) has completed and published a survey of imported produce items. The survey, begun in 1999, included a number of items of fresh produce. Among the samples taken were some fresh herbs. The survey determined the presence of certain pathogens, including *E. coli* 0157:H7, *Salmonella,* and *Shigella*. The USFDA (USFDA-CFSAN, 2001) also began a survey of domestic produce in 2000. Partial results of that study are available. The results indicate that pathogens are present on the fresh produce in small but significant numbers. The contamination is present on both domestic and imported products.

16.5 RECALLS AND OUTBREAKS

The potential presence of pathogens on spices and herbs could cause potential health consequences (USFDA-CFSAN, 2002a). In 2002 the FDA had a number of recalls of various spices because of their contamination with pathogens (Vij et al., 2006). The usual contamination with dried spices has been *Salmonella*. However, *Listeria* contamination of a fresh bay leaf resulted in a recall of that product.

A summary of some of the recent food poisoning outbreaks (CDC, 1997) involving herbs and spices show that a number of different vehicles were involved. The outbreaks involved a variety of organisms, and the case size involves a few to a great many people. Some of these cases involve a single incident, and others involve a large number.

Some recent outbreaks in the United States involving primarily fresh herbs have caused some major problems. An outbreak of cyclosporiasis involving over 300 cases occurred in 1997 (CDC, 1999). The outbreak involved two states and the District of Columbia. Fresh basil was implicated as the cause of the infection. A company, that catered food and had a number of stores, each with a retail outlet and a production kitchen, was implicated. People involved complained of diarrhea, nausea, vomiting, and/or abdominal cramps. The incubation period was anywhere from 1 to 14 days, with a median of 8 days. The illness lasted 1 to 10 days, with a median of 5 days. Laboratory confirmation from stools was obtained.

An outbreak of *Shigella sonnei* was observed on parsley (Campbell et al., 2001). The outbreak occurred from July through August 1998. Almost 500 people in four states and two Canadian provinces were involved, and they had diarrhea or loose stools accompanied by fever. Incubation time for the onset of illness is about 2 to 4 days. There was laboratory confirmation of the organism in stool samples. PFGE analysis confirmed that in five of the locations, similar patterns were identified. The food was served primarily in restaurants, although other locations, such as a food fair, were implicated. The vehicle was uncooked parsley. Tracebacks showed that the product could have been imported or could have come from domestic farms. An investigation of one of the farms showed poor water quality and poor sanitation practices by workers due to inadequate sanitary facilities. Investigation also found that the parsley was usually washed before preparation. However, the parsley was usually chopped in the morning, left at room temperature, then used during the day.

An outbreak of *Salmonella* Thompson was observed on cilantro (Campbell et al., 2001). The outbreak occurred in March 1999 in one state. Approximately 40 people had diarrhea, nausea, vomiting, and abdominal cramps. The incubation period was usually 8 to 72 hours, and the illness was usually of short duration, lasting 2 to 5 days. Laboratory confirmation by stool culture and PFGE analysis helped confirmed the organism. *S.* Thompson is not an organism usually found in food-poisoning incidences. The cilantro was served in restaurants usually as part of a fresh salsa. Traceback studies were not able to determine all of the farms from which the product was obtained. From some of the records available, it was determined that some of the product was imported. All of the restaurants involved washed the cilantro and chopped the product with a knife. The chopped product was held from 1 to 7 days after chopping. The restaurants all indicated that the product was held under refrigeration until use.

Wu et al. (2000) studied the growth of *S. sonnei* on parsley. They found that whole leaves inoculated with 10^3 CFU/g had an increase of about 1 log within 1 day at 21°C, whereas chopped parsley with the same inoculum level increased 3 log within 2 days at 21°C. When held at 4°C the number of organisms decreased slowly with time. However, less than a 1-log decrease was observed over 4 days, and survivors were still found after 14 days.

Campbell et al. (2001) studied the growth of *S.* Thompson on cilantro. They found that whole leaves held at room temperature increase about 1 log when inoculated with 10^4 CFU/g within 2 days, whereas chopped cilantro with the same inoculum increased 3 log within only one day when incubated at 26°C. No growth was observed when the cilantro was held at 4°C.

16.6 CONTROL PROCEDURES

Herbs and spices are agricultural products that are consumed with minimal processing and often are consumed fresh. Thus, the producers of these products should be looked upon as food processors, not just as growers of agricultural products. Because it is important to control contamination from farm to table, all entities along the food chain need to do their part to minimize contamination of the food. One way to do this is through good agricultural practices (GAPs) (ICMSF, 1998). The agricultural industry provided a guidance document in the summer of 1997. This was followed by voluntary guidelines from the U.S. Food and Drug Administration in 1998 (USFDA-CFSAN, 1998). The guidance was designed to help improve food safety from farm to table. The guidance is based on seven basic principles:

1. Prevent contamination rather than correct following contamination.
2. Minimize food safety hazards and practice good agricultural and management practices.
3. Fresh produce can be contaminated at any point in the food chain.
4. Water quality dictates contamination potential.
5. Animal manure or municipal biosolid wastes should be used with care.
6. Worker hygiene and sanitation practices are critical.
7. Follow all applicable laws and regulations.

Implementation of these practices on the farm and by produce buyers and distributors will assist greatly in improving the overall food safety of the foods we consume. In addition, there is a need for good record keeping of where the product was grown and who distributed what product to whom. Without this type of information, product traceback in case of illness is difficult.

The use of hazard analysis of critical control points (HACCP) is important to be able to evaluate the potential safety hazards present during many of the steps involved in bringing the product from farm to table. The use of HACCP principles makes it possible to evaluate areas that are critical to food safety. Hazard analysis is a critical step in this process. As part of the process, limits need to be determined and set for the process. A critical step needs to be operated within known limits. Once the limits are set, procedures need to be in place so that operation within the limits can be verified. The limits also need to be validated periodically. If the limits are not being met, a deviation has occurred and the deviation needs to be corrected. If this correction requires a change in the plan, such a change needs to be documented appropriately.

If one were to look at the parsley incident, one would note that two areas of concern would be the washing of the parsley and the keeping of the chopped parsley for an extended period of time at room temperature. Washing the parsley in good-quality water will help in removing contaminants. Wu et al. (2000) found that washing the parsley in a dilute solution of vinegar or in chlorinated water (>150 ppm) greatly reduced the contamination with *S. sonnei*. As noted earlier, they also found that growth of *S. sonnei* on chopped parsley occurred rapidly at room temperature but not at refrigeration temperatures. They also found that growth occurred slowly on whole parsley. Thus, washing the parsley in chlorinated water and keeping it uncut in the refrigerator until use would greatly reduce the probability of a food-poisoning incident.

Similarly, a strategy for reducing the probability for cilantro would indicate that cilantro should not be cut until ready for use, and that it should be refrigerated to retard growth of *S.* Thompson. Additionally, studies by Brandl and Mandrell (2002) showed that *S.* Thompson had the ability to colonize the surface of cilantro leaves. Thus, contamination of the cilantro during growth or harvest could play a role in food safety. This emphasizes the need for good agricultural practices as an important feature in the food safety chain from farm to table.

16.7 CONCLUSIONS

Spices and herbs are growing in use. Their growth is based on the concept that they provide flavor and aroma to foods and are good for you. Although they have some antimicrobial properties, the basis for their use in foods is the flavor and aroma that they provide. There is natural contamination which if not controlled could provide a vehicle for spoilage or illness to occur. There are procedures such as GAP and/or HACCP, which can help to maintain and improve food safety in the food chain. To be able to sell product in the current environment, it will be necessary to provide a consistent quality product that meets food safety requirements.

REFERENCES

Aguilera MO, Stagnitta PV, Micalizzi B, Stefanini de Guzmán AM (2005): Prevalence and characterization of *Clostridium perfringens* from spices in Argentina. *Anaerobe.* 11:327–334.

ASTA (American Spice Trade Association) (2001): *The American Spice Trade Association Report Spice Statistics 2000*. ASTA, Washington, DC.

Azzouz MA, Bullerman LB (1982): Comparative antimycotic effects of selected herbs, spices, plant components and commercial antifungal agents. *J Food Prot.* 45:1298–1301.

Banerjee S, KrPanda Ch, Das S (2006): Clove (*Syzygium aromaticum* L.), a potential chemopreventive agent for lung cancer. *Carcinogenesis.* 27:1645–1654.

Brandl MT, Mandrell RE (2002): Fitness of *Salmonella enterica* serovar Thompson in the cilantro phyllosphere. *Appl Environ Microbiol.* 68:3614–3621.

Bullerman LB, Lieu FY, Seier SA (1977): Inhibition of growth and aflatoxin production by cinnamon and clove oils: cinnamic aldehyde and eugenol. *J Food Sci.* 42:1107–1116.

Burnett AB, Beuchat LR (2001): Comparison of sample preparation methods for recovering *Salmonella* from raw fruits, vegetables, and herbs. *J Food Prot.* 64:1459–1465.

Burt S (2004): Essential oils: their antibacterial properties and potential applications in foods—a review. *Int J Food Microbiol.* 94:223–253.

Campbell JV, Mohle-Boetani J, Reporter R, et al. (2001): An outbreak of *Salmonella* serotype Thompson associated with fresh cilantro. *J Infect Dis.* 183:984–987.

CDC (Centers for Disease Control and Prevention) (1997): Outbreak of cyclosporiasis—northern Virginia–Washington, D.C.–Baltimore, Maryland, metropolitan area, 1997. *MMWR Morb Mortal Wkly Rep.* 46:689–691.

——— (1999): Outbreaks of *Shigella sonnei* infection associated with eating fresh parsley—United States and Canada, July–August 1998. *MMWR Morb Mortal Wkly Rep.* 48:285–289.

Cho SH, Lee CH, Jang MR, et al. (2008): Aflatoxins contamination in spices and processed spice products commercialized in Korea. *Food Chem.* 107:1283–1288.

Conner DE, Beuchat LR (1984): Effects of essential oils from plants on growth of food spoilage yeasts. *J Food Sci.* 49:429–434.

Dababneh BFA, Al-Delaimy KS (1984): Inhibition of *Staphylococcus aureus* by garlic extracts. *Lebensm Wiss Technol.* 17:29–31.

De Boer E, Spiegelenberg WM, Janssen FW (1985): Microbiology of spices and herbs. *Antonie Van Leeuwenhoek.* 51:435–438.

DeWit JC, Notermans S, Gorin N, Kampelmacher EH (1979): Effect of garlic oil or onion oil on toxin production by *Clostridium botulinum* in meat slurry. *J Food Prot.* 42:222–224.

Fazekas B, Tar A, Kovacs M (2005): Aflatoxin and ochratoxin A content of spices in Hungary. *Food Addit Contam.* 22:856–863.

García S, Iracheta F, Galvan F, Heredia N (2001): Microbiological survey of retail herbs and spices from Mexican markets. *J Food Prot.* 64:99–103.

Hitokoto H, Morozumi S, Wauke T, Sakai S, Kurata H (1980): Inhibitory effects of spices on growth and toxin production of toxigenic fungi. *Appl Environ Microbiol.* 39:808–822.

Huhtanen CN (1980): Inhibition of *Clostridium botulinum* by spice extracts and aliphatic alcohols. *J Food Prot.* 43:195–196.

ICMSF (International Commission on Microbiological Specifications for Foods) (1998): *Microorganisms in Foods*, Vol. 6, *Microbial Ecology of Food Commodities*. Blackie Academic and Professional, London.

Ismaiel AA, Pierson MD (1990): Inhibition of germination, outgrowth, and vegetative growth of *Clostridium botulinum* 67B by spice oils. *J Food Prot.* 53:755–758.

Johnson MG, Vaughn RH (1969): Death of *Salmonella typhimurium* and *Escherichia coli* in the presence of freshly reconstituted dehydrated garlic and onion. *Appl Microbiol.* 17 (6): 903–905.

Juven BJ, Kanner J, Schved F, Weisslowicz H (1994): Factors that interact with the antibacterial action of thyme essential oil and its active constituents. *J Appl Bacteriol.* 76: 626–631.

Karaioannoglou PG, Mantis JW, Panetsos AG (1977): The effect of garlic extract on lactic acid bacteria (*Lactobacillus plantarum*) in culture media. *Lebensm Wiss Technol.* 10:148–150.

Karapinar M, Aktuğ ŞE (1987): Inhibition of foodborne pathogens by thymol, eugenol, menthol and anethole. *Int J Food Microbiol.* 4:161–166.

Kim JM, Marshall MR, Cornell JA, Preston JF III, Wei CI (1995): Antibacterial activity of carvacrol, citral, and geraniol against *Salmonella typhimurium* in culture medium and on fish cubes. *J Food Sci.* 60:1364–1374.

Kneifel W, Berger E (1994): Microbiological criteria of random samples of spices and herbs retailed on the Austrian market. *J Food Prot.* 57:893–901.

Kris-Etherton PM, Hecker KD, Bonanome A, et al. (2002): Bioactive compounds in foods: their role in the prevention of cardiovascular disease and cancer. *Am J Med.* 113: 71–88.

Kyung KH, Park KS, Kim YS (1996): Isolation and characterization of bacteria resistant to the antimicrobial activity of garlic. *J Food Sci.* 61:226–229.

Mantis AJ, Karaioannoglou PG, Spanos GP, Panetsos AG (1978): The effect of garlic extract on food poisoning bacteria in culture media *I. Staphylococcus aureus*. *Lebensm Wiss Technol.* 11:26–28.

McKee LH (1995): Microbial contamination of spices and herbs: a review. *LWT-Food Sci Technol.* 28:1–11.

Pafumi J (1986): Assessment of the microbiological quality of spices and herbs. *J Food Prot.* 49:958–963.

Romagnoli B, Menna V, Gruppioni N, Bergamini C (2007): Aflatoxins in spices, aromatic herbs, herb-teas and medicinal plants marketed in Italy. *Food Control.* 18:697–701.

Saleem ZM, Al-Delaimy KS (1982): Inhibition of *Bacillus cereus* by garlic extracts. *J Food Prot.* 45:1007–1009.

Shan B Cai YZ Brooks JD Corke H (2007): The in vitro antibacterial activity of dietary spice and medicinal herb extracts. *Int J Food Microbiol.* 117:112–119.

Shelef LA, Naglik OA, Bogen DW (1980): Sensitivity of some common foodborne bacteria to the spices sage, rosemary, and allspice. *J Food Sci.* 45:1042–1044.

Ueda S, Yamashita H, Kuwabara Y (1982): Inhibition of *Clostridium botulinum* and *Bacillus* sp. by spices and flavouring compounds. *Nippon Shokuhin Kogyo Gakkaishi.* 29:389–392.

Ultee A, Kets EPW, Smid EJ (1999): Mechanisms of action of carvacrol on the food-borne pathogen *Bacillus cereus*. *Appl Environ Microbiol.* 65:4606–4610.

USFDA (U.S. Food and Drug Administration) (2002a): *Enforcement report, recalls, and field corrections: foods–class I.* www.fda.gov/bbs/topics/enforce/2002/enf00762.html. Accessed May 2008.

——— (2002b): CFR 21 182.10. Spices and other natural seasonings and flavorings. http://edocket.access.gpo.gov/cfr_2002/aprqtr/21cfr182.10.htm. Accessed May 2008.

——— (2008): Foods; labeling of spices, flavorings, colorings and chemical preservatives. Electronic Code of Federal Regulations, 21 CFR 101.22. http://ecfr.gpoaccess.gov/cgi/t/text/text-idx?c=ecfr&sid=37c16f32511a18ed0d0f22743dd35d85&rgn=div8&view=text&node=21:2.0.1.1.2.2.1.1&idno=21. Accessed May 2008.

USFDA-CFSAN (U.S. Food and Drug Administration–Center for Food Safety and Applied Nutrition) (1998): *Guide to Minimize Microbial Food Safety Hazards for Fresh Fruits and Vegetables*. HFS-342. Food Safety Initiative Staff, USFDA, Washington, DC.

——— (2001): FDA survey of imported fresh produce FY 1999 field assignment. Office of Plant and Dairy Foods and Beverages. http://www.cfsan.fda.gov/. Accessed October 2003.

USDA-FAS (U.S. Department of Agriculture–Foreign Agricultural Service) (2002): FASonline. http://www.fas.usda.gov/ustrade/. Accessed June 2008.

Vij V, Ailes E, Wolyniak C, Angulo FJ, Klontz KC (2006): Recalls of spices due to bacterial contamination monitored by the U.S. Food and Drug Administration: the predominance of salmonellae. *J Food Prot*. 69:233–237.

Webster's Third New International Dictionary (1961): Merriam-Webster, Springfield, MA.

Wu FM, Doyle MP, Beuchat LR, Wells JG, Mintz ED, Swaminathan B (2000): Fate of *Shigella sonnei* on parsley and methods of disinfection. *J Food Prot*. 63:568–572.

Zaika LL (1988) Spices and herbs: their antimicrobial activity and its determination. *J Food Saf*. 9:97–118.

CHAPTER 17

FOOD SAFETY ISSUES AND THE MICROBIOLOGY OF MAYONNAISE, SALAD DRESSINGS, ACIDIC CONDIMENTS, AND MAYONNAISE-BASED SALADS

LARRY R. BEUCHAT

17.1 INTRODUCTION

Mayonnaise, salad dressings, and acidic condiments such as mustard, ketchup, relish, and salsa are consumed in various forms. The low pH of these products, achieved by the use of vinegar, lemon juice, or less often, other acidulants as ingredients, is the major factor depended upon to prevent or retard the growth of most microorganisms. Lactobacilli are the major group of bacteria involved in spoilage of mayonnaise, salad dressings, and acidic condiments (Smittle and Flowers, 1982). Acid-tolerant yeasts, particularly strains of *Zygosaccharomyces bailii* are capable of metabolizing benzoate; *Pichia, Torulopsis,* and *Debaryomyces* also contribute to spoilage of these products (Deak and Beuchat, 1996). Spoilage by these microorganisms, although not a public health concern, does cause economic losses to the industry.

It is the behavior of pathogenic bacteria such as *Salmonella,* enterohemorrhagic *Escherichia coli, Listeria monocytogenes*, and *Staphylococcus aureus* in mayonnaise, dressings, condiments, and salads, sandwiches, and other ready-to-eat foods containing these ingredients that are of concern. These products are often intended for repeated use from the same container over a period of several days in food service or home settings. This situation creates opportunities for contamination with foodborne pathogens, followed by an interval of time that may allow growth. Even if growth does not occur in contaminated products, upon combining with other ingredients, which may have a buffering effect on the acidic pH, growth of the pathogens may ensue.

Microbiologically Safe Foods, Edited by Norma Heredia, Irene Wesley, and Santos García

In this chapter we briefly review the survival and growth characteristics of foodborne pathogenic bacteria in mayonnaise, salad dressings, acidic condiments, and ready-to-eat foods containing these ingredients. The reader is referred to other reviews that cover the subject more extensively (Michels and Koning, 2000; Radford and Board, 1993; Smittle, 2000; Smittle and Flowers, 1982). In addition to describing microbiological safety aspects of these products, the influence of physical structure and ingredient composition on survival and growth of pathogens, as well as spoilage microorganisms, is covered in some depth in these reviews.

17.2 MAYONNAISE

17.2.1 *Salmonella*

The influence of pH and temperature on the behavior of *Salmonella* Enteritidis in homemade mayonnaise has been studied (Perales and Garcia, 1990). Mayonnaise was adjusted to pH 3.6, 4.0, 4.5, and 5.0 using wine vinegar or lemon juice, inoculated with *S.* Enteritidis at populations up to 6 log CFU/g, and stored for up to 5 days at 4, 24, or 35°C. Inactivation was more rapid in mayonnaise made with vinegar (acetic acid) rather than lemon juice (citric acid) and at higher temperature, regardless of the acidulant (Table 1). The pathogen grew at 24°C and 35°C in mayonnaise (pH 4.5 and 5.0) made with lemon juice but not in mayonnaise made with wine vinegar. To prevent salmonellosis transmission by homemade mayonnaise, it was recommended that vinegar be used as an acidulant in order to achieve a pH between 3.6 and 4.0 and that mayonnaise be stored in a warm place. The effects of temperature on survival of *S.* Enteritidis and spoilage microorganisms in homemade mayonnaise (pH 4.4) held at 5 and 25°C for 8 days was studied by Roller and Covill (2000). Mayonnaise prepared using lemon juice (1.2%) as an acidulant supported growth at 25°C, whereas the pathogen was inactivated in mayonnaise prepared with acetic acid (0.16%). At 5°C, the population of *S.* Enteritidis did not change in mayonnaise containing lemon juice, but death occurred in mayonnaise acidified with acetic acid. The addition of

TABLE 1 Behavior of *Salmonella* in Homemade Mayonnaise as Affected by pH and Acidulant at 24°C

		Log CFU/mL at pH:			
Acidulant	Time (h)	3.6	4.0	4.5	5.0
Vinegar	0	6.2	6.2	6.2	6.2
	2	1.3	6.1	6.1	6.1
	48	<1.0	3.0	6.1	6.0
Lemon juice	0	6.2	6.2	2.4	2.4
	2	6.2	6.2	3.3	4.2
	48	5.9	5.7	8.2	7.3

Source: Adapted from Perales and Garcia (1990).

TABLE 2 Death of *Salmonella* Enteritidis at 20°C in Mayonnaise Made with Various Oils

	Log CFU/mL			
Oil	0 h	24 h	48 h	72 h
Italian extra virgin olive	3.8	2.6	1.2	0.1
Greek extra virgin olive	3.9	2.7	1.9	0.1
Blended olive	4.0	3.3	3.0	2.8
Sunflower	4.2	4.1	3.9	3.7

Source: Adapted from Radford et al. (1991).

chitosan to mayonnaise accelerated the inactivation of *S*. Enteritidis, but only after 6 days at 5°C.

The influence of various types of oils on the death rate of *S*. Enteritidis in homemade mayonnaise was investigated by Radford et al. (1991). Mayonnaise containing sunflower oil, a blend of olive oils, extra virgin Italian olive oil, or extra virgin Greek olive oil was adjusted to pH 4.3 using acetic acid as an acidulant, inoculated with *S*. Enteritidis at about 4 log CFU/g, and held at 20°C. Populations of *S*. Enteritidis were determined at 0, 24, 48, and 72 h. Death of the pathogen was more rapid in mayonnaise made with extra virgin olive oils than in mayonnaise made with sunflower oil or a blend of olive oils (Table 2). The more rapid inactivation rates in mayonnaise containing extra virgin olive oils were attributed to their higher acid and phenolic contents compared to the other test oils.

Lock and Board (1994) determined the fate of *S*. Enteritidis in commercial mayonnaise. Thirty mayonnaises ranging in pH from 2.6 to 4.8 were inoculated with *S*. Enteritidis at about 6 log CFU/g and stored at 4 or 20°C for up to 4 days before analyzing. The pathogen died more rapidly as the pH became more acid, especially in products containing acetic acid as the acidulant. A looseness of the correlation of death rates with pH in the range 4.0 to 4.8 may have reflected the contribution of ingredients other than acids to anti-*Salmonella* activity. It was evident, as in other studies, that storage at a refrigeration temperature protected *Salmonella* against inactivation.

Glass and Doyle (1991) investigated the effects of different concentrations of acetic acid on the fate of an eight-serotype mixture of *Salmonella* in a reduced-calorie mayonnaise and a cholesterol-free, reduced-calorie mayonnaise. Both products were produced by a commercial manufacturer. The reduced-calorie mayonnaise was modified to contain 0.1, 0.3, 0.5, or 0.7% acetic acid in the aqueous phase; the cholesterol-free, reduced-calorie mayonnaise contained 0.3 or 0.7% acetic acid. The pH was adjusted to 3.9 to 4.3 by adding hydrochloric acid. Inoculated at a population of about 6 log CFU/g and held at 23.9°C, *Salmonella* was not detected in 100-g samples of either mayonnaise made with 0.7% acetic acid and stored for 48 h. Populations in mayonnaise containing other concentrations of acetic acid decreased during storage, and at 2 weeks the pathogen was not detected in 100-g samples containing 0.3% acetic acid in the aqueous phase. It was concluded that properly acidified (pH < 4.1) reduced-calorie mayonnaise containing 0.7% acetic acid in the aqueous phase is a microbiologically safe product. The authors pointed out that it is incumbent on the manufacturer to verify the microbiological safety of such formulations of reduced-calorie mayonnaise and salad dressings that deviate substantially from the acid and/or pH requirements.

The fate of a 14-strain mixture of *S.* Enteritidis in four commercial mayonnaise products was studied by Erickson and Jenkins (1991). Products were inoculated, stored at 26.6°C, and analyzed daily for 10 days and at 14 days, if needed. Reductions of 8 log CFU/g or more occurred within 3 days in sandwich spread (initial pH 3.3), real (regular, full-calorie) mayonnaise (pH 3.9), reduced-calorie mayonnaise dressing (pH 3.9), and cholesterol-free reduced-calorie mayonnaise dressing (pH 3.9). Rates of inactivation were similar in all four products. These observations are in general agreement with those of other researchers, showing that *Salmonella* is rapidly inactivated in various mayonnaise formulations held at ambient temperature (Glass and Doyle, 1991; Perales and Garcia, 1990; Wethington and Fabian, 1950).

A standardized laboratory-scale procedure to prepare mayonnaise for the purpose of studying the behavior of *S.* Enteritidis has been developed (Leuschner and Boughtflower, 2001). The objective of the work was to simulate naturally contaminated mayonnaise in a reproducible manner to be able to investigate the effects of formulation, processing, and storage conditions on the survival and growth of *Salmonella*. Liquid egg was inoculated with *S.* Enteritidis at populations giving 1 to 3 log CFU/g in the final product. The pathogen had increased stability in mayonnaise when cells were subjected to low pH in two stages, first to pH 5.8 and afterward to pH 4.5 before addition to the mayonnaise. The pH of the mayonnaise was 4.2 to 4.5 over a 4-week period at 4°C during which populations of *S.* Enteritidis remained stable.

17.2.2 *Escherichia coli* O157:H7

Survival and growth characteristics of *E. coli* O157:H7 in three different lots of commercial mayonnaise (pH 3.6 to 3.9) stored at 5 and 20°C were reported by Zhao and Doyle (1994). Products were inoculated at a population of 3.8 log CFU/g. The pathogen did not grow at either temperature but survived for 34 to 55 days at 5°C and for 8 to 21 days at 20°C. Higher populations survived in real mayonnaise than in reduced-calorie mayonnaise. It was suggested that reduced-calorie mayonnaise contained an ingredient(s) with anti-*E. coli* O157:H7 properties that was not present in real mayonnaise. It was concluded that commercial mayonnaise produced under good manufacturing practices is not a health concern. Rather, abusive handling of mayonnaise resulting in contamination after containers are opened is the principal basis for concern.

Weagant et al. (1994) studied the survival of three strains of *E. coli* O157:H7 in commercially prepared mayonnaise (pH 3.65) held at 7 and 25°C. The initial population (ca. 8 log CFU/g) decreased at 25°C to an undetectable level within 3 days. When inoculated mayonnaise was stored at 7°C, the pathogen was detectable for up to 35 days. It was concluded that mayonnaise and possibly other acidic foods could serve as conveyances of *E. coli* O157:H7 infection when stored at refrigeration temperatures.

The influence of temperature on the rate of death of *E. coli* O157:H7 in commercially manufactured full-fat (real) and reduced-calorie mayonnaise dressings was also studied by Hathcox et al. (1995). Survival of low initial populations (0.23 to 0.29 log CFU/g) in the two products stored at 5°C was studied. The pathogen did not grow in either formulation, regardless of the inoculum level or storage temperature. The rate of inactivation increased with an increase in temperature. Populations in reduced-calorie and full-fat real mayonnaise formulations inoculated with low numbers of *E. coli* O157:H7 and held at 30°C were reduced to undetectable levels within 1 and 2 days, respectively; viable cells were not detected after 1 day at 20°C. When inoculated at a population of 2.2 log CFU/g of mayonnaise, *E. coli* O157:H7 was not detected after 4 days at 30°C or 7 days at 20°C. Survival was greater in full-fat mayonnaise than in reduced-calorie mayonnaise dressing at all storage temperatures. When *E. coli* O157:H7 was inoculated at populations of 5.9 to 6.3 log CFU/g, it was not detected in reduced-calorie mayonnaise dressing held at 5°C for 58 days and was approaching undetectable levels in full-fat mayonnaise after 93 days. Changes in populations of the pathogen in both types of mayonnaise inoculated with 5.9 to 6.3 log CFU/g and held at 5, 20, and 30°C for up to 28 days (Table 3) illustrate the behavior of *E. coli* O157:H7 in these products.

Reductions of more than 6 log CFU/g were reported for two strains of *E. coli* O157:H7 in a commercial mayonnaise (pH 3.91) stored at 22°C for 3 days (Raghubeer et al., 1995). In the same study, *E. coli* O157:H7 was inactivated less rapidly in ranch salad dressing (pH 4.51). The greater antimicrobial effect of mayonnaise was attributed in part to its lower pH and the lysozyme in egg white used in the formulation. These and other studies (Zhao and Doyle, 1994) show that *E. coli* O157:H7 dies when inoculated into mayonnaise that is prepared commercially using good manufacturing practices. Death of *E. coli* O157:H7 is most rapid at temperatures at which mayonnaise is stored, distributed, and offered for sale at retail. If subsequent cross-contamination of mayonnaise occurs at some point after containers of commercially processed products are opened, the pathogen may survive for several weeks.

TABLE 3 Fate of *Escherichia coli* O157:H7 in Commercial Full-Fat (pH 3.86 to 3.97) and Reduced-Calorie (pH 4.08) Mayonnaise as Affected by Temperature

		Log CFU/g			
Type	Temp. (°C)	0 days	4 days	14 days	28 days
Full-fat	5	6.3	5.0	3.3	3.6
	20	6.3	4.6	2.0	<0.1
	30	6.3	0.5	<0.1	
Reduced-calorie	5	5.9	5.5	5.0	4.5
	20	5.9	4.8	<0.1	
	30	5.9	<0.1		

Source: Adapted from Hathcox et al. (1995).

17.2.3 *Listeria monocytogenes*

The survival characteristics of *L. monocytogenes* in commercial reduced-calorie mayonnaise containing 0.3 and 0.7% acetic acid in the aqueous phase and cholesterol-free, reduced-calorie mayonnaise made with 0.1, 0.3, 0.5, and 0.7% acetic acid have been described (Glass and Doyle, 1991). Products inoculated with a six-strain mixture of *L. monocytogenes* at 6 log CFU/g were stored at 23.9°C for up to 14 days. The pathogen was not detected in 100-g samples at 10 or 14 days post-inoculation of reduced-calorie and cholesterol-free, reduced-calorie mayonnaise, respectively. Reductions of more than 4 log CFU/g occurred within 3 days in mayonnaise (initial pH 3.9) containing 0.7% acetic acid in the aqueous phase. *L. monocytogenes* was more resistant to the harsh pH and acidulant conditions imposed by the two types of mayonnaise than was *Salmonella* exposed to the same experimental conditions. It was concluded that properly acidified (pH < 4.1) reduced-calorie mayonnaise containing 0.7% acetic acid in the aqueous phase is microbiologically safe.

The viability of *L. monocytogenes* in sandwich spread (pH 3.3), real mayonnaise (pH 3.9), reduced-calorie mayonnaise (pH 3.9), and cholesterol-free, reduced-calorie mayonnaise dressing stored at 26.6°C has been investigated (Erickson and Jenkins, 1991). Inactivation rates were directly correlated with the aqueous-phase acetic acid concentration (i.e., sandwich spread $\geq$ real mayonnaise $>$ cholesterol-free, reduced-calorie mayonnaise dressing $>$ reduced-calorie mayonnaise dressing $>$ reduced-calorie mayonnaise dressing). Populations of *L. monocytogenes* decreased about 3 and 5 log CFU/g of reduced-calorie and cholesterol-free, reduced-calorie dressing, respectively. The higher antilisterial activity in the cholesterol-free formulation was attributed in part to egg white lysozyme. It was concluded that commercial mayonnaise, including reduced-calorie mayonnaise dressing varieties, represent a negligible consumer safety risk.

17.2.4 *Staphylococcus aureus*

Wethington and Fabian (1950) were among the first researchers to study the behavior of foodborne pathogens in mayonnaise. Three strains of enterotoxigenic *Staphylococcus* inoculated at a population of about 7.5 log CFU/g survived for at least 80 h in mayonnaise (pH 4.0) stored at room temperature (37°C). This compares to similar reductions of six serotypes of *Salmonella* within 22 h, indicating that salmonellae are substantially more sensitive to the acid pH and other antimicrobial factors characteristic of mayonnaise.

Factors affecting enterotoxin production by *S. aureus* in homemade mayonnaise have been described (Gomez-Lucia et al., 1987). Ten enterotoxigenic strains producing one or more enterotoxin types (A, B, C, or D) were inoculated at levels of 4 to 5 log CFU/g of homemade mayonnaise adjusted at pH values initially ranging from 4.0 to 5.8. Samples were stored at 37°C for up to 7 days. In mayonnaise at pH $\leq$ 4.9, the *S. aureus* population decreased to about 2 log CFU/g; at pH 5.0 the population reached about 5 log CFU/g, and at pH $\geq$ 5.15 it was about 7 log CFU/g. Enterotoxin was detected only in mayonnaise at initial pH $\geq$ 5.15 and when the pH after storage of inoculated mayonnaise for 7 days was not less than 4.7. The observation that mayonnaise containing *S. aureus* at populations as high as 8 log CFU/g did not undergo sensorial changes enhances the possibility of its consumption, with subsequent enterotoxication.

17.3 SALAD DRESSINGS AND SAUCES

The rates of death of *Salmonella, E. coli* O157:H7 and *L. monocytogenes* in commercial shelf-stable, dairy-based, pourable salad dressings have been reported (Beuchat et al., 2003). Three full-fat ranch dressings, three reduced-fat ranch dressings, two full-fat blue cheese dressings, and two reduced-fat blue cheese dressings were inoculated with two populations (2.4 to 2.5 log CFU/g and 5.3 to 5.9 log CFU/g) and stored at 25°C for up to 15 days. *Salmonella* was not detected by enrichment (<1 CFU/25 mL) in any of the salad dressings stored for 1 day, and *E. coli* O157:H7 and *L. monocytogenes* were reduced to undetectable levels between 1 and 8 days and 2 and 8 days, respectively. Overall, the type of salad dressing (i.e., ranch versus blue cheese) and the level of fat in dressings did not markedly affect the rate of inactivation of pathogens. Based on these observations, it was concluded that commercially manufactured shelf-stable, dairy-based, pourable ranch and blue cheese salad dressings manufactured by three U.S. companies and stored at 25°C do not support the growth of either *Salmonella, E. coli* O157:H7, or *L. monocytogenes* and should not be considered as potentially hazardous foods as defined by the U.S. Food and Drug Administration Food Code (USFDA-CFSAN, 2001).

Inactivation rates of *E. coli* O157:H7 in blue cheese dressing (pH 4.44) and Thousand Island dressing (pH 3.76) held at 5°C were determined by Weagant et al. (1994). An initial population of about 8 log CFU/g decreased to about 5 log CFU/g of blue cheese dressing and about 2.5 log CFU/g of Thousand Island dressing within 35 days. The inactivation rate in Thousand Island dressing was similar to that in mayonnaise (pH 3.65) stored at 7°C. An initial population of *E. coli* O157:H7 at about 6 log CFU/g of commercial ranch salad dressing (pH 4.51) decreased by about 5 log CFU/g during storage at 4°C for 17 days (Raghubeer et al., 1995). Death of the same test strains was more rapid when cells were inoculated into a commercial mayonnaise (pH 3.91). The pathogen decreased to undetectable levels between 3 and 4 days at 4°C.

Erickson et al. (1995) conducted a study to determine the survival characteristics of a four-strain mixture of *E. coli* O157:H7 in five commercial mayonnaise-based products. Included in the study were sandwich spread (pH 3.21), tartar sauce (pH 3.16), reduced-fat tartar sauce (pH 3.16), reduced-fat and/or cholesterol-free mayonnaise dressing (pH 3.94), and reduced-fat mayonnaise dressing (pH 3.52). The pathogen was inoculated at a population of about 6 log CFU/g and products were stored at 25°C. The most rapid inactivation occurred in products with pH ≤ 3.52, resulting in ≥ 6 log CFU/g decreases within 3 days. Inactivation was attributed to synergistic interactions between acidic pH, undissociated sorbate, and lysozyme originating from the egg whites.

Enterotoxigenic *Staphylococcus* is more resistant than several serotypes of *Salmonella* to the harsh stresses imposed by salad dressing (pH 3.20) (Wethington and Fabian, 1950). Reductions of about 7.5 log CFU/g occurred for *Staphylococcus* within 36 h, compared to similar reductions in salmonellae within 8 h when inoculated dressing was stored at room temperature or 37°C.

17.4 ACIDIC CONDIMENTS

Survival of *Salmonella* in ketchup (pH 3.6), mustard (pH 3.1), and sweet pickle relish (pH 2.8) was studied by Tsai and Ingham (1997). An initial population of about 6.5 log CFU/g was reduced to undetectable levels within 1 h. The death rate was less rapid in ketchup than in relish. Acid-adapted cells of two of three strains survived for 1 day but not 2 days when ketchup was stored at 23°C. Death of nonadapted cells occurred between 6 and 24 h. This compares to survival of acid-adapted cells but not nonadapted cells of two strains for at least 2 days at 5°C. The study also revealed that, in general, *Salmonella* was more sensitive than *E. coli* O157:H7 to stresses imposed by the acid pH and perhaps other constituents in ketchup.

The ability of *E. coli* O157:H7 to survive in various brands of commercial Dijon, yellow, and deli-style mustard, pH ranging from 3.17 to 3.63, has been evaluated (Mayerhause and Benckiser, 2000). Mustards were inoculated with 6 log CFU/g and stored at refrigerated and room temperatures. *E. coli* O157:H7 survived in Dijon mustard for 6 h at room temperature and 2 days at refrigerated temperature. The pathogen was not detected in yellow or deli-style mustards beyond 1 h. Overall, survival was greater at refrigerated temperatures. The rapid death of *E. coli* O157:H7 in mustards indicates that these products are not likely to be vectors of *E. coli* O157:H7 in foodborne illness.

The viability of *E. coli* O157:H7 inoculated into a mayonnaise–mustard sauce (pH 3.68) has been studied (Weagant et al., 1994). The pathogen, initially at about 8 log CFU/g, decreased to an undetectable level within 3 days when the sauce was held at 5°C. Inactivation was much more rapid in the mayonnaise-mustard sauce than in mayonnaise (pH 3.65) held at 7°C, indicating that lethality was attributable to anti-*E. coli* O157:H7 components in the mustard.

Tsai and Ingham (1997) examined the effects of temperature and adaptation to acid on survival of *E. coli* O157:H7 in ketchup (pH 3.6), mustard (pH 3.1), and sweet pickle relish (pH 2.8). Cells of three strains exposed to pH 5.0 in trypticase soy broth were inoculated into test products at a population of about 5 log CFU/g and stored at 5 and 23°C. Two of the three strains survived in ketchup stored at 23°C for 1 day but none was detected on day 2; one strain survived for at least 7 days at 5°C. Acid-adapted cells survived longer than do nonadapted cells. The pathogen was not detected in mustard or sweet pickle relish within 1 h after inoculation.

L. monocytogenes dies rapidly in ketchup at 5 and 21°C (Beuchat and Brackett, 1991). An initial population of about 6.4 log CFU/g decreased to < 1 log CFU/g in ketchup (pH 3.6 to 3.9) within 8 days at 5°C. Death was more rapid at 21°C, undetectable levels occurring within 4 days after inoculation. The rapid death of

L. monocytogenes in ketchup compared to tomato juice (pH 4.21) and tomato sauce (pH 4.07 to 4.18) was attributed to a lower pH and to a higher concentration of acetic acid.

17.5 SALADS, SANDWICHES, AND OTHER READY-TO-EAT FOODS CONTAINING MAYONNAISE AND ACIDIC CONDIMENTS

17.5.1 *Salmonella*

Several outbreaks of salmonellosis have been associated with consumption of salads containing homemade mayonnaise (Radford and Board, 1993). The source of *Salmonella* is probably the raw eggs used in mayonnaise. An outbreak caused by *S.* Enteritidis involved 404 of 965 patients in a hospital in the United States (Telzak et al., 1990). Raw eggs used to make mayonnaise were the *Salmonella* source implicated. In the UK, at least 351 cases of salmonellosis in six outbreaks were associated with homemade mayonnaise prepared by caterers (Anonymous, 1989). Waldorf salad, coleslaw, salmon cornets with cucumber mousse, curried eggs, and tartar sauce, all containing homemade mayonnaise, were potential vehicles of *S.* Typhimurium in an outbreak involving 88 infected people (Mitchell et al., 1989).

Epidemiologic investigation has implicated an egg-based sauce as the vehicle of *S.* Enteritidis infection of 173 people at a wedding in Denmark (Stevens et al., 1989). Four hundred cases of salmonellosis among passengers on flights from the Canary Islands to Denmark and Germany were linked to the consumption of items containing egg mayonnaise (Davies, 1976). Sandwiches containing mayonnaise were associated with 68 cases of salmonellosis in the UK (Ortega-Bentio and Langridge, 1992). Isolates from patients and the flock of one of the suppliers of eggs used to make the mayonnaise contained *S.* Typhimurium DT4.

Several studies have been conducted to determine survival and growth characteristics of *Salmonella* and other foodborne pathogens in mayonnaise-based salads. Doyle et al. (1982) determined survival and growth characteristics of *S.* Typhimurium and *S. aureus* in meat salads that contained varying amounts of mayonnaise (Table 4). Chicken and ham salads were inoculated with pathogens and stored at 4, 22, and 32°C for up to 24 h. Very little growth occurred in meat salads stored at 4°C whether or not mayonnaise was present. At 22 and 32°C there was an increase of less than 1 log CFU/g within 5 h, with the greatest increase occurring in salads containing no mayonnaise. Increasing the concentration of mayonnaise in the salads retarded the growth of *S.* Typhimurium and *S. aureus*. It was cautioned that mayonnaise should not be considered as a substitute for refrigeration for preserving meat salads from growth of foodborne pathogens.

Survival and growth of a 12-strain mixture of *Salmonella* in chicken and macaroni salads prepared with real mayonnaise, reduced-calorie mayonnaise, and reduced-fat, reduced-calorie mayonnaise dressings were investigated by Erickson et al. (1993). The initial population of *Salmonella* was about 3.5 log CFU/g. Salads stored at 4 and 12.8°C were analyzed for *Salmonella* at 1- to 3-day intervals for up to 10 days.

TABLE 4 Fate of *Salmonella* Typhimurium and *Staphylococcus aureus* in Cooked Chicken and Ham and in Mayonnaise-Based Chicken and Ham Salads as Affected by Temperature

				Log CFU/g (24 h)		
Pathogen	Meat	Mayonnaise	pH	4°C	22°C	32°C
S. Typhimurium	Chicken	No	6.4	3.2	6.5	7.7
		Yes	6.1	2.6	5.5	6.7
	Ham	No	5.9	3.0	6.5	7.9
		Yes	5.6	2.7	5.6	6.5
S. aureus	Chicken	No	6.4	3.0	5.5	7.0
		Yes	6.1	2.6	4.3	6.9
	Ham	No	5.6	3.6	4.3	6.6
		Yes	5.2	3.0	3.1	5.1

Source: Adapted from Doyle et al. (1982).

The pathogen decreased by about 2 log CFU/g in both salads held for 10 days at 4°C. *Salmonella* grew at 12.8°C in chicken salad, reaching about 7 log CFU/g within 2 days, but decreased by about 3 log CFU/g of macaroni salad. This behavior was attributed in part to differences in the pH of chicken salad (pH 5.65 to 5.78) compared to macaroni salad (pH 4.54 to 4.62). Changes in populations were not affected by the type of mayonnaise used to make the salads.

Swaminathan et al. (1981) monitored populations of *S*. Typhimurium in sandwiches containing sliced turkey breast meat, with and without commercially manufactured mayonnaise. Sandwiches were kept at 4, 21, and 30°C and samples were analyzed at 4, 8, and 24 h. Significant increases in population occurred in sandwiches containing turkey meat within 8 h at 30°C and 24 h at 21°C. The presence of mayonnaise in sandwiches had a significant inhibitory effect on the rate of growth of *S*. Typhimurium but did not inhibit growth in sandwiches stored at 21 or 30°C for 8 or 24 h. It was concluded that sandwiches containing mayonnaise and sliced turkey may be stored at 21°C for periods not exceeding 4 h without significant growth of *S*. Typhimurium. It was recommended, however, that the best protection against growth would be to store sandwiches at 4°C until consumption.

Factors affecting survival and growth of *S*. Enteritidis and spoilage microorganisms in mayonnaise-based shrimp salad have been described (Roller and Covill, 2000). Mayonnaise (pH 4.4), shrimp, and ketchup were combined at a ratio of 16 : 8 : 1 (w/w/w), inoculated with *S*. Enteritidis (5 to 7 log CFU/g), and stored at 5 and 25°C for up to 8 days. Populations were maintained or increased rapidly at these temperatures.

17.5.2 *Escherichia coli* O157:H7

E. coli O157:H7 is capable of growing in roasted beef salad made with mayonnaise (Addul-Raouf et al., 1993). Ground beef salads containing up to 40% mayonnaise were inoculated with a five-strain mixture of *E. coli* O157:H7 and stored at 5, 21, and 30°C for up to 3 days. There was no change in population in salad (pH 5.40 to 6.07) containing up to 40% mayonnaise when it was stored at 5°C. At 21 and 30°C significant increases in populations occurred in salads (pH 5.55 to 5.94) containing 16 to 32% mayonnaise between 10 and 24 h of storage. Death was more rapid as the pH of salads stored at 5°C was decreased from 5.98 to 4.70. Acidification of beef with acetic acid was more effective than acidification with citric or lactic acids in controlling the growth of *E. coli* O157:H7. These findings show that *E. coli* O157:H7 can grow in beef salads with a mayonnaise content commonly used in salad recipes. Caution should be taken to handle cooked beef in a manner that prevents cross-contamination with *E. coli* O157:H7 during marketing and handling in food service establishments and in the home.

The fate of *E. coli* O157:H7 in two commercial coleslaw preparations (pH 4.3 and 4.5) held at 4, 11, and 21°C for 3 days was studied by Wu et al. (2002). An initial population of 5.3 log CFU/g decreased by 0.1 to 0.5 log CFU/g within 3 days at all three temperatures. Reductions of 0.4 to 0.5 log CFU/g occurred at 21°C, whereas decreases at 4 and 11°C were 0.1 to 0.2 log CFU/g. Results suggest that acid tolerance of *E. coli* O157:H7, not temperature abuse, is a major factor influencing its survival in restaurant-prepared coleslaw.

Skandamis and Nychas (2000) developed a model to predict the survival of *E. coli* O157:H7 in homemade eggplant at various temperatures, pH values, and oregano essential oil concentrations. Salads containing 0, 0.7, 1.4, and 2.1% (v/w) oregano essential oil were adjusted to pH 4.0, 4.5, and 5.0, inoculated with *E. coli* O157:H7, and stored at 0, 5, 10, and 15°C for up to 25 h. Populations decreased by more than 1 log CFU/g in all cases. Inactivation was enhanced as the pH was decreased and the oregano essential oil concentration and storage temperature were increased. The development of polynomial models, based on Baranyi model estimates of survival kinetics, appeared to predict responses of *E. coli* O157:H7 in eggplant salad.

17.5.3 *Listeria monocytogenes*

Survival and growth of *L. monocytogenes* in ham salad and potato salad as affected by mayonnaise pH and temperature has been studied (Hwang, 2005). The initial pH (ca. 3.8) of mayonnaise was adjusted to 4.2 or 4.6 with sodium hydroxide. Mayonnaise and ham or cooked potato cubes (1 × 1 × 1 cm) were combined at a ratio of 1 : 3 (mayonnaise/ham or potato), inoculated with *L. monocytogenes* at a population of about 2 log CFU/g, and stored at 4, 8, and 12°C. Results showing the behavior of *L. monocytogenes* in cooked potatoes and mayonnaise-based potato salad stored at 8°C for up to 12 days are summarized in Table 5. The pathogen grew in ham salad held at all three temperatures but was inactivated in potato salad. The rates of growth in ham salad and death in potato salad increased as the storage temperature decreased. The pH of mayonnaise did not have a consistent effect on rates of growth of death. Since potatoes alone supported the growth of *L. monocytogenes*, inactivation in potato salad was due to the presence of mayonnaise. The lack of buffering capacity, coupled

TABLE 5 Fate of *Listeria monocytogenes* in Cooked Potatoes and Mayonnaise-Based Potato Salad Stored at 8°C for Up to 12 Days

		Log CFU/g			
Substrate	pH	0 days	3 days	6 days	12 days
Cooked potatoes	5.9	2.0	4.2	5.8	7.0
Mayonnaise-based	3.8	2.2	4.1	0.9	<0.1
potato salad	4.6	2.1	2.2	1.8	1.5

Source: Adapted from Hwang (2005).

with the low nutrient content of potatoes, probably contributed to lethality to *L. monocytogenes*.

The behavior of *L. monocytogenes* in homemade chicken salad and macaroni salad prepared with real mayonnaise, reduced-calorie mayonnaise dressing, and reduced-calorie, reduced-fat mayonnaise dressing was investigated by Erickson et al. (1993). The initial population of *L. monocytogenes* was about 3.5 log CFU/g and salads were stored at 4 and 12.8°C for up to 10 days. The pathogen grew in chicken salad but not in macaroni salad. Behavior was not affected by the type of mayonnaise used to prepare the salads. Growth in chicken salad was attributed to a higher pH (5.65 to 5.78) than that of macaroni salad (pH 4.54 to 4.62). The microbiological shelf life of chicken and macaroni salads was subjectively judged to be 5 and 7 days, respectively. It was concluded that under proper refrigeration and good hygienic practices, salads made with commercial real mayonnaise and mayonnaise dressings represent negligible microbial health risks to consumers.

REFERENCES

Abdul-Raouf UM, Beuchat LR, Ammar MS (1993): Survival and growth of *Escherichia coli* O157:H7 in ground, roasted beef as affected by pH, acidulants, and temperature. *Appl Environ Microbiol*. 59:2364–2368.

Anonymous (1989): *Salmonella in Eggs*, Vol. 2. Minutes of evidence and appendices. House of Commons Session 1988-89 (U.K.). Agriculture Committee. First report. Her Majesty's Stationery Office, London.

Beuchat LR, Brackett RE (1991): Behavior of *Listeria monocytogenes* inoculated into raw tomatoes and processed tomato products. *Appl Environ Microbiol*. 57:1367–1371.

Beuchat LR, Adler BB, Harrison MD (2003): Death of *Salmonella, Escherichia coli* O157:H7, and *Listeria monocytogenes* in salad dressings. In Proc. International Association for Food Protection Annual Meeting, *Baltimore*, August 14–17.

Davies RF (1976): *Salmonella* Typhimurium foodborne outbreak. *Wkly Epidemiol Rec*. 51:75.

Deak T, Beuchat LR (1996): *Handbook of Food Spoilage Yeasts*. CRC Press, Boca Raton, FL.

Doyle MP, Bains NJ, Schoeni JL, Foster EM (1982): Fate of *Salmonella* Typhimurium and *Staphylococcus aureus* in meat salads prepared with mayonnaise. *J Food Prot*. 45:152–156.

Erickson JP, Jenkins P (1991): Comparative *Salmonella* spp. and *Listeria monocytogenes* inactivation rates in four commercial mayonnaise products. *J Food Prot.* 54:913–916.

Erickson JP, McKenna DN, Woodruff MA, Bloom JS (1993): Fate of *Salmonella* spp., *Listeria monocytogenes*, and indigenous spoilage microorganisms in home-style salads prepared with commercial real mayonnaise or reduced calorie mayonnaise dressings. *J Food Prot.* 56:1015–1021.

Erickson JP, Stamer JW, Hayes M, McKenna DN, Van Alstine LA (1995): An assessment of *Escherichia coli* O157:H7 contamination risks in commercial mayonnaise from pasteurized eggs and environmental sources, and behavior in low-pH dressings. *J Food Prot.* 58:1059–1064.

Glass KA, Doyle MP (1991): Fate of *Salmonella* and *Listeria monocytogenes* in commercial, reduced-calorie mayonnaise. *J Food Prot.* 54:691–695.

Gomez-Lucia E, Goyache J, Blanco JL, Garayzabal JFF, Orden JA, Suarez G (1987): Growth of *Staphylococcus aureus* and enterotoxin production in homemade mayonnaise prepared with different pH values. *J Food Prot.* 50:872–875.

Hathcox AK, Beuchat LR, Doyle MP (1995): Death of enterohemorrhagic *Escherichia coli* O157:H7 in real mayonnaise and reduced-calorie mayonnaise dressing as influenced by initial population and storage temperature. *Appl Environ Microbiol.* 61:4172–4177.

Hwang C-A (2005): Effect of mayonnaise pH and storage temperature on the behavior of *Listeria monocyctogenes* in ham and potato salad. *J Food Prot.* 68:1628–1634.

Leuschner RC, Boughtflower MP (2001): Standardization laboratory-scale preparation of mayonnaise containing low levels of *Salmonella enterica* serovar Enteritidis. *J Food Prot.* 64:623–629.

Lock JL, Board RG (1994): The fate of *Salmonella* Enteritidis PT4 in deliberately infected commercial mayonnaise. *Food Microbiol.* 11:499–503.

Mayerhause CM, Benckiser R (2000): Survival of enterohemorrhagic *Escherichia coli* O157:H7 in retail mustard. In Proc. International Association for Food Protection Annual Meeting, *Atlanta*, GA, August 6–9.

Michels MJM, Koning W (2000): Mayonnaise, dressings, mustard, mayonnaise-based salads, and acid sauces. In: Lund BM, Baird-Parker TC, Gould GW (Eds.). *The Microbiological Safety and Quality of Food*, Vol. 1. Aspen Publishers, Gaithersburg, MD, pp. 807–835.

Mitchell E, O'Mahoney M, Lynch D, et al. (1989): Large outbreak of food poisoning caused by Salmonella Typhimurium definitive type 49 in mayonnaise. *Br Med J.* 298:99–101.

Ortega-Bentio JM, Langridge P (1992): Outbreak of food poisoning due to *Salmonella* Typhimurium DT4 in mayonnaise. *Public Health.* 106:203–208.

Perales I, Garcia MI (1990): The influence of pH and temperature on the behavior of *Salmonella* Enteritidis phage type 4 in home-made mayonnaise. *Lett Appl Microbiol.* 10:19–22.

Radford SA, Board RG. (1993): Review: fate of pathogens in home-made mayonnaise and related products. *Food Microbiol.* 10:269–278.

Radford SA, Tassou CC, Nychas G-JE, Board RG (1991): The influence of different oils on the death rate of *Salmonella* Enteritidis in homemade mayonnaise. *Lett Appl Microbiol.* 12:125–128.

Raghubeer EV, Ke JS, Campbell ML, Meyer RS (1995): Fate of *Escherichia coli* O157:H7 and coliforms in commercial mayonnaise and refrigerated salad dressing. *J Food Prot.* 58:13–18.

Roller S, Covill N (2000): The antimicrobial properties of chitosan in mayonnaise and mayonnaise-based shrimp salads. *J Food Prot.* 63:202–209.

Skandamis PN, Nychas G-TE (2000): Development and evaluation of a model predicting the survival of *Escherichia coli* O157:H7 NCTC 12900 in homemade eggplant salad at various temperatures, pHs, and oregano essential oil concentrations. *Appl Environ Microbiol.* 66:1646–1653.

Smittle RB (2000): Microbiological safety of mayonnaise, salad dressings and sauces produced in the United States: a review. *J Food Prot.* 63:1144–1153.

Smittle RB, Flowers RS (1982): Acid tolerant microorganisms involved in the spoilage of salad dressings. *J Food Prot.* 45:977–983.

Stevens A, Joseph C, Bruce J, et al. (1989): A large outbreak of *Salmonella* Enteritidis phage type 4 associated with eggs from overseas. *Epidemiol Infect.* 103:425–433.

Swaminathan B, Howe JM, Essling CM (1981): Mayonnaise sandwiches and *Salmonella*. *J Food Prot.* 44:115–117.

Telzak EE, Budnick LD, Greenberg MSZ, et al. (1990): Nosocomial outbreak of *Salmonella* Enteritidis infection due to the consumption of raw eggs. *N Engl J Med.* 323:394–397.

Tsai Y-W, Ingham SC (1997): Survival of *Escherichia coli* O157:H7 and *Salmonella* spp. in acidic condiments. *J Food Prot.* 60:751–755.

USFDA-CFSAN (U.S. Department of Agriculture–Center for Food Safety and Applied Nutriton) (2001): Food Code, *FDA Good Guidance Practices Regulations.* 21 CFR 10.115, 65 FR 56468, September 2005. http://www/cfsan.fda.gov/~dms/fc01-toc.html, pp. 12–13.

Weagant SD, Bryant JL, Bark DH (1994): Survival of *Escherichia coli* O157:H7 in mayonnaise and mayonnaise-based sauces at room and refrigerated temperatures. *J Food Prot.* 57:629–631.

Wethington MC, Fabian FW (1950): Viability of food-poisoning staphylococci and salmonellae in salad dressing and mayonnaise. *Food Res.* 15:125–134.

Wu FM, Beuchat LR, Doyle MP, Garrett V, Wells JG, Swaminathan B (2002): Fate of *Escherichia coli* O157:H7 in coleslaw during storage. *J Food Prot.* 65:845–847.

Zhao T, Doyle MP (1994): Fate of enterohemorrhagic *Escherichia coli* O157:H7 in commercial mayonnaise. *J Food Prot.* 57:780–783.

CHAPTER 18

FOOD SAFETY ISSUES AND THE MICROBIOLOGY OF CHOCOLATE AND SWEETENERS

NORMA HEREDIA and SANTOS GARCÍA

18.1 INTRODUCTION

Traditionally, chocolate and other confectionery products have been regarded as microbiologically stable and safe to eat. Due to the inherent low water content of chocolate, this substance is unlikely to support the growth and proliferation of bacterial pathogens, and thus the risk of a foodborne illness associated with chocolate consumption is low. However, occasional outbreaks of salmonellosis have occurred throughout the world in association with the consumption of chocolate and chocolate products contaminated with *Salmonella*.

18.2 NORMAL FLORA OF RAW AND FERMENTED COCOA BEANS

Filamentous fungi are common components of the microflora of commercial cocoa beans, although relatively few xerophilic (prefers dry environments) species have been identified (Martin, 1987). In fact, the only xerophilic species isolated in an early study of the microflora of cocoa beans was *Aspergillus glaucus*, an anamorph of the genus *Eurotium* (ICMSF, 2005).

The contribution of bean fermentation to the quality of chocolate has been recognized for more than 100 years, and numerous studies have been conducted to determine the microbial species associated with this process (Schwan et al., 1995). Fermentation of cocoa beans typically results from the succession of microbial populations. Yeasts conduct the alcoholic fermentation via the sequential growth of *Kloeckera* and its teleomorphic form *Hanseniaspora, Saccharomyces, Candida, Pichia*, and *Kluyveromyces* species (Ardhana and Fleet, 2003). The lactic acid bacteria

Microbiologically Safe Foods, Edited by Norma Heredia, Irene Wesley, and Santos García

also ferment pulp sugars and utilize citric acid. This process involves the growth of *Lactobacillus, Leuconostoc*, and *Lactococcus* species. Acetic acid bacteria (*Acetobacter* and *Gluconobacter* spp.) grow eventually. Finally, *Bacillus* spp. develop when the pH of the bean mass becomes less acidic (4.9), and the temperature increases to 40 to 50°C due to heat generated by the fermentation process (Ardhana and Fleet, 2003). Fermented beans are frequently dried in the sun with little or no protection from environmental contamination. The microflora of the fermented and dried beans consists primarily of members of the genus *Bacillus*.

Bacteria can also permeate the shell and contaminate the meat of the dicotyledonous seed (D'Aoust, 1977). The internal microflora of cocoa beans demonstrated the presence of mold, yeast, and bacteria. The total bacterial content ranged from 10^3 to 10^8 CFU/g. These cocoa beans contained similar populations of yeast and fungi, principally from the *Penicillum* and *Aspergillus* genera (D'Aoust, 1977). Dry roasting of raw cocoa beans (145 to 150°C for 30 to 40 min) reduced the initial levels of contamination by two orders of magnitude. Following this heat treatment, only *Bacillus stearothermophilus* and *B. coagulans* could be detected (Barrile et al., 1971). This finding offers an explanation for the presence of *Bacillus* and *Micrococcus* in chocolate powder (Douglas et al., 2000).

Analyzing chocolate milk, Douglas et al. (2000) detected gram-negative rods in 14% of samples. The majority of these gram-negative organisms were *Pseudomonas* spp., and approximately 73% were catalase-positive, oxidase-negative, spore-forming, gram-positive rods, which were identified as *Bacillus* spp.

18.3 SPOILAGE AND SHELF LIFE OF CHOCOLATE

In the past, food spoilage has been regarded as merely a minor inconvenience for the food industry, whereas contamination of food with pathogens has obviously been regarded as extremely important. Currently, food spoilage is actually becoming a major focus of the food industry, due to the considerable scale of food and beverage production via modern food-processing technologies. In addition, attempts to reduce the use of preservatives and limit processing of food are causing changes in the methods and formulations of foods (Loureiro and Querol, 1999). The shelf life of chocolate and sweeteners is influenced by the number and species composition of microflora present in the raw product as well as by the processing and storage conditions (Douglas et al., 2000).

Some xerophilic fungi have been isolated from manufactured chocolate products: *Bettsia alvei* (teleomorph of *Chrysosporium farinicola*) and *Chrysosporium xerophilum* from spoiled hazelnut chocolate, *Neosortorya glabra* from spoiled chocolate confectionery (Hocking et al., 1994), and *Chrysosporium farinicola* from chocolate (Kinderlerer, 1997).

Chocolate and other flavored milks have recently increased the market of milk products. *Rahnella aquatilis* has been detected in chocolate milk stored at acceptable refrigeration temperatures (5°C/40°F) and at unsafe temperatures. At these higher temperatures, this organism produces guaiacol, a product of metabolized vanillin that is a major component of the flavoring of chocolate milk (Jensen et al., 2001). The presence of this bacterium in some chocolate milk products causes spoilage through the development of an unacceptable odor. Although *R. aquatilis* is not considered to be a public health threat, a gene encoding for a heat-labile toxin has been identified from a single strain isolated from fish (Lindberg et al., 1998).

Contamination of industrial plants and products with aerobic endospore-forming organisms is a widespread problem, especially since endospores are much more resistant than vegetative forms to heat, chemicals, irradiation, and desiccation. The ubiquitous presence of these endospore-forming bacteria, which are nutritionally versatile and form endospores at a wide range of pH's and temperatures, makes this group of bacteria an ever-present problem in these industries. Members of the *Bacillus cereus* group, *B. licheniformis*, *B. coagulans*, *B. fumarioli*, *B. badius*, *B. subtilis*, *Brevibacillus agri*, *Alicylobacillus acidocaldarius*, and *Paenibacillus cokkii* have been implicated in food spoilage (De Clerck et al., 2004).

18.4 PATHOGENS IN CONFECTIONERY PRODUCTS

Even though confectionery products are not as significant in the transmission of foodborne illness as other foods, such as poultry or meat, these products have been involved sporadically in outbreaks around the world. Although unable to grow in chocolate because of the low water activity, *Salmonella* spp. are able to survive for periods of up to 13 years in chocolate stored at ambient temperatures (Barrile et al., 1970; Tamminga et al., 1977). *Salmonella* infections following consumption of contaminated chocolate, although rare, were identified as early as the 1960s. Conceivably, the ingredients present in chocolate protect *Salmonella* against the acidic conditions of the stomach. Thus, the few *Salmonella* present in the finished product survive digestion to colonize the lower gastrointestinal tract and produce clinical symptoms (D'Aoust, 1977). All *Salmonella* epidemics related to chocolate contamination were widely distributed temporally and geographically, and affected large numbers of people, predominantly children (Table 1).

Additionally, similar to *Salmonella*, *E. coli* O157:H7 can survive in these confectionery products. This bacterium showed similarities with *Salmonella* in both survival and infective dose (Baylis et al., 2004). *Listeria monocytogenes* has also been detected in commercially produced chocolate, although its behavior in these products has not been fully described (Kenney and Beuchat, 2004). Dalton et al. (1997) reported an outbreak in which chocolate milk served at a picnic was found to be contaminated with *L. monocytogenes*. From this contaminated chocolate milk, 45 people were affected and four died.

18.5 SOURCES OF CONTAMINATION

L. monocytogenes has been isolated from chocolate factories (Kenney and Beuchat, 2004), and coconuts or nuts that are added to chocolates could be the source of contamination. In addition, inadequate sanitary controls during harvesting and

TABLE 1 Overview of *Salmonella enterica* Contamination of Chocolate

Year	Country	Serovar	Vehicle	Source of Contamination	Number of Persons Affected
1970	Sweden	Durham	Chocolate products	Cocoa powder	110
1973–1974	United States, Canada	Eastbourne	Chocolate balls from Canada	Cocoa beans	200
1982	England, Wales	Napoli	Chocolate bars from Italy	Cocoa beans or cross-contamination (pipework)	272
1985–1986	Canada	Nima	Chocolate coins from Belgium	Unknown	Unknown
1987	Norway, Finland	Typhimurium	Chocolate products from Norway	Avian contamination speculated	349
2001–2002	Germany, other European countries	Oranienburg	Two chocolate brands from Germany	Unknown	439

Source: Modified from Gordon (2006), Werber et al. (2005).

processing of coconut contribute to *Salmonella* contamination of desiccated coconut (Schaffner et al., 1967).

The stability of high-sugar products depends on the a_w (water activity) value, pH, presence of preservatives, and temperature. At a_w values between 0.61 and 0.75, the growth rate of yeast that causes spoilage is very low. As a result, spoilage may only become apparent after many months. If high-sugar products are stored in high relative humidity, the a_w increases due to hygroscopy, and these conditions support a significantly faster growth rate for yeast (Martorell et al., 2005).

Identification of specific vehicles of foodborne outbreaks is quite difficult if the exposure is common. In multinational outbreaks, international collaboration provides an important means of identifying the common source of infections, particularly when the contaminated food is very popular.

Microbiological contamination of primary ingredients must be controlled because failure to minimize contamination constitutes a potential health hazard to plant personal as well as to the consumer. The presence of *Chrysosporium* has been reported in cocoa beans and in chocolate crumb, suggesting that soil contamination occurs either after pollination of the flowers or during fermentation and then carried along during manufacturing to the finished product (Kinderlerer, 1997). Confectionery ingredients such as sugar, salt, vanillin, and lecithin are not likely sources of pathogenic bacteria; however, Carmine Red, which is used as a food additive, was previously identified as the cause of a nosocomial outbreak and the source of *Salmonella cubana* contamination in candy coatings (Lennington, 1967).

Contamination of finished chocolate products results from contaminated cocoa nibs and liquor, which stem from the lack of separation of raw bean rooms from other processing areas and from nonbactericidal roasting of cocoa beans (D'Aoust, 1977). Furthermore, in some parts of the world, such as Mexico, chocolate is commonly sold without wrapping, and this practice may affect the final microbiological quality of the product (Torres-Vitela et al., 1995).

In conclusion, contamination routes of chocolate and sweeteners by pathogenic bacteria and organisms causing spoilage include the use of contaminated raw materials, contamination during manufacturing, deviations from good manufacturing practices, or pest control failure.

18.6 FACTORS THAT INFLUENCE SURVIVAL AND GROWTH OF PATHOGENS AND SPOILAGE ORGANISMS

Microorganisms require moisture, food, and suitable temperatures for growth. Nutrition sources are in abundance in food-processing facilities, particularly in areas inaccessible to routine cleaning and sanitation, such as structures that are not routinely taken apart for cleaning. The numbers and types of organisms capable of tolerating the environmental conditions present in chocolate and confectionery plants increase dramatically as organisms gain the ability to resist preservative measures (Mortorell et al., 2005). Environmental temperatures in manufacturing plants are often in a range suitable for microbial growth. Other factors, such as oxidation–reduction potential, presence or absence of inhibitors, and interaction between microbial populations, further affect the growth of these microbes. Nonetheless, moisture control in the factory environment is considered to be the most critical factor influencing microbial growth (Kornacki, 2006).

Taken together, the following indicates that the chocolate and sweeteners industry faces a difficult situation:

1. Raw ingredients (e.g., cacao beans, milk powder, gelatin) carry pathogens such as *Salmonella* spp. or spoilage organisms such as *Bacillus* or related endospore-forming bacteria (De Clerck et al., 2004).
2. Low water activity and high fat content in chocolate increases the thermal resistance of microbes so that temperatures reached during chocolate production do not necessarily destroy pathogenic microorganisms (ICMSF, 2005).
3. Contamination by a small number of certain pathogens such as *Salmonella* and *L. monocytogenes* may be sufficient to cause disease.
4. Low levels of contamination may affect a large number of persons (often children) scattered over a wide geographic area and thus have the potential to cause serious public health consequences (Werber et al., 2005).

Furthermore, chocolate milk production involves steps such as the addition of flavoring and subsequent mixing and pumping that create additional opportunities for bacterial contamination. *L. monocytogenes* has been reported to grow to high levels in chocolate milk (Kenney and Beuchat, 2004).

18.7 MAINTAINING PRODUCT QUALITY AND REDUCING MICROBIAL NUMBERS

Several technologies have been used to ensure the microbiological purity of confectionery products. Ethylene and propylene oxide fumigation have been used to reduce the endogenous flora of nutmeats and to decontaminate cocoa powder (Shenkel, 1972). Ethylene oxide, however, is no longer permitted in the United States, due to the possible formation of toxic chlorohydrins (Wesley et al., 1965). Irradiation may, in fact, prove to be an effective and economical measure for the control of contamination in both raw and finished products. Doses of approximately 0.45 megarad were required to disinfect coconut and cocoa powder (D'Aoust, 1977), although the technique was found to be of limited application due to adverse effects on the organoleptic characteristics of both products (D'Aoust, 1977).

Cocoa inhibits the growth of various microorganisms, including *Salmonella* spp. (Busta and Speck, 1968), *L. monocytogenes* (Pearson and Marth, 1990), and *E. coli* O157:H7 (Takahashi et al., 1999). In addition, cocoa limits the verocytotoxin production of this *E. coli* strain (Takahashi et al., 1999). These antimicrobial properties have been attributed to two components of cocoa, caffeine and theobromine (Kenney and Beuchat, 2004).

Rosenow and Marth (1987) found that the addition of cocoa to milk decreased the relative generation time of *L. monocytogenes* and that populations were highest in samples containing all chocolate milk ingredients (cocoa, sugar, and carrageenan) after 8 days at 13°C. Casein was hypothesized to mask the potential bactericidal effect of cocoa, and cocoa was suggested to add nutrients for growth of *L. monocytogenes* (Pearson and Marth, 1990). These authors also speculated that addition of carrageenan, a common stabilizer used in chocolate milk, further reduced *L. monocytogenes* generation time by maintaining the cocoa in solution.

Preventing contamination is the only effective way to secure a safe product. Adherence to sound manufacturing practices is critical for ensuring a product free of contamination. Raw ingredients should preferably be purchased on specification from reputable suppliers who are conscious of microbial contamination and thus maintain rigorous quality control. Raw materials should always be isolated from other plant operations (D'Aoust, 1977). The importance of maintaining a dry work environment should be emphasized. Water condensates from cold water pipes, refrigerator coils, and cooling tunnels easily facilitate contamination by pathogenic bacteria (Kleinert, 1976). Trimmings and damaged items should not be added to fresh batches of chocolate as this practice may prolong contamination and increase the possibility of massive plant contamination (D'Aoust, 1977). Fortunately, food safety controls in much of the food industry have been greatly improved by the widespread adoption of quality assurance approaches and the implementation of hazard analysis of critical control point (HACCP) systems to prevent or reduce the likelihood of microbiological contamination. This preventive approach is focused primarily on operational procedures and is less dependent on quality control procedures (Betts and Blackburn, 2002). In addition, formal microbiological risk assessment, a part of HACCP and other risk-based approaches used by food manufacturers, has become a useful tool for improving food safety.

18.8 MICROBIOLOGICAL METHODS FOR DETECTION AND QUANTIFICATION

The heterogeneous distribution of organisms throughout the food and the overall low numbers of microorganisms present indicates that every isolation of *Salmonella* from chocolate through routine testing must be treated as a major cause of concern. In addition, relying on numbers as a measure of risk to the consumer may be misleading. In fact, some outbreaks of salmonellosis have been linked to the consumption of chocolate containing only a few cells of the pathogen (D'Aoust and Pivnick, 1976). Therefore, a technique capable of detecting very small amounts of *Salmonella* is necessary to analyze chocolate reliably. Classically, the fluorescent antibody (FA) technique, which has been recognized by the Association of Official Analytical Chemists (AOAC) as suitable for the examination of food in which the incidence of the pathogen is suspected of being low, has been reported as satisfactory in detection of *Salmonella* in chocolate and chocolate products (Fantasia et al., 1975).

Microbes that are isolated from dry fatty matrices require specialized treatment to ensure survival after rehydration. Direct inoculation into selective media provides poor recovery unless a suitable period of resuscitation in a nonselective medium is included in the protocol (Gordon, 2006). Thus, classical standard methods for *Salmonella* testing generally recommend pre-enrichment of samples in nonselective broth, followed by enrichment in tetrathionate, selenite, or other selective media and then plating in differential agar media. Pre-enrichment of chocolate samples in reconstituted skim milk powder with added brilliant green is preferred because the casein in milk powder neutralizes anthocyanins, which may exhibit antimicrobial activity (Zapatka et al., 1977). Although the International Office of Cocoa and Chocolate and the International Sugar Confectionery Manufacturers' Association recommend mannitol broth for pre-enrichment (IOCC/ISCMA, 1973), pre-enrichment in reconstituted milk powder actually increases the sensitivity of the method (D'Aoust and Sewell, 1984). Significant advances have been made in the last two decades in the development of rapid methods for the recovery of small amounts of *Salmonella* in foods. Chapter 27, which covers rapid methods for detection of foodborne pathogens, may be useful to the reader.

18.9 REGULATIONS

Although the feasibility of microbiological standards for products such has chocolate has been questioned, recalls of contaminated confectioneries and outbreaks resulting from these products emphasize the past underestimation of foodborne pathogens in confectioneries and underscore the importance of controls for all aspects of production. The International Cocoa Organization (ICCO) was established in 1973 under the auspices of the United Nations. Currently, this organization is comprised of 41 members divided between producing and consuming countries. This organization has suggested methods for testing the microbiological quality of this type of product. The goal of this group is to ensure the safety of the products, especially since children are a major confectionery-consuming population and are also a population especially susceptible to foodborne pathogens (IOCC/ISCMA, 1973).

REFERENCES

Ardhana MM, Fleet GH (2003): The microbial ecology of cocoa bean fermentations in Indonesia. *Int J Food Microbiol*. 86:87–99.

Barrile JC, Cone JF, Keeney PG (1970): A study of salmonellae survival in milk chocolate. *Manuf Confectioner*. 50:34–39.

Barrile JC, Ostovar K, Keener PG (1971): Microflora of cocoa beans before and after roasting at 150°C. *J Milk Food Technol*. 34:369–371.

Baylis CL, MacPhee S, Robinson AJ, Griffiths R, Lilley K, Betts RP (2004): Survival of *Escherichia coli* O157:H7 and O26:H11 in artificially contaminated chocolate and confectionery products. *Int J Food Microbiol*. 96:35–48.

Betts RP, de W Blackburn C (2002): Detecting pathogens in food. In: de W Blackburn C, McClure PJ (Eds.). *Foodborne Pathogens, Hazards, Risk Analysis and Control*. Woodhead Publishing, Cambridge, UK, pp. 13–52.

Busta FF, Speck ML (1968): Antimicrobial effect of cocoa on *Salmonella*. *Appl Microbiol*. 16 (2):424–425.

Dalton CB, Austin CC, Sobel J, et al. (1997): An outbreak of gastroenteritis and fever due to *Listeria monocytogenes* in milk. *N Engl J Med*. 336:100–105.

D'Aoust, JY (1977): *Salmonella* and the chocolate industry. *J Food Prot*. 40:718–727.

D'Aoust JY, Pivnick H (1976): Small infectious doses of *Salmonella*. *Lancet*. 1:1196–1200.

D'Aoust JY, Sewell A (1984): Efficacy of an international method for detection of *Salmonella* in chocolate and cocoa products. *J Food Prot*. 47:111–113.

De Clerck E, Vanhoutte T, Hebb T, Geerinck J, Devos J, De Vos P (2004): Isolation, characterization, and identification of bacterial contamination in semifinal gelatin extract. *Appl Environ Microbiol*. 70:3664–3672.

Douglas SA, Gray MJ, Crandall AD, Boor KJ (2000): Characterization of chocolate milk spoilage patterns. *J Food Prot*. 63:516–521.

Fantasia LD, Schrade JP, Yager JF, Debler D (1975): Fluorescent antibody method for the detection of *Salmonella*: development, evaluation and collaborative study. *J AOAC*. 58:828–844.

Gordon K (2006): *Salmonella* in high fat, low moisture foods: a recurring issue. *World Food Reg Rev*. 16:22–25.

Hocking AD, Charley NJ, Pitt JL (1994): *FRR Culture Collection Catalogue*. North Ryde, NSW, Australia: CSIRO Division of Food Science and Technology.

ICMSF (International Commision on Microbiological Specifications for Foods) (2005): Cocoa, chocolate and confectioneries. In: Roberts TA, Pitt JI, Farkas J, Grau FH (Eds.). *Microorganisms in Foods: Microbial Ecology of Food Commmodities*, Vol. 6. Kluwer Academic, New York, pp. 379–389.

IOCC/ISCMA (International Office of Cocoa and Chocolate/International Sugar Confectionery Manufacturers' Association) (1973): *Microbiological Examination of Chocolate and Other Cocoa Products*, IOCC/ISCMA, Brussels, Belgium.

Jensen N, Varelis P, Whitfield FB (2001): Formation of guaiacol in chocolate milk by the psychrotrophic bacterium *Rahnella aquatilis*. *Lett Appl Microbiol*. 33:339–343.

Kenney SJ, Beuchat L (2004): Survival, growth, and thermal resistance of *Listeria monocytogenes* in products containing peanut and chocolate. *J Food Prot*. 67:2205–2211.

Kinderlerer JL (1997): *Chrysosporium* species, potential organisms of chocolate. *J Appl Microbiol*. 83:771–778.

Kleinert J (1976): Rheology of chocolate In: De Man JM, Voisey PW, Rasper VF, Stanley DW (Eds.). *Rheology and Texture in Food Quality*. AVI Publishers, Wesport, CT, pp. 445–473.

Kornacki JJ (2006): Microbial sampling in the dry food processing environment. *Food Safety Mag*. February–March.

Lennington KR (1967): FDA looks at the *Salmonella* problem: ever-present threat to the industry. *Manuf Confectioner*. 47:31–33.

Lindberg AM, Ljungh A, Lofdahl S, Molin G (1998): *Enterobacteriaceae* found in high numbers in fish, minced meat and pasteurized milk or cream and the presence of toxin encoding genes. *Int J Food Microbiol*. 39:17–23.

Loureiro V, Querol A (1999): The prevalence and control of spoilage yeasts in foods and beverages. *Trends Food Sci Technol.* 10:356–365.

Martin RA (1987): Chocolate. *Adv Food Res.* 31:211–342.

Mortorell P, Fernández-Espinar MT, Querol A (2005): Molecular monitoring of spoilage yeast during the production of candied fruit nougats to determine food contamination sources. *Int J Food Microbiol.* 101:293–302.

Pearson LJ, Marth EH (1990): Inhibition of *Listeria monocytogenes* by cocoa in a broth medium and neutralization of this effect by casein. *J Food Prot.* 53:38–46.

Rosenow EM, Marth EH (1987): Addition of cocoa powder, cane sugar and carrageenan to milk enhances growth of *Listeria monocytogenes. J Food Prot.* 50:716–729.

Schaffner CP, Mosbach K, Bibit VS, Watson CH (1967): Coconut and *Salmonella* infection. *Appl Microbiol.* 15 (3):471–475.

Schwan RF, Cooper RM, Wheals AE (1995): Microbial fermentation of cocoa beans, with emphasis on enzymatic degradation of the pulp. *J Appl Bacteriol.* 79 (Symp Suppl): 96S–107S.

Shenkel J (1972): Mikrobiologische fragen bei der susswarenherstellung and notwendige betriebshygienische forderungen. *Int Rev Sugar Confect.* 25:300–305.

Takahashi T, Taguchi H, Yamaguchi H, et al. (1999): Antibaterial effects of cacao mass on enterohemorrhagic *Escherichia coli* O157:H7. *Kansenshogaku Zasshi.* 73:694–701.

Tamminga SK, Beumer RR, Kampelmacher EH, van Leusden FM (1977): Survival of *Salmonella typhimurium* in milk chocolate prepared with artificially contaminated milk powder. *J Hyg.* 79:333–337.

Werber D, Dreesman J, Fil F, et al. (2005): International outbreak of *Samonella* Oranienburg due to German chocolate. *BMC Infect. Dis.* 5:7.

Wesley F, Rourke R, Darbishire O (1965): The formation of persistent toxic chlorohydrins in foodstuffs by fumigation with ethylene oxide and with propylene oxide. *J Food Sci.* 30:1037–1042.

Zapatka FA, Varney GW, Sinskey AJ (1977): Neutralization of the bactericidal effect of cocoa powder on salmonellae by casein. *J Appl Bacteriol.* 42:21–25.

PART IV

PREVENTION AND CONTROL STRATEGIES

CHAPTER 19

MICROBIAL RISK ASSESSMENT

MARIANNE D. MILIOTIS and ROBERT L. BUCHANAN

19.1 INTRODUCTION

Global changes such as increase in population growth, urbanization, poverty, international trade in food and animal feed, and international travel, as well as newly emerging pathogens, the role of food-processing operations, and the aging population, are the major factors influencing the incidence and profiles of foodborne illness (Miyagishima and Käferstein, 2003). The combination of these factors has created major new challenges, elevating the risk of contamination of raw and ready-to-eat foods worldwide. Strategies developed to prevent these illnesses rely increasingly on science-based approaches. This includes an increased role for risk assessment as a systematic rationale for integrating the many factors that must be considered to develop consistent, science-based standards for international trade (WHO, 1995).

19.1.1 Food Safety as a Risk Management Activity

A typical diet in many countries consists of a wide variety of fresh and processed foods that are derived from raw ingredients acquired both domestically and internationally. Foods are prepared and consumed both within the home and at millions of food service establishments. Few foods are commercially sterile and all require care in production, processing, distribution, marketing, preparation, and consumption. With such a highly complex, interdependent activity, it is important that everyone understand that food safety is based on the pragmatic management of a vast array of potential risks. This is reflected in the two primary means for controlling food safety risks: good hygienic practices (GHPs) and the hazard analysis of critical control point (HACCP) system. The latter is a risk management system based on an evaluation of hazards that are reasonably likely to occur, followed by the implementation of mitigations to control those hazards to an acceptable level.

Microbiologically Safe Foods, Edited by Norma Heredia, Irene Wesley, and Santos García

As food safety systems have become more complex, with multiple approaches and technologies available for controlling hazards, it has become increasingly important to be able to evaluate the relative effectiveness or equivalence of controlling hazards. This includes being able to consider effectively the wide diversity in the food industry, which typically ranges from multinational corporations to family-operated establishments. Microbiological risk assessment (MRA) techniques are providing new tools to measure and compare the risks presented by specific microbiological hazards in specific foods (Lammerding and Paoli, 1997). Increasingly, quantitative microbial risk assessments are being requested to provide information that assists in making risk-based management decisions (Buchanan and Whiting, 1998). This includes developing more transparent tools for establishing standards for food in international trade (FAO/WHO, 2002). Similarly, microbial risk assessment techniques are being used increasingly to augment HACCP approaches. The integration of MRA with HACCP has great potential for relating food manufacturing operations to public health goals (Buchanan and Whiting, 1998) and thereby providing a more objective means for establishing the critical limit that needs to be achieved at a critical control point.

Although the original goal of MRAs was to assist in decision making, the use of MRAs has evolved and expanded to include:

- Collecting and objectively evaluating information on a risk issue
- Facilitating channels of communication between groups affected
- Assisting in the understanding of complex processes to make them more manageable
- Providing a tool that can assist in the evaluation of proposed management. strategies, such as measuring the risk reduction potential of various risk control options
- Highlighting data and information gaps and identifying research needs

19.1.2 Risk and How It Is Measured

Risk is defined as the possibility of suffering harm or loss. Risk assessment, as defined by *Codex Alimentarius* in 1995, is "the estimation of the severity and likelihood of harm or damage, resulting for exposure to hazardous agents or substances" (FAO/WHO, 1995). In microbial risk assessment, the hazardous agents or substances are the microorganisms and/or their toxins. Risk is measured using data and analytic models that estimate the extent of human exposure to a pathogenic microorganism and the probability and severity of human response to that exposure.

19.1.3 History of MRA

Throughout history, attempts have been made to assess and manage risk-related to hazards. Many of these have been informal evaluations but are still valuable and effective (Kindred, 1996). In 1983 the National Research Council in the United States recommended that risk assessment methods be applied to strengthen the scientific basis of risk-based decision making. A report on how federal agencies should evaluate and control risk entitled *Risk Assessment in the Federal Government: Managing the Process*, was published (NRC, 1996). This report, known as "The Red Book," focused largely on consideration of carcinogens. It was precedent setting because it formalized, for the first time, a number of basic risk assessment concepts. These concepts served as a model for several studies in the 1980s and early 1990s on the risk of foodborne illness, such as inspection programs for meat and poultry, beef, and seafood.

In the mid-1990s, increased awareness of the public health impact of microbial foodborne disease, in terms of both severity of illness and economic cost to society and industry prompted regulators worldwide to consider new strategies to reduce foodborne illness. This was accelerated by the increasing importance and growth of global food trade and the concomitant establishment of the World Trade Organization and the signing of the Sanitary and Phytosanitary Agreement and the Technical Barriers to Trade Agreement, which emphasized the role of risk assessment in resolving international trade disputes (WHO, 1995). One of these strategies is the use of microbial risk assessment to assist in evaluating foodborne illness and in managing the safety of the food supply.

Microbial risk assessments generally use the same conceptual framework as that developed for chemical risk assessments. Although there are many similarities between chemical and microbiological risk assessments, there are also several important differences. A major difference is that with microbiological hazards, an acute illness typically results from a single exposure. Although there are concerns with acute toxicity with certain chemicals, most toxicological concerns associated with foods are chronic chemical hazards that result from low-level, continual, or multiple exposures. A second major difference is that, often, microbes can grow and multiply in a food whereas chemicals do not. Thus, the level of microorganisms in a food (or other environments) can change drastically over a short period, whereas chemical concentrations usually remain constant. Such changes in microbial levels must be accounted for in a microbial risk assessment model.

In 1996 the FAO/WHO Joint Expert Consultation published a document on principles and guidelines for risk assessment for the Codex Committee on Food Hygiene (CCFH, 1996). About the same time, the International Life Sciences Institute (ILSI) also independent of the CCFH, developed a framework for conducting microbial risk assessments (ILSI, 2000). Since then, several quantitative microbiological food safety risk assessments have been conducted by industry groups, national governments, and international organizations and MRAs are now a standard component in the effort to protect public health and facilitate free trade (Schroeder et al., 2007).

19.2 RISK ASSESSMENT FRAMEWORK

Microbial risk assessment is a component of the entire risk analysis paradigm, which consists of risk management, risk assessment, and risk communication (Fig. 1). Risk management is the process of weighing policy alternatives in light of results or risk assessment, and if required, selecting and implementing appropriate control options,

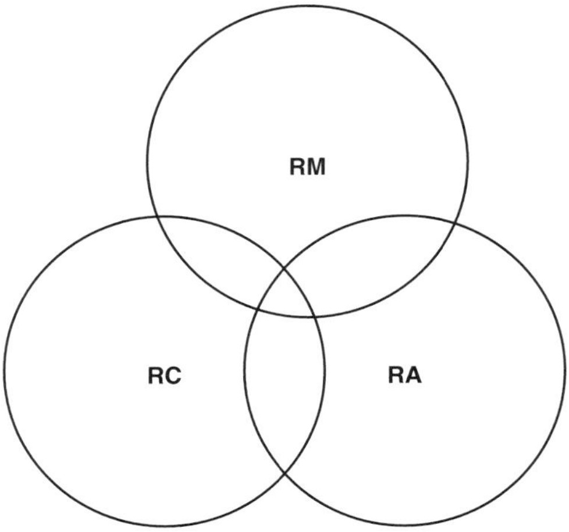

FIG. 1 The three components of risk analysis: risk management (RM), risk assessment (RA), and risk communication (RC).

including regulatory measures if warranted. Risk assessment is the scientific evaluation of known or potential adverse health effects resulting from human exposure to hazards. Risk communication is the interactive exchange of information and opinions concerning risk and risk management among risk assessors, managers, consumers, industry, and other interested parties. It is important to note that risk assessments often benefit from public input and are most effective when they consider the range of science and value judgments (NRC, 1996). The risk assessment process consists of hazard identification, exposure assessment, hazard characterization (dose–response), and risk characterization (FAO/WHO, 1999).

19.2.1 Hazard Identification

Hazard identification identifies, by a thorough review of available information, the pathogen that may be present in a particular food and the adverse health effects that can potentially occur as a result of its presence (CDC, 2005). Thus, a hazard characterization will typically consist of three components: a pathogen, a disease manifestation, and a food product(s) (e.g., *Vibrio parahaemolyticus*/gastroenteritis/raw oysters).

19.2.2 Hazard Characterization

Hazard characterization (dose–response) assesses the relationship between the level of intake (dose) and the nature, severity, and frequency of illness or other adverse health effects (response). This assessment may be qualitative or quantitative. One cannot discuss dose–response without mentioning the disease triangle. The prediction of illness depends on three components: pathogen, host, and environment (food vehicle and microbial competitors present in the food) (Fig. 2) (Coleman and Marks, 1998).

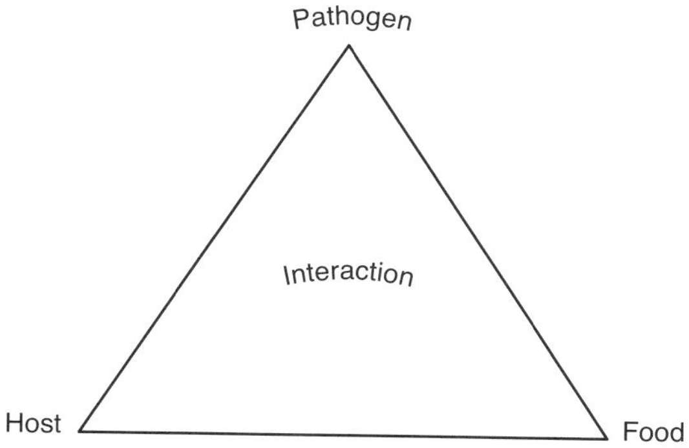

FIG. 2 Disease triangle showing interactions among pathogen, host, and food environment.

In other words, changes in the pathogen, host, or environment may have a substantial impact on the incidence and severity of illness predicted (Coleman and Marks, 1998).

19.2.3 Exposure Assessment

Exposure assessment is the qualitative or quantitative evaluation of the total intake of a hazard that is likely to occur. Potentially, this could involve multiple routes of entry (e.g., oral, respiratory, dermal) and vehicles (e.g., food, water, person-to-person contact), but in general the acute nature of most infectious diseases has led to risk assessments that consider a primary route of entry and a primary vehicle or related class of vehicles (e.g., ready-to-eat refrigerated foods). For exposure assessment, transmission of the hazard involved is often modeled through the food pathway, a chain of processes from a source of the raw ingredients (e.g., the farm) to the moment of consumption. Such evaluations have followed the prevalence and the concentration of the hazard along the consecutive processes of the food pathway, taking into account the variability and uncertainty attending this transmission (Nauta, 2000). The food pathway is typically subdivided into unit operations, which describe treatments to which the ingredients are being subjected as they are being converted to a food, and the impact that these operations have on the hazard. For each step, the input–output relationship is then described. Such relationships are identified through direct observation (surveillance studies measuring the changes in hazards or surrogates in a production environment), by laboratory experimentation (simulation in the laboratory of the processes occurring during manufacturing), or by mathematical modeling based on established physicochemical principles (e.g., thermodynamic relationship associated with a heat process) (Notermans et al., 1998).

19.2.4 Risk Characterization

Risk characterization integrates the previous steps (i.e., hazard identification, hazard characterization, and exposure assessment) to produce a risk estimate, the likelihood of illness or death from exposure to a particular microorganism, as well as the uncertainty associated with the estimate. The influence of inputs and assumptions of a model is described by standard evaluation techniques such as sensitivity and uncertainty analyses. The technical issues and methodologies in developing the models and interpreting the output are often complex. Therefore, an additional aspect of the risk characterization is to provide a context around which the risk estimate should be interpreted and the limitations associated with the analysis of which the reader must be cognizant, including the potential consequences of extrapolating the results beyond the limits of the original analysis. There are several modeling techniques for assessing the relative importance of factors contributing to risk and its uncertainty:

1. *Sensitivity analysis*. Sensitivity analysis is conducted to determine which model input factors have the strongest influence on the outcome predicted, such as probability of illness.
2. *Uncertainty analysis (or sensitivity analysis of uncertainty)*. Uncertainty analysis is conducted to determine which factor(s) contributed most to the uncertainty of the predicted outcome.
3. *Validation*. One of the most difficult problems facing risk assessors is determining whether their model is an accurate representation of the "real world" (i.e., they need to validate the risk assessment model). Typically, this is done by comparing predicted results with data that have not been incorporated into the risk assessment. For example, one of the validation approaches used in the USFDA *Vibrio parahaemolyticus* risk assessment was to compare the levels of total *V. parahaemolyticus* in retail oysters predicted by the exposure assessment model against data obtained by the ISSC/FDA 1998–1999 retail survey (USFDA-CFSAN, 2005). The risk assessment was also able to validate at least parts of its risk characterization by comparing predictions against a new set of CDC data on regional and seasonal incidences of *V. parahaemolyticus* infections.

19.3 RISK ASSESSMENT ANALYTICAL TOOLS

Microbial risk assessment is a systematic analytical approach intended to support the understanding and management of microbial risk issues. It evaluates scientific data to estimate the likelihood and magnitude of the occurrence of an adverse human health effect after exposure to a pathogenic microorganism. Within the models described above, specific tools exist that are used to perform risk assessments (Notermans and Mead, 1996; van Gerwen et al., 2000).

Statistical packages such as SAS and SPSS are used in model development for experimental design, data handling, prediction, and confidence intervals (Wijtzes, 2002). Other widely used tools for performing probabilistic modeling include the @RISK and Crystal Ball risk analysis packages, which are associated with Excel spreadsheets, and use of the Monte Carlo simulation technique. Additional tools can be found at http://www.foodrisk.org. Monte Carlo simulation is a type of spreadsheet simulation that continuously generates values for uncertain variables randomly to simulate a model. A simulation calculates multiple scenarios of a model by repeatedly sampling values from the probability distributions for the uncertain variables and using those values for the cell. For each uncertain variable (one that has a range of possible values), you define the possible values with a probability distribution. The type of distribution you select is based on the conditions surrounding that variable (e.g., normal, triangular, uniform, lognormal). Each step in the risk assessment framework described above is modeled differently.

19.4 QUALITATIVE VS. QUANTITATIVE RISK ASSESSMENTS

Risk assessments can be qualitative or quantitative. However, regardless of type, the process is the same: The risk pathway must be identified, the data collected, and the risk assessed (Snary et al., 2004). Qualitative risk assessment is a descriptive form of risk assessment that is frequently used in microbial risk decision making (Fazil et al., 2005). It provides an estimate of risk in words, such as high, medium, and low, and utilizes all relevant data, including numerical data, in obtaining a conclusion. Quantitative risk assessments describe the risk using mathematical modeling techniques, and therefore the estimate of risk is expressed as a mathematical statement such as "risk per serving," which is the risk of a person becoming ill after consuming a single serving of a particular contaminated food, or as "risk per annum," which is the number of illnesses per year that is predicted. This number is determined by multiplying the mean predicted risk per serving by the number of servings consumed. The benefit of a structured risk assessment process lies in the ability to synthesize data and information, represent complex relationships, describe the probability and severity of adverse events, and inform the decision-making process (Fazil et al., 2005).

19.4.1 Qualitative Methods

When scientific evidence is limited or incomplete or if time and resources are not available to conduct a quantitative risk assessment, information obtained from the literature and/or experts is used to conduct a qualitative risk assessment. Qualitative assessments are often carried out before quantitative assessments and require fewer mathematical resources. The results generated from them can indicate whether or not further quantitative assessment is required or possible (Snary et al., 2004). Most qualitative risk assessments are semiquantitative because of the propensity of risk assessors to attempt to convert qualitative statements into frequencies for the purpose of averaging or describing the frequency of response. As soon as responses are assigned a numerical value, the assessment is no longer strictly qualitative. A qualitative risk assessment in itself, because of its speed and simplicity, can also provide sufficient information to aid in decision making (Fazil et al., 2005). One example of a qualitative method is that conducted by Anderson et al. (2001), where data generated by expert opinion were used to estimate the intensity of illness from the ingestion of *Campylobacter jejuni*. It is worth noting that a well-designed expert elicitation can be a highly sophisticated risk assessment tool that includes an assessment of the expertise of the experts (Martin et al., 1995; WHO, 1999).

19.4.2 Quantitative Methods

Quantitative risk assessments typically rely on mathematical expressions or models to describe the probable occurrence of an adverse event. A model is a simplified representation of a part of reality (Coleman and Marks, 1998). Depending on the scope of the risk assessment and the data sets that are available, two types of mathematical models are combined: exposure assessment models, which determine the level of a hazard ingested by consumers, and dose–response models, which relate the exposure to the incidence of an adverse effect. With dose–response models, several mathematical functions and approaches have been used in the different quantitative MRAs to relate exposure levels to the frequency and severity of biological effects. Two broad approaches to dose–response modeling are used: empirical and mechanistic models.

Empirical models are based on experimental data and describe experimental observations as a mathematical relationship (Wijtzes, 2002). Most currently available dose–response models are empirical. For example, the dose–response models used by FAO/WHO for their *Listeria monocytogenes* and *Salmonella* risk assessments were based on describing available outbreak and related public health data using non-threshold mathematical functions (FAO/WHO, 2000; Miyagishima and Käferstein, 2003). It is important to note that empirical models are valid only for the data set on which they are based, and any extrapolation of the model to other microorganisms or disease manifestations should be viewed with caution.

Mechanistic models are built on a conceptual understanding of the behavior of microbes and the mechanisms through which they cause disease. They offer a stronger scientific rationale for predicting dose–response relations, but not necessarily more accurate predictions. However, a well-designed mechanistic model should provide greater opportunity for extrapolating beyond the range of the experimental data. Potentially, mechanistic models would be more flexible since they focus on specific physiological or chemical attributes. For example, Buchanan et al. (2001) outlined a simple three-compartment mechanistic dose–response model for foodborne salmonellosis. The model compartments were survival in the stomach, attachment and colonization in the intestine, and invasion of body tissues or production of toxins.

Quantitative models are also used extensively for performing quantitative exposure assessments. The key to a successful exposure assessment is accurate estimation of the levels of the microorganism that are actually ingested by the consumer. This can be a significant challenge considering how rapidly microbiological populations can change (e.g., growth, inactivation) and the limited locations along the food chain where microbiological data are collected. Modeling techniques are critical to taking data from a specific location in the food chain and, through the use of models, predicting the level actually consumed. This relies heavily on predictive microbiology modeling techniques, which are described below and in more detail in Chapter 30.

Risk assessment models are also either deterministic or probabilistic. Deterministic models provide outcomes as point estimates for the microbial load at different time points (Poschet et al., 2003). Probabilistic models take a more random approach and provide a range of outcomes. Poschet et al. (2003) demonstrated that a more probabilistic approach using Monte Carlo analysis can be generated from experimental observations and a deterministic growth model.

In a study by Walls and Scott (1997) in which the potential risk of foodborne illness from a cooked meat product contaminated with *Staphylococcus aureus* and hamburger contaminated with *Salmonella* was estimated, point estimates were used as opposed to distributions of data, which may have accounted for the higher-than-expected number of infections predicted. A more stochastic approach using a range of cooking times and temperatures might have provided a more accurate measure of the temperature gradient during the cooking of hamburger (Walls and Scott, 1997).

19.5 TYPES OF RISK ASSESSMENT

There are basically four general types of risk assessments: risk–risk, risk ranking, product pathway analysis, and geographic pathway/risk of introduction.

19.5.1 Risk–Risk Assessments

Risk–risk assessments are analyses that consider trading-off one risk for another; that is, reducing the risk of one hazard increases the risk of another. An example of this would be a determination of the impact on public health of treating drinking water with a chemical (risk associated with by-products of drinking-water disinfection) versus the impact of exposure to pathogenic organisms such as *Cryptosporidium parvum* in untreated water.

19.5.2 Risk-Ranking Assessments

Risk-ranking assessments compare the relative risk among several hazards or foods. These types of assessment techniques might involve a single pathogen associated with multiple foods, a single food that has multiple pathogens, or multiple pathogens and multiple foods. Risk-ranking assessments can help establish regulatory program priorities and identify critical research needs. The FDA/USDA *Listeria monocytogenes* risk assessment is an example of a risk-ranking assessment (USFDA/USDA, 2003). The food categories are divided into five overall risk designations, which are likely to require different approaches to controlling foodborne listeriosis. The resulting rankings—very high, high, moderate, low, and very low risk—are illustrated in Fig. 3, which compares the relative risks among the different food categories and population groups considered in the assessment. As shown in Fig. 3, the exposure

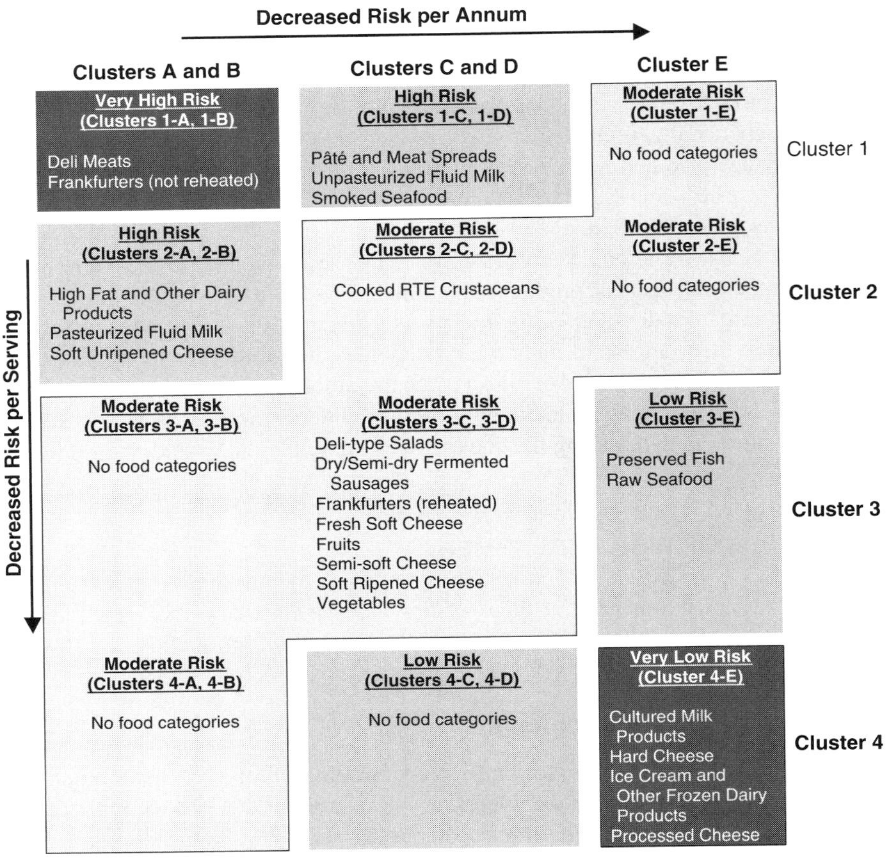

FIG. 3 Two-dimensional matrix of food categories based on cluster analysis of predicted per serving and per annum relative rankings. (From USFDA/USDA, 2003.)

models and accompanying what-if scenarios identify broad factors that affect consumer exposure to *L. monocytogenes* at the time of food consumption:

1. Amounts and frequency of consumption of a ready-to-eat food
2. Frequency and levels of *L. monocytogenes* in a ready-to-eat food
3. Potential of the food to support growth of *L. monocytogenes* during refrigerated storage
4. Refrigerated storage temperature

19.5.3 Product Pathway Analyses

Product pathway analyses are assessments that examine the factors that influence the risk associated with specific food–hazard pairs. Ideally, assessment starts at the farm and ends with consumption. These types of assessment techniques help identify the key factors that affect exposure, including the impact of potential mitigation or intervention strategies on the risk predicted. The FDA *Vibrio parahaemolyticus* risk assessment and the USDA *Escherichia coli* O157:H7 risk assessments are examples of product pathway analyses (USFDA-CFSAN, 2005; USDA-FSIS, 2001).

19.5.4 Geographic Risk Assessments

Geographic risk assessments examine the factors that either limit or allow a risk to occur. The risk of introduction of disease agents through food animals or animal products (e.g., intentionally as in bioterrorism, or unintentionally) can be examined. For example, the risk of introduction of variant Creutzfeldt–Jacob disease in humans by the transmission of BSE from cattle through meats and animal product pathways might be examined using a geographical approach.

19.6 PREDICTIVE MICROBIOLOGY

To estimate the risk for foodborne infections, risk assessors need information on the number of microorganisms present in food at the time of consumption (Ross and McMeekin, 2003). However, this is one of the difficulties associated with microbial risk assessment. Numbers of bacteria in food can change at all stages of food production and processing, depending on the nature of the food and the way it is handled, stored, and processed. Predictive microbiology can be used to estimate changes in bacterial numbers. The term *predictive microbiology* describes the scientific discipline of predicting microbial behavior (e.g., growth, survival, inactivation) as a function of environmental factors (McMeekin et al., 1993). It is a means of generating exposure data and establishing critical limits for hazard analysis of critical control point (HACCP) plans (Hathaway and Cook, 1997). The primary tool for doing so is the development of mathematical models that describe the characteristics of microorganism growth and other behaviors under different environmental conditions. Predictive microbiology provides a means of modeling the impact that different steps of production, processing, marketing, and preparation pathway have on the concentration of a microorganism (see Chapter 30). This enables both estimation of changes in bacterial numbers, providing an exposure assessment of a person to a pathogen, and assists in evaluating intervention strategies in risk management (Foegeding, 1997). The availability of predictive microbiology models such as the U.S. Department of Agricultures/Agricultural Research Services Pathogen Modeling Program (COMBASE) (USDA-ARS, 2006) has proven integral to the successful development of microbiological risk assessments. Examples of how predictive microbiology has been effectively incorporated in risk assessments are described below.

Whiting and Buchanan (1997) demonstrated a dynamic approach to modeling risk which assists in identification and setting critical control points and assessing the impact of altering food formulations or processes in their quantitative risk assessment model for a *Salmonella* Enteritidis infection from thermally processed liquid whole eggs made into mayonnaise in the home. Dose–response models for infectivity were integrated with predictive microbiology models for growth and inactivation (thermal and nonthermal) using a stochastic simulation approach, data on the frequency of pathogens in raw ingredients. The risk assessment not only indicated that pasteurization provides sufficient consumer protection from a high incidence of infected birds and from temperature abuse between the farm and the egg breakers, but, by simulating different scenarios, it also showed the consequences of inadequate pasteurization temperatures and/or temperature abuse during storage.

19.7 USING RISK ASSESSMENT TO MAKE RISK MANAGEMENT DECISIONS

The primary reason for conducting health risk assessments in a regulatory environment is to assist in decision making. In other words, quantitative MRA is intended to answer specific questions to assist in protecting public health. The scientific evaluations and mathematical models developed for the various microbial hazards can assist the risk managers to evaluate the effectiveness of interventions to reduce or prevent foodborne illness, weigh policy alternatives, and develop appropriate action plans. Below are some examples of different risk assessments and their application in decision making and some examples of risk assessments conducted by regulatory agencies within the United States.

1. *USDHHS/FDA quantitative risk assessment on the public health impact of* V. parahaemolyticus *in raw oysters* (VPRA). The VPRA is an example of a risk assessment with the potential to be a useful tool. The risk assessment showed that strategies aimed at reducing various levels of the pathogen by different magnitudes reduced illness accordingly (USFDA-CFSAN, 2005). For example, strategies aimed at reducing *V. parahaemolyticus* levels by 100-fold reduced illness by 100-fold. When levels were reduced about 10,000-fold, illness was reduced to a point where it would be difficult to detect. Immediate refrigeration of the oysters after harvest would reduce illness by about 10-fold. The VPRA also demonstrated that reducing time to refrigeration also reduced illness (Fig. 4).

2. *USDHHS/FDA–USDA/FSIS quantitative risk ranking risk assessment on* Listeria monocytogenes (LMRA) *in ready-to-eat foods*. The LMRA is a good example of using a risk assessment to develop an action plan to reduce foodborne illness due to this microbe (USFDA/USDA, 2003; USDHHS/USFDA, 2005). The LMRA was a joint effort led by the Food and Drug Administration's Center for Food Safety and Applied Nutrition (USFDA-CFSAN) in collaboration with the USDA's Food Safety and Inspection Service (FSIS), in consultation with the U.S. Centers for Disease Control and Prevention (CDC). The LMRA was commissioned in response to a presidential request for federal agencies to develop control plans to reduce listeriosis by 50% by the year 2005 (USFDA/USDA, 2003). The purpose of the assessment was to identify which foods should receive the most regulatory attention in an effort to improve public health. From Fig. 2, which compares the relative risks among the various food categories and population groups considered in the assessment, the risk assessment

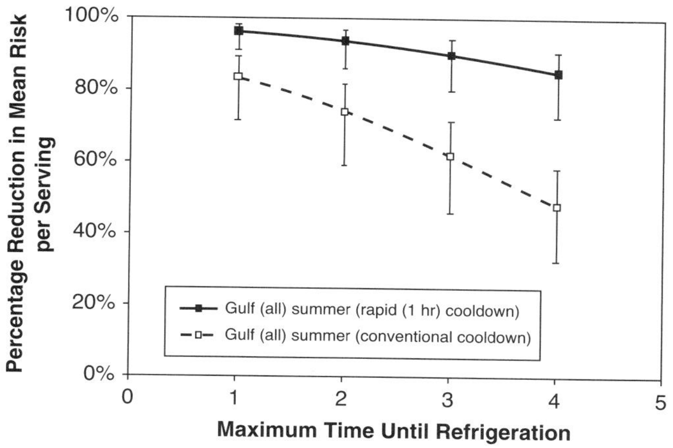

FIG. 4 Predicted effectiveness of rapid versus conventional cooling on *Vibrio parahaemolyticus* risk for Gulf coast summer harvest. (From USFDA-CFSAN, 2005.)

should prove to be a useful tool in focusing control strategies and ultimately improving public health through effective risk management. For example, very high risk foods, such as deli meats and unheated frankfurters, would be consistent with the need for immediate attention in relation to the national goal for reducing the incidence of foodborne listeriosis. Likely activities include the development of new control strategies and/or consumer education programs suitable for these products. Some high-risk foods, such as smoked seafood, pâté, and meat spreads are priority candidates for new control measures. Other high-risk foods, such as unpasteurized milk, might call for continued avoidance. Although high-risk foods such as high-fat and other dairy products (e.g., pasteurized milk, soft unripened cheeses) have low rates of contamination and correspondingly low predicted per serving relative risks, they are consumed often by a large percentage of the population, resulting in their elevated predicted relative risks. These foods would require advanced epidemiologic and scientific investigations to either confirm predictions of the risk assessment or to identify factors not captured by the current models that would reduce the relative risk predicted.

The risks associated with foods that are of moderate risk, such as cooked ready-to-eat crustaceans, deli salads, fruits, vegetables, and some soft cheeses (Fig. 3), appear to be associated primarily with product recontamination, which, in turn, is dependent on continued vigilant application of proven control measures.

Low-risk foods such as preserved fish and raw seafood have moderate contamination rates but include conditions (e.g., acidification) or a short shelf life that limit *L. monocytogenes* growth. When manufactured consistent with current good manufacturing practices, these are not likely to be a major source of foodborne listeriosis.

Very low risk foods, such as cultured milk products, hard cheese, ice cream, and other frozen dairy products, and processed cheese, which are all subjected to bactericidal treatment, have very low contamination rates and possess an inherent characteristic that either inactivates *L. monocytogenes* (e.g., cultured milk products, hard cheese) or prevents its growth (e.g., ice cream and other frozen dairy products, processed cheese), are highly unlikely to be a significant source of foodborne listeriosis.

In addition, the what-if scenarios modeled in this risk assessment provide insight to the impact on public health of limiting storage times, avoiding high-temperature refrigeration storage, and reducing contamination levels.

Based on the results of the risk assessment, the FDA, in consultation with the CDC, developed an action plan with several objectives (USDHHS/USFDA, 2005). These include developing and/or revising guidance for processors, retail and food service providers, and institutional establishments; developing and delivering training and technical assistance for industry and food safety regulatory employees; and enhancing educational efforts. Other key outcomes that resulted from the LMRA include redirection of field assignments and recognition of a need for product pathway analysis to further study potential mitigation during processing and manufacture. This has led to the initiation of a risk assessment on smoked finfish.

3. *USDA-FSIS risk assessment on Escherichia coli* O157:H7 (ECRA) *in ground beef*. Another example of a risk assessment that has been used as a tool in regulatory decision making is the ECRA. Like the VPRA, this risk assessment is an example of product pathway analysis. The ECRA was used to determine the effect of various mitigations in the slaughterhouse on the risk of illness from *E. coli* O157:H7. Results from the ECRA provided the basis for the subsequent ruling that *E. coli* O157:H7 is reasonably likely to occur in ground beef.

REFERENCES

Anderson SA, Yeaton Woo RW, Crawford LM (2001): Risk assessment of the impact on human health of resistant *Campylobacter jejuni* from fluoroquinolone use in beef cattle. *Food Control*. 12:13–25.

Buchanan RL, Whiting RC (1998): Risk assessment: a means for linking HACCP plans and public health. *J Food Prot*. 61:1531–1534.

Buchanan RL, Smith JL, Long W (2001): Microbial risk assessment: dose–response relations and risk characterization. *Int J Food Microbiol*. 58:159–172.

CCFH (Codex Committee on Food Hygiene) (1996): *Principles and Guidelines for the Application of Microbiological Risk Assessment*. Codex Committee on Food Hygiene Discussion Paper 1.

CDC (Centers for Disease Control and Prevention) (2005): Preliminary FoodNet data on the incidence of infection with pathogens transmitted commonly through food—10 sites, United States, 2005. *MMWR Morb Mortal Wkly Rep*. 54:352–356.

Coleman M, Marks H (1998): Topics in dose–response modeling. *J Food Prot*. 61:1550–1559.

FAO/WHO (Food and Agriculture Organization/World Health Organization) (1995): Guidance on the applications of the principles of risk assessment and risk management to food hygiene including strategies for their application. CX/FH 95/8. *Codex Alimentarius*. FAO/WHO, Geneva.

——— (1999): Expert consultation: risk assessment of microbiological hazards in foods, Geneva, Switzerland. http://www.fao.org/DOCREP/005/Y4392E/y4392e07.htm. Accessed June 2008.

——— (2000): *Listeria monocytogenes* in ready-to-eat foods: report of the Joint FAO/WHO Expert Consultation on Risk Assessment of Microbiological Hazards in Foods. http://www.fao.org/ag/agn/jemra/listeria_en.stm. Accessed January 2008.

——— (2002): Risk assessments of *Salmonella* in eggs and broiler chickens, Geneva. http://www.fao.org/DOCREP/005/Y4392E/Y4393E00. Accessed June 2008.

Fazil A, Paoli G, Lammerding AM, Davidson V, Isaac-Renton J, Griffiths M (2005): Microbial Risk assessment as a foundation for informed decision-making: a needs, gaps and opportunities assessment (NGOA) for microbial risk assessment in food and water. http://www.uoguelph.ca/crifs/NGOA/Finalupdates/NGOAfinalreport.pdf. Accessed March 2007.

Foegeding PM (1997): Driving predictive modeling on a risk assessment path for enhanced food safety. *Int J Food Mcrobiol.* 36:87–95.

Hathaway SC, Cook RL (1997): A regulatory perspective on the potential uses of microbial risk assessment in international trade. *Int J Food Microbiol.* 36:127–133.

ILSI (International Life Sciences Institute) (2000): Revised framework for microbial risk assessment: ILSI Risk Science Institute Report. http://www.ilsi.org/file/mrabook.pdf. Accessed January 2008.

Kindred TP (1996): Risk analysis and its application in FSIS. *J Food Prot.* Suppl: S24–S30.

Lammerding AM, Paoli GM (1997): Quantitative risk assessment: an emerging tool for emerging foodborne pathogens. *Emerg Infect Dis.* 3:483–484.

Martin SA, Wallsten TS, Beaulieu ND (1995): Assessing the risk of microbial pathogens: application of a judgement-encoding methodology. *J Food Prot.* 58:289–295.

McMeekin TA, Olley J, Ross T, Ratkowsky DA (1993): *Predictive Microbiology: Theory and Application.* Wiley, New York.

Miyagishima K, Käferstein, FF (2003): The WHO agreement on the application of sanitary and phytosanitary measures: an international trade agreement with implications for national and international food safety standards. In: Miliotis MD, Bier JW (Eds.). *International Handbook of Foodborne Pathogens.* Marcel Dekker, New York, pp. 745–752.

Nauta MJ (2000): Separation of uncertainty and variability in quantitative microbial risk assessment models. *Int J Food Microbiol.* 57:9–18.

Notermans S, Mead GC (1996): Incorporation of elements of quantitative risk analysis in the HACCP system. *Int J Food Microbiol.* 30:157–173.

Notermans S, Nauta MJ, Jansen J, Jouve JL, Mead GC (1998): A risk assessment approach to evaluating food safety based on product surveillance. *Food Control.* 9:217–223.

NRC (National Research Council) (1996): *Understanding Risk: Informing Decisions in a Democratic Society.* National Academy of Sciences. National Academies Press, Washington, DC.

Poschet F, Geeraerd AH, Scheerlinck N, Nicolaï BM, Van Impe JF (2003): Monte Carlo analysis as a tool to incorporate variation on experimental data in predictive microbiology. *Food Microbiol.* 20:285–296.

Ross T, McMeekin TA (2003): Modeling microbial growth within food safety risk assessments. *Risk Anal.* 23:179–197.

Schroeder CM, Jensen E, Miliotis M, Dennis SB, Morgan KM (2007): Microbial risk assessment. In: Simjee S (Ed.): *Foodborne Diseases*. Humana Press, Totowa, pp. 435–456.

Snary EL, Kelly LA, Davison HC, Teale CJ, Wooldridge M (2004): Antimicrobial resistance: a microbial risk assessment perspective. *J Antimicrob Chemother.* 53:906–917.

USDA-ARS (U.S. Department of Agriculture–Agriculture Research Service) (2006): New database helps monitor food pathogens. http://wyndmoor.arserrc.gov/combase/default.aspx. Accessed January 2008.

USDA-FSIS (U.S. Department of Agriculture–Food Safety and Inspection Service) (2001): Risk assessment of the public health impact of *Escherichia coli* O157:H7 in ground beef. http://www.fsis.usda.gov/OPPDE/rdad/FRPubs/00-023N/00-023NReport.pdf. Accessed March 2007.

USDHHS/USFDA (U.S. Department of Health and Human Services/U.S. Food and Drug Administration) (2005): Current FDA activities related to the *Listeria monocytogenes* action plan. http://www.foodsafety.gov/~dms/lmr2pla2.html. Accessed June 2008.

USFDA-CFSAN (U.S. Food and Drug Administration–Center for Food Safety and Applied Nutrition) (2005): Quantitative risk assessment on the public health impact of pathogenic *Vibrio parahaemolyticus* in raw oysters. http://www.cfsan.fda.gov/~dms/vpra-toc.html. Accessed March 2007.

USFDA/USDA (U.S. Food and Drug Administration/U.S. Department of Agriculture) (2003): Quantitative assessment of relative risk to public health from foodborne *Listeria monocytogenes* among selected categories of ready-to-eat foods. http://www.foodsafety.gov/~dms/lmr2-toc.html. Accessed March 2007.

van Gerwen SJC, te Giffel MC, van't Riet K, Beumer RR, Zwietering MH (2000): Stepwise quantitative risk assessment as a tool for characterization of microbiological food safety. *J Appl Microbiol.* 88:938–951.

Walls I, Scott VN (1997): Use of predictive microbiology in microbial food safety risk assessment. *Int J Food Microbiol.* 36:97–102.

Whiting RC, Buchanan RL (1997): Development of a quantitative risk assessment model for *Salmonella enteritidis* in pasteurized liquid eggs. *Int J Food Microbiol.* 36:111–125.

WHO (World Health Organization) (1995): *Application of Risk Analysis to Food Standards Issues*. Report of the Joint Food and Agricultural Organization of the United Nations and World Health Organization. WHO/FNU/FOS/95.3.

——— (1999): *Principles and Guidelines for the Conduct of Microbiological Risk Assessment*. CAC/GL-30. WHO, Geneva, Switzerland.

Wijtzes T (2002): Tools for microbiological risk assessment. In: Brown M, Stringer M (Eds.). *Microbiological Risk in Food Processing*. Woodhead Publishing, Cambridge, UK, pp. 193–213.

CHAPTER 20

GOOD MANUFACTURING PRACTICES

OLGA I. PADILLA-ZAKOUR

20.1 INTRODUCTION

Good manufacturing practices (GMPs) are used to manufacture human food that is safe to eat and is produced in keeping with good public health practices. In the United States, GMPs are defined in the *Code of Federal Regulations*, Title 21, Part 110, which regulates the production of all types of foods. This ordinance covers all aspects of food manufacturing, including personnel and facilities. GMPs protect food from microorganisms, pests (insects, rodents, and others) and foreign material both physical and chemical (USFDA, 2006a). To understand the elements of GMPs, it is necessary to understand the following selected terms as they are defined by the U.S. Food and Drug Administration (USFDA, 2006b):

- *Acidified* foods are foods with an equilibrium pH of 4.6 or lower.
- *Blanching* (except for tree nuts and peanuts) is a prepackaging heat treatment of foodstuffs for a sufficient time and at a sufficient temperature to partially or completely inactivate naturally occurring enzymes and to result in other physical or biochemical changes in the food.
- A *critical control point* is a point in a food process where there is a high probability that improper control may cause, allow, or contribute to contamination or decomposition of the final food.
- *Food-contact surfaces* are those that contact human food and those surfaces from which drainage onto the food or onto surfaces that contact the food ordinarily occurs during the normal course of operations. Included are utensils and food-contact surfaces of equipment.
- *Microorganisms* are organisms both harmful and beneficial, such as yeasts, molds, parasites, bacteria, and viruses and include species having public health significance. The term *undesirable microorganisms* includes those

Microbiologically Safe Foods, Edited by Norma Heredia, Irene Wesley, and Santos García

microorganisms that are of public health significance, that subject food to decomposition, that indicate that food is contaminated with filth, or that otherwise may cause food to be adulterated within the meaning of the regulation.

- *A pest* is any objectionable animal or insect, including birds, rodents, flies, and larvae.
- *A plant* is the building or facility or parts thereof, used for or in connection with the manufacture, packaging, labeling, or holding of human food.
- A *quality control operation* is a planned and systematic procedure for taking all actions necessary to prevent food from being adulterated (within the meaning of the act).
- *A safe-moisture level* is a level of moisture low enough to prevent the growth of undesirable microorganisms in the finished product under the intended conditions of manufacturing, storage, and distribution. The maximum safe moisture level for a food is based on its water activity (a_w). An a_w value will be considered safe for a food if adequate data are available that demonstrate that at or below the given a_w, the food will not support the growth of undesirable microorganisms.
- *To sanitize* is to treat food-contact surfaces by a process that is effective in destroying vegetative cells of microorganisms of public health significance, and in substantially reducing numbers of other undesirable microorganisms, without adversely affecting the product or its safety for the consumer.
- *Water activity* (a_w) is a measure of the free moisture in a food that could be used by microorganisms to grow, and is the quotient of the water vapor pressure of the substance divided by the vapor pressure of pure water at the same temperature.

20.2 PERSONNEL

Personnel who take part in the manufacture of food should be healthy. Anyone who is, or even appears to be, sick should not participate in food manufacturing until he or she is well. Even a minor sore throat or cough represents a risk. Workers can spread *Salmonella* and hepatitis A long after they are symptom-free. Respiratory infections such as influenza are transmitted through coughing and sneezing (Gravani et al., 1997). If employees have open lesions or wounds, including sores and blisters, these must be covered or cured appropriately so that the person is no longer a potential source of contamination. Even healthy employees carry sizable numbers of bacteria such as *Staphylococcus* and *Streptococci*, and intestinal bacteria such as *Shigella* and *Escherichia coli*. Bacteria are present on the lips, nose, mouth, and hair. Proper, clean attire and intact gloves and hair nets must be worn to ensure that these bacteria are not transferred to food products or equipment (Gravani et al., 1997; Marriott, 1999).

All personnel who work in food processing must maintain adequate personal cleanliness so that they and their clothing do not contaminate the food or food-processing equipment. Clothing must not be loose and must be clean. The company may provide uniforms, aprons, and other outer garments. Figure 1 shows a healthy,

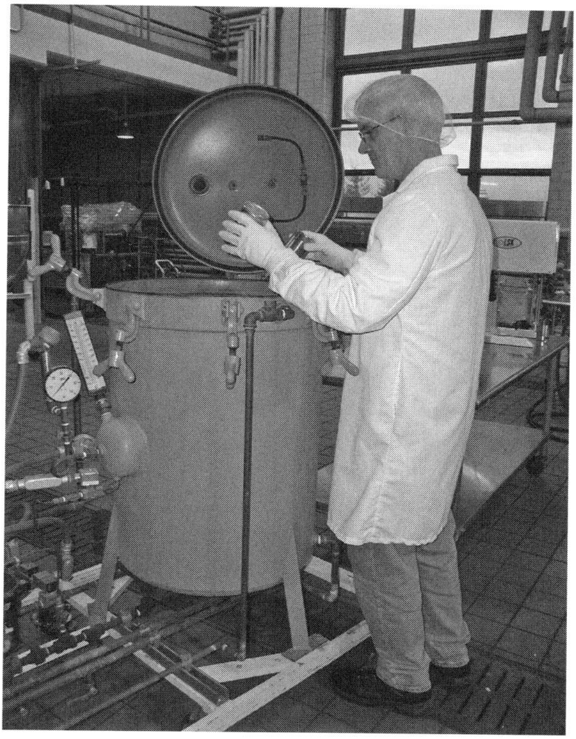

FIG. 1 Food manufacturing employee in a canning plant demonstrating proper use of hair net, clean coat, and gloves.

properly clothed employee in a canning facility. Hair and beard nets and other hair restraints, such as headbands and hats, must be worn to prevent hair from coming into contact with food. Outer garments such as aprons or coats must be removed before using the restroom, to avoid contamination. All touching or itching of the head should be avoided. If necessary, retouching hair and itching should be done in restroom, away from food processing, and hair must be adequately restrained before the employee returns to the processing area after proper hand washing. This prevents hair from falling into the food and bacteria from the hair contaminating hands and gloves, and then foods (Gravani et al., 1997). Because they also pose a contamination risk, all jewelry and personal ornaments must be removed prior to working in a food manufacturing area. Any hand jewelry that cannot be removed must be covered with gloves so that it does not contaminate the food.

Hands must be washed frequently, adequately, and in stations provided for hand washing, not in sinks used to prepare foods. Figure 2 shows a sensor-activated sink used by employees to wash their hands after using the bathroom. Water for hand washing should be as hot as the hands can stand, about 43°C. After moistening hands and exposed portions of the arms, soap thoroughly and rub together for at least 20 s,

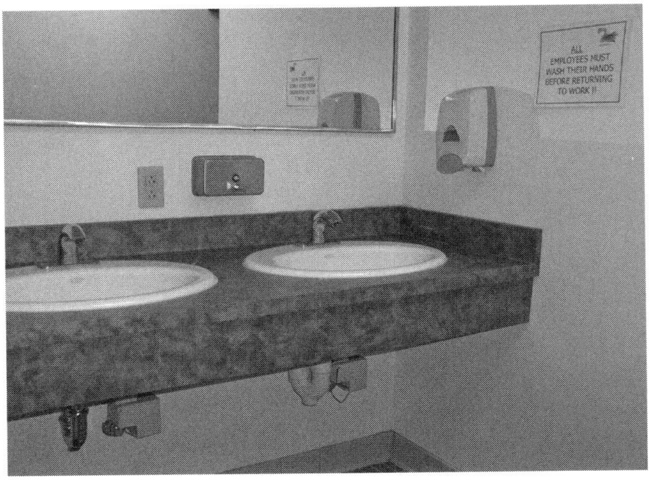

FIG. 2 Sensor-activated sink, liquid soap dispenser, and posted reminder for employees to wash hands after using the bathroom.

paying particular attention to areas between the fingers and under the nails (Staff of J.J. Keller & Assoc., 2000). Rinse thoroughly with clean water and dry the hands using individual disposable towels, a hot-air dryer, or continuous towel system which the operator keeps supplied with clean towels. Hands must be washed after using the toilet; after touching hair, body, or clothing; after handling garbage; when moving to another section of the food-processing facility; after handling soiled work surfaces, equipment, or materials; and after eating or drinking.

Gloves should be worn at all times if required for processing food. They should be impenetrable and be maintained intact in a clean and sanitary fashion. Latex gloves are quite common and are an excellent example. If the gloves are pierced or ripped, they should be disposed of and an intact pair used (Gravani et al., 1997; Staff of J.J. Keller & Assoc., 2000).

Food-processing businesses must provide education and training in cleanliness and established procedures to all personnel so that everyone understands what is required and why. Pre-employment health examinations may be required and are a good way to stress the importance of personal hygiene (Marriott, 1999). In addition, a supervisor who is responsible for personnel cleanliness must be clearly assigned. Employees who are sick or have open wounds must not be allowed to work in food preparation areas and, if necessary, could be assigned to perform office work.

20.3 BUILDINGS AND FACILITIES

GMPs for buildings and facilities can be classified as pertaining to grounds or to plant construction and design.

20.3.1 Grounds

Food may be contaminated by the area around the processing plant. The operator must ensure proper storage of equipment, such as equipment used in the loading of product into trucks for distribution. Pests should be controlled on the premises through the removal of litter and waste and by cutting weeds and grass within the vicinity of the processing facility (USFDA, 2006b). Ideally, pea gravel or similar material should be laid around the building over polyethylene or equivalent to discourage rodents. Doing so eliminates breeding and habitat areas that harbor such pests as mice, cockroaches, and flies. For the same reason, adequate drainage should be provided: for example, removing or emptying containers that collect rainwater. Such places are breeding grounds for mosquitoes, harbor *Listeria monocytogenes*, and may attract birds, which naturally carry *Campylobacter* and *Salmonella* (Marriott, 1999). Drainage also eliminates the possibility of foot-borne contamination. Finally, drainage eliminates the possibility that contaminated water may seep into the food-processing facility (USPHS, 2005).

The operator of the facility should maintain roads, yards and parking areas so that they do not pose a contamination threat to any food that is exposed to them, such as during the shipping process or via employees who move from outdoor to indoor facilities.

Operating systems for waste treatment and disposal must be provided. Waste should never come into contact with food or processing equipment and should be disposed of in keeping with good public health procedures. Waste from food processing is generally high in organic matter, which is ideal for microbial growth. Solid waste may be removed to a dump, rendered, composted, or dried and used as feed for livestock. Pretreatment of liquid waste, including the often high amount of wastewater from processing, is often required before it can enter the municipal waste system. Liquid waste contains spent sanitizers and cleaning compounds and has a high organic content. Pretreatment conducted at the plant may include flow equalization, screening, and skimming to separate larger solids, floatable matter, and material that settles to the bottom within 1 h when tested. Further waste treatment will depend on cost, local regulations, and municipal capacity to treat the volume of waste produced, and may include the use of aerobic and anaerobic lagoons, and specialized filtering systems (Marriott, 1995, 1999).

20.3.2 Plant Construction and Design

An enclosed building must be used for food processing. There should be sufficient space within the building for staff, equipment, and the storage of materials. Aisles between equipment and materials should be provided so that movement is easy and unobstructed, and cleaning is easily performed (USPHS, 2005).

Precautions to prevent contamination within the building must be taken, for instance through the separation of operations so that the food processing operation occurs in isolated stages that correspond to physical locations within the facility. Ideally, raw materials and adjuncts enter the process near the receiving area, move through preparation, process, and packaging areas, and proceed to storage (Imholte, 1984; Jowitt, 1980; Marriott, 1999). All effort must be made to prevent finished product from coming into contact with unprocessed product and raw materials, since doing so may contaminate the finished product.

Floors, walls, and ceiling surfaces must be easy to clean, smooth, nonabsorbent, durable, and kept in good repair. The joints between floors and walls must be sealed to prevent dirt from collecting in the seam. Insulation must be properly installed and free from cracks that attract dirt, are a breeding ground for pathogens, and offer an entry point for pests. Studs, joists, and rafters must not be exposed in areas with moisture. All fixtures, light sockets and switches, vents, fans, decorative items, and so on must be easily cleanable and kept clean. Be aware of condensation potential, take measures to prevent condensation or drips from contaminating food or equipment, and use adequate ceiling and covers.

Adequate ventilation must be provided to control odors and vapors and to protect food from contamination. Air should flow through the facility in such a way as to eliminate the possibility of it contaminating food or equipment. Ventilation of toilet facilities and locker rooms should be exhausted directly to the outside.

There must be adequate lighting so that operation and cleaning can be carried out properly, including toilets and hand-washing facilities. Toilets and hand-washing stations must be provided. Toilet facilities should be kept in good repair, have self-closing doors, and should not be accessed directly from the food-processing area. Figure 3 represents an example of a self-flushing toilet activated by infrared sensors. Hand-washing facilities should be located within convenient reach of employees at multiple stages in the food-processing area and in areas where equipment or utensils are washed (USPHS, 2005). Hand cleanser (soap) and hand drying in the form of individual disposable towels or heated air drying must be provided. Figure 4 shows two commonly used dispensers for liquid soap and for disposable paper towels.

The water supply must be sufficient and from an adequate, protected source (municipal or treated). Water should be tested regularly to evaluate its suitability. Protect water with backflow and antisiphoning devices: air gap, vacuum breaker, or check valve. Water additives and treatments must be food grade and cannot contaminate food. Water temperature should be checked regularly at all locations where hot water is needed.

Plumbing should be up to code for health and safety. Floors must drain properly through adequate drainage systems. In general, one 10-cm drain inlet should be provided for every 36 m^2 of wet processing area. Floors should be sloped to the drains at about 1 to 2% linear slope. Backflow-prevention devices must be in place and checked regularly. Plumbing for liquid waste must meet design requirements and have adequate capacity. The same is true for the sewage system (Imholte, 1984; Shapton, 1991).

There must also be protection from glass breakage; light bulbs must be shielded with plastic covers so that breakage will not result in glass fragments in the food. Windows should be in good condition and if allowed to open, fitted with metal screens (18 mesh) to impede the entrance of pests (Imholte, 1984; Shapton, 1991).

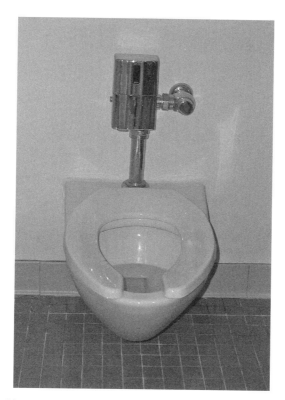

FIG. 3 Self-flushing toilet (infrared sensor) installed in employees' bathroom to minimize contamination.

20.4 SANITATION

Cleaning is the physical removal of soil from surfaces. There are several cleaning options available, depending on the type of operation: manual, soaking, spray methods, cleaning in place, foaming, and high-pressure cleaning (Gould, 1994; Marriott, 1995, 1999). Sanitizing destroys pathogens. Sanitizing treatments must be safe for food products and consumers. GMPs require that all food contact surfaces, including utensils and equipment, must be cleaned as frequently as necessary to protect against contamination of food. All must also be sanitized either by application of heat or by use of sanitizers. A sanitizer is a substance that reduces the microbial load to safe levels as determined by public health requirements (USFDA, 2006b; USPHS, 2005). Chemical sanitizers which have commonly been used in food-processing facilities include chlorine compounds, iodine compounds, and quaternary ammonium compounds (Quats). Other sanitizers now approved for use in food production for specific purposes include peroxyacetic acid, hydrogen peroxide, activated sodium bromide, ozone, and ultraviolet light. Ozone and ultraviolet light are commonly used

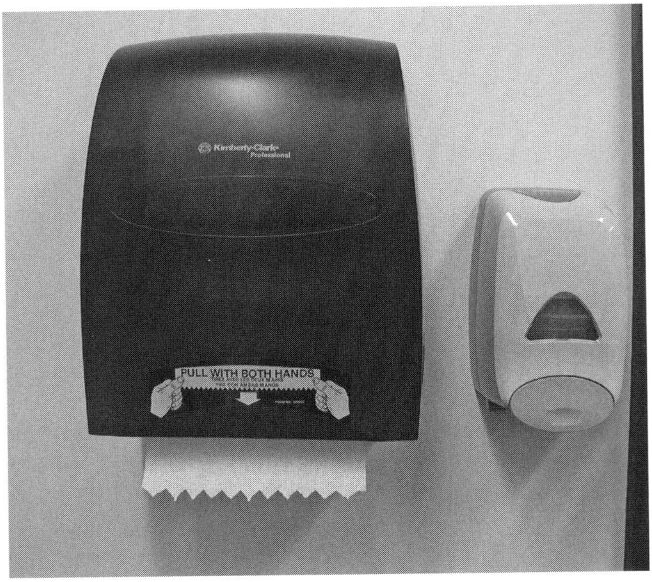

FIG. 4 Commonly used dispensers for liquid soap and disposable paper towels at employee hand wash stations.

to disinfect water. The correct application of a sanitizer is critical to achieve proper disinfection of a cleaned surface, which is dependent on concentration, temperature, exposure time, pH, and the presence of interfering substances (Wedding, 2007).

Chlorine is still the most used sanitizer in the food industry, due to its low cost, fast germicidal action, ease of use, and availability. Typical concentrations for sanitizing surfaces are 50 to 200 ppm. Disadvantages of chlorine-based sanitizers include the fact that it is unstable, breaks down with heat, is less effective if organic matter is present, may corrode stainless steel and metals, and is irritating to skin, eyes, and throat. Iodine compounds are commonly used as skin sanitizers, as they do not irritate skin and have good germicidal effects at 25 ppm. Quats are suitable for porous surfaces and are often used for sanitizing floors, walls, and equipment, due to their stability with time, and when heated do not react with organic matter and do not irritate skin, although they are less effective than chlorine against bacteria (Marriott, 1995; Weddig, 2007).

Sanitizing may also be accomplished with heat, utilizing hot water or steam, typically at 71 to 100°C. It is commonly used as the final step during dish and glassware washing. The surface of dishes and glassware must reach 71°C to be sanitized effectively. Utensils and small pieces of equipment may be manually washed, rinsed, and then sanitized by immersion in water at 77°C or above for 30 s (Marriott, 1999; USPHS, 2005).

A comprehensive cleaning cycle for manual sanitation includes the following steps: prerinse; application of detergent solution; manual scrubbing and cleaning;

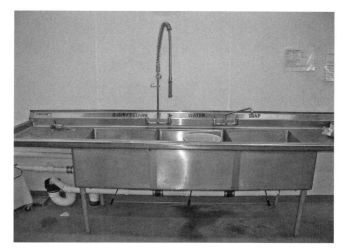

FIG. 5 Three-compartment stainless steel sink installed in food production area for hand washing and sanitizing of utensils and small equipment.

rinse; sanitizing rinse; and optional potable water rinse. Use of a three-bay, stainless steel sink is normally required by law to discourage recontamination between steps (see Fig. 5).

The U.S. Food Code stipulates that utensils and food-contact surfaces must be cleaned and sanitized before each use with a different type of raw animal food (beef, fish, poultry, etc.), between working at different processing stages, between use with raw fruits and vegetables and potentially hazardous foods, and at any time when contamination may have occurred (Gravani et al., 1997; USPHS, 2005).

Toxic materials must be limited to cleaners, sanitizers, laboratory reagents, and plant maintenance and operation materials. It is imperative to store toxic and cleaning materials properly. Use chemicals only as labeled and only when safe. Do not store chemicals above or next to food, ingredients, and packaging materials. Make sure that all chemical containers are labeled properly. Use of chemical sanitizers by employees should only be done by employees trained in their use, with proper precautions taken. The company must provide employees with protective gear when sanitizing solutions are prepared and applied. Employees should wear boots to protect feet from water and spray, gloves, and goggles. Sanitizers should be used only in a well-ventilated area. Employees may have to wear face masks in some cases to prevent them from inhaling sanitizers (Gould, 1994; Marriott, 1999; USFDA, 2006b; USPHS, 2005).

20.5 PEST CONTROL

Flies and cockroaches may transmit *Campylobacter*, *Clostridium botulinum*, *Clostridium perfringens*, *Salmonella*, *Shigella*, *Streptococcus*, *Staphylococcus*, and others. Rodents are sources of *Salmonella* and parasites. Birds are hosts for a

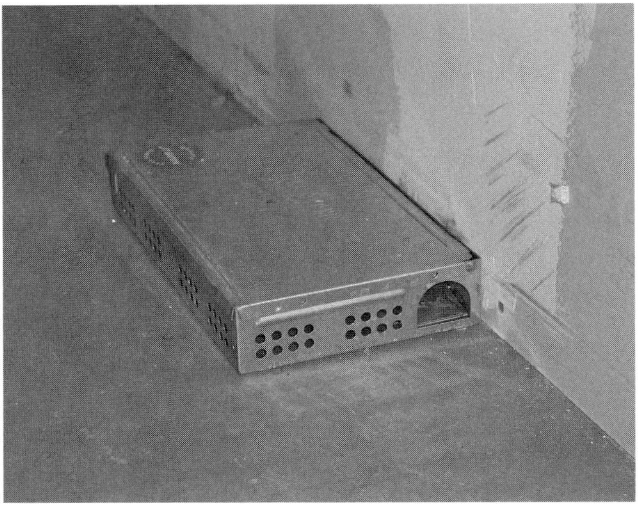

FIG. 6 Rodent trap located against the wall in areas adjacent to food production.

variety of pathogens, such as *Campylobacter*, *Salmonella*, and *Listeria*. Insecticides and rodenticides are permitted only under precautions and restrictions to protect food from contamination, so no pest should be allowed in any portion of the facility, and effective measures must be taken to prevent access (Marriott, 1995; USFDA, 2006b; USPHS, 2005).

Birds and rodents must not be able to get into the processing plant via the vents or ventilation stacks. Screening should be installed to prevent pests from entering through vents, ventilation stacks, and windows. Metal screens with less than 6-mm openings are necessary for rodents, as they can easily break cloth screens. Walls should be examined for holes that provide access and nesting places to rodents (Shapton, 1991). Locker and staff rooms for eating and congregating must be easily cleaned. Garbage must be disposed of properly and promptly. Doors and windows must close tightly and doors must not be left open. Air curtains and truck seals discourage pest entry through loading docks. Finally, incoming supplies should be checked thoroughly to make sure that they do not contain any pests (Marriott, 1995; USFDA, 2006b; USPHS, 2005).

If pests do enter a processing facility, control methods may be used, including trapping (see Figs. 6 and 7) and ultrasonic devices that prevent pests from accessing an area. The best way to control pests, however, is through prevention.

20.6 EQUIPMENT

Equipment defines an article used in the operation of a food plant, such as a freezer, grinder, meat block, oven, refrigerator, or table. Equipment includes thermometers, vents, and hoods as well as pH meters and similar testing devices.

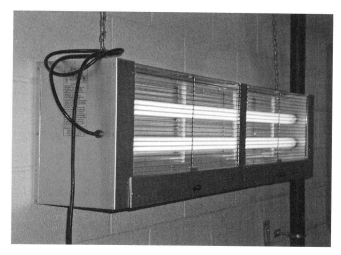

FIG. 7 Insect light trap to attract flies and to eliminate them by electrocution, installed near the receiving door of a food plant.

Equipment used in food-processing facilities must be made from food-grade materials. These materials must be durable, corrosion-resistant, nonabsorbent, and resist chipping, pitting, scratching, and distortion. They should have smooth, easily cleaned surfaces and allow proper maintenance. Use stainless steel when possible and select type 304 for general equipment and type 316 for applications involving heating high-acid foods, as it is more corrosion resistant, due to its lower carbon content. Similarly, food contact surfaces must be easy to clean, free of breaks, open seams, chips, and other imperfections, and have smooth, finished welds and joints (Imholte, 1984; Jowitt, 1980; USPHS, 2005).

Cast iron may be used only for food cooking surfaces and in utensils that are used through the uninterrupted process of cooking through service. Lead in such items as china, pewter, solder, and flux may be present only in minute percentages and is best avoided altogether. Copper may not be used in processing food with a pH below 6, such as vinegar or wine. This includes cooking ware as well as fittings for tubing. Galvanized metal may not be used at any time for food equipment or utensils. Nonstick coatings may be used only with the proper nonscoring, nonscratching utensils (USPHS, 2005). Only hard woods such as maple may be used, and only for cutting boards, baker's tables, rolling pins, salad bowls and chopsticks, and paddles in confectionery operations when processing confections at a temperature at or above 110°C. Fruit and nuts may be kept in their wooden shipping containers until processed (USPHS, 2005).

Avoid any adulteration of food with lubricants, fuel, metal fragments, contaminated water, or any other contaminants from equipment use, maintenance, and sanitation. Bearings and gearboxes for equipment must be leakproof. Vents must be adequate to prevent grease and condensation from building up on walls and food-contact surfaces and must not drip grease or condensate. Sponges must never be used for any purpose since they are very difficult to clean and nearly impossible to sanitize (Marriott, 1995; USFDA, 2006b; USHSP, 2005).

Temperature-measuring devices such as thermometers must be easy to read. They must have sensors placed in the warmest location in refrigeration equipment and the coolest place in heating equipment. Equipment that will hold potentially hazardous foods must have a dedicated temperature-measuring device. Temperature-measuring devices for food and water on ware-washing equipment must have a numerical scale, printed record, or digital readout in increments of no more than 1°C in the intended range of use (USFDA, 2006b; USPHS, 2005).

20.7 OPERATIONS

All operations must be conducted to avoid or eliminate the possibility of contamination of food stuffs. This includes receiving, inspecting, transporting, segregating, preparing, manufacturing, packaging, and storing food, all of which must be done with adequate sanitation. In addition, there must be appropriate quality control to ensure that food is suitable for human consumption and that packaging materials are safe and suitable (USFDA, 2006b).

Raw materials for food processing must be acquired from a reputable, commercial source. Raw materials should be inspected when they arrive at the facility and any tests carried out to ensure that they are clean and suitable for processing into food. Inspection includes ascertaining whether the packing crates and boxes are intact or whether they have contributed to contamination or deterioration of the raw materials inside. Materials should be washed as necessary in clean, potable water to remove soil. Raw materials must then be held in bulk in containers which will prevent contamination by pests, undesirable microorganisms, and extraneous material. Frozen materials must be kept frozen and thawed as necessary in a manner that prevents adulteration (USFDA, 2006b; USPHS, 2005).

Raw materials must not contain harmful microorganisms or toxins such as aflatoxin. If they do, materials should either be destroyed, pasteurized, or treated to make sure that they no longer pose a threat. Suppliers' guarantees or certification are often evidence of compliance with this requirement and should be incorporated into the company's specifications.

All manufacturing and storage must be done under controls that minimize the potential for microbial growth. Control may be established by monitoring the physical qualities of the product at several points: for instance, pH, a_w, humidity, temperature, time, and flow rate for continuous processes.

Manufacturing operations such as freezing, dehydration, acidification, heat processing and refrigeration are also control points. Records of controls and tests to verify their adequacy must be maintained for at least a period of time that represents the shelf life of the finished product. Food that can easily become contaminated or which has a high likelihood of undesirable microbial growth must be stored in a way that prevents such growth. Frozen foods must be kept frozen. Refrigerated foods must be held at 5°C or lower. Hot foods must be maintained at 60°C or higher (Gravani

TABLE 1 Thermal Processes for the Production of Hot-Packed Shelf-Stable Acid and Acidified Foods

Product pH	Minimum Lethality: $F_{93.3C}$ (min)[a]	Hot-Fill Temperature for 3-min Hold (°C)
4.4, 4.5	20.0	—
4.3, 4.4	10.0	99
4.2, 4.3	5.0	96
4.1, 4.2	2.5	93
4.0, 4.1	1.0	90
3.9, 4.0	0.5	87
<3.9	0.1	81

Source: Adapted from Pflug (1998).

[a] $F_{93.3C}$ = equivalent time in minutes at 93.3°C to achieve commercial sterility, with a z-value of 8.9°C. z-value = indicates the change of death rate based on temperature; it is the number of degrees to achieve 90%.

et al., 1997; USFDA, 2006b). Acid or acidified foods must be heat-treated to kill vegetative microorganisms of pathogens such as *E. coli* and *Clostridium botulinum* when the foods are to be held in hermetically sealed containers at room temperature (Pflug, 2003). Table 1 indicates the hot-fill temperature required for a hot-fill hold treatment as a function of pH to manufacture shelfstable acid and acidified foods.

When required by the manufacturing process, heat blanching must be done by holding the food at the required temperature and time and then either chilling it rapidly to prevent microbial growth or moving it without delay through the processing steps. Batters, breadings, sauces, gravies, and dressings must be held in a way that prevents contamination by (1) using ingredients that are not contaminated; (2) employing adequate heat processes where applicable; (3) using adequate time and temperature controls; (4) providing adequate physical prevention of contamination through drips, or splatters; (5) cooling to an adequate temperature, and (6) disposing of batters, and the like at appropriate intervals to prevent contamination. These intervals may be determined by time, temperature, pH, or other appropriate factors (USFDA, 2006b).

Filling, assembling, and packaging must be completed in accordance with proper controls to prevent contamination. This may be accomplished through strict adherence to a hazard analysis of critical control point (HACCP) plan (see Chapter 22). In addition, adequate cleaning and sanitizing of food contact surfaces must take place. Materials for food containers and packaging must be safe and suitable, sanitary handling measures must be taken, and food must be protected from contamination, particularly from air-borne contaminants. If reduced oxygen packaging (ROP), such as vacuum packaging, is used to extend the shelf-life of a product, food must meet regulations to protect the product against pathogens such as *Clostridium botulinum* and *Listeria monocytogenes*. Multiple barriers that are currently in used for ROP foods are pH control below 4.6, low a_w (below 0.93), refrigeration temperatures of 5 to 3.3°C or lower depending on the product, and use-by-date labeling (USPHS, 2005).

If the food is a_w-controlled for microbial growth, a_w must be monitored and records kept. Nonhazardous foods require an a_w of 0.85 or below. Soluble solids must be controlled in ratio to the water in the finished food product. Finished food must be protected from condensates by use of a moisture barrier package or other means (USFDA, 2006b; USPHS, 2005).

If the food is acid or acidified or relies on the control of pH as a control, the pH must be tested and records kept. This includes monitoring the pH of raw ingredients as well as the finished product to ensure that the final pH does not exceed 4.6. The amount of acid or acidified food added to a low-acid food must also be monitored (USFDA, 2006b; Wedding, 2007).

Any food product that may be contaminated must be destroyed or reworked. The determination of whether to destroy or rework a food product depends on the HACCP plan, the level and type of contamination, and the methods required to put the food into compliance. If raw materials are adulterated and capable of being reconditioned, they should be reconditioned using methods that are proven effective. Before the raw material is reincorporated in the food-manufacturing process, it must be examined and found to be unadulterated. Reconditioned materials or materials that have been removed from processing for reasons other than sanitation is called rework. Rework should be stored in bulk in food-appropriate containers separate from raw materials and finished product. Rework may be reincorporated in food processing if is found to be unadulterated upon examination, or if it is reconditioned through processing (USFDA, 2006b).

20.8 WAREHOUSING AND DISTRIBUTION

Storage and transportation of finished foods must be conducted under conditions that protect against physical, chemical, and microbial contamination and against deterioration of the food and the container. Finished food products that are warehoused prior to distribution must be separated to prevent contamination from raw materials. For this reason, raw materials should never be received at a time when finished product is being loaded into vehicles for distribution. Alternatively, two separate loading docks may be provided. If finished product is stored in the same location that also stores raw materials, raw materials must be kept strictly segregated.

If food for human consumption is manufactured in a plant that also manufactures materials consumed by animals, food for humans must never come into contact with animal food. All care must be taken to protect the human food from contamination by the animal food.

The FDA also establishes and periodically updates the maximum level of natural or unavoidable defects in foods that represent no health hazard for humans, as in many cases it is impossible to manufacture defect-free products even when following good manufacturing practices (GMPs) (USFDA, 2004). Examples of defect action levels are presented in Table 2.

20.9 SANITATION STANDARD OPERATING PROCEDURES

SSOP stands for *sanitation standard operating procedure*. It addresses sanitation conditions and practices before, during, and after processing. An SSOP is a written

TABLE 2 Maximum Defect Action Levels for Selected Food Products

Food Product	Maximum Defect Action Level
Allspice (ground)	Average of 30 or more insect fragments per 10 g.
	Average of 1 or more rodent hairs per 10 g.
Broccoli (frozen)	Average of 60 or more aphids, thrips, and/or mites per 100 g.
Cocoa beans	More than 4% of beans by count are moldy.
	More than 4% of beans by count are insect-infested or insect-damaged.
	More than 6% of beans by count are insect-infested or moldy. (*Note*: Level differs when both filth and mold are present.)
	Average of 10 mg or more mammalian excreta per pound.
Pitted olives	Average of 1.3% or more by count of olives with whole pits and/or pit fragments 2 mm or longer measured in the longest dimension.
Pineapple juice	Average mold count of 15% or more.
	Mold count of any one subsample is 40% or more.
Tomatoes (canned)	Average of 10 or more fly eggs per 500 g.
	5 or more fly eggs and 1 or more maggots per 500 g.
	2 or more maggots per 500 g.

Source: USFDA (2004).

document with detailed information and responsibilities regarding all aspects of the food processing being done and addressing most aspects of GMPs. An effective way to determine if a food company is in compliance with all the different aspects covered by GMPs is to conduct periodic self-evaluations using the inspection forms used by FDA inspectors (see Fig. 8).

The eight key sanitation conditions and practices for SSOPs described earlier are the safety of water; condition and cleanliness of food-contact surfaces, prevention of cross-contamination, maintenance of hand washing, hand sanitizing and toilet facilities; protection of the food from adulterants; labeling, storage, and proper use of toxic compounds, employee health conditions, and the exclusion of pests (Marriott, 1999; Shapton, 1991).

The SSOP is a document which indicates the practices to be adhered to in order to accomplish the eight key components. In other words, food processors do not simply know they must wash their hands or that a certain number of toilet facilities are to be provided. Such information is written down and followed. Procedures for cleaning and sanitation are written down in the SSOP as well as procedures for processing the food, including all steps and stages. SSOPs are an integral part, and prerequisites to, the hazard analysis of critical control points (HACCP) plan. HACCP is a systematic approach to food safety which identifies, evaluates, and controls food safety hazards. The hazards may be physical, biological, or chemical agents that are likely to contaminate food and cause illness or injury if not controlled. HACCP aims to prevent food contamination or lower it to an acceptable level before it reaches the consumer. Potential problems are identified before production begins, enabling effective and efficient monitoring during production to ensure that the problems have not occurred. The practice of identifying and observing potential areas of concern

DEPARTMENT OF HEALTH AND HUMAN
FOOD GMP INSPECTION REPORT

FOOD AND DRUG ADMINISTRATION

1. ESTABLISHMENT NAME AND ADDRESS *(Include ZIP code)*	2. DATE INSPECTED
	3. PRODUCT(S) INSPECTED
	4. STATE LICENSE OR PERMIT NUMBER
5. NAME AND TITLE OF RESPONSIBLE PLANT OFFICIAL	6. TELEPHONE NUMBER *(Include Area Code)*
7. NAME AND TITLE OF RESPONSIBLE CORPORATE OFFICIAL	8. TELEPHONE NUMBER *(Include Area Code)*

INSTRUCTIONS:
Answer the following questions by checking the appropriate box. Explain "No", answers on continuation sheet(s). Precede each explanation with the item number. Use "N/A" where questions are Not Applicable.

INSPECTION CRITERIA

NO.	PLANTS AND GROUNDS	YES	NO
1.	Are premises free of harborages and/or breeding places for rodents, insects and other pests	☐	☐
2.	Is adequate drainage provided to avoid contamination of facilities and products	☐	☐
3.	Is sufficient space provided for placement of equipment, storage of materials and for production operations	☐	☐
4.	Are floors, walls and ceilings constructed of easily cleanable materials and kept clean and in good repair	☐	☐
5.	Are food and food contact surfaces protected from contamination from pipes, etc., over working areas	☐	☐
6.	Are food processing areas effectively separated from other operations which may cause contamination of food being processed	☐	☐
7.	Are food products and processing areas protected against contamination from breakage of light bulbs and other glass fixtures	☐	☐
8.	Is air quality and ventilation adequate to prevent contamination by dust and/or other airborne substances	☐	☐
9.	Are doors, windows and other openings protected to eliminate entry by insects, rodents and other pests	☐	☐
	EQUIPMENT AND UTENSILS		
10.	Are all utensils and equipment constructed of adequately cleanable materials and suitable for their intended uses	☐	☐
11.	Is the equipment designed and used in a manner that precludes contamination with lubricants, contaminated water, metal fragments, etc.	☐	☐
12.	Is the equipment installed and maintained so as to facilitate the cleaning of equipment and adjacent areas	☐	☐

FIG. 8 FDA inspection form 2966 for evaluation of a food company's compliance with good manufacturing practices.

INSPECTION CRITERIA			
NO.	**SANITARY FACILITIES AND CONTROLS**	**YES**	**NO**
13.	Is the water supply adequate in quantity and quality for its intended uses	☐	☐
14.	Are the water temperatures and pressures maintained at suitable levels for its intended use	☐	☐
15.	Is the sewage disposal system adequate	☐	☐
16.	Is the plumbing adequately sized, designed, installed and maintained in a manner to prevent contamination	☐	☐
17.	Are adequate toilet rooms provided, equipped and maintained clean and in good repair	☐	☐
18.	Are adequate handwashing and/or sanitizing facilities provided where appropriate	☐	☐
19.	Is all refuse properly stored and protected where necessary from insects, rodents and other pests and disposed of in an adequate manner	☐	☐
	SANITARY OPERATIONS		
20.	Is the facility kept clean and in good physical repair	☐	☐
21	Is cleaning of facilities and equipment conducted in such a manner as to avoid contamination of food products	☐	☐
22.	Are detergents, sanitizors, hazardous materials and other supplies used in a safe and effective manner	☐	☐
23.	Are cleaning compounds and hazardous materials kept in original containers, stored separate from raw materials	☐	☐
24.	Are the processing areas maintained free of insects, rodents and other pests	☐	☐
25.	Are insecticides and rodenticides used and stored so as to prevent contamination of food	☐	☐
26.	Are all utensils and equipment cleaned and sanitized at intervals frequent enough to avoid contamination of food products	☐	☐
27.	Are single service articles stored, handled, dispensed, used and disposed of in a manner that prevents contamination	☐	☐
28.	Are utensils and portable equipment stored so as to protect them from splash, dust and other contamination	☐	☐
	PROCESSES AND CONTROLS		
29.	Is responsibility for overall plant sanitation specifically assigned to an individual	☐	☐
30.	Are raw materials and ingredients adequately inspected, processed as necessary and stored to assure that only clean, wholesome materials are used	☐	☐
31.	Is ice (where used) manufactured from potable water and stored and handled in a sanitary manner	☐	☐
32.	Is food processing conducted in a manner to prevent contamination and minimize harmful microbicilogical growth	☐	☐
33.	Are chemical microbiological or extraneous material testing procedures used where necessary to identify sanitation failures of food contamination	☐	☐
34.	Are packaging processes and materials adequate to prevent contamination	☐	☐
35.	Are only approved food and/or color additives used	☐	☐
36.	Are products coded to enable positive lot identification, and are records maintained in excess of expected shelf-life	☐	☐
37.	Are weighing and measuring practices adequate to ensure the declared quantity of contents	☐	☐

FIG. 8 (*Continued*)

INSPECTION CRITERIA			
NO.	PROCESSES AND CONTROLS	YES	NO
38.	Are labels of products covered during inspection in compliance (submit violative labels as exhibits)	☐	☐
39.	Are finished products stored and shipped under conditions which will avoid contamination and deterioration	☐	☐

DETAILS OF MANUFACTURING PROCEDURES AND CONTROLS

Provide brief description of manufacturing processes and controls for product(s) inspected. Where appropriate, report times, temperatures, and other critical processing steps. If microbiological or any other type of contamination is suspected or encountered, fully describe the relationship between the routes of contamination and the process. Use flow charts where appropriate. If more space is needed, use continuation sheet.

NO.	PERSONNEL	YES	NO
40.	Are personnel with sores, infections, etc., restricted from handling food products	☐	☐
41.	Do employees wear clean outer garments, use adequate hair restraints and remove excess jewelry when handling food	☐	☐
42.	Do employees thoroughly wash and sanitize hands as necessary	☐	☐
43.	Do employees refrain from eating, drinking and smoking and observe good food handling techniques in processing areas	☐	☐

FIG. 8 *(Continued)*

CORRECTIONS AND SAMPLES

If any corrections were made as a result of this inspection or made as a result of a previous inspection (*including voluntary destructions, capital improvements, etc.*), complete Voluntary Correction section of cover sheet Form FDA 481 (E) CG.

If any samples were collected, list sample numbers and briefly describe samples.

DISCUSSIONS WITH MANAGEMENT

Indicate individual with whom inspection was discussed. Identify official (*name and title*) having authority to authorize corrections. Record any recommendations/warnings given, and management's response.

CONTINUATION SHEET

(Use additional sheets as appropriate.)

SIGNATURE OF INSPECTOR	DATE

FIG. 8 *(Continued)*

allows a company to recognize and correct food safety issues in real time (Gravani et al., 1997; Marriott, 1999).

Acknowledgments

The author thanks Elizabeth Keller for assistance provided in the preparation of this chapter.

REFERENCES

Gould WA (1994): *Current Good Manufacturing Practices: Food Plant Safety*, 2nd ed. CTI Publications, Baltimore.

Gravani RB, Rishoi DC, Tauer JR (1997): *Food Safety Handbook*. Chain Store Publishing, New York.

Imholte, TJ (1984): *Engineering for Food Safety and Sanitation*. D.C. Thompson, London.

Jowitt R (Ed.) (1980): *Hygienic Design and Operation of Food Plant*. AVI Publishing, Westport, CT.

Marriott NG (1995): *Essentials of Food Sanitation*. Springer, New York.

——— (1999): *Principles of Food Sanitation*. 4th ed. Aspen Publishers, Gaithersburg, MD.

Pflug IJ (1998): *Microbiology and Engineering of Sterilization Processes*, 9th ed. Environmental Sterilization Laboratory, University of Minnesota, Minneapolis, MN.

——— (2003): *Microbiology and Engineering of Sterilization Processes*, 11th ed. Environmental Sterilization Laboratory, University of Minnesota, Minneopolis, MN.

Shapton DA (1991): *Principles and Practices for the Safe Processing of Foods*. CRC Press, Boca Raton, FL.

Staff of J.J. Keller & Assoc. (2000): *Food Safety Handbook for Foodservice Employees*. J.J. Keller & Associates, Neenah, WI.

USFDA (U.S. Food and Drug Administration) (2004): Good manufacturing practices (GMPs) for the 21st century: food processing. http://www.cfsan.fda.gov/~dms/gmp-1.html. Accessed December 2007.

——— (2006a): Guidance for industry: questions and answers regarding food allergens, including the Food Allergen Labeling and Consumer Protection Act of 2004, 4th ed.: final guidance. http://www.cfsan.fda.gov/~dms/alrguid4.html. Accessed December 2007.

——— (2006b): 21 CFR Ch 1 110. Current good manufacturing practice in manufacturing, packing, or holding human food. http://www.cfsan.fda.gov/~lrd/cfr110.html. Accessed December 2007.

USPHS (U.S. Public Health Service) (2005): *Food Code*. U.S. Department of Health and Human Services, College Park, MD.

Weddig LM (2007): *Canned Foods: Principles of Thermal Process Control, Acidification and Container Closure Evaluation*, 7th ed. GMA Science and Education Foundation, Washington, DC.

CHAPTER 21

CLEANING AND SANITIZING OPERATIONS

KEVIN KEENER

21.1 INTRODUCTION

The only constant in cleaning and sanitizing operations is change. Cleaning and sanitizing operations are always changing with constantly increasing demands by the consumer and regulatory agencies. In addition, high turnover in plant sanitation personnel and language barriers further complicate a sanitation program's effectiveness. These challenges can be overcome, and many food companies have been very successful in developing effective sanitation programs. This chapter provides recommendations on developing a successful sanitation program, along with a list of references for additional information. If cleaning and sanitizing operations are a plant priority, all departments must commit to this effort and make it a priority. Success can be achieved through constant effort and attention to detail.

21.2 FOOD SANITATION

The focus of this chapter is to describe the requirements (U.S. regulations) for sanitation programs, the attributes of a successful food sanitation program, and potential consequences of a sanitation failure. The sanitation program requirements encompass four major elements: people, facility, equipment, and maintenance. All need appropriate consideration in order to develop a successful sanitation program.

21.3 FOOD REGULATIONS

Food regulations in the United States are a patchwork of rules and regulations that have developed over time. For a single food, numerous government agencies have

Microbiologically Safe Foods, Edited by Norma Heredia, Irene Wesley, and Santos García

inspection roles. At the federal level, the primary agencies with regulatory responsibilities are the U.S. Food and Drug Administration (FDA), an agency within the Department of Health and Human Services, and the Food Safety Inspection Service (FSIS) an agency within the U.S. Department of Agriculture. The FDA has the responsibility of ensuring the safety of all foods under the Federal Food Drug and Cosmetic Act of 1938 with the exceptions of meat, poultry, and egg products. Federal Food, Drug, and Cosmetic Act Section 201(f) (USFDA-FFDCA, 2006) defines *food* as articles used for food or drink for man or other animals, chewing gum, and articles used for components of any such articles. The FSIS has primary responsibility for meat, poultry, and egg products under the Meat Product Inspection Act (1906) (USDA-FSIS, 2006c), Poultry Product Inspection Act (1957) (USDA-FSIS, 2006d), and Egg Product Inspection Act (1970) (USDA-FSIS, 2006e). Other agencies have supporting roles in various commodities and provide grading and export inspection services. These are identified in proceeding commodity sections as appropriate.

21.4 SANITATION PROGRAMS

All meat, poultry, and egg-processing plants are required to have a written sanitation program. Sanitation is the creation and maintenance of hygienic and healthful conditions in food-processing plants. Sanitation involves an applied science that has the overall goal of providing a clean environment and preventing food product contamination during processing. The universal goal of sanitation is to protect the food supply. An effective sanitation program includes positives such as:

- Microbial and chemical monitoring
- Control of food spoilage, and lower consumer complaints
- Increased storage life of the product
- Improved employee morale
- Reduced public health risks

Specific sanitation requirements vary for each commodity. FSIS has sanitation requirements for meat, poultry, and egg products in Title 9, Part 416 of the *Code of Federal Regulations* (USDA-FSIS, 2006a). For FDA-inspected food processors there are also sanitation requirements. These are detailed in the current good manufacturing practices (cGMP's) in Title 21, Part 110 of the *Code of Federal Regulations* (USDA-FSIS, 2006b). In addition, the FDA has developed specific GMPs for some food processes, such as bottled water, baby food, and seafood. These regulations are minimum sanitation requirements; many food processors exceed these requirements.

21.4.1 Sanitation Requirements

Sanitation requirements for meat, poultry, and egg products are listed in Title 9, Part 416 (USDA-FSIS, 2006a) and subdivided into two parts. Sections 416.1–416.6 are referred to as the sanitation performance standards (SPSs) and Sections 416.11–416.17 are referred to as the sanitation standard operating procedures (SSOPs). (*Note*: There are no sections between 416.7 and 416.10.)

21.4.2 Sanitation Performance Standards

Sanitation performance standards describe specific areas that inspection personnel will evaluate regarding sanitation performance. Establishments must comply with the regulatory performance standards for sanitation cited below, but may do so by whatever means they determine to be appropriate. No specific sanitary practices are required; FSIS inspection personnel will verify that official establishments comply with the performance standards. Section 416.1 (USDA-FSIS, 2006a), known as the General Rules, requires that "each official establishment must be operated and maintained in a manner sufficient to prevent the creation of insanitary conditions and to ensure that product is not adulterated." Section 416.2 describes specific concerns regarding buildings and grounds and pest control. The information on buildings and grounds includes criteria for construction, ventilation, lighting, plumbing, sewage disposal, and water. The facility must also be designed to allow management of pest (flies, rodents, birds, etc.).

It should be noted that pest control substances must be approved by the EPA (U.S. Environmental Protection Agency) for use in food-processing environments and be used in a manner that does not adulterate product or create unsanitary conditions. Under the Federal Insecticide, Fungicide, and Rodenticide Act (FIFRA), the EPA reviews pesticides, cleaners, sanitizers, antimicrobials, and so on, their formulations, intended use, and other information; registers all pesticides, sanitizers, antimicrobials, and so on, for use in the United States; and prescribes labeling, use, and other regulatory requirements to prevent unreasonable adverse effects on the environment, including humans, wildlife, plants, and property. Any meat or poultry establishment using a pesticide, cleaner, sanitizer, or antimicrobial must follow the FIFRA requirements.

Section 416.3 (USDA-FSIS, 2006a) describes the appropriate selection of equipment and utensils and their respective installation and maintenance. Section 416.4 details the requirements for cleaning and sanitizing of food-contact and non-food-contact surfaces and utensils. Section 416.5 describes the requirements for management of employee hygiene practices, including the person and their respective practices to prevent product adulteration. If any equipment, utensils, rooms, or compartments are found to be unsanitary, the inspector (FSIS/state) will place a tag on the equipment ("U.S. rejected"). The equipment, utensil, room, or compartment cannot be used until corrective action has taken place to produce sanitary conditions.

21.4.3 Sanitation Standard Operating Procedures

Minimum requirements for sanitation operating procedures are stated in Title 9, Sections 416.11–416.17 (USDA-FSIS, 2006a). Each official establishment is required (shall) to develop, implement, and maintain written standard operating procedures for sanitation (Section 416.11). "The SSOPs shall describe all procedures an official establishment will conduct daily, before and during operations, sufficient to prevent direct contamination or adulteration of product(s)" (Section 416.12). The SSOPs cover the entire establishment and all shifts of operation. These procedures include at a minimum: frequency of cleaning, cleaning procedures, and designated plant personnel. SSOPs must be signed and dated by the "overall authority" usually the owner or plant manager. The FSIS also requires compliance with preoperational SSOPs prior to production and other SSOPs as written.

Monitoring procedures must be established by plant personnel to verify implementation of the SSOPs (Section 416.13). The written SSOPs must be reviewed routinely and the effectiveness assessed. Revisions are required (shall) as necessary to keep them effective and current with respect to changes in facilities, equipment, utensils, operations, or personnel (Section 416.14). The establishment must also maintain daily records sufficient to document the implementation and monitoring of the SSOPs and any corrective action taken (section 416.16). The establishment is required to maintain 6 months of written records, and they must be available to FSIS upon request if within the most recent 48 h of plant operation, or within 24 h.

It is the establishment's responsibility to implement the procedures as they are written in the SSOPs. If the establishment or FSIS determines that the SSOPs fail to prevent direct contamination or adulteration of product, the establishment must implement corrective actions that include the appropriate disposition of product, restoration of sanitary conditions, and measures to prevent recurrence. It is also required that SSOPs describe the procedures that the establishment will take to prevent direct contamination or adulteration of product (Section 416.15).

FSIS has the responsibility to verify that the establishment is conducting the SSOPs as written. Specifically, they will verify the adequacy and effectiveness of the sanitation SOPs and the procedures specified therein by determining that they meet the requirements of this part (section 416). Such verification may include:

1. Reviewing the sanitation SOPs
2. Reviewing the daily records documenting implementation of the SSOPs and the procedures specified therein and any corrective actions taken or required to be taken
3. Direct observation of the implementation of the SSOPs and the procedures specified therein and any corrective actions taken or required to be taken
4. Direct observation or testing to assess the sanitary conditions in the establishment

21.4.4 Current Good Manufacturing Processes

The FDA requires that all foods (excluding meat, poultry, and egg products) meet the cGMPs. The cGMPs regulations are printed in Title 21, Part 110 of the *Code of Federal Regulations* (USDA-FSIS, 2006b). The cGMP regulations are general sanitation requirements. They are subdivided into specific plant requirements. Within

21 CFR 110, definitions of food processes and products (Section 110.3) are stated along with the specific definition of adulteration. Specific requirements for plant personnel are found in Section 110.10 and plant and grounds in Section 110.20. In brief, these specific regulations dictate that plant (building), grounds, and plant personnel must be constructed and managed in a sanitary manner so as not to lead to adulteration of food processed in the facility.

Section 110.35 (USDA-FSIS, 2006b) describes sanitary operation requirements for the facility, such as required cleaning of food-contact and non-food-contact surfaces, cleaners, and sanitizers. Sanitary facilities and controls (Section 110.39) dictate requirements for sanitary water, plumbing, toilet and hand-washing station requirements, floor drain requirements, and placement of signs instructing employees in required hygiene practices. Design of equipment and utensils (Section 110.40) for food contact are required to be constructed of nontoxic, corrosive-resistant materials. "The design, construction, and use of equipment and utensils shall preclude the adulteration of food with lubricants, fuel, metal fragments, contaminated water, or any other contaminants." Each freezer and cold storage cooler is required to have a thermometer with an automatic control system or alarm system if under manual operation. All instruments and controls must be designed and maintained so as not to adulterate food. Any gases (e.g., air, nitrogen) introduced into the food or used to clean food contact surfaces or equipment must be treated appropriately so as to not adulterate the food.

> All operations in the receiving, inspecting, transporting, segregating, preparing, manufacturing, packaging, and storing of food shall be conducted in accordance with adequate sanitation principles (Section 110.80) (USDA-FSIS, 2006b). Appropriate quality control operations shall be employed to ensure that food is suitable for human consumption and that food-packaging materials are safe and suitable. Overall sanitation of the plant shall be under the supervision of one or more competent individuals assigned responsibility for this function. All reasonable precautions shall be taken to ensure that production procedures do not contribute contamination from any source. Chemical, microbial, or extraneous-material testing procedures shall be used where necessary to identify sanitation failures or possible food contamination.

All food that has become contaminated to the extent that it is adulterated should be rejected, or if permissible, treated or processed to eliminate the contamination. Finished food products should be stored and transported appropriately so as to protect against product adulteration or container damage (Section 110.93).

Some foods when processed under cGMPs contain natural or unavoidable defects that are at low levels and are not hazardous to health. The FDA establishes a maximum level of each defect in a food produced under cGMPs that is called the defect action level (DAL) (Section 110.110) (USDA-FSIS, 2006b). DALs are established as needed and change as new technology and processing practices become available. DALs do not excuse the food from being adulterated by noncompliance with cGMPs, even when its effect produces defects below the DAL. In addition, the mixing of food exceeding a DAL with food below the DAL is not allowed (even if the final product does not exceed the DAL), and the final product would be deemed adulterated (USDA-CFSAN, 2001). A complete list of current DALs for natural or unavoidable defects in food for human use that present no health hazard may be obtained upon request from the Center for Food Safety and Applied Nutrition (HFS-565), Food and Drug Administration, 5100 Paint Branch Pkwy., College Park, MD 20740.

Note: Maximum levels for pesticide residues in raw agricultural products are determined by the EPA under FIFRA. FDA's DAL for pesticide residues are EPA's limits unless an allowance is made for a higher level. Many food processes concentrate food products, and thus pesticides may cause the product to be considered adulterated if the DAL of pesticide residue is exceeded in the finished product. In addition, if the product is a ready-to-eat product, it may not be blended to lower the pesticide residue. For example, the DAL for aflatoxin (a carcinogen produced by certain molds) in peanuts and peanut products is 20 ppb. A finished peanut or peanut product must contain less than 20 ppb aflatoxin if it is to be sold for human consumption. If the amount of aflatoxin exceeds 20 ppm in dry roasted peanuts, they cannot be sold for human consumption. Also, these dry roasted peanuts cannot be blended with dry roasted peanuts containing a lower level of aflatoxin to lower the overall level of aflatoxin. In addition, if peanuts containing less than 20 ppb aflatoxin were used to produce peanut butter and the peanut butter (finished product) had an aflatoxin level above 20 ppb, this product could not be sold for human consumption. Also, this peanut butter could not be blended with peanut butter containing less than 20 ppb aflatoxin to lower the overall concentration below 20 ppb.

In addition to the regulatory requirements, there are many voluntary sanitation programs, such as the National Shellfish Sanitation Program (USFDA-CFSAN, 2003) and the National Good Agricultural Practices Program for fruits and vegetables (Cornell University Law School, 2006). These programs are voluntary programs supported by government and industry. They provide educational training and inspections of sanitation programs.

21.4.5 Sanitation Failure Case Study: Green Onions and Hepatitis A

In December 2004 an economics study on food safety was performed by the U.S. Department of Agriculture's Economic Research Service on hepatitis A outbreaks linked to green onions from Mexico and the associated economics. Further details on this report may be obtained from the USDA-ERS (Calvin et al., 2004).

In fall 2003, a series of hepatitis A outbreaks occurred in the United States. Hepatitis A is a virus found in fecal material and usually results from an infected person contaminating food, or food contacting fecal-contaminated water. Symptoms appear 2 to 4 weeks after contracting the virus and may include nausea, diarrhea, fever, jaundice, fatigue, and loss of appetite. Hepatitis A is a liver disease and in most cases symptoms are mild and recovery is usually within 2 to 4 weeks. There is no known treatment for hepatitis A.

In 2003, 87% percent of all green onions consumed in the United States came from Mexico. Green onions are a labor-intensive crop and as many as nine persons may contact the onions during harvesting and packing.

On November 15, 2003, FDA issued a notice that hepatitis A outbreaks from green onions had occurred in September 2003 in Tennessee, North Carolina, and Georgia. FDA noted that the green onions "appeared" to be from Mexico. One person died from hepatitis A in these outbreaks. Further testing confirmed that the Tennessee and Georgia outbreaks were caused by green onions from Mexico. During the October – November 2003 period, another large outbreak occurred at a Pennsylvania restaurant, with over 500 persons contracting hepatitis A, and three deaths. Epidemiological and traceback evidence confirmed green onions from 4 out of 27 packers in Mexico. FDA announced this second outbreak and results on November 20–21. These four companies produced a small share of the green onions exported to the United States. It should be noted that the incubation period for hepatitis A is up to 50 days. Thus, the onions in question were harvested in the July–September time frame. During the winter, onions are harvested from Mexicali in Baja California and in Sonora, and in summer the onions are harvested from the cooler western coastal range (Ojos Negros, Valle de la Trinidad, El Condor, and Valle de Guadalupe). Unfortunately, consumers are not knowledgeable about onion harvesting.

The Impact: After the first announcement on November 15, 2003, the demand for green onions dropped and the price of green onions fell 72%. This resulted in a $10 million dollar loss in sales for the last two weeks of November 2003. In addition, 182 ha (450 acres) were left unharvested. Shipments of green onions to the United States dropped 42% during this 2-week period. Prices rebounded and demand increased after December 10 and returned to normal by December 21, 2003.

The exact cause of the outbreak was never determined; however, sanitation deficiencies were found at one of the four packers identified. The economic loss to the onion growers and packers, although due to a few minor companies with poor sanitation programs, was considerable. Their failures stained the entire industry and everyone suffered because of it. Ironically, those hurt the most were the least involved. The green onions suspected were harvested in late summer and fall, but the FDA announcements did not begin until November, at which time different producers were supplying the United States. Thus, these growers suffered severe economic hardship because someone 6 months earlier had an inadequate sanitation program. The point is that a proper sanitation program is everyone's business. Your company's sanitation program reflects not only on your company, but on the industry as a whole.

21.5 SANITATION PROGRAM DEVELOPMENT

Whether one is slaughtering chickens or packing fruit and vegetables for export, there is need for a sanitation program. Such a program is a process that requires continuous improvement. As processes change, the sanitation program needs to be reviewed and updated. There are many challenges in food plant sanitation, including minimally processed food, ready-to-eat food, a global marketplace, emerging food pathogens, and food allergens. Historically, food was canned and cooked for many hours to kill any bacteria and spores present. Currently, many consumers prefer the taste and flavor of fresh and raw food. Thus, the sanitation program for minimally processed and ready-to-eat food must be designed accordingly to prevent cross-contamination or post-package contamination since a terminal heat treatment is no longer standard practice.

Since transportation systems and many food companies are global, the food business is a global marketplace. The challenge in sanitation regarding global marketplace is that shelf-life and spoilage concerns need to be minimized. For example, a U.S. meat processor ships boneless hams to Japan. To do so, the processor guarantees a 45-day shelf life on the product. Currently, the average ham shelf life in the United States is around 28 days. In order to capitalize on this market, this processor's sanitation program and process produces an almost "sterile" raw pork product. The sanitation challenge is to clean the facility thoroughly every day.

Food allergies are an increasing problem in the U.S. population. It has been estimated that up to 8% of children have some form of food allergy. The eight primary allergens are peanuts, tree nuts, milk, eggs, fish, shellfish, soybeans, and wheat. Here again, the challenge is to clean and sanitize the facility and equipment properly to prevent cross-contamination between two dissimilar foods produced in the same facility, such as peanut butter cookies and chocolate chip cookies. As food processes change, the potential organisms of interest may also change. For example, in the United States, canned foods are not refrigerated and are stored at warehouse temperatures (50 to 90°F/10 to 32°C). Many of these foods have a shelf life of more than 1 year. However, recently a company started shipping canned goods to the Middle East, where warehouse temperatures range from 100 to 130°F (38 to 54°C). Containers started swelling because of thermophilic (heat-resistant) the growth of spoilage bacteria in the containers. These thermophilic bacteria are found on raw products and in the environment. This company needed to redesign their process and sanitation program to target these spoilage bacteria.

There are a number of challenges in developing a successful sanitation program:

- Sanitation is non-revenue generating.
- A sanitation failure can bankrupt business.
- No two products or processes are alike.
- Third-shift personnel, who usually carry out the work, are the lowest-paid and newest hires.
- Sufficient management endorsement is needed for sanitation and maintenance programs.
- Sanitation workers lack proper training and are usually trained on the job.

These challenges must be balanced with the fact that sanitation is the foundation on which a food company is built. A poor sanitation program is similar to a ship taking on water. If the hole is not plugged, eventually the ship will sink, regardless of how fast the boat moves. To develop a successful sanitation program, there are seven steps and four areas of emphasis. The seven steps are addressed below.

21.5.1 Seven Steps in Establishing an Effective Sanitation Program (Marriott and Gravani, 2006)

1. Start with a company policy statement that includes a standard for the plant's sanitation program and post it for all to see. This is necessary because it puts sanitation in front of everyone, making it a company priority, not just the priority of one or two people.
2. Collect all local, state, FDA, USDA, and EPA regulations applicable to the specific product(s) being produced. It is necessary to know the regulatory requirements for a food-processing facility: who will inspect, how often, documentation requirements, training requirements, and so on.
3. Develop a sanitation team with all necessary departments represented (e.g., quality control, engineering, maintenance, production, management, sanitation). Survey the entire plant for incoming material, including raw ingredients, packaging materials, water, and equipment parts, to determine possible sources of contamination, and identify key areas that require extra attention. Many facilities are not properly documented. When the food-processing facility was originally built, blueprints were made and followed. Since that time (which may be 40 or 50 years ago), things have gradually changed (e.g., plant expansion, equipment upgrading), much of which has not been adequately documented. To develop a successful sanitation program, one needs to see clearly all processes, equipment, and utilities. Thus, one must survey the facility and develop accurate flow diagrams for people, processes, and utilities.
4. The sanitation team should establish written procedures for preventive sanitation using SSOPs, a workable HACCP (hazard analysis of critical control points) program, regulations, and the survey described above, including a written maintenance program. It is necessary to have a comprehensive team of experts as to plant operations. In particular, management and maintenance are critical. Sanitation program success cannot be achieved without management buy-in and maintenance support. Sanitation programs cost money and management needs to be willing to invest. Maintenance personnel know the problem areas in the plant and need to communicate these to the sanitation team.
5. Establish a daily written record-keeping system for the sanitation program so that inspections are thorough, with all pertinent items checked, all deviations with corrective actions documented, and other remarks necessary for management or other departments recorded. Daily records are necessary because a food-processing plant is a dynamic environment where things change constantly. Unless written records are generated daily, or preferably hourly, potential problems may be forgotten in the daily chaos, until the next crisis arises.
6. Establish a written training program to teach new employees the sanitation program, continually improve current employee's knowledge of sanitation, and establish a sanitation incentive program. Proper training is a necessary cost, and a potential cost savings. Improperly trained sanitation workers can

cost a company two to three times their annual salary in water consumption and wastewater generation, not to mention the potential for unsanitary conditions. A hot-water spigot left on 8 h per day can cost a plant \$10,000 per year in hot water. If the water is not shut off over a weekend, for example, this could a cost plant \$100,000 per year.

7. Develop a written assessment for an established sanitation program. In a food-processing plant, conditions are maintained or improve only when given priority. Without continual review and constant scrutiny, sanitation programs will slowly degrade and become a serious problem rather than a point of pride. Even if no serious sanitation failure occurs, employee pride and product quality will suffer as the sanitation program deteriorates, and regulatory action will increase.

21.5.2 Areas of Emphasis: People, Facility, Equipment, and Preventive Maintenance

When developing a sanitation program, there are four areas of emphasis: people, equipment, facility, and preventive maintenance. The following truisms have been observed:

- Properly trained people cannot clean poorly designed equipment.
- Poorly trained people cannot clean properly designed equipment.
- Properly trained people, properly designed equipment, and poorly designed facility equals disaster.
- Properly trained people, properly designed equipment, properly designed facility, and poor maintenance program equals high costs and potential disaster.

People People are the most important part of a successful food sanitation program. Properly trained persons can make the difference between success and failure of a sanitation program. Sanitation workers usually work second or third shift and receive minimal pay compared to other processing plant personnel. Thus, there is usually high turnover (>40% per year) and minimal supervision. A challenge in training a sanitation crew is in educating them on sanitary principles and practices. They may be unfamiliar with Western culture, such as proper hand washing. They may not speak or understand English. Proper training requires instruction in their native language. Detailed instructions must be provided, both verbal and written, regarding specifics for cleaning and sanitizing specific process lines and individual pieces of equipment. On-the-job-training is important, but unless written instructions are available, sanitation procedures will slowly change to the quickest and easiest approach rather than continuing the most effective. Appropriate safety training should also be provided. Many of the sanitation crew may be unfamiliar with proper safety (e.g., protective eyewear, rubber boots, rubber gloves, respirators, cleaning at elevated heights). Sanitation is one of the most dangerous jobs in the United States, and proper safety training can prevent injuries and deaths.

To retain sanitation workers, an incentive program is an effective tool. These could include performance bonuses or idea awards that can lead to reduced sanitation costs. Once trained and adequately skilled, a sanitation worker is in high demand. It is estimated that a properly trained sanitation worker can save a company between \$5000 and \$10,000 per year in retraining and in waste and water consumption. In a facility with 100 sanitation personnel, the company could save more than \$500,000 per year if employees are retained.

Personnel Training People need to be trained — one does not "intuitively know" how to clean and sanitize. In my experience, 60% of the problems are linked to the personnel training program, 20% are linked to poor facility design, and 20% are linked to equipment. Of the equipment problems, 19% are caused by a poor or nonexistent maintenance program. Sanitation program problems cost a lot of money. Proper training of sanitation personnel in dry cleanup and providing incentive programs for sanitation workers can yield hundreds of thousands of dollars in cost savings per year. The simple practice of one worker using a sanitation hose as a water broom to sweep solid waste into drains can cost a processing plant \$50,000 or more per year.

An estimated 25 to 50% of a plant's waste and water use can be eliminated by proper sanitation training, saving greater than \$1,000,000 per year in a large processing plant. There are seven key points in a sanitation training program:

1. Written program with assessment. Workers need to be instructed by written procedures and hands-on training. There is no substitute for hands-on experience. In addition, an assessment procedure must be written and followed. This should detail validation procedures and consequences for failure or incentives for a job well done.
2. Sanitation workers need to understand how to meet GMPs or SSOPs, and part of the assessment needs to address this proficiency.
3. The Occupational Safety and Health Administration (OSHA) requires workers to perform sanitation safely. It is important that all workers receive training in appropriate safety procedures and be assessed in their understanding.
4. In cooperation with equipment manufacturers and chemical suppliers, written cleaning and sanitation procedures and sanitation records should be developed.
5. Selection of cleaners and sanitizers should be done in consultation with chemical supplier(s). Many factors need to be considered in selecting cleaners and sanitizers, including type of debris, water chemistry, and equipment construction.
6. Record keeping is a necessary requirement. Under FSIS interpretation, if written records are not made, the sanitation activity did not occur and the product is deemed adulterated.
7. A successful sanitation personnel training program requires a goal for the worker. Although properly cleaning and sanitizing a piece of equipment and plant area is valuable for a plant, individual workers may require added

incentives to feel valued by the plant. Successful sanitation personnel training programs contain such rewards or incentives as a pay bonus, time off, company store discounts, and educational training to achieve a track record of excellent sanitation performance. This helps sanitation workers feel valued and focused on their task.

Facility Design Food-processing facility design has not always received adequate consideration. Historically, any vacant building was converted into a food-processing facility. As more space became needed, a wall was removed and another wing was added to the facility. This worked well for many years, but with the recent requirements for sanitation verification and HACCP programs, these approaches have proven problematic. Specifically, if a food-processing facility has inadequate design features (e.g., ventilation, lighting, drains, traffic, entrances and exits), it becomes very difficult to create and maintain a sanitary environment. Poor ventilation can lead to condensation and fomite migration from insanitary to sanitary areas and equipment. Many post-product contamination (*Listeria*) issues result directly from poor facility design. To better design food-processing facilities, the American Meat Institute organized a facility design task force with industry, regulators, and academicians. This committee developed eleven principles of sanitary facility design (Bricher, 2005):

1. *Distinct hygienic zones are established in the facility.* To control fomite movement and pathogen transfer from air and persons, specific hygienic zones are established and appropriate barriers installed to prevent movement of dirty air to cleaner parts of the plant.
2. *Personnel and material flows are controlled to reduce hazards.* Entrances and exits into the distinct hygienic zones are limited and materials flow from raw/dirty area to clean/hygienic areas.
3. *Water accumulation is controlled inside the facility.* Water is a necessary element for biological activity. It can also be a safety hazard. Therefore, it important to have sufficient drains, flow controls, and flow monitors on water systems in the plant.
4. *Room temperature and humidity are controlled.* Temperature and humidity are important elements in pathogen control. High humidity can result in condensation in low-airflow areas of the plant. In addition, a warm plant can be uncomfortable for workers and also provide optimum growing temperatures for pathogenic bacteria present on raw meat, fruits, and vegetables.
5. *Room airflow and quality are controlled.* Movement of contaminated from "dirty" locations in the plant to "clean" locations is a primary cause for cross-contamination of food. To minimize this problem it is recommended that a food-processing facility be designed under positive air pressure. This air pressure control should be regulated so that all air moves, such as through doors opening and closing, from the cleanest locations (e.g., packaging) to

the dirtiest (e.g., receiving). The quality of this air should also be controlled with filters and treatment systems to remove odors and any contaminants.

6. *Site elements should facilitate sanitary conditions.* The facility should be located with consideration given to maintaining sanitary conditions. For example, a food-processing facility was built in an open field and trees were planted in front as part of the landscaping. Over the years, the trees grew up and began harboring wild birds. The birds defecated on the sidewalks, loading docks, and periodically found their way into the plant. This facility found that they had a *Salmonella* problem. It was determined not to be from the raw product they were receiving but from the wild birds outside the facility. The trees were cut down and replaced with smaller bushes, eliminating the *Salmonella* problem.
7. *The building envelope facilitates sanitary conditions.* This requires that the grass be mowed, all trashed picked up, all trash cans periodically cleaned and covered, and the foundation periodically checked and cracks sealed to prevent rodent or insect infiltration.
8. *Interior spatial design promotes sanitary conditions.* Space utilization is designed appropriately to prevent persons from tracking through dirty areas to reach clean areas and to keep aerosols generated during cleaning from contaminating areas already cleaned.
9. *Building components and construction facilitate sanitary conditions.* The interior walls and ceiling need to be made of nonporous, water-resistant materials that can be cleaned and sanitized easily. Preferably no wood is exposed, and if possible, no wood is used in the construction.
10. *Utility systems are designed to prevent contamination.* All utilities are accessible and easily assessed. This includes plumbing, heating, ventilation, refrigeration, and electrical systems. Often, these are accessible and easily accessed when facilities are built, but with plant expansions are often overlooked.
11. *Sanitation is integrated into facility design.* A food-processing plant needs to be designed with appropriate consideration given to cleaning and sanitizing the facility and equipment. Floor drains must be sized appropriately for the large volumes of water generated during cleaning. A sufficient number of hot-water and steam access points for hoses and equipment connections must be provided. Floors need to be sloped adequately to allow water to reach drains and prevent pooling. All walls, ceilings, and floors need to be sealed appropriately to prevent infiltration of water. Ventilation systems need to remove excess moisture generated during sanitation.

These 11 principles provide specific guidance when designing a food-processing facility. Although it is very useful for all persons involved to understand these principles, it is recommended that only qualified engineering and architectural firms design and construct food-processing plant facilities.

Equipment Design The American Meat Institute recently assembled an equipment design task force that developed a list of 10 principles recommended for sanitary equipment design (AMI, 2005):

1. *Cleanable to a microbiological level.* This requires that equipment be manufactured such that every point of food contact be accessible and that periodic microbial testing be performed to ensure sanitary condition.
2. *Made of compatible materials.* Compatible materials are those materials that are not extremely different. For example, a stainless steel auger in a polypropylene trough is incompatible. The extreme hardness of the auger compared to the soft plastic sleeve will cause considerable scoring and wear in the sleeve, which may produce insanitary conditions.
3. *Accessible for inspection, maintenance, cleaning, and sanitation.* This implies that all equipment be manufactured such that it can be assessed visually for cleanliness and maintenance.
4. *No product or liquid collection.* Equipment should be designed with adequate drainage to prevent accumulation of food materials, cleaners, or sanitizers.
5. *Hollow areas should be hermetically sealed.* There should be no open areas that are inaccessible to cleaning. For example, if hollow legs (tubular) are present, these need to be sealed off (welded) to prevent bacteria from colonizing in inaccessible areas.
6. *No niches.* Cracks, crevices, and sharp angles should be avoided because these are very difficult areas to clean.
7. *Sanitary operational performance.* The equipment can be operated in a sanitary manner, meaning that when equipment is functioning properly, it is producing a sanitary product with no contamination from lubricants or wearing parts.
8. *Hygienic design of maintenance enclosures.* All equipment must be completely accessible for maintenance. Covers and shields on pulleys, belts, augers, grinders, and so on, must be made of suitable material so that they can be properly cleaned and sanitized.
9. *Hygienic compatibility with other plant systems.* All systems in the facility must accommodate cleaning and sanitizing. For example, if a piece of equipment must be washed down, it should not be located near a dry storage area.
10. *Validate cleaning and sanitizing protocols.* All procedures used for cleaning and sanitizing need to be written and appropriate verification and validation performed to ensure sanitary conditions. This typically includes visual supervision during sanitation and microbiological testing upon completion.

Equipment Design Standards In addition to these guidelines there are a few equipment design standard organizations and some recommended equipment lists for specific commodities. In the United States the 3-A Sanitary Standards Organization and P3-A Pharmaceutical Standards Organization develop written standards for dairy processing equipment and pharmaceutical manufacturing. The 3-A Standards Organization includes equipment fabricators, processors, milk regulatory officials (sanitarians), representatives from academia, USDA dairy programs, FDA, and other sanitarians, consumers, and others, who all work collaboratively to develop equipment standards. Required primarily in dairy processing, the 3-A Standards Organization currently has 70 3-A standards for equipment design. In addition, they will provide third-party verification (TPV) as required under the National Conference of Interstate Milk Shippers (NCIMS) regulations.

For other commodities, different organizations provide equipment certification. For example, the USDA Agricultural Marketing Service provides review and certification of meat and poultry processing equipment. The International Fresh-Cut Produce Association (IFPA) has a Sanitary Equipment Design Buying Guide and Checklist for those working in fresh produce. The NSF (formerly National Sanitation Foundation) is another organization that provides equipment review and certification.

In Europe, equipment is manufactured according to the European Hygienic Engineering and Design Group (EHEDG) recommended practices. These are recommendations developed for specific plant processes which have been adopted by most European countries. Thus, in many countries these are equivalent to the equipment design regulations. They include a number of specific documents that can be obtained from www.ehedg.org. A few examples of these are listed below for reference and can be accessed through their website www.ehedg.org.

Doc 1	Microbiologically safe continuous pasteurization of liquid foods, 1992
Doc 3	Microbiologically safe aseptic packing of food products, 1993
Doc 8	Hygienic equipment design criteria, 2004
Doc 10	Hygienic design of closed equipment for the processing of liquid food, 1993
Doc 11	Hygienic packing of food products, 1993
Doc 16	Hygienic pipe couplings, 1997
Doc 17	Hygienic design of pumps, homogenizers, and dampening devices, 2004
Doc 18	Passivation of stainless steel, 1998
Doc 22	General hygienic design criteria for the safe processing of dry particulate materials, 2001
Doc 30	Air handling in the food industry

Preventive Maintenance Preventive maintenance is an often overlooked aspect of food-processing plant operations. It is a hidden cost that is not usually tracked. For a food-processing plant to run efficiently, a preventive maintenance program needs to be developed. The maintenance program is the grease that keeps the wheel from squeaking. In a processing plant expected to run 16 hours per day 360 days per year, equipment must be in top running order. Frequent inspections and servicing prevent equipment breakdowns and plant shutdowns. Programs such as statistical process control and documented visual inspections can be used to track processing conditions (i.e., meat slicing thickness). As equipment wears, variations are seen visually and in recorded product data. Machine adjustments or equipment repair can be undertaken before product quality is affected. Statistical process control and frequent visual inspection are two tools that can be used to prevent 90% of plant shutdowns. The total cost for 1 h of down time in a large food-processing plant can exceed $100,000.

21.6 CRISIS MANAGEMENT: HOW TO SURVIVE A RECALL

One needs to expect that a sanitation failure will happen at their plant, and they need to be prepared. The question is not "if" but "when," and we need to determine whether adequate preparations are in place. Five steps should be considered in preparing for a sanitation failure:

1. Develop a recall team with all departments represented (e.g., quality conrol, engineering, maintenance, production, management, sanitation, legal representation).
2. Develop a written recall plan and record-keeping system that facilitates product tracking. This will detail what lots might be affected, who received this product, and what they (customers) should do with the product. Should it be returned to you directly? Disposed of immediately? Returned to the point of purchase? These decisions will depend on what type of failure occurred and what, if any, alternatives exist for the suspect product.
3. A spokesperson needs to be selected as a point of contact to answer customer concerns. This person needs instruction from legal counsel on what can and cannot be stated.
4. A mock recall needs to be performed and changes to the recall plan should be made as needed.
5. Annual reviews of the recall program need to be performed, including updating representatives, recall procedures, and mock recall training. It is important that one recognize that a recall is a traumatic event and that written plans need to be in place. Decisions need to be made quickly and appropriate information provided to customers, the media, and government officials. The processor's and the industry's reputation is in the spotlight and "on the line." A poorly conducted recall can have a significantly negative impact on the entire industry, as in the case of the green onions.

21.7 EDUCATIONAL AND TRAINING RESOURCES

There are many educational and training resources for sanitation programs. The following list is a starting point and by no means complete. The resources are subdivided into four areas: government agencies, professional organizations, magazines, and university links.

21.7.1 Government Agencies

- U.S. Department of Agriculture Agricultural Marketing Service: www.ams.usda.gov
- U.S. Department of Agriculture Food Safety Inspection Service: www.fsis.usda.gov
- U.S. Department of Health and Human Services Food and Drug Administration: www.fda.gov
- U.S. Department of Health and Human Services Food and Drug Administration, Center for Food Safety and Applied Nutrition: www.cfsan.fda.gov
- U.S. Environmental Protection Agency: www.epa.gov/ebtpages/humafoodsafety.html
- SSOPs: www.access.gpo.gov/nara/cfr/waisidx_06/9cfr416_06.html
- SPSs: www.fsis.usda.gov/OPPDE/rdad/frpubs/SanitationGuide.htm

21.7.2 Professional Organizations

- 3-A Sanitary Standards: www.3-a.org
- American Meat Institute: www.meatami.com/
- European Hygienic Engineering Design Group: www.ehedg.org
- Food Products Association: www.fpa-food.org/
- Grocery Manufacturers Association: www.gmaonline.org/
- National Cattlemen's Beef Association: www.beefusa.org/
- National Pork Producers Council: www.nppc.org
- National Sanitation Foundation: www.nsf.org
- United Fresh Produce Association (United Fresh): www.unitedfresh.org/

21.7.3 Magazines

- *Food Engineering*: www.foodengineeringmag.com/
- *Food Processing*: www.foodprocessing.com/resource_centers/production_operations/safety_sanitation.html
- *Food Protection Trends*: www.foodprotection.org/publications/fpt.asp
- *Food Safety Magazine*: www.foodsafetymagazine.com
- *Journal of Food Protection*: www.foodprotection.org/publications/jfp.asp
- *Meat & Poultry*: www.meatpoultry.com/

21.7.4 Universities

- North Carolina State University, Department of Food Science: www.ces.ncsu.edu/depts/foodsci/distance/

- Oklahoma State University, Food and Agricultural Products Research and Technology Center: www.fapc.okstate.edu/
- Penn State University, Department of Food Science: foodsafety.cas.psu.edu/sanitation_links.htm
- Purdue University, Department of Food Science: www.foodsci.purdue.edu/news/
- Texas A&M University, Department of Meat Science: meat.tamu.edu/
- University of California Davis, Department of Food Science and Technology: seafood.ucdavis.edu/Pubs/99resources.htm
- University of Guelph, Department of Food Science: www.foodscience.uoguelph.ca/home/
- University of Nebraska Lincoln, Food Processing Center: fpc.unl.edu/Entrepreneur/index.shtml
- Virginia Tech, Department of Food Science and Technology: www.fst.vt.edu/graduate/courses.html

REFERENCES

AMI (American Meat Institute) (2005): AMI fact sheet: sanitary equipment design. American Meat Institute, Arlington, VA.

Bricher JL (2005): Equipped for excellence: a blueprint for success. *Food Safety Mag.* 10:56–62.

Calvin L, Avendano B, Schwentesius R (2004): The economics of food safety: the case of green onions and hepatitis A outbreaks. Outlook report VGS30501. http://www.ers.usda.gov/Publications/vgs/nov04/VGS30501/. Accessed May 2008.

Cornell University Law School (2006): *U.S. Code Collection*. Legal Information Institute, Cornell Law School, Ithaca, NY. http://www.law.cornell.edu/uscode/. Accessed May 2008.

Marriot NG, Gravani RB (2006): *Principles of Food Sanitation*. Springer, New York.

USDA-FSIS (U.S. Department of Agriculture–Food Safety and Inspection Service) (2006a): Animals and animal products: sanitation. 9 CFR 416. http://www.access.gpo.gov/nara/cfr/waisidx_05/9cfr416_05.html. Accessed May 2008.

——— (2006b): Food and drugs: current good manufacturing practices in manufacturing, packing, or holding human food. 21 CFR 110. http://www.cfsan.fda.gov/~lrd/cfr110.html Accessed May 2008.

——— (2006c): Meat Products Inspection Act. http://www.fsis.usda.gov/Regulations_&_Policies/Federal_Meat_Inspection_Act/index.asp. Accessed May 2008.

——— (2006d): Poultry Products Inspection Act. http://www.fsis.usda.gov/Regulations_&_Policies/Poultry_Products_Inspection_Act/index.asp. Accessed May 2008.

——— (2006e): Egg Products Inspection Act. http://www.fsis.usda.gov/Regulations_&_Policies/Egg_Products_Inspection_Act/index.asp. Accessed May 2008.

USFDA-CFSAN (U.S. Food and Drug Administration – Center for Food Safety and Applied Nutrition) (2001): Action levels for poisonous or deleterious substances in human food and animal feed. http://vm.cfsan.fda.gov/~lrd/fdaact.html. Accessed May 2008.

——— (2003): National shellfish sanitation program. guide for the control of molluscan shellfish. http://www.cfsan.fda.gov/~ear/nss2-toc.html. Accessed May 2008.

USFDA-FFDCA (U.S. Food and Drug Administration – Federal Food, Drug, and Cosmetic Act) (2006): Memorandum of understanding between the Environmental Protection Agency and the Food and Drug Administration. http://www.fda.gov/oc/mous/domestic/225-79-2001.html Accessed May 2008.

CHAPTER 22

HAZARD ANALYSIS OF CRITICAL CONTROL POINTS

MARTIN W. BUCKNAVAGE and CATHERINE NETTLES CUTTER

22.1 INTRODUCTION

Prior to the implementation of the seven principles of hazard analysis of critical control points (HACCP), food manufacturers relied heavily on inspection-based systems to manage food safety. To guarantee the safety of their products, manufacturers adopted HACCP as a scientific-based, risk-related approach to ensure safety. Using a systematic approach, potential biological, chemical, or physical hazards associated with the food process can be identified and analyzed at each step in the process.

After a manufacturer determines potential hazards within the process, those with any significant risk are identified (also known as hazard analysis principle 1). Next, the establishment determines if there are points within the process where these potential hazards can be eliminated, prevented, or controlled. These are called critical control points (CCPs; principle 2). At these points, critical limits (CLs) or parameters are identified to maintain control of the hazard (principle 3). When a CL has been identified, the establishment identifies procedures (who, when, where, frequency) for monitoring each of the CCPs (principle 4). If the CL has not been met, establishments identify corrective actions to ensure that the deviation is corrected and no adulterated product enters commerce (principle 5). Once the procedures are in place, record-keeping procedures for documenting the monitoring of CCPs are established (principle 6). And finally, establishments should verify their HACCP plan periodically to ensure that it is working as intended (principle 7). When all seven principles are applied successfully, in conjunction with good hygienic practices and other prerequisite programs, the establishment has the tools necessary to ensure the safety of foods they produce.

Microbiologically Safe Foods, Edited by Norma Heredia, Irene Wesley, and Santos García

In this chapter we provide an overview of the seven principles of HACCP, review the interaction of government and industry in the realm of HACCP, and discuss the challenges faced by the meat and poultry industry and regulatory agencies in implementing HACCP.

22.2 HACCP FUNDAMENTALS

22.2.1 Historical Perspective of HACCP

The concept of HACCP was launched with the early stages of the space program in the 1950s (Stevenson, 2006a). The Pillsbury Company, the U.S. Army Laboratory in Natick, Massachusetts, and the National Aeronautical and Space Association (NASA) developed the foundation of HACCP as a way to ensure the safety of food produced for astronauts. Given the impracticality of testing all of the foods produced and using inspection-based systems that could not guarantee safe food 100% of the time, this coalition introduced the approach of building safety into the food manufacturing process in 1971 (Stevenson, 2006a). Although there was interest throughout the 1970s, it was not until 1985 when the National Academy of Sciences (NAS) subcommittee on Food Protection recommended the use of HACCP by industry as well as regulators as an effective and efficient way to assure the safety of foods. In 1988, the National Advisory Committee on the Microbiological Criteria for Foods (NACMCF, 1989) adopted the recommendations of the NAS subcommittee and further defined and clarified the concept of HACCP. This 1989 NACMCF report applied the seven principles of HACCP to food-processing operations with two revisions, issued in 1992 and 1997 (NACMCF, 1997).

Throughout the 1990s, HACCP was adopted voluntarily by individual companies throughout the United States. However in the 1990s, regulatory agencies required companies within entire sectors of the food supply to have HACCP systems in place. In 1995, the U.S. Food and Drug Administration (FDA) issued its *Procedures for the Safe and Sanitary Processing and Importing of Fish and Fishery Products (21 CFR 123 and 1240)*, requiring mandatory HACCP programs for all facilities that processed seafood products for human consumption to be in place by December 1997 (Stevenson, 2006a). In 1996, the U.S. Department of Agriculture–Food Safety Inspection Service (USDA-FSIS) issued *Pathogen Reduction: Hazard Analysis and Critical Control Point (HACCP) Systems (9 CFR 304, req.)*, also known as the "mega reg," which mandated that all USDA-FSIS-inspected meat- and poultry-processing facilities have HACCP-based systems by 2000. In 2004, the FDA mandated HACCP for fruit juice processing in *Hazard Analysis and Critical Control Point (HACCP): Procedures for the Safe and Sanitary Processing and Importing of Juice* (21 CFR 120). To date, these three examples are the only federally mandated HACCP regulations enforced in the United States.

The Codex Alimentarius Committee on Food Hygiene provides international food safety standards (FAO/WHO, 2003). In 2006, the European Union (EU) mandated that all food operators adopt procedures based on the seven principles of HACCP.

Recently, Mexico has mandated HACCP for seafood. Additionally, HACCP has been adopted in Canada, Australia, and Japan and is being considered by the food industry in China as well as Central and South America (Castillo, 2002; Stevenson, 2006a; WHO, 1999).

22.2.2 Current Status of HACCP

In the United States there is widespread voluntary adoption of HACCP programs by the food industry except in smaller companies where there is no government mandate or customer requirements. These smaller companies often lack the financial resources and training opportunities to develop and implement such food safety systems. An incentive is the requirement by customers for their suppliers to have a HACCP system in place for the products they purchase. For foods entering the U.S., the exporter must meet all regulatory requirements, including HACCP, before food products enter the country.

Recently, HACCP has eclipsed the traditional food-processing industries and penetrated the retail, food service, equipment, packaging, and agricultural sectors. Food service and retail operators face the challenge of designing HACCP systems to control multiple and varied processes in one location. Equipment and packaging manufacturers are finding that implementation of HACCP programs is a requirement for doing business with their food industry customers. In the agricultural sector, HACCP is in place in larger agricultural businesses and/or it is a customer requirement. There are limited HACCP-type programs for on-farm or production sectors (Scott and Stevenson, 2006).

For many establishments that must operate under mandatory HACCP systems imposed by regulatory agencies, there also is the challenge of uniting the seven principles of HACCP with the requirements of government agencies. This concept is referred to as regulatory HACCP. Food-processing establishments have the additional task of incorporating HACCP and other food safety requirements of their customers. This concept is referred to as business HACCP. It is important to differentiate between these two concepts and scientific HACCP, which applies science to an establishment's HACCP plan. In some cases, food establishments must incorporate these political and customer expectations into their HACCP plan even though they may not be truly science-based.

22.2.3 Overview of HACCP Plan Development and Implementation

In the planning and implementation stages of HACCP programs, several preliminary tasks must be completed: designating a HACCP coordinator, forming the HACCP team, describing the food and its distribution, and then developing and verifying a flow diagram. Before initiating the HACCP process, the food establishment must also have implemented several prerequisite programs, such as standard operating procedures (SOPs), good manufacturing practices (GMPs), and sanitation standard operating procedures (SSOPs) (Bernard et al., 2006).

22.2.4 Preliminary Tasks

Assembling the HACCP Coordinator and Team Overall responsibility for the development and management of the HACCP program should be assigned to the HACCP coordinator, who should demonstrate good organizational skills and an in-depth understanding of the operations (Stevenson, 2006b). The HACCP coordinator should ensure that prerequisite programs are in place and monitored as required, the HACCP program is operational, CCPs are monitored, and documentation is reviewed and maintained in an organized fashion.

From a regulatory aspect, a HACCP coordinator should to be formally trained and certified in HACCP from an approved educational provider. From a technical standpoint, the HACCP coordinator must understand the manufacturing process and the potential hazards associated with the product. While consultants may augment the technical capabilities of the HACCP coordinator or HACCP team, they may not be present on a daily basis. In the event there is a deviation in the HACCP plan, it is important that a designated person with overall responsibility of the HACCP program be present and be adequately trained in HACCP to react appropriately to a variety of circumstances.

The HACCP coordinator position may be independent of or associated with quality assurance (QA) or quality control (QC) (Stevenson, 2006b). In smaller companies where there are no technical specialists such as a QA or QC manager, the tendency is to assign HACCP coordinator responsibilities to a production supervisor or quality technician. In either case, that person should possess the organizational capabilities and have the technical acumen to handle the requirements demanded by HACCP (Stevenson and Barach, 2006).

Once the HACCP program is in place, the HACCP coordinator will have ongoing responsibilities, including records review, internal audits, and ensuring that prerequisite programs adequately support the HACCP program. In the event of a deviation, the HACCP coordinator also should determine the cause of a given deviation and implement changes to eliminate that cause (Stevenson and Barach, 2006).

For the proper implementation of HACCP, the coordinator should supervise team members who come from various departments within the establishment (Stevenson and Barach, 2006). Departments with representation on the HACCP team should include maintenance, engineering, quality assurance/control, production, purchasing, supply chain management, and/or product development. Having persons with a variety of skills and knowledge of the operation will strengthen the HACCP team in its ability to correctly determine all the inputs, the process flow, hazard analyses, and the CCPs. When certain gaps exist within the team, assistance can be drawn from consultants, suppliers, and departmental groups within the establishment. Assistance in the development of the HACCP plan also can be found through research by the HACCP team in the scientific literature, textbooks, equipment manuals, trade journals, the Internet, regulatory publications, processing authorities, and so on. (Stevenson and Barach, 2006).

Along with the technical skills, HACCP team members must have organizational and supervisory skills for implementation and management of the HACCP program (Stevenson and Barach, 2006). Team members are responsible for identifying and training employees for monitoring and process control tasks and may draft and review procedures and checklists related to the HACCP documentation of these control points. While a HACCP coordinator oversees the day-to-day review of HACCP records, other team members may have HACCP assignments, including daily verification procedures. In cases where team members have extensive responsibilities in developing, implementing, or managing the HACCP plan, it may be beneficial for them to receive formalized HACCP certification. The HACCP team should be involved in the decision-making process when new proposals are reviewed and in revalidating the HACCP plan to incorporate this change (Stevenson and Barach, 2006).

Management should support the HACCP team and endorse the transition to HACCP-based food safety programs via open communication to company employees. Management should empower employees who have HACCP-related responsibilities to be actively involved in all phases of HACCP plan. Participation includes team members who develop, implement, and oversee the day-to-day operations of the HACCP program, employees who are charged with monitoring CCPs, persons who perform prerequisite tasks, and supervisors who take corrective actions when deviations occur.

Management provides the necessary resources to develop, implement, and manage HACCP (Stevenson and Barach, 2006). This includes providing additional equipment to control the process properly, allowing time for the HACCP team to meet and training for team members and line employees. Although training members of upper management is not normally required, their knowledge of HACCP and food safety will benefit their decision-making responsibilities.

After management designates the HACCP coordinator and team members, management should work with that team to schedule HACCP plan development and implementation. During this time, management should receive regular status updates to ensure that the goals for HACCP implementation are on schedule and that the team is not encountering delays in implementing HACCP.

Describing the Food, Its Distribution, and Flow Diagram With the HACCP team in place, the process of describing the product and process flow can begin. Figure 1 outlines the process that is used to analyze the food product(s) for which the HACCP plan is being developed. Important elements of the product description are product properties: whether it is frozen, refrigerated, or shelf stable; the type of storage and distribution required; the shelf life of the product; the intended customer of the product; labeling requirements; ingredients; and how the product is processed. The potential for mishandling by the customer should also be determined. Each of these elements should be appraised thoroughly while developing the product description and should written out in detail (Stevenson, 2006b).

Next, a flow diagram should be drawn, detailing the process from raw ingredient through to finished product and distribution. Each stage of the process is listed, with identification of inputs, raw ingredients, rework, packaging, and the process control steps that occur along the way (Fig. 2).

The process flow diagram should incorporate all steps that have an impact on the process and product. If a process has a conveyor that moves product from a grinder

PRODUCT DESCRIPTION

1 Product name(s)	All beef hot dogs.
2 Process type	Heat processed, stuffed meat product.
3 Product properties	Contains meat and other non meat ingredients (including preservatives).
4 How is the product to be used (intended use) and who is the inteneded consumer?	Intended for general public. Although label description is for reheating, may be eaten without reheating.
5 Type of packaging	Vacuum packed in plastic packaging then into corrugated boxes.
6 Shelf-life	60 days at refrigeration temperature.
7 Where will the product be sold?	Retail stores.
8 Labeling instructions	Keep refrigerated, contains nitrites.
9 Special distribution control	Store below 40 degree F.

Approved: Dave Smith **Date:** 11/08/09

FIG. 1 Product description for all-beef hot dogs. (Adapted from Scott and Stevenson, 2006.)

to a cooker, this lesser step may be grouped with a larger process step, provided that the lesser step does not affect the safety of the product. However, if it affects food safety in some other way, in that the conveyor speed controls the throughput through that cooker, that conveyor should be part of the flow diagram. In general, the more detailed the process flow, the better able the HACCP team will be to capture all important information at each and every step. Once the process flow has been drafted,

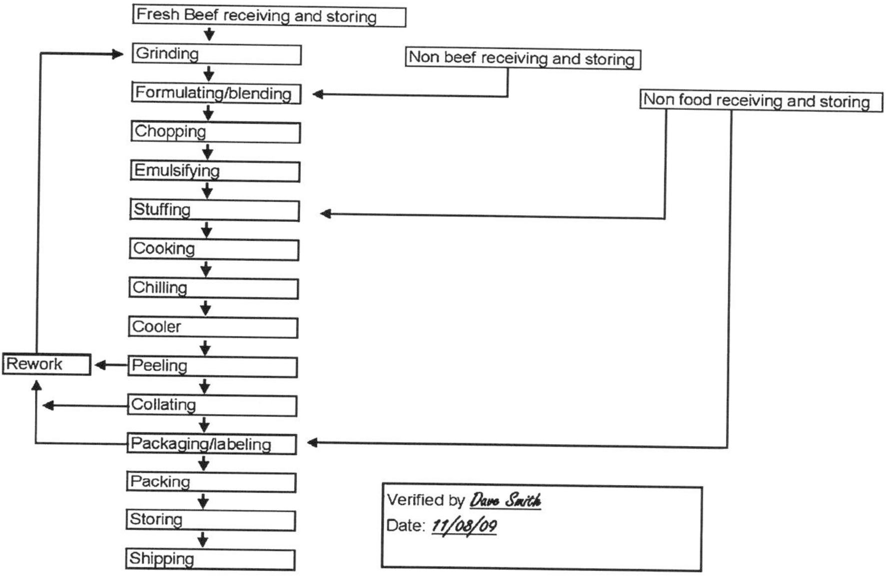

FIG. 2 Process flow for all-beef hot dogs. (Adapted from Scott and Stevenson, 2006.)

the HACCP team must verify that the process is correct. Therefore, the diagram must be taken out to the production floor, evaluated for accuracy, and additional input gathered from knowledgeable employees (Surak and Wilson, 2007).

22.2.5 Prerequisite Programs

Prerequisite programs help control elements outside the process so that they do not contribute to unforeseen hazards. They address topics such as ensuring that the processing environment is clean, that the people working on the process do not contaminate the food, and that the raw materials do not introduce hazards that are not accounted for in the HACCP plan. Prerequisite programs that are recognized and mandated by regulatory agencies include good manufacturing practices (GMPs), sanitation standard operation procedures (SSOPs), and/or standard operating procedures (SOPs) (Bernard et al., 2006).

GMPs are the basic requirements for the sanitary processing of foods to ensure wholesomeness and safety and are detailed in Chapter 20. SOPs are protocols that clearly describe a process, task, or activity (Surak and Wilson, 2007). An example of an SOP is shown in Fig. 3.

For USDA-FSIS-inspected meat and poultry establishments, there is a regulatory requirement for sanitation standard operating procedures (SSOPs) (USDA-FSIS, 1996). SSOPs are the detailed cleaning and sanitizing procedures required for all equipment, surfaces, and processing environment (see Chapter 20). These procedures should be written clearly in detail sufficient to allow personnel to properly clean and

Raw, Ground Model

SOP for Tempering/Thawing of Frozen Materials

1. Place frozen product in a tempering room or cooler that is maintained at 50°F or cooler and allow product to thaw or reach desired level of tempering. The following additional time guideline will be followed:
   - If the room temperature is greater than 41°F but not above 50°F, thawed product must be colder to 41°F or cooler within 8 hours of thawing.
2. Alternatively, frozen ground beef or whole chicken may tempered or thawed at a temperature greater than 50°F but not greater than normal room temperature (72°F), with the following restrictions:
   - Ground beef portions of at least 1 pound in size may be tempered/thawed for up to 9 hours.
   - Whole chicken of at least 3.7 pounds in size may be tempered/thawed for up to 9 hours.
   - Thawed product must be cooled to 41°C or colder within 2 hours of thawing.
3. Tempering/thawing conditions warmer than 72°F must be evaluated to ensure that the pathogenic bacterial growth will not occur on the products.
4. The tempering/thawing product will be monitored on a scheduled basis to prevent product drip and loss of package integrity, and to ensure that product drip does not contaminate other products.
5. The product surface temperature will be monitored and documented on a scheduled basis to ensure that the guidelines listed above are met.
6. When possible, the outer layer of trim and/or pieces being thawed will be removed and refrigerated. This process will be repeated as often as necessary to ensure that the outer surface of the thawing mass is not held for an unsafe time at temperatures that could allow pathogen growth.
7. The lot code of frozen product that has been purchased from an outside vendor will be recorded on a batch sheet or production log (before tempering/thawing) for use in product tracking if the vendor institutes a recall.

01/26/2006 Version; Supersedes all other versions.

FIG. 3 Example of an SOP. (Courtesy of the University of Wisconsin Center for Meat Process Validation.)

sanitize the equipment, surfaces, and environment. Documentation for the cleaning, as well as the verification that it was completed, should be recorded on a daily basis (Jantschke and Chen, 2006).

Allergen control programs identify and control all allergen-containing ingredients throughout the process and in the finished product (Surak and Wilson, 2007). These protocols describe the handling and introduction of raw materials that contain allergens, processing aids, and finished product through SOPs, labeling, and/or segregation. The programs may set up scheduling restrictions and/or cleaning protocols to prevent cross-contamination of products with different allergen profiles. For example, an establishment may fabricate two different hot dog formulations: one with soy protein and one without. For hot dog formulations made without soy protein, employees should produce the hot dogs at the beginning of the day when the equipment is clean, sanitized, and free of soy protein. Conversely, hot dogs made with soy protein should be made at the end of the day and then the equipment cleaned and sanitized. In these instances, thorough sanitation of equipment between the production of the two formulations should prevent cross-contamination of the soy between the two separate batches.

Supplier control programs are used by manufacturers to assure that suppliers have effective food safety programs in place (Surak and Wilson, 2007). The goal of these programs is to ensure that the supplies received by the establishment do not contain hazards that compromise the establishment's HACCP plan. These programs may list the criteria by which a supplier and their products are to be evaluated and the process by which new suppliers are approved.

Chemical control programs define the receipt, storage, and use of all potentially hazardous chemicals in the processing establishment (Surak and Wilson, 2007). The goal of a chemical control program is to reduce the likelihood that these potentially hazardous chemicals contaminate the process through misuse. Chemical control programs should describe where chemicals are stored, how they are secured, procedures for use, and often entail an accounting and tracking system to ensure that unauthorized use has not occurred.

Integrated pest management programs prevent and control pests (rodents, insects, birds, etc.) and their nutrient sources within and/or in close proximity to the establishment (Bernard et al., 2006). Pests such as rats and roaches can contaminate food with bacterial pathogens as well as destroy facilities and equipment. If contamination does occur, then established procedures using approved chemicals or entrapment can be used to rid the establishment of the pest(s).

Environmental and end-product testing can be employed by establishments to verify that procedures taken by employees have been successful. Environmental testing for contaminants such as bacterial pathogens and allergens ensures that the sanitation processes have been performed adequately. Finished product testing verifies that the HACCP system, as well as other prerequisite programs, has yielded a product that meets established food safety criteria (Bernard et al., 2006; Surak and Wilson, 2007).

Product traceability and recall programs trace back all raw materials and track finished product in order to conduct product retrieval in the event of potential contamination either from within the establishment or from the supplier (Bernard et al., 2006). Lot information on incoming materials should be recorded and ingredients tracked as they are utilized within the process. Lot information from finished product should be tracked as it is distributed. A component of such programs is conducting a mock recall which verifies that the tracking system is capable of retrieving distributed product to each and every customer within a specified time frame.

Food defense and/or biosecurity programs should be in place to prevent the intentional contamination of food, as described in Chapter 29. Establishments should evaluate their operations and instigate measures to reduce the risk of an intentional threat. Securing facilities, improving hiring practices, training employees, and restricting access to outsiders are just some of the precautions that can be taken (USDA-FSIS, 2007).

One critical component for the success of any HACCP program is employee education and training. Those establishments that employ HACCP should educate employees in the basic elements of HACCP, train these people in their respective roles, and have these employees apply those elements to their operation on a daily basis. The training materials used are based on established, standardized materials from the Food Products Association (Scott and Stevenson, 2006) and the International HACCP Alliance (International HACCP Alliance, updated annually).

Employee training, offered during orientation and then on a regular basis, instructs personnel in processing, food safety, and HACCP. Training should be delivered in an understandable language and in sufficient detail for employees to complete assigned tasks successfully. Once trained, a system should be in place to verify that the employee has acquired the knowledge needed to complete these tasks. The system should require documentation of both the training and verification processes. For example, if QA/QC personnel undergo GMP training, management should document employee training and provide regular updates (Gravani et al., 2006).

Receiving, storage, and distribution prerequisite programs control the receipt, handling, storage, and shipping of raw materials, in-process materials, and finished product (Surak and Wilson, 2007). These procedures are established to ensure that the items are held at the proper temperature to prevent degradation, put in proper location to prevent cross-contamination, and are rotated to keep items fresh. "First-in, first-out" policies, labeling, and lot coding are other important elements of these types of prerequisite programs.

Preventive maintenance programs ensure that manufacturing equipment is operational, thereby reducing food safety issues that may result during an unexpected breakdown (Surak and Wilson, 2007). Maintenance safety programs should also be in place to prevent unintentional contamination by the maintenance personnel, their equipment, and/or parts. Properly maintained equipment is also less likely to introduce physical hazards such as metal fragments into the flow, process, or food.

Customer complaint programs alert the manufacturer to possible issues associated with food products. Typically, establishments will track consumer complaints and use the information to scan for potential health or safety issues in the field. This information should be reviewed daily or weekly to identify any sudden increase in complaints or the existence of a serious complaint and to ensure that someone from management addresses the complaints in a timely manner (Bernard et al., 2006).

For a HACCP program to be effective, prerequisite programs must be in place, documented, verified on a regular basis, and deemed to be operating effectively. Several types of prerequisite programs have the potential to keep hazards from becoming serious enough to adversely affect the safety of the foods produced. That is, they keep potential hazards or low risk from becoming a classification of "likely to occur."

Sanitation and the associated SSOPs are one part of the prerequisite programs that requires additional attention (see Chapter 20). In addition to having a large impact on food safety, these prerequisite programs often are an undervalued part of manufacturing operations. One important consideration is the difference in regulatory requirements for sanitation records. Under FDA regulations, written SSOPs are not required of the manufacturer. However, FDA has identified eight areas that should be recorded and monitored: safety of water; condition of food-contact surfaces; prevention of cross-contamination to food, packaging, and food-contact surfaces; maintenance of hand-washing and rest room facilities; protection against chemical contamination; proper labeling, storage, and use of toxic compounds; control of employee health conditions; and exclusion of pests from the food establishment (Bernard and Ward, 2001; Jantschke and Chen, 2006; USFDA-CFSAN, 2004).

USDA-FSIS requires meat and poultry establishments comply with Sanitation Performance Standards (SPS) and written SSOPs (Jantschke and Chen, 2006; USDA-FSIS, 1996). SPS are sanitary expectations of the establishment and process and specifically address five areas: grounds and facilities; equipment and utensils; sanitary operations; employee hygiene; and tagging of unsanitary equipment, utensils, rooms, or components used in the manufacture of food that are deemed unacceptable.

Given a comparison of the FDA and USDA-FSIS requirements, it is best for facilities to exceed the regulatory requirements and have written procedures for all areas of sanitation, recorded documentation that the procedures have been complete, and documentation demonstrating the effectiveness of the procedures. In addition to daily cleaning, facilities should have a master sanitation schedule (MSS) established for the cleaning of nonroutine areas such as overhead areas, drains, and refrigeration coils. Procedures and documentation for task completion should be established for each entry on the MSS.

Cleaning and sanitizing should also be addressed during employee training so that employees understand the potential risks of product contamination associated with an inadequate sanitation program (Marriott and Gravani, 2006). With the preliminary tasks complete and prerequisite programs in place, the HACCP team can move toward developing the HACCP plan.

22.2.6 Three Categories of Hazards

The hazards to be addressed by HACCP plans are divided into three categories: biological, chemical, and physical. Biological hazards are comprised of bacteria, viruses, and parasites that cause illness through infection and/or intoxication (see Chapter 2). Improper storage and holding temperatures, inadequate cooking temperature(s), poor personal hygiene, cross-contamination, and improper reheating facilitate the growth of foodborne bacterial pathogens and spoilage organisms (Bernard and Ward, 2001; CDC, 2007; Scott, 2006; USDA-FSIS, 1999).

Control of biological hazards begins with the prevention of contamination in raw materials. For a food-processing establishment, control may be met through receipt of a certificate of analysis, letter of guarantee, or another form of assurance issued by the supplier. Numerous process control procedures (e.g., cooking, cooling, or changing product characteristics through drying or fermentation.) may be employed subsequently to eliminate or control biological hazards in the food product. Process validation studies ensure that a given process will achieve the results expected. For example, if a given process is set to achieve a 6-log reduction by heating the product, the process must be tested or validated to ensure that it is indeed capable of affecting a 99.999% kill of the pathogen. Under these circumstances, it may be necessary to test different pathogens in different phases of growth to ensure that the worst-case scenario will be represented. Predictive modeling is effective in simulating conditions for growth and destruction of pathogens and spoilage organisms (see Chapter 30).

Chemical hazards include naturally occurring chemicals, intentionally added chemicals, and unintentionally added chemicals (Jantschke and Barach, 2006). Naturally occurring chemicals are usually associated with incoming raw materials and may include histamine, ciguatoxin, and other seafood-related toxins, mycotoxins from grains, or allergens. Chemicals added intentionally can be associated with raw materials or used as an ingredient or an aid in processing. Chemicals such as pesticides, fungicides, fertilizers, or antibiotics may be added to the raw products during production or growth, and if not controlled, can become a hazard with that raw material. Ingredients such as preservatives, coloring agents, additives, processing aids, and some vitamins may become a hazard when their addition to the process is not controlled. Chemicals added unintentionally are those that are used within the process and are added to foods accidentally. Primary among this group are machine lubricants, cleaning and sanitizing chemicals, and other maintenance-related chemicals.

Allergens and their control deserve special attention in prerequisite programs and HACCP plans since they affect many food items as either a direct addition or as potential cross-contaminants. Establishments often handle more than one allergen and have numerous product formulations, each with a different allergen makeup. These establishments need to adopt more complicated control systems, including labeling, storage, scheduling, and cleaning practices to prevent allergen cross-contamination. Some facilities will use color-coded tags or scoops for easy identification of a given allergen or equipment used to transport it within the plant (Surak and Wilson, 2007).

Because of the diversity of the chemicals, a chemical control program should be in place to address chemicals at each phase of the operation, from sourcing, to receiving, and through production to distribution (Jantschke and Barach, 2006). The control program must identify where any of these toxic chemicals have a likelihood of contaminating the food produced and then identify measures to prevent unintentional inclusion. Possible preventive methods may include the requirement of a certificate of analysis to verify control by the supplier, storage of chemicals in a restricted area to prevent accidental use, proper labeling to prevent misidentification, or product formulation control to prevent overaddition. For example, if an establishment uses sodium nitrite in some of its formulations, that chemical must be labeled and stored in a place where it will not be accidently misidentified. It must have strict procedures for addition as well as verification through analysis that the right amount was added. Adding this chemical to the wrong product or overusing it in the formulation may result in a health issue.

Physical hazards are typically hard or sharp objects that result in injury to the person who consumes the product. The most common examples of these hazards are glass, metal, plastic, stones, shells, wood, and bones. The USFDA has established a compliance policy guide that provides further information on the classification of physical hazards (Jantschke and Elliot, 2006). In this guidance document, a sharp or hard foreign object is considered to be a hazard if it measures between 7 and 25 mm in any dimension (provided that it is not intended for infants, where there are more restrictions). Prerequisite programs such as GMPs, glass control program, or metal control programs often can be used for the control of physical hazards.

With an understanding of the types of hazards associated with foods, the team develops their HACCP plan. It is important for the HACCP team to take a broad look at the process to determine the hazards that can be associated with the product, especially those that can be associated with a supplier-specific raw material. For example, a supplier may grow a spice that is treated with a pesticide. Since the literature may not indicate any pesticide association with that particular spice, it may be missed by the team during the hazard analysis.

22.2.7 Seven Principles of HACCP

To develop and implement a HACCP plan, one must follow the seven principles of HACCP systematically: complete a hazard analysis; determine the critical control points (CCPs) required to control the identified hazards; establish the critical limits that must be met at each identified CCP; establish procedures to monitor the CCP(s); establish corrective actions to be taken when there is a deviation identified by monitoring a given CCP; establish effective record-keeping systems; and establish procedures for verification. There are many excellent sources of information to assist food manufacturers with the planning and implementation of HACCP programs (Bernard and Ward, 2001; Scott and Stevenson, 2006; USDA-FSIS, 1999; USFDA-CFSAN, 2004; WHO, 1999).

Once the product description and a verified process flow diagram are complete and there are well-functioning prerequisite programs in place, the HACCP team can begin to address the seven principles necessary for the development and implementation of HACCP. Below is a brief overview of steps involved in the development of a HACCP plan.

Conduct the Hazard Analysis The goal of conducting a hazard analysis is to assess potential hazards that present a significant health risk to the consumer at every step in the process. This will identify all potential hazards for a given step and evaluate each hazard to determine if it is a significant risk based on the probability of occurrence and the severity of its health effects.

The HACCP team should review all the available scientific information associated with raw materials, process, manufacturing equipment, storage and distribution, and intended use by the consumer. This information can be obtained online, in government and university publications, in scientific and trade journals, and from equipment and ingredient suppliers. A list of potential biological, chemical, and physical hazards that may be introduced, increased, or controlled at each step in the process should be collected by the HACCP team during this part of the assessment (Fig. 4). The HACCP team will determine if the hazards cause injury (i.e., severity) and if there is a likelihood of occurrence in the product based on plant history or scientific evidence (i.e., outbreak data).

Prerequisite programs, food preparation methods, storage conditions, and consumer handling instructions can all affect the risk of a hazard. In any case where a high degree of control is needed, one or more CCP(s) may be needed within the process. Control measures may not prevent the hazard, but may only control the hazard to some degree. In some cases, more than one control measure may be needed for a hazard. In other cases, one control measure may control more than one hazard in the process (Bernard et al., 2006).

Determine the Critical Control Point(s) In the first step, the HACCP team will have conducted a hazard analysis in order to identify hazards of significant risk at each step in the process of manufacturing food. Once the hazard analysis is completed, each step in the process should be evaluated to determine the control measures where the identified hazards can be prevented, eliminated, or reduced to an acceptable level. These control measures are the CCPs. A CCP is differentiated from a control point (CP) in that a CP is any step at which a hazard is controlled, but is not necessarily essential to the safety of the product. In other words, loss of control at a CCP will result probably in an unsafe product.

The hazard analysis should assist in determining CCPs since significant hazards must be controlled at one or more CCPs within the process. It is common for HACCP teams to identify too many CCPs. One repercussion of too many CCPs in a HACCP plan is an increase in monitoring and record-keeping procedures without any additional benefit regarding the safety of the system. Using decision trees (Fig. 5), the HACCP team should assess whether the step is sufficient to control the hazard or if another step(s) in the process will accomplish this task (Weddig, 2006a).

All CCPs do not result in elimination of the hazard but may maintain it at an acceptable level (Weddig, 2006a). For example, in making hot dogs, a CCP should be identified that eliminates enteric pathogens (e.g., *E. coli* O157:H7, *Listeria monocytogenes*, *Salmonella*) associated with the raw meat. Heat lethality treatments that raise the internal temperature to 170°F (77°C) are sufficient to kill the pathogens. Conversely, fresh refrigerated raw ground meat that is sold in retail operations has no heating step to eliminate the pathogens, so cooking of the ground meat by the consumer is the only point where the pathogens are destroyed. In these scenarios, the establishment will want to minimize growth of pathogens associated with the product while it is under their control by implementing carcass washes with antimicrobials or maintaining an internal product temperature below 40°F (4°C) during or after grinding.

Establish the Critical Limits With each CCP, the critical limits (CLs) must be established to determine when that CCP is "in" or "out" of control. The HACCP team

HAZARD ANALYSIS FOR: All Beef Hot Dogs PRODUCT: Weiner Line PROCESS

Ingredient or Processing Step	Potential hazards introduced or enhanced at this step	Does this potential hazard need to be addressed in HACCP plan? (Yes or No)	Why? (Justification for decision made in previous column)	What measure can be applied to prevent, eliminate or reduce the hazards being addressed in your HACCP plan?	Is this step a Critical Control Point (CCP)?
Grinding	BIOLOGICAL Growth of vegetative pathogens present in raw beef	NO	Period of time at this step is short, opportunity of pathogen growth not reasonably likely to occur.		
	CHEMICAL Excessive sanitizers	NO	Excessive sanitizers residues no likely to occur due to effective sanitation program with SSOPs NRLTO		
	Allergens from species contamination	NO	Research has indicated that allergic reaction to spices contamination is relatively mild. Allergens present in the meat are unstable to heat. NRLTO. Established rework SOP has historically prevented the mixing of species into all-beef products.		
	PHYSICAL Bone chips	NO	The final grinder is equipp ed with a bone collection system. The grinder will not function without the bone collector system in place		
	Metal fragments	Yes	The potential for metal contamination from grinder exists, fragments co uld result in mild to moderate injury	Periodic inspection of equipment	Yes (CCP 1(P)

FIG. 4 Excerpt from hazard analysis for hot dogs. (Adapted from Scott and Stevenson, 2006.)

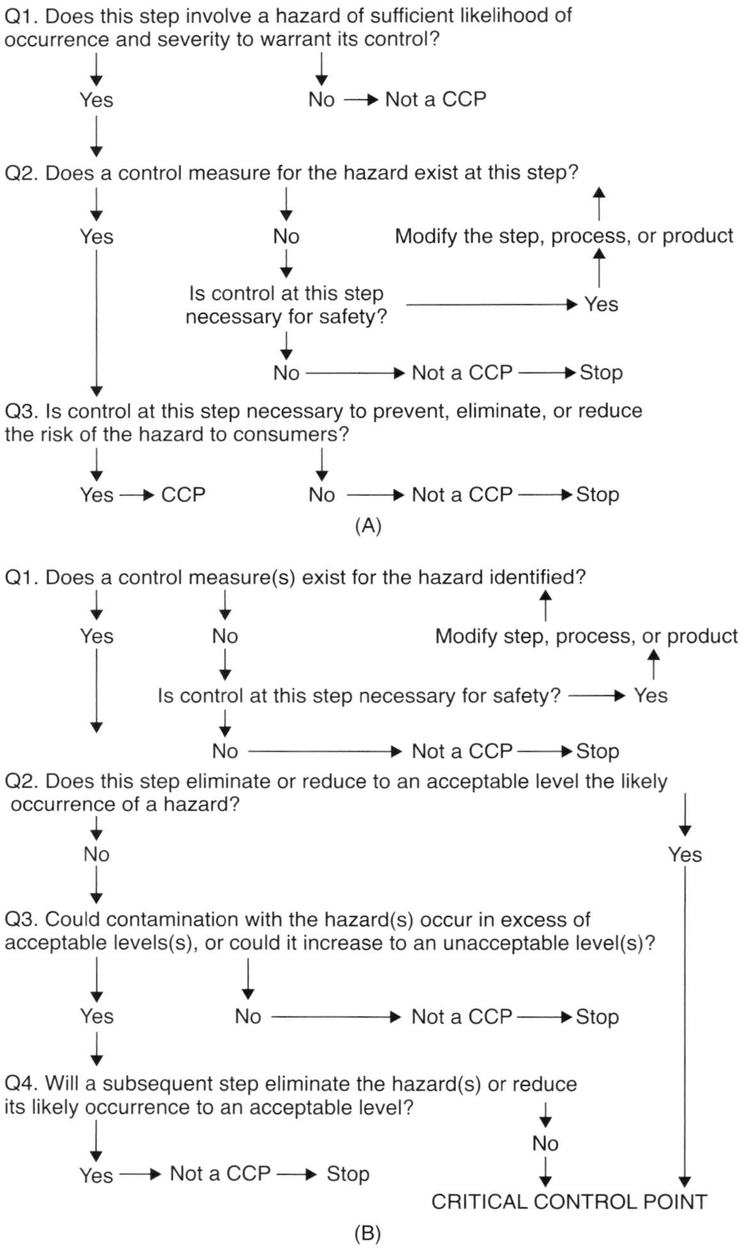

FIG. 5 (A) National Advisory Committee for the Microbiological Criteria for Food (NACMCF) and (B) *Codex Alimentarius* (Codex) decision trees for determination of CCPs in HACCP plans. (Adapted from Scott and Stevenson, 2006.)

should determine the maximum or minimum value to which the hazard is prevented, eliminated, or reduced to an acceptable level. The HACCP team must decide on the CLs to determine when a product is compliant with the HACCP plan, and what point constitutes a process deviation. CLs can be either the measurement of a given parameter or an observation at some point in the process. The CL that is chosen should be capable of being monitored instantaneously, supply a result in real time, and be recordable. The CL chosen also should have sufficient accuracy and precision to detect deviations (Weddig, 2006b).

To control a process, immediate feedback is essential. If results take too long (as is seen with microbiological testing), it may not capture "out of control" data in order to prevent a hazard from occurring. Examples of instantaneous CLs are temperature measurements, pH measurements, and/or sanitizer concentration. Each establishment will have to determine the CL that works best for its product and process. A common example of a measured CL is the destruction of vegetative bacterial cells in poultry at 165°F (74°C) for 15 s. If heating the product does not achieve the 165°F internal temperature, the CL is not met and the resulting situation is considered a process deviation.

CLs may be garnered from the scientific literature or in regulatory publications. If limits are not formally established, establishments should conduct in-house research to validate the processing parameters at the CCP designated. An example of such a situation is when the type of process is new or novel, as has been seen in the application of high-pressure processing for ready-to-eat meats or pulsed electric fields for beverage processing (see Chapter 23). Similarly, when a processing parameter is different from an established or regulatory processing standard, the establishment will need to generate data to support their choice of a CL. For example, if it took longer than 6 h to reduce the temperature of a cooked meat product from 135°F (57°C) to 41°F (5°C), but the establishment determined that the addition of antimicrobials (i.e., nitrites) in the product would prevent the outgrowth of spore-forming, pathogenic organisms, the establishment should present data, research, or predictive models to substantiate that claim.

Establishments may contract food-testing laboratories to simulate the conditions of the plant and food product under laboratory-controlled experiments to determine if a process is sufficient to prevent, reduce, or eliminate a hazard (e.g., a spore-forming pathogen) to an acceptable level. Known as challenge studies, these experiments are done off-site to prevent the introduction of pathogens into the establishment, but can be expensive to conduct.

Similarly, experiments can be performed in-house to generate data and/or research reports that can support the decision-making process. In these cases, variables such as microbial indicator organisms (i.e., aerobic/standard plate counts, lactic acid bacteria, generic *E. coli*, etc.) can be monitored before, during, and after the CCP and data captured, much as in a laboratory setting. However, no pathogens are used. The establishment should summarize the research findings into a concise and clear document with supporting records and include this information in the HACCP plan as support for the CL.

As is often is the case, it is difficult to measure a CCP related directly to a product attribute such as internal temperature. It would be virtually impossible to monitor the internal temperature of every product going through the process. Instead, processing parameters that affect the internal temperature should be considered. An establishment that produces cooked ground beef patties may set CLs based on more than one parameter: patty thickness (less than $\frac{1}{4}$ in.), cooker temperature (350°F/177°C), and cooker line speed (3 f/min). In these instances, the establishment would determine how each of the individual and collective parameters affects the final internal temperature (160°F/71°C). As such, in-plant generated data would be needed to establish the proper settings (patty thickness, cooker temperature, line speed) to ensure that the ground beef patty reaches an internal temperature of 160°F. Establishments should not only collect these types of data initially for inclusion in the HACCP plan, but again periodically, to ensure that the CLs are still valid over time (Weddig, 2006b).

Establish the Monitoring Procedures The monitoring procedures determine and document whether the CLs are being met. The HACCP team must answer the questions of what will be monitored, how it will be monitored, when it will be monitored, and who will monitor it. With regard to what will be monitored, regulatory requirements state that all CCPs must be monitored and CLs be identified (see principle 3). The frequency at which the parameter is measured must be set in order to detect deviations that have the potential to occur within the process. The person measuring the parameter should be capable of completing the activity and documenting the process, as well as reacting appropriately to out-of-control measurements (Gombas et al., 2006).

An important characteristic of monitoring is whether it is continuous or discontinuous. For example, the temperature of product in an oven could be checked to see if it has reached the proper temperature. This discontinuous monitoring procedure does give an accurate assessment of the product temperature, but it may be difficult in a continuous-flow oven. Rather, the oven temperature and product flow could be monitored continuously to ensure that conditions are maintained for the product to reach the proper internal temperature. In this case, the oven parameters would need to be validated for their ability to produce the proper internal product temperature. For discontinuous monitoring, as in the example above, a sampling regimen must be established and validated to ensure that the worst-case scenario is captured. In cases where process variability is high, continuous monitoring may be preferred. An observation used for monitoring a CCP is an example of a discontinuous monitoring procedure. Examples of the use of observations for monitoring may be a visual check of a certificate of analysis, or watching an employee to ensure that a preservative was added into the formulation.

Procedures for monitoring of a CCP must be written clearly. The monitoring task must be completed at its set frequency by the person designated to perform it. If a task is too difficult or if the person is not able to perform it at the specified times, the resulting lapses will constitute a process deviation. Figure 6 gives an example of the particulars associated with monitoring.

PRODUCT : All Beef Hot Dogs PROCESS: Fully cooked not shelf stable

Critical Control Point (CCP)	Hazard(s) to be addressed in the HACCP Plan	Critical limits for each control measure	Monitoring				Corrective action	Verification activities	Record-Keeping procedures
			What	How	Frequency	Who			
CCP 2 (B) Cooking	Vegetative pathogens such as *Salmonella, E. coli* O157:H7 and other enteric pathogens, and *Listeria monocytogenes*.	Minimum internal product temperature150°F	Temperature of this product	Manual thermometer	Once per batch	Oven operator	Continue cooking batch until critical limit is met	QA Manager will conduct reshipment review of records	Oven log
							If cook cannot be completed, hold product	QA verifies accuracy of thermometer at start-up and end of shift. Recalibrates as needed, puts product on hold if needed	Calibration records
							Evaluate safety of product	QA manager or designee observes oven Operator take temperature once per shift	Oven Validation Report
							Requirements of 9CFR417.3 will be met	Validate operation of oven at least once per year	Corrective action log

FIG. 6 Excerpt from HACCP plan summary for hot dogs. (Adapted from Scott and Stevenson, 2006.)

Establish Corrective Actions Written corrective action (CA) procedures address potential deviations at each CL. The CA procedures should not only detail the disposition of the product, but also what should be done to correct the situation that caused the deviation. It is important to document the deviations within the HACCP program and the subsequent CA procedures that do occur. CA procedures should spell out how the deviated product will be handled: whether it is to be reprocessed or destroyed. CA procedures also must ensure that no unsafe product reaches distribution.

Typically, the corrective actions for a deviation would entail the following steps. First, the process would be stopped and the product diverted. The CCP would be brought back into control and any product produced during the deviation would be segregated and held from shipment into normal channels. A decision on the product's disposition would be made by a responsible person with proper authority and knowledge of the HACCP plan, such as the HACCP coordinator or designated HACCP team member. The cause of the deviation would be investigated, rectified, and recorded. It is often difficult to address every possible product deviation, but the better detailed the CA procedures, the easier it is for employees to react and correct deviations when they do occur (Stevenson and Taylor, 2006).

Establish Validation and Verification Procedures Validation is focused on the supporting documentation and on scientific and technical evidence which indicates that the HACCP plan will control the hazards effectively. Validation is completed initially when the HACCP plan is being developed for determination of the potential hazards, determination of the CCPs, and identification of CLs used in the HACCP plan. Validation support of these HACCP principles may include scientific and trade reports, regulatory publications, validation studies, and in-plant data. Validation also occurs at implementation of the HACCP plan to ensure that everything is functioning as intended, including monitoring and record keeping.

Validation should also be completed when any changes are made to the process that can affect the HACCP plan or when new technical information becomes available that has the potential to affect the initial validation. Items that can affect the HACCP plan and require revalidation include changes in the prerequisite programs, raw materials, product formulations, equipment, and rework. Regulatory agencies such as the USDA-FSIS also require revalidation and immediate modification anytime that the HACCP plan is found to be inadequate in its ability to control hazards.

Verification consists of various reviews and audits which ensure that the HACCP plan is operating as intended. Verification is completed on the prerequisite programs through record review and quality audits to ensure that the procedures are compliant with HACCP and that they are being completed as required within the precepts of that particular program. Pre-shipment record review is mandated by the USDA-FSIS and should occur daily in all federally inspected establishments before product is shipped off-site. Verification of CL monitoring activities ensures day-to-day compliance at each CCP. This review should include information such as calibration of equipment used for monitoring the CL, monitoring as described by the HACCP plan, and CAs taken when necessary. If there are no changes to the process, verification of the

HACCP plan should occur at least yearly. This all-encompassing review evaluates the HACCP plan, the prerequisite programs, the product description and process flow, monitoring and calibration records, and corrective action reports.

Verification can be completed by internal as well as external parties. The HACCP team should conduct an internal review of the HACCP plan on a regular (yearly) basis or as deemed necessary. External parties are often used to perform annual, third-party audits of the HACCP plan to ensure system integrity (Scott et al., 2006).

Establish Record-Keeping and Documentation Procedures Records are an essential part of a HACCP plan. Procedures must be established for ensuring that the appropriate records are maintained properly and are available for inspection. Records provide auditable evidence that the HACCP-related procedures and processes are being followed. In addition to having the monitoring records as part of HACCP records, the HACCP plan with product description, product flow diagram, hazard analysis, the HACCP plan summary, and the supporting documentation are important elements of the HACCP records.

There are four types of HACCP records: summary of the hazard analysis, the HACCP plan, the supporting documentation, and the daily operational records. With regard to the HACCP plan, it should include a list of the HACCP team, description of the food, a verified flow diagram, and the HACCP plan summary listing the CCPs along with their critical limits, monitoring actions, corrective actions, verification activities, and record-keeping system (Fig. 6). Support documentation must show how the CCPs and associated CLs were established. Daily operational records include CCP monitoring data, calibration records, corrective action reports, and prerequisite program records.

The FSIS requires that HACCP records contain dates and times, operator signatures, actual observations or data, and reviewers' signatures. Records must undergo review prior to the shipment of that product from the facility. This review should be completed by a trained person. All records pertaining to the food processed under a HACCP plan must be kept a minimum of 1 year for fresh, refrigerated items and 2 years for frozen, ready-to-eat, or shelf-stable items. These records must be available for review upon request of the regulatory agency. In the event of a recall, outbreak, or other legal matter, having accurate record-keeping procedures in place as well as clear, concise documentation are critical (Weddig and Stevenson, 2006).

22.3 CONCLUSIONS

The use of HACCP by food establishments as a methodology to assure the safety of food is increasing worldwide. Although the fundamentals of HACCP have been constant, the application of HACCP continues to be refined to meet the challenges of a dynamic food system. These changes can be seen in the impact on government regulations affecting the industry. Establishments must then work with the government agencies to define how these regulatory actions will impact their operations and refine what they do in order to comply.

While training and education systems must provide an understanding of HACCP fundamentals to industry personnel, these systems must also stay up to date with continuous regulatory changes by incorporating these changes into a regular training regimen. This is can be a complex task, given that regulated mandates are often subject to interpretation and lack detail for specific implementation. The key to a robust HACCP education and training system is to train personnel from all levels in the organization to improve decision making, ensure that training occurs on a regular basis so that personnel are aware of recent changes, and involve regulators in the training initiatives to achieve a single message. Government personnel and educational providers should pay special attention to the needs of the small and very small establishments that may lack the resources and/or technical expertise to react adequately to changing requirements (International HACCP Alliance, 2005).

REFERENCES

Bernard DT, Parkinson NG, Chen Y (2006a): Prerequisites to HACCP, Chapter 2. In: Scott VN, Stevenson KE (Eds.) *Hazard Analysis and Critical Control Point (HACCP): A Systematic Approach to Food Safety*, 4th ed. The Food Products Association, Washington, DC.

Bernard DT, Stevenson KE, Scott VN (2006): Hazard analysis, Chapter 8. In: Scott VN, Stevenson KE (Eds.) *Hazard Analysis and Critical Control Point (HACCP): A Systematic Approach to Food Safety*, 4th ed. The Food Products Association, Washington, DC.

Bernard D, Ward D (2001): *HACCP: Hazard Analysis and Critical Control Point Training Curriculum*, 4th ed. National Seafood HACCP Alliance, University of Florida/IFAS, Gainesville, FL.

Castillo A (2002): HACCP experiences worldwide. http://www.fsis.usda.gov/OPPDE/rdad/FRPubs/02-006N/P2Castillo/Castillo.PPT. Accessed January 2008.

CDC (Centers for Disease Control and Prevention) (2007): Food safety. http://www.cdc.gov/foodsafety/. Accessed January 2008.

FAO/WHO (Food and Agriculture Organization/World Health Organization) (2003): Hazard analysis and critical control point (HACCP) system and guidelines for its application. Codex Alimentarius Annex to the Recommended International Code of Practice General Principles of Food Hygiene CAC/RCP 1-1969, Rev. 4-2003. FAO/WHO Codex Alimentarius Commission, Rome.

Gombas DE, Stevenson KE, Bernard DT (2006): Monitoring critical control points, Chapter 11. In: Scott VN, Stevenson KE (Eds.) *Hazard Analysis and Critical Control Point (HACCP): A Systematic Approach to Food Safety*, 4th ed. The Food Products Association, Washington, DC.

Gravani RB, Weddig LM, Taylor BT, Bernard DT (2006): HACCP training, Chapter 17. In: Scott VN, Stevenson KE (Eds.) *Hazard Analysis and Critical Control Point (HACCP): A Systematic Approach to Food Safety*, 4th ed. The Food Products Association, Washington, DC.

Hontz LR, Scott VN (2006): HACCP and the regulatory agencies, Chapter 16. In: Scott VN, Stevenson KE (Eds.) *Hazard Analysis and Critical Control Point (HACCP): A Systematic Approach to Food Safety*, 4th ed. The Food Products Association, Washington, DC.

International HACCP Alliance (2005): Strategic plan for improving small and very small establishments' food safety programs to further protect public health and ensure regulatory compliance. http://www.haccpalliance.org/alliance/StrPlanSmVSmPlants.pdf. Accessed December 2007.

——— (updated annually): Alliance approved curricula for an introductory course for development of HACCP plans. http://www.haccpalliance.org/alliance/training.html. Accessed January 2008.

Jantschke M, Barach JT (2006): Chemical hazards and controls, Chapter 5. In: Scott VN, Stevenson KE (Eds.) *Hazard Analysis and Critical Control Point (HACCP): A Systematic Approach to Food Safety*, 4th ed. The Food Products Association, Washington, DC.

Jantschke M, Chen Y (2006): Sanitation and sanitation standard operating procedures, Chapter 2. In: Scott VN, Stevenson KE (Eds.) *Hazard Analysis and Critical Control Point (HACCP): A Systematic Approach to Food Safety*, 4th ed. The Food Products Association, Washington, DC.

Jantschke M, Elliot PH (2006): Physical harzards and controls, Chapter 6. In: Scott VN, Stevenson KE (Eds.) *Hazard Analysis and Critical Control Point (HACCP): A Systematic Approach to Food Safety*, 4th ed. The Food Products Association, Washington, DC.

Marriott NG, Gravani RB (2006): *Principles of Food Sanitation*, 5th ed. Springer Science + Business Media, New York.

NACMCF (National Advisory Committee on the Microbiological Criteria for Food) (1989): *HACCP Principles for Food Production*. USDA-FSIS, Washington, DC.

——— (1997): *Hazard Analysis and Critical Control Point Principles and Application Guidelines*. USDA-FSIS, Washington, DC. http://www.fsis.usda.gov/Regulations_&_Policies/National_Advisory_Committee_on_Microbiological/index.asp. Accessed January 2008.

Scott VN (2006): Biological hazards and controls, Chapter 4. In: Scott VN, Stevenson KE (Eds.) *Hazard Analysis and Critical Control Point (HACCP): A Systematic Approach to Food Safety*, 4th ed. The Food Products Association, Washington, DC.

Scott VN, Stevenson KE (Eds.) (2006): *Hazard Analysis and Critical Control Point (HACCP): A Systematic Approach to Food Safety*, 4th ed. Food Products Association, Washington, DC.

Scott VN, Stevenson KE, Gombas DE (2006): Verification procedures, Chapter 13. In: Scott VN, Stevenson KE (Eds.) *Hazard Analysis and Critical Control Point (HACCP): A Systematic Approach to Food Safety*, 4th ed. The Food Products Association, Washington, DC.

Stevenson KE (2006a): Introduction to hazard analysis and critical control point systems, Chapter 1. In: Scott VN, Stevenson KE (Eds.) *Hazard Analysis and Critical Control Point (HACCP): A Systematic Approach to Food Safety*, 4th ed. The Food Products Association, Washington, DC.

Stevenson KE (2006b): Initial tasks in developing HACCP plans, Chapter 7. In: Scott VN, Stevenson KE (Eds.) *Hazard Analysis and Critical Control Point (HACCP): A Systematic Approach to Food Safety*, 4th ed. The Food Products Association, Washington, DC.

Stevenson KE, Barach JT (2006): Organizing and managing HACCP programs, Chapter 15. In: Scott VN, Stevenson KE (Eds.) *Hazard Analysis and Critical Control Point (HACCP): A Systematic Approach to Food Safety*, 4th ed. The Food Products Association, Washington, DC.

Stevenson KE, Taylor BT (2006): Corrective action, Chapter 12. In: Scott VN, Stevenson KE (Eds.) *Hazard Analysis and Critical Control Point (HACCP): A Systematic Approach to Food Safety*, 4th ed. The Food Products Association, Washington, DC.

Surak JG, Wilson S (Eds.) (2007): *The Certified HACCP Auditor Handbook*. ASQ Quality Press, Milwaukee, WI.

USDA-FSIS U.S. Department of Agriculture–Food Safety Inspection Service(1996): Pathogen reduction: hazard analysis and critical control point (HACCP) systems; final rule. *Fed Reg*. 61: 3806–3898, July 25.

——— (1999): Guidebook for the preparation of HACCP plans. http://www.fsis.usda.gov/PPDE/nis/outreach/models/HACCP-1.pdf. Accessed January 2008.

——— (2007): Food defense and emergency response website. http://www.fsis.usda.gov/Food_Defense_&_Emergency_Response/index.asp. Accessed January 2008.

USFDA-CFSAN (U.S. Food and Drug Administration–Center for Food Safety and Applied Nutrition) (2004): Juice HACCP hazards and controls guidance. http://www.cfsan.fda.gov/~dms/juicgu10.html. Accessed January 2008.

Weddig LM (2006a): Critical control points, Chapter 9. In: Scott VN, Stevenson KE (Eds.) *Hazard Analysis and Critical Control Point (HACCP): A Systematic Approach to Food Safety*, 4th ed. The Food Products Association, Washington, DC.

Weddig LM (2006b): Critical limits, Chapter 10. In: Scott VN, Stevenson KE (Eds.) *Hazard Analysis and Critical Control Point (HACCP): A Systematic Approach to Food Safety*, 4th ed. The Food Products Association, Washington, DC.

Weddig LM, Stevenson (2006): Record keeping, Chapter 14. In: Scott VN, Stevenson KE (Eds.) *Hazard Analysis and Critical Control Point (HACCP): A Systematic Approach to Food Safety*, 4th ed. The Food Products Association, Washington, DC.

WHO (World Health Organization) (1999): Strategies for Implementing HACCP in Small and/or Less Developed Businesses, WHO Consultation. The Hague, The Netherlands, June 16–19.

CHAPTER 23

TRADITIONAL AND HIGH-TECHNOLOGY APPROACHES TO MICROBIAL SAFETY IN FOODS

TATIANA KOUTCHMA

23.1 INTRODUCTION

Preservation is a process by which chemical agents or physical treatments prevent biological deterioration of a substance. Microbial growth in foods is one of the leading causes of food spoilage, with the subsequent development of undesirable sensory characteristics. The pathogenicity of certain microorganisms is a major safety concern in the processing of foods. A wide range of physical treatments and chemical agents is employed to preserve foods with high quality and safety level. Based on the mode of action, major food preservation techniques can be categorized as (1) inhibiting chemical deterioration and microbial growth; (2) directly inactivating bacteria, yeasts, molds, or enzymes; and (3) avoiding recontamination before and after processing. Methods of impeding microbial growth include refrigeration and freezing, reduction of water activity, acidification, adding preservatives, and adding or removing gases (oxygen or carbon dioxide). Direct inactivation can be performed during blanching, cooking, frying, pasteurization, and sterilization. Packaging, hygienic processing, and storage are the common approaches to avoiding recontamination.

However, of the many techniques used to preserve foods, only pasteurization and sterilization rely on killing the most resistant pathogens of public health concern. As defined by the U.S. Food and Drug Administration (FDA), sterilization is a process to remove or destroy all viable forms of microbial life, including bacterial spores. Pasteurization was defined as a process of mild heat treatment to reduce significantly or kill the number of pathogenic and spoilage microorganisms. In September 2004, the U.S. Department of Agriculture (USDA) National Advisory Committee on Microbiological Criteria for Foods redefined the term *pasteurization*. The rationale was that new physical methods of treatment are emerging as a result of current consumer

Microbiologically Safe Foods, Edited by Norma Heredia, Irene Wesley, and Santos García

demands for foods that are more fresh, natural, or minimally processed and additive-free. The use of thermal treatment leads to overcooking, an undesirable cooked flavor, and nutritional deterioration.

To satisfy these demands, traditional preservation techniques have been modified. However, the definition of a traditional pasteurization process relied only on thermal treatment, since this was the most widely used process in the category. The new definition of pasteurization includes "any process, treatment, or combination thereof, that is applied to food to reduce the most microorganism(s) of public health significance to a level that is not likely to present a public health risk under normal conditions of distribution and storage" (Sugarman, 2004). Cooking, steam and hot water treatments, microwave processing, ohmic/inductive heating, high-pressure processing, ultraviolet (UV) radiation, irradiation, pulsed electric fields, pulsed light, infrared processing, nonthermal plasma, oscillating magnetic fields, ultrasound, and filtration have been reviewed (Sugarman, 2004) Similarly, microbial death kinetics, including calculations of F-values (unit of measurement used to compare relative sterilizing effects of different procedures, equal to 1 min at 121.1°C) have been described (Pflug and Zeghman, 1985). The commercial challenge to produce safe minimally processed foods provides the incentive to establish process requirements for novel high technologies and to evaluate their efficiency and their equivalency for their application to pasteurization and sterilization processes.

The objective of this chapter is to survey emerging high-technology preservation techniques for their potential use by the food industry for pasteurization and sterilization. The techniques include ionizing irradiation, UV radiation, microwave and radio-frequency heating (MW/RF) and high-pressure processing (HPP). The engineering aspects of these technologies have advanced such that commercialization may now be possible. The knowledge of physical nature of the process as well as a resistance of microorganisms is essential for establishing preservation processes. The efficiency of the process is dependent on a number of parameters that are unique to each technology, which are described in this chapter.

23.2 THERMAL VS. NONTHERMAL TECHNOLOGY

Since the emergence of new preservation techniques, the argument between nonthermal and thermal effects has existed. Nevertheless, it is necessary for food processors to know and understand those different scenarios in order to meet process and regulations requirements and, if possible, to predict processing values under specified conditions.

First, what characterizes thermal, athermal or nonthermal, enhanced or specific biological effects of physical treatments should be clearly defined. The review of Stuerga and Gaillard (1996) has provided some definitions for use in biological studies. These are based on irradiation or power flux density expressed in watts per square meter (W/m^2) or specific absorption rate in watts per kilogram (W/kg) and do not involve any assumptions relating to mechanisms of interaction. The threshold selected for the standard definition of biological metabolism corresponds to 4 W/kg of living matter: (1) *thermal effects* were defined for irradiation power density greater than 4 W/kg, when the organism cannot dissipate the energy supplied by the irradiation; (2) *athermal effects* correspond to density between 0.4 and 4 W/kg. In such conditions, the thermoregulation system is able to compensate for the effect of irradiation.

Traditionally, the macroscopic thermal effect is characterized by increasing temperature within the material. What characterizes nonthermal effects? According to Risman (1996), any nonthermal effect must not be explicable by macroscopic temperatures, time–temperature histories, or gradients. This means that any effects that can be explained by applying verified theories to experimental data and macroscopic temperatures are *not* nonthermal (e.g., microwave heating, adiabatic heat of compression). Cases where physical treatment gives a particular time–temperature profile and gradients which cannot be achieved by other means are only *process-specific*.

Nonthermal effects under the application of electromagnetic radiation (Fig. 1) refer to lethal effects not involving a significant rise in temperature, as, for example, in the case of ionizing radiation. One of the effects of such high-energy photons is breakage of chemical bonds. Roughly the energy of one electron volt (eV) will break a covalent bond in a molecule and produce one ion pair; this is referred to as a direct nonthermal effect. Electromagnetic radiation with frequency above 2500×10^6 MHz, which possesses such a capability, is generally referred to as ionizing radiation (e.g., x-rays, gamma rays). As the wavelength increases and frequency decreases, there is not enough energy to break chemical bonds. Ultraviolet, visible, and possibly infrared rays may have enough energy to break weak hydrogen bonds.

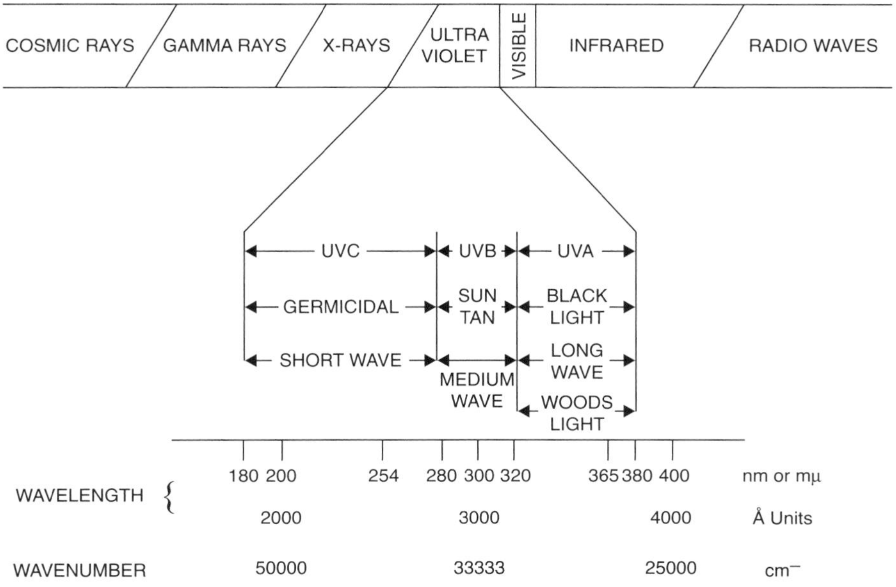

FIG. 1 Electromagnetic radiation spectrum.

The radio-frequency (RF) band of the electromagnetic spectrum covers a broad range of high frequencies, typically either in the kilohertz range (3 kHz $< f <$ 1 MHz) or the megahertz range (1 MHz $< f <$ 300 MHz). Microwaves (MWs), which are somewhat similar to RF waves in heating behavior, are in a still higher frequency range, between 300 MHz and 300 GHz. Both RF and MW are considered to be part of nonionizing radiation because they do not have sufficient energy (less than 10 eV) to ionize biologically important molecules or to break any chemical bonds.

Even though the majority of researchers found that microwave treatment destroys bacteria solely due to heat generated in the volume of the products, Gedye (1988, 1991) found that microwave reactions could produce different products than from reactions achieved using conventional techniques. According to Gedye, microwave heating does not alter the reaction but simply provides a much faster and more efficient (higher temperature) method of carrying out organic reactions. These effects were defined as *enhanced microwave effects*.

Heat can be generated as an intrinsic factor during application of some other physical treatment, such as pulsed electric field (PEF), high-pressure processing, and sonication and may contribute to the process lethality. The total effect of those treatments can be an enhanced or combined effect of a bactericidal action of the physical agent itself (pressure, electric field, cavitations) plus release of heat. As an example, pressurization of compressible substances such as food products during high-pressure treatment results in a temperature increase due to adiabatic heating (a process that happens without loss or gain of heat), which depends on food parameters and setup conditions. This temperature increase can be desirable or undesirable, depending on the food to be treated. In addition, the contribution of the temperature increase to inactivation kinetics should be defined properly and addressed in any process design and validation.

23.3 ESTABLISHMENT OF SPECIFICATIONS FOR PRESERVATION

For the design of a preservation specification of a thermal pasteurization or sterilization process, processing time F_p is traditionally defined by the initial load of resistant organisms (N_O), the endpoint of the process (N_F), and the logarithmic resistance of target bacteria under defined conditions (D_T):

$$Fp = D_T(\log N_O - \log N_F) = \text{SLR} \times D_T$$

Three approaches are used to define the treatment level or sterility assurance level (Heldman and Newsome, 2003). References are available for more in-depth discussion of the kinetics of microwave heating (Lin and Sawyer, 1988) and the lethal action of irradiation or exposure to irradiation (Farber, 2000).

23.4 TECHNOLOGIES BASED ON THERMAL EFFECTS

23.4.1 Heat Treatment

Thermal processing is the most frequently used treatment in pasteurization and sterilization as well as in combination with other physical agents, such as UV and ionizing radiation, ultrasound, and chemical and biological agents. Establishment of the traditional thermal process for foods has been based on two main factors: (1) knowledge of the thermal inactivation kinetics of the most heat-resistant pathogen of concern for each specific food product, and (2) determination of the nature of heat transfer properties of the food system. Thus, these two factors are well established for thermal processes and should be used for establishing and validating scheduled new thermal processes based on thermal effects.

23.4.2 Microwave and Radio-Frequency Heating of Foods

In addition to microbial inactivation by conventional methods of heating, microwave (MW) and radio-frequency (RF) heating are also considered to be heat-based processes that can inactivate microorganisms by thermal effects. MW and RF heating are attractive for heating of foods, due to their volumetric propagation (i.e., heat is generated within the product), fast temperature rise, and controllable heat deposition and easy cleanup.

Three types of electronic heating are commonly encountered: ohmic, dielectric (RF and MW), and induction microwave. Ohmic or electric-resistant heating relies on direct ohmic conduction losses in a medium and requires the electrodes to contact the medium directly. Ohmic heating gives direct heating because the product acts as an electrical resistor. The heat generated in the product is the loss in resistance. Since the heating effect depends on the eddy currents induced in the material, this type of heating works well with conductors.

In the various electronic heating methods, it is important to recognize the interaction between the electromagnetic field at the frequency in question and the material being subjected to the energy. Unlike conventional systems where heat energy is transferred from a hot medium to a cooler product and results in large temperature gradients, MW and RF heating involves the transfer of electromagnetic energy directly into the product by selective absorption and dissipation, initiating volumetric heating due to frictional interaction between molecules. MW and RF heating are accomplished as a combination of dipole rotation (i.e., when polar molecules try to align themselves in response to applied alternating electric field and interact with neighboring molecules, resulting in lattice and frictional losses as they rotate) and electric resistance heating resulting from movement of the dissolved ions.

MW and RF waves lie in the radar range and can interfere with communication systems; only selected frequencies are permitted for domestic, industrial, scientific, and medical applications. These frequencies are 13.56, 27.12, and 40.68 MHz (RF), and 915 MHz, 2450 MHz, 5.8 GHz, and 24.124 GHz (MW). Microwave energy is generated by special oscillator tubes, magnetrons, or klystrons and can be transmitted to an applicator or antenna through a waveguide or coaxial transmission line. The output of such tubes tends to be in a range from 0.5 to 100 kW. Microwaves are primarily guided radiation phenomenon, and they are able to radiate into a space, which could be the inside of the oven or cavity. Microwave ovens incorporate a waveguide to deliver MW energy to cook food in a cavity. In the microwave frequency range, the dielectric heating mechanism dominates up to moderated temperatures. The water content of the foods is an important factor for the microwave heating performance. For wet foods, the penetration depth from one side is approximately 1 to 2 cm at 2450 MHz. The physical basis of microwave technology has been described (Mechenova and Yakovlev, 2004)

RF heating is also known as high-frequency dielectric heating or capacitative dielectric heating (Piyasena et al., 2003). During RF heating, the product to be heated forms a dielectric between two capacitor plates, which are then charged alternately positive and negative by a high-frequency alternating electric field. Because RF uses longer wavelengths than MW, electromagnetic waves in the RF spectrum can penetrate deeper into the product so there is no surface overheating or hot or cold spots, a common problem with MW heating. RF heating also offers simple uniform field patterns as opposed to the complex nonuniform standing-wave patterns in a microwave oven. RF heating involves the heating of poor electrical conductors. It is also characterized by freedom from electrical and mechanical contact with the food. RF heating involves the application of a high-voltage alternating electric field to a food sandwiched between two parallel electrodes. Typically, RF heaters generate heat by means of an RF generator that produces oscillating fields of electromagnetic (EM) energy, and consists of a power supply and control circuitry, a hydraulic press and parallel plates, and a system for supporting processed material.

Commercial Applications Microwave heating has gained attention as an alternative to traditional pasteurization of liquid foods, such as milk, citrus, orange, and other juices. Higher product quality and extended shelf life can be achieved with microwave heating due to reduced processing times compared to conventional thermal processes. Microwave processing systems can be more energy efficient; the system can be turned on and off instantly so operation is easily controllable. It can be cleaned easily and there is no problem of product fouling on the surface of the equipment. Numerous studies document the effectiveness of microwave heating on pathogenic microorganisms (USFDA-CFSAN, 2000b). A range of potential pathogens and spoilage microorganisms and enzymes has been inactivated by microwave heating of food products (Ramaswamy et al., 2000). As an example, Nikdel et al. (1993) reported the complete inactivation of *Lactobacillus plantarum* and pectin methylesterase in orange juice without changing the taste by microwave heating in a continuous lab-scale pasteurizer. Microwave treatment is a mild and efficient way of providing milk with satisfactory microbial and sensory qualities without causing extensive heat damage (Lopez-Fandino et al., 1996).

Microwaves can rapidly provide the thermal energy required to eliminate *Salmonella* Enteritidis and drastically reduce the come-up time in existing pasteurization processes of in-shell eggs. Conventional pasteurization processing in a water bath for in-shell eggs can take more than 30 min. Microwave heating can significantly reduce pasteurization time and minimize quality deterioration (Rehkopf and Koutchma, 2005). Because of the larger penetration depth and more uniform heat, RF heating could be an attractive alternative to MW heating for processes involving pasteurization and sterilization of large and thick foods, due to such advantages as lower investment cost and easier temperature control. Early studies on RF pasteurization of meats were conducted in the 1950s. Pircon et al. (1953) described a process for sterilizing boned ham at 9 MHz using an industrial model of a 15-kW oscillator and reported that a 56.6% energy conversion efficiency was achieved and that 2.7 kg of meat could be heated to 80°C in about 10 min. Bengtsson et al. (1970) developed continuous RF pasteurization of cured hams packaged in Cryovac casings at 35 MHz. A conveyor fed the material between the electrodes of the load capacitor with a 1-kW output generator. For a 0.91-kg lean ham, the treatment time was reduced to one-third of its initial value by heating in a capacitor tunnel at 60 MHz to achieve a desired center temperature of 80°C. Houben et al. (1994) performed continuous RF pasteurization of coagulated-type sausage emulsion at 27 MHz using two power generators at 25 and 10 kW. In the final configuration, the time taken to bring the temperature of the sausage emulsion from 15°C to 80°C at a mass flow rate of 120 kg/h was about 2 min. A heating rate up to 40°C/min was achieved, compared to about 1°C/min at the center of a 50-mm-diameter sausage during conventional heating. It was concluded that RF heat treatments have a lethal effect on the test organism at least comparable to conventional hot-water treatments at the same pasteurization values F_p. MW and RF heating offer the potential for continuous pasteurization of solid foods that are more than a few centimeters thick. One important consideration in such processes is to provide uniform temperature distribution in the product. The development of temperature profiles in pasteurizing processes is less critical than for sterilizing processes, and temperature control can be determined by modeling the respective MW or RF application to optimize proper combinations of food and process parameters.

Modeling of MW and RF Systems Traditionally, industry has relied on the use of waveguides, stirrers, and turntables to achieve uniformity in the electromagnetic field within the MW cavity. These usually do not result in uniform temperature distribution within the product. Improving the design of MW systems by enhancing the design of the cavity in relation to food composition should lead to a better processing system. The modeling approach permits more even power distribution and improved process control. It will also greatly facilitate studies on the effects of heating parameters as influenced by applicator design and the size and shape of the food product. Recent progress in numerical methods, software development, and computer hardware has made possible advanced computer-aided design of MW systems. The finite-difference time-domain (FDTD) method has been recognized as a powerful technique for modeling of the electromagnetic component of MW heating processing (Yakovlev, 2001, 2004; Yakovlev and Celuch, 2003). Figure 2 demonstrates typical results of FDTD simulation of a microwave oven. The oven is excited by a rectangular waveguide (78 × 18 mm) and contains a glass shelf (of 6 mm thickness and 227 mm diameter located at 15 mm from the bottom) with a bread (dielectric permittivity $\varepsilon' = 4.17$,

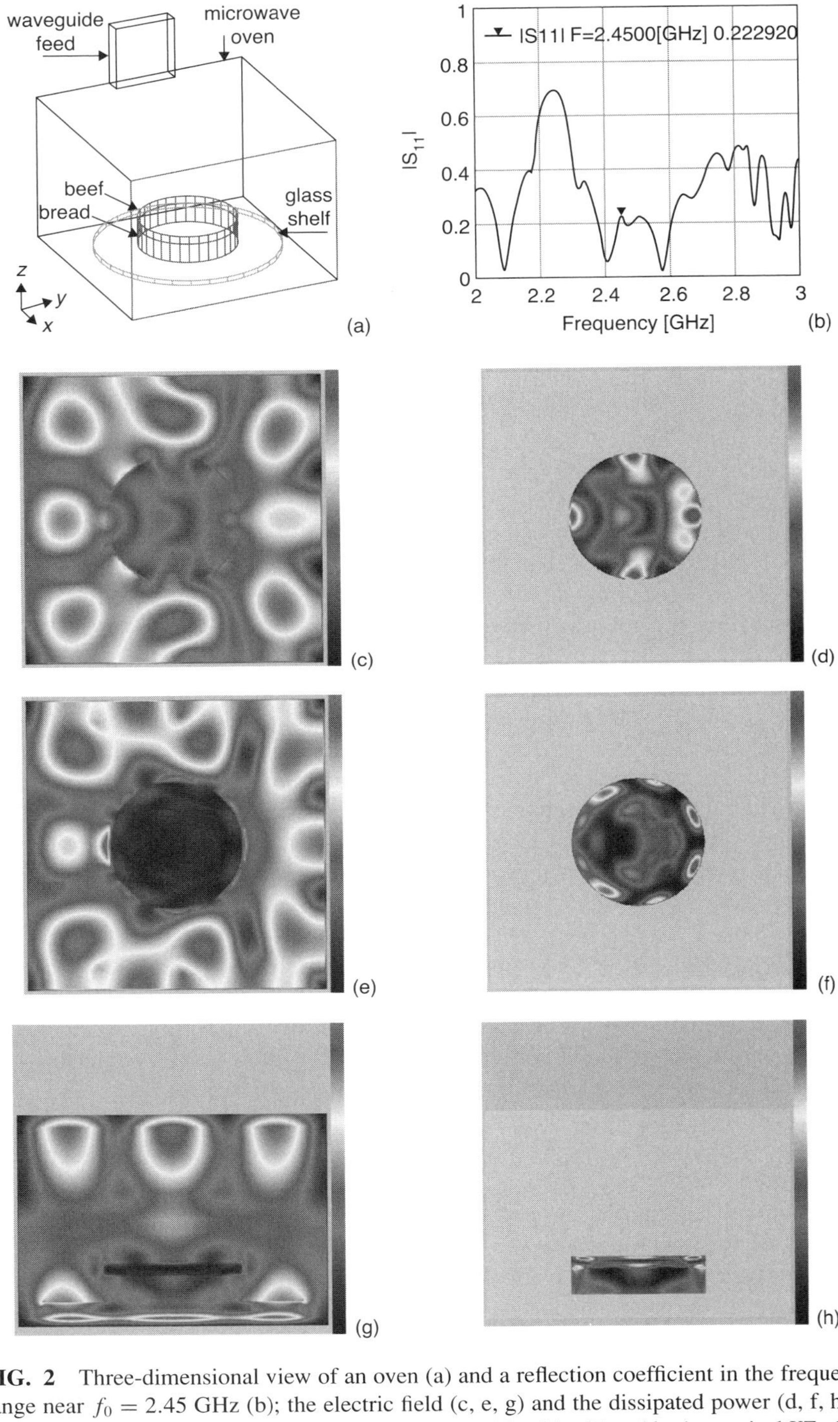

FIG. 2 Three-dimensional view of an oven (a) and a reflection coefficient in the frequency range near $f_0 = 2.45$ GHz (b); the electric field (c, e, g) and the dissipated power (d, f, h) in the horizontal XY-plane (c-f) [through bread (c, d) and beef (e, f)] and in the vertical YZ-plane (g, h) (through the center of the food load). (Courtesy of V. V. Yakovlev.)

loss factor $\varepsilon'' = 0.21$) and hamburger ($\varepsilon' = 48.2$, $\varepsilon'' = 2.19$) sandwich. The MW system is characterized by sufficiently high efficient coupling (about 95%). However, the food load is not heated uniformly: Both components are characterized by the hot spots on the edges, and more energy is released in the hamburger.

23.4.3 High-Pressure Processing

HPP has the potential to deliver a thermal equivalent of pasteurization or sterilization with reductions in process time, while ensuring the safety of the product without appreciable changes in color, flavor, and texture. The effects of high pressure are instantaneous throughout a food product and are independent of product composition, size, mass, or geometry. The inactivation mechanism of HPP proceeds through low energy and does not promote the formation of unwanted new chemical compounds as "radiolytic" by-products, or free radicals that can result when foods are irradiated. The effects of HPP on microboial food safety and quality have been summarized eloquently (Considine et al., 2008).

Food items, with or without packaging, can be subjected to pressures between 400 and 800 MPa. Pressurization of compressible substances like a food product results in a mild temperature increase related to pressure increase as shown in Fig. 3. Pressure (P), temperature (T), and time (t) are critical process parameters for establishing preservation process specification to effectively inactivate target pathogenic and spoilage bacteria. The process temperature range can be specified from 0°C to

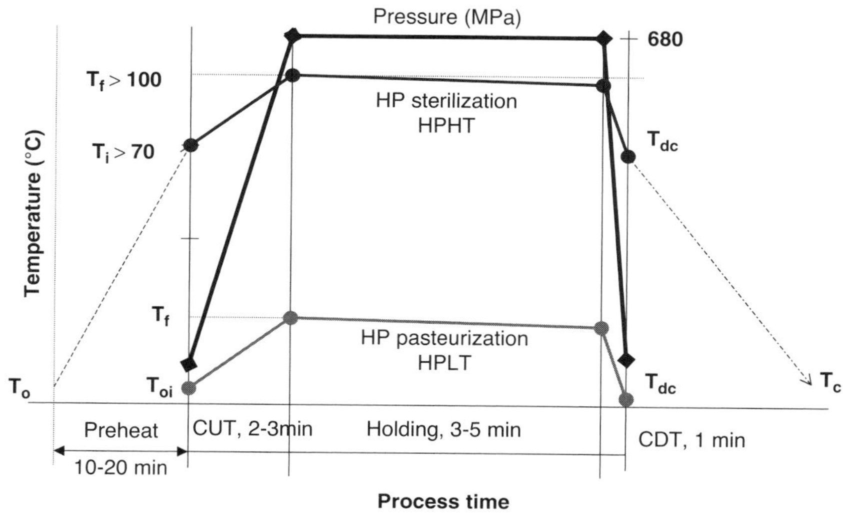

FIG. 3 High-pressure cycle of pasteurization and sterilization processes T_0, initial temperature of product before preheating; T_i, initial process temperature; T_f, process temperature; T_{dc}, temperature after decompression; T_c, temperature after cooling; T_{oi}, initial temperature after preheating; CUT, come-up time; CDT, come-down time.

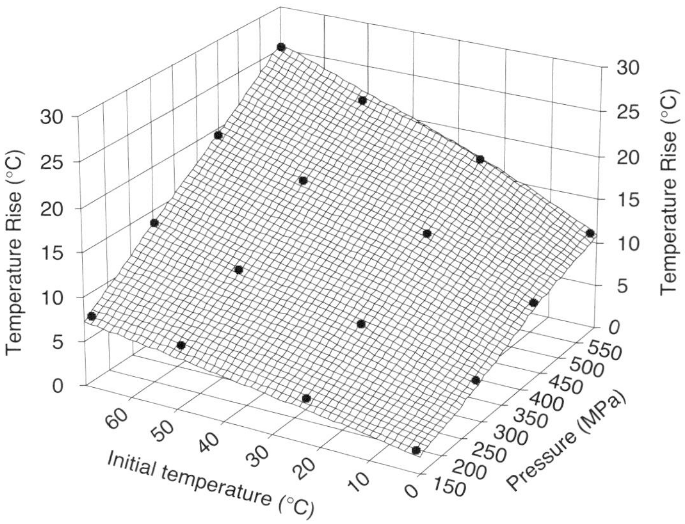

FIG. 4 Temperature increase in water as a function of pressure and initial temperature. (From Patazca et al., 2006.)

temperatures higher than 100°C. The extent of temperature rise depends on the pressure (P), initial temperature (T_0), thermal physical properties, and dimensions of the tested food. Figure 4 depicts temperature increase in the water associated with different pressure levels and initial temperatures. Heating of the product due to adiabatic compression depends on intrinsic factors, including heat capacity and compressibility of the foodstuff under consideration. Under the usual processing conditions of foods that have a high water content, a temperature increase of less than 20°C at a maximum pressure of 800 MPa can be expected. The initial temperature of the samples (T_i) before processing can be determined by subtracting the temperature increase attributed to the compression heating from the final process temperature desired. Preheating or precooling and temperature equilibration are important steps in HPP to achieve required process temperature. Immediately after pressure release, the product returns to its initial temperature. The fast cooling capacity of HHP is of most interest in the production of high-quality foods. Commercial exposure times can range from a 1-ms pulse to over 20 min.

Compression Heating Compression or decompression is an adiabatic isotropic process in which a food product undergoes a transient temperature increase or decrease, ΔT (°C), related to pressure increases or decreases, ΔP (Pa). Temperature increase is directly proportional to thermal expansivity and inversely proportional to the density and heat capacity of the product (Knorr and Heinz, 2001). Composition of food is another important factor that affects the magnitude of compression heating (CH). Water, carbohydrates, fats, and proteins are the main components of the complex food matrix that respond uniquely under compression. Bridgman (1931) studied the CH behavior of water extensively. Rasanayagam et al. (2003) reported values of compression heating of selected fatty foods and some model food materials during HPP. It appeared that water had the lowest CH, about 3°C per 100 MPa at $T = 25°C$, while fats had the highest CH values, up to 6.7 to 8°C per 100 MPa. Nevertheless, limited information is available on the CH of real foods with complex compositions. Patazca et al. (2007) studied the compression heating of selected food substances. Significant difference in compression heating behavior was observed in foods with a high oil or fat content, such as vegetable oil, cheese, and mayonnaise, and a high water content, such as milk, gravy, and eggs. Foods with a high water content experienced a temperature increase to pressure change similar to that of water (polar component), in the range of 3°C per 100 MPa (Fig. 5A). Another pattern of behavior under HP was found for the group of foods that have a significant proportions of nonpolar components, such as fats such as cheese, mayonnaise, and vegetable oil. The magnitude of CH decreased with the pressure for oil and mayonnaise and did not change significantly for cheese (Fig. 5B). Similarly, the CH of foods that are a rich source of proteins, such as meats (beef and chicken breast), did not deviate significantly from waterlike products.

High-Pressure Equipment The main components of high-pressure units are thick-walled vessels with sealed plugs and compression systems for pressure-transmitting fluids (e.g., H_2O). The volume contraction of water, which is the main constituent of most foodstuffs under isothermal compression up to 800 MPa at 20°C is about 17%. The design of the HP vessel, the type and temperature of the pressure medium, and the pressurization rate are the primarly factors that affect heat loss through the walls and also regulate the magnitude of the CH or cooling. The use of a heating element or insulation sleve placed inside a pressure chamber can compensate for the temperature loss throughout an HP vessel and may be necessary to achieve process uniformity.

The commercial Quintus 35-L Food Press (Avure Technologies, Kent, Washington) operates at pressures up to 700 MPa; temperatures can vary between 4 and 40°C. The processing cycle time can vary from 3 to 15 min, excluding load and unload time. The typical high-pressure processing cycle shown in Fig. 6 includes the following steps: (1) the packaged food items are placed in the pressure vessel; (2) the vessel is sealed and filled with water; (3) a pump forces more water into the vessel, to creat hydrostatic pressure (pressure is transmitted isostatically by the fluid medium); (4) the vessel pressure is maintained for a predetermined period of holding time; (5) when the cycle is completed, the vessel is quickly depressurized, and temperatures return to the starting temperature; and (6) the HP vessel is opened and product is removed.

The 35-L HP unit Quintus QFP 35-L S Press, designed for sterilization, operates at pressures up to 690 MPa and temperatures up to 130°C. The system was designed and built in the Avure Vasteras plant in Sweden. The system has multiple subsystems, including a preheating tank, a cooling tank, a wirewound vessel, a low-pressure fill system, a high-pressure pump, and a control system. The temperature-controlled

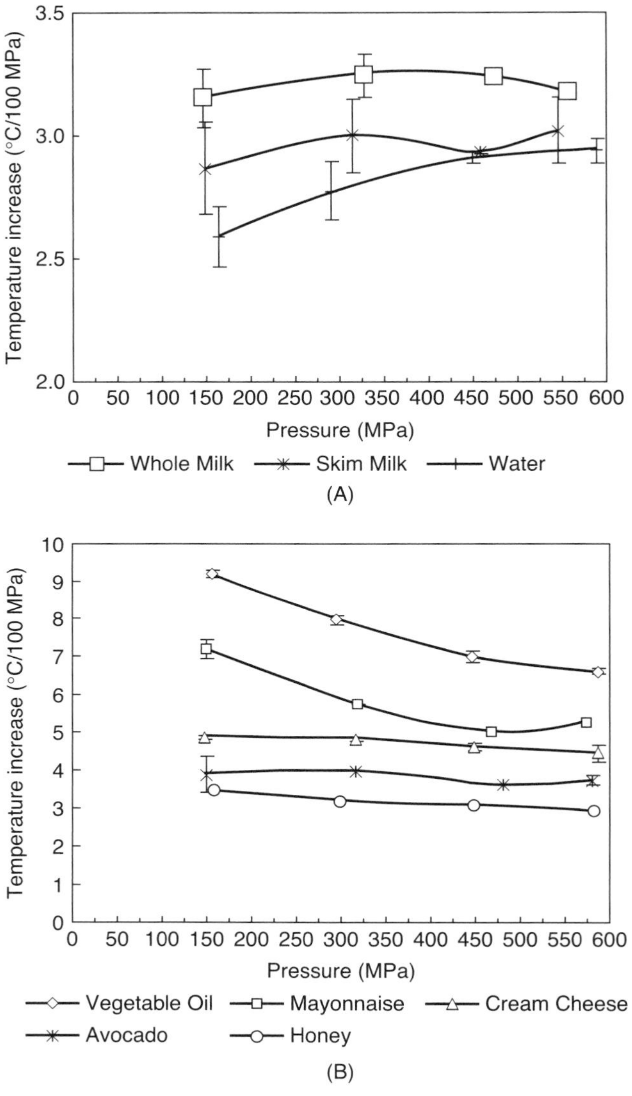

FIG. 5 Adiabatic heat of compression of selected foods.

preheating tank is used to maintain the minimum initial temperature of the product. The cooling tank has a refrigeration system for cooling the water to the desired temperature. Rapid cooling maintains product quality by minimizing detrimental chemical reactions.

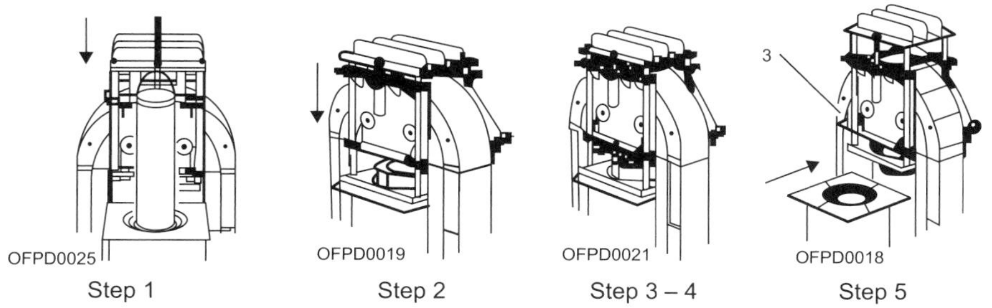

FIG. 6 Vessel close and open sequences. (Courtesy of Avure Technologies, Kent, WA.)

Commercial Applications: High-Pressure Pasteurization The beneficial effects of HPP on the sensorial characteristics of foods is of special interest to food processors. Since 1990, a variety of pressure-treated fruit juices, toppings, jams, and tenderized meats have been sold in Japan. In 1997, sliced cooked ham became available in Spain. HPP's capacity to increase the shelf life of guacamole, chicken products, and cold cuts and to ensure safer seafood (oysters) has been demonstrated and accepted by the retail market in the United States (Table 1). HP technology has a great potential to deliver new and improved products: to provide extended-shelf-life ready-to-eat meats; to extend the shelf-life of minimally processed foods; to implement mild processing of some potentially hazardous foods; to accelerate enzymatic processes; and to create products with unique textures by pressure-induced gelation and denaturating of proteins. The USDA has approved HPP as a post-packaging lethality treatment for *Listeria* in prepackaged ready-to-eat meat products.

TABLE 1 Commercially Available HP-Treated ESL Foods in the United States

Category of Product	Company	Product/Brand
Ready-to-eat meat products	Hormel	Parma Brand prosciutto ham
	Perdue	Shortcuts, carved chicken breasts
Ready-to-eat meals	Avomex	Menu-fresh meat kits
Seafood	Avotec	Ceviche salad
	Motivatit Oyster	Oysters
Beverages	Avomex	Solo Frutta carrot and apple fruit purees
	Orchand House	Seriously fresh juices and seriously smooth smoothies
Value-added fruits and vegetables	Avomex	Salsa, guacamoles
	Winsoms of Walla Walla	Chopped onions

Source: Adapted from Considine et al. (2008).

The post-lethality treatment is applied to the final product or sealed package to eliminate *Listeria* resulting from contamination from post-lethality exposure.

High-Pressure Sterilization Spore inactivation is important for the safety of shelf-stable, low-acid foods (e.g., ready-to-eat meals, dairy-based sauces, vegetables), and in particular, it is essential to inactivate *Clostridium botulinum* spores, the bacterium that causes botulism. HP technology holds promise for the sterilization of low-acid foods. However, heat combined with HPP is required for effective destruction of bacterial spores. Establishment of process criteria for HP sterilization processes requires optimization of process temperature and pressure to inactivate target pathogenic and spoilage spore-forming bacteria based on knowledge of food behavior under pressure.

The concept of defining the thermal process specification by describing the outcome or "endpoint of a preservation process" as the probability of nonsterile unit (PNSU), introduced by Pflug and Zeghman (1985), and can be adapted for determining the F_O-value for the high-pressure, high-temperature sterilization of foods. A spoilage failure rate of 10^{-6} was selected for mesophilic spores represented by *Clostridium sporogenes* PA3679 and 10^{-3} for the thermophilic spores. *Geobacillus stearothermophillus* is the critical species of nonpathogenic thermophilic bacteria that is traditionally used in establishing thermal process specification. Patazca et al. (2006) and Koutchma et al. (2005a) demonstrated that log-linear models are suitable to predict the microbial inactivation of both classical surrogates used in thermal processing, such as *G. stearothermophilus* and *C. sporogenes* PA3679. The linear relationships or thermal resistance curves are presented graphically for both spore-forming species in Figs. 7 and 8. The F_O-values shown were calculated for a of 7-log reduction for PA 3679 spores and a 5-log reduction for *G. stearothermophilus* spores based on the assumption of Pflug and Zeghman (1985). The calculations showed that a delivered process of 3.2 min at 121°C at pressures of 600 or 700 MPa or 1.5 min at 800 MPa and 121°C will be adequate to prevent spoilage by mesophilic and thermophilic spore-forming organisms using HP-HT process. When HP-HT sterilization process is compared with the 27 min of heat sterilization that would be required in order to achieve commercial sterility in terms of spoilage spore-formers, it is apparent that the length of the HP-HT process is drastically reduced. According to the *D*-value differences between HP-HT and classic thermal sterilization, combining temperature with pressure reduces the process times. Nevertheless, the design of HP-HT processes to make foods safe from a public health point of view requires knowledge of *D*-values of *C. botulinum* spores at similar high-pressure conditions.

23.5 TECHNOLOGIES BASED ON NONTHERMAL EFFECTS

23.5.1 Irradiation

Food irradiation has proven to be a safe and effective process for increasing food safety and extending product shelf life (O'Bryan et al., 2008). Nearly 50 countries have

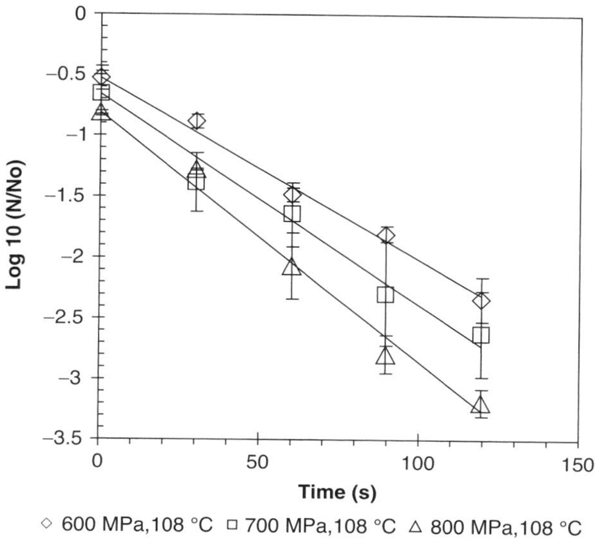

FIG. 7 Survivors' curves of *C. sporogenes* PA 3679 spores at 600, 700, and 800 MPa and 108°C process temperature. (From Koutchma et al., 2005.)

approved or allow food irradiation, although the foods and doses differ by country. In the United States, all fruits and vegetables, poultry, red meat, and spices/seasonings are approved for irradiation at specified maximum dose levels (USFDA-CFSAN 2000a). There are petitions under review by the FDA for irradiation treatment of

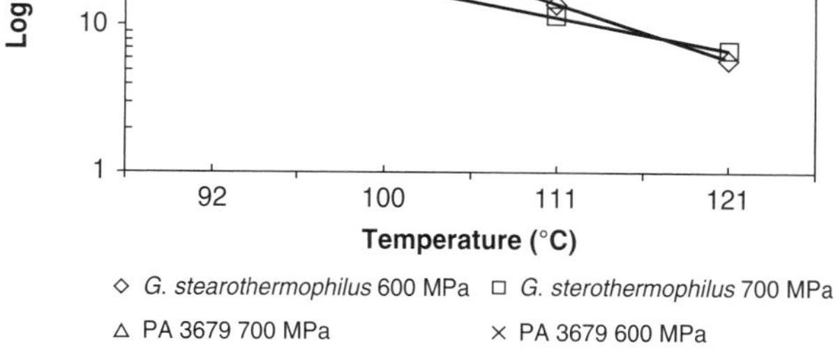

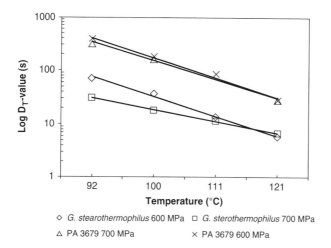

FIG. 8 Thermal resistance curves of *C. sporogenes* PA 3679 and *G. stearothermophillus* spores at 600 and 700 MPa. (From Koutchma et al., 2005; Patazca et al., 2006.)

TABLE 2 Comparison of Typical Radiation Processing Parameters

	Gamma	X-Ray	E-Beam
Typical power source	3.5 MCi[a]	25 kW	35 kW
Processing speed at 4 kGy (tons/h)	12	10	10
Source energy (MeV)	1.33	5	5–10
Penetration depth (cm)	80–100	80–100	8–10
Dose homogeneity	High	High	Moderate
Dose rate (kGy/h)	Low	High	Higher
Best application	Bulk processing of large boxes; palletized product in shipping cartons	Bulk processing of large boxes; palletized product in shipping cartons	Primary packaged products in-line

[a]1 MCi ≈ 15 kW of power.

processed meats (hot dogs, deli meat), processed vegetables (including fruit juices), molluskan shellfish, and crustaceans.

Irradiation can be accomplished with three available technologies: gamma-ray processing, x- ray, and high-energy electrons, also known as electron-beam or E-beam processing. The FDA has approved the use of gamma rays from decaying isotopes of cobalt-60 or cesium-137, x-rays with a maximum energy of 5 million electron volts (MeV), and electrons with a maximum energy of 10 MeV. Comparison of the radiation technologies, which involves examination of the radiation dose yield, dose rate, related biological effects, and post-irradiation storage and radiolytic effects, can be helpful for understanding their performance. Three typical radiation parameters are compared in Table 2.

Factors Affecting Irradiation Inactivation High-energy electrons and gamma and x-rays can kill or inactivate bacteria, fungi, and insects by breaking molecular bonds in the microbial DNA. It has been suggested that there are differences in the effects of these technologies on microbial inactivation due to the differences in free-radical formation, but the comparison was inconclusive, due to differences in doses used. Lethality of irradiation depends on the target microorganism, the condition of the treated item, and environmental factors. Addition or removal of salt or water, time and temperature of the treatment, and the presence of oxygen are factors that will influence the antimicrobial effect of irradiation.

Two processes have been used to define the extent of pathogen reduction by irradiation. Radiation pasteurization refers to the destruction of pathogenic non-spore-forming foodborne bacteria with a medium dose requirement of 1 to 10 kGy to reduce the microbial population, including pathogens of concern. Sterilization irradiation is used for radiation processes that will render the food commercially sterile or for foods that are both sterile and shelf stable. In this case, sterilization must ensure elimination of the most resistant pathogen (spores of *C. botulinum*). To achieve

TABLE 3 Current Applications of Irradiation for Foods

Benefit	Dose (kGy)	Products
	Low Dose (Up to 1 kGy)	
Inhibition of sprouting	0.05–0.15	Potatoes, onions, garlic, root ginger, yams
Insect disinfestation and parasite disinfection	0.15–0.5	Fresh and dried fruits, dried fish, and meat, fresh pork
Delay of physiological processes (e.g., ripening)	0.25–1.0	Fresh fruits and vegetables
	Medium Dose (1 –10 kGy)	
Extension of shelf life	1.0–3.0	Fresh fish, strawberries, mushrooms
Elimination of spoilage and pathogenic microorganisms	1.0–7.0	Fresh and frozen seafood, raw or frozen poultry and meat, in-shell eggs
Improving technological properties of food	2.0–7.0	Grapes (increasing juice yield), dehydrated vegetables (reducing cooking time)
	High Dose (10–15 kGy)	
Industrial sterilization (in combination with mild heat)	30–50	Meat, poultry, seafood, prepared foods, sterilized hospital diets, frozen meats for astronauts
Decontamination of certain food additives and ingredients	10–50	Spices, enzyme preparations, natural gum

this, doses up to 50 kGy, higher then those currently permitted for commercial foods (up to 10kGy), are needed.

Ionizing radiation is used as a means of extending the shelf life of produce. A summary of current applications of irradiation for foods is given in Table 3. However, foods currently allowed to be irradiated are very limited. As with other technologies, organoleptic changes in the food need to be considered.

Dosimetry For elimination of selected pathogens, establishment of critical limits for preservation by food irradiation can be accomplished on the basis of D_{10}-values reported in the literature for various types of foods. The effectiveness of the technology needs to be validated for the specific applications. Process control monitoring in food irradiation is well known. The standard dosimetry techniques are now sufficiently established to provide one of the most reliable means of quality control. Post-irradiation dosimetry is a part of the validation process and is necessary in order to find optimal irradiation conditions and to know about radiolytic effects in foods.

Analytical techniques for the identification of irradiated foods are well developed and based on irradiation-mediated chemical, physical, or biological changes in the foods.

Low-Energy Pulsed Electron-Beam Irradiation Food irradiation by high-energy electrons with energy up to 5 MeV has proven to be a safe and effective process for increasing food safety and extending product shelf life. The kinetic energy for low-energy electron beams or "soft electrons" is less than 300 keV. Low-energy electrons have a depth of penetration into food products of a few hundred micrometers. This type of radiation treatment can be considered as a surface treatment. Biological effects of low-energy electron-pulsed electron beams are less studied.

To evaluate the effect of pulsed low-energy electron irradiation, *E. coli* bacteria and *B. pumilus* spores were exposed to low-energy electron beams on the surfaces of filters. *B. pumilus*, a producer of radioduric spores, and *E. coli* K12 (ATCC 25253) were selected as test specimens. Irradiation experiments were carried out with a culture at initial inoculation levels of 5 and 3 log CFU. The number of pulses varied from 1 to 20 for *E. coli* and was increased to 50 and 100 pulses for *B. pumilus* spores. For each exposure, two filters were used in a layered structure: film dosimeter/inoculated filter/Lexan plastic/dosimeter/inoculated filter.

The effect of the number of pulses of electron-beam irradiation on *E. coli* and *B. pumilus* is illustrated in Fig. 9. A significant reduction of *E. coli* was found after exposure to three pulses or 0.9 kGy. Complete inactivation of *E. coli* at an initial concentration of 10^3 CFU was observed on the surface of both filters after 15 pulses or exposure to 4.5 kGy. To inactivate 10^3 spores of *B. pumilus,* more than 50 pulses or 15 kGy were needed. The frequency of 25 Hz was the most effective in destroying *E. coli* and *B. pumilus* spores. Data presented here demonstrate that pulsed low-energy electron-beam irradiation of 150 keV inactivated *E. coli* bacteria and *B. pumilus* spores on filter surfaces in the layered structure. Under the conditions of this study, electron-beam treatment was more effective at reducing *E. coli* than at reducing *B. pumilus* spores, and high pulse frequencies resulted in higher kill rates.

Use of soft electrons can supplement food irradiation technology by opening a door to novel sanitary treatments. Low-dose electrons can be used as alternatives

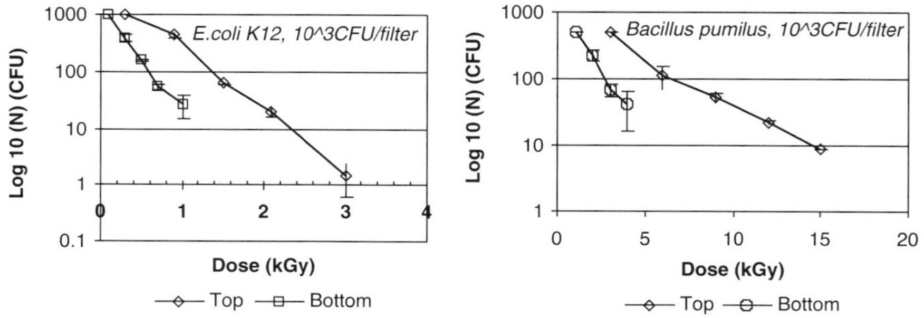

FIG. 9 Effect of the number of electron-beam pulses (1 pulse = 0.3 kGy) on survival of *E. coli* and *B. pumilus* spores.

to steam or chemicals for elimination of microorganisms on the surface of grains, dehydrated vegetables, spices, and tea leaves, with little quality loss. This can include the heat-resistant bacterial spores that frequently contaminate the surface of dry food ingredients.

Continuous UV Light Ultraviolet light processing is a nonthermal method for eliminating or reducing the levels of undesirable microorganisms in foods and beverages. Among the well-known nonthermal processing technologies, UV treatment is one of the least exploited methods of treatment. Compared to heat pasteurization, UV treatment may have the added benefits of retention of product quality, simplicity of operation, and lower operating costs. UV light is the term given to the portion of the electromagnetic spectrum between visible light and x-rays, in the region between 100 and 380 nm. UV wavelengths in the vicinity of 260 nm are the most effective for inactivating microorganisms, mainly by damaging DNA, as they coincide closely to the peak of DNA absorptivity.

A number of commercially produced sources emit energy in the UV range. These include mercury vapor, metal halide, antimony, and xenon sources. Low-pressure mercury sources are highly efficient in inactivating microbial cells and have a number of other advantages; they emit most of their UV energy at 253.7 nm, are relatively inexpensive, have reasonably long service lives (thousands of hours), and can run at a low surface temperature of 60°C. The longer wavelength (UVA) is generated from medium-pressure mercury lamps.

In pulse UV treatment, which has received less attention, pulses of microsecond duration with very high intensity and wide-spectrum wavelengths are usually applied. The literature indicates that lower doses may be required with pulsed UV compared to continuous UV. The pulse UV technology is developed for surface treatment of solid foods; however, future applications in the treatment of juices and other liquid foods are possible.

The FDA approved UV light as an alternative to thermal pasteurization of fresh juice products (USFDA-CFSAN, 2000b). The performance criterion defined by the FDA for fruit and vegetable juice processing is a 5-log reduction in the number of target pathogens of concern. The exposure of microorganisms to UV light or residence time in the UV reactor should be sufficient to achieve target pathogen inactivation. The effects of physical and optical properties of juice such as absorptivity and turbidity, viscosity, and density on the UV treatment must be considered in UV process design. UV light has very little transmission through fresh juice products, due to the presence of colored compounds, organic solutes, or suspended matter, and this alters the performance efficiency of the UV pasteurization process. In addition, the combination of physical variables such as fluid density, viscosity, and velocity, reactor design, and dimensions need to be considered to meet the required performance standard.

Absorptive and Physical Properties of Liquid Foods The Beer–Lambert law defines the UV absorption effects of liquids by incorporating an absorption coefficient: the absorbance divided by the path length. As evident from Fig. 10, UV absorptivity of fresh juices varies considerably. Lillikoi juice had the least

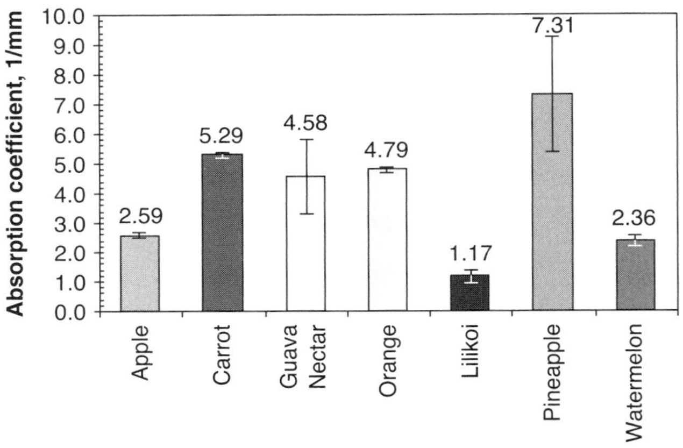

FIG. 10 Absorption coefficient of fruit and vegetable juices. (From Koutchma et al., 2005.)

absorptivity, with an absorption coefficient from 1.1 mm^{-1} followed by watermelon and apple juice (Koutchma et al., 2005b) . Orange and guava juices had somewhat similar absorbencies of 4.6 to 4.8 mm^{-1}, whereas carrot and pineapple juices were almost opaque blends of juices containing particulate, pulpy materials. Turbidity of juices due to the presence of suspended solids was in the range from 1000 NTU for apple and lillikoi juices to 4000+ NTU for guava, carrot, orange, and pineapple juices. The effect of suspended particles on turbidity and absorption coefficient of caramel model solutions was reported by Koutchma and Parisi (2004). An apparent increase in absorbance due to light scattering by particles was observed. The juices studied also represent different °Brix and pH levels with varying viscosities (Fig. 11). Lillikoi and apple juice represented less viscous, high-acidity products. Watermelon and guava juice are less acidic and have viscosities typical of Newtonian liquids.

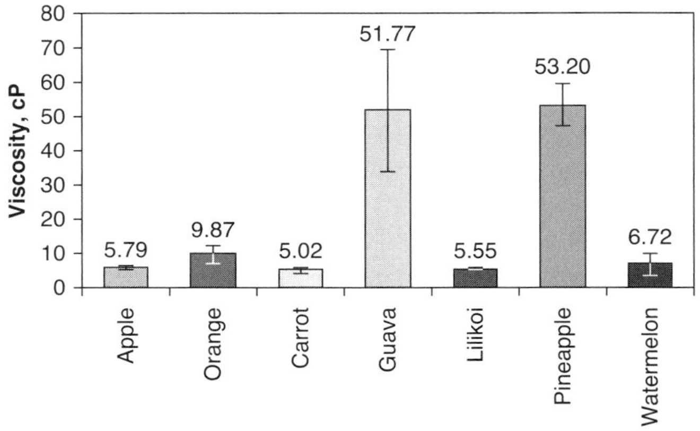

FIG. 11 Viscosity of fruit and vegetable juices. (From Koutchma et al., 2005.)

The distinguishing characteristics of pineapple and orange juices were their high acidity and viscosities: more than 10 times greater than the viscosities of apple and watermelon juices typical of non-Newtonian liquids.

Reactors Used for UV Treatment of Liquid Foods Different types of reactors can be used for UV treatment of liquid foods. However, the correct choice of UV reactor design can reduce the interference of high UV absorptivity and turbidity associated with fresh juices and ciders and improve inactivation efficiency. The flow pattern inside a UV reactor strongly influences the summed dose since the position and residence time of the microorganisms in certain regions of the irradiation field can vary significantly. Another reason for establishing flow characteristics is to obtain an indication of the mixing behavior of the fluid and how it can affect inactivation.

Currently, continuous-flow UV rectors are being evaluated for use in fresh juice pasteurization. The first approach uses an extremely thin film UV reactor to decrease the path length and thus avoid problems associated with lack of penetration. Thin-film reactors are characterized by laminar flow with a parabolic velocity profile. Maximum velocity of the liquid is observed in the center, and this velocity is twice as fast as the average velocity of the liquid and results in nonuniform processing conditions (Koutchma and Parisi, 2004). The two laminar flow designs shown in Fig. 12 are a thin-film CiderSure UV reactor (FPE Inc., Macedon, New York) and a Taylor–Couette flow reactor (Forney et al., 2004). In the CiderSure unit (Fig. 12A), low-pressure mercury arc lamps are mounted within a quartz sleeve running centrally through the reactor. Apple juice or cider is pumped from a reservoir through a 0.08-cm annular gap between the inner surface of the chamber and the outer surface of the quartz sleeve. Forney et al. (2004) developed a UV reactor that pumps fluid through

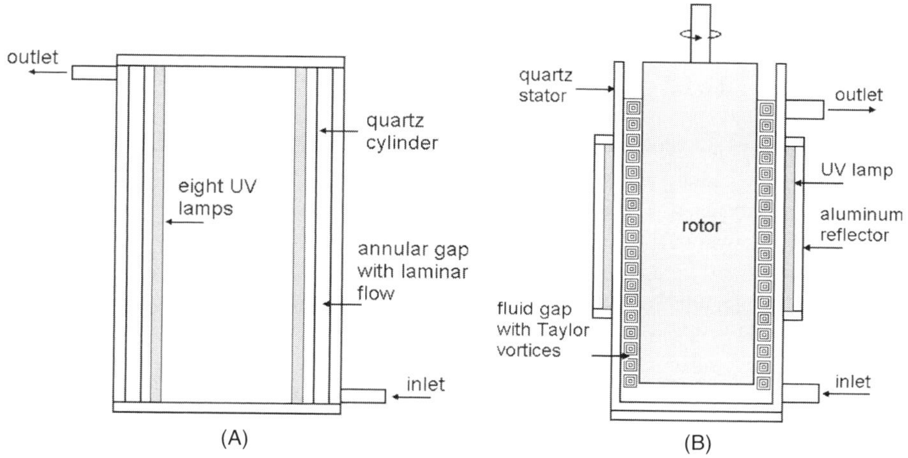

FIG. 12 (A) laminar thin-film reactor (Cider Sure); (B) laminar Taylor–Couette UV reactor. (From Koutchma et al., 2004; Forney et al., 2004.)

the annular gap between two concentric cylinders (Fig. 12B) to provide sufficient exposure and to reduce the fluid boundary layer thickness next to the radiation source contained within the outer stationary cylinder. The smaller inner cylinder consists of laminar vortices that both fill the annular gap of several millimeters and circumscribe the inner cylinder.

The second approach is to increase the turbulence within a UV reactor to bring all material into close proximity with UV light during treatment. The higher flow rates achieved under turbulent conditions improve the homogeneity of the flow when the fastest-flowing particle travels 1.1 to 1.2 times faster than the volume-averaged particle, and each volume of the product will be exposed to UV light due to better mixing.

The current 21 CFR 179 (USFDA-CFSAN, 2000b) food additive regulation stipulates the use of turbulent flow for UV-light reactors used to treat fresh juices. The presence of dead spaces in the reactor may affect the average residence time of the fluid in the reactor and require tracer analysis to measure the residence-time distribution. A desirable design for UV reactors is pure plug flow, which indicates that every element of liquid resides in the reactor for the same time period and that all microorganisms would receive an equivalent UV dose if the UV irradiance were equal at all points. However, it is important to recognize that treatment of some high-viscosity fluids, such as sucrose or fluids with pulp such as orange juice, will be incompatible with some reactor designs.

Process Behavior Commercial UV reactors are flow-through systems which have a distribution of exposure time (RTD) and light irradiance distribution (LID) due to attenuation following the Beer–Lambert law. Consequently, there is a variation in UV doses (a product of LID and RTD) to which any given microorganism is exposed, and this can alter the performance of the reactor. The delivery of a UV dose within a reactor at full scale is one of the challenges to achieving a 5-log reduction in numbers of the most resistant pathogens in fresh juices. For the UV pasteurization process, this indicates that detailed knowledge of microbial UV inactivation and complete representation of radiation irradiance and velocity fields are required in the development of the UV process.

Measurement of Absorbed UV Dose Although currently, no practical method is available for measuring the dose distribution delivered by a UV reactor, biodosimetry is commonly used. Biodosimetry/bioassay is a biological approach in which the relationship between UV dose and log survival of the target bacteria is developed using a collimated beam, low-pressure, static UV system. *E. coli* K12 can be used as a target bacterium for biodosimetry in juice products since it is a surrogate of *E. coli* O157:H7. UV irradiance on the surface of the object can be determined using a calibrated radiometer, and used for UV dose calculations. Then the count of surviving target bacteria in a UV reactor is determined, and the effective germicidal dose is back-calculated knowing the decimal reduction (D_{10}) dose, which is obtained from the dose–response curve constructed using a collimated beam UV system. The dose value measured is termed the reduction equivalent dose (RED). The RED value lies between the minimum and average doses. The drawbacks of this method are that the results are presented as the most probable results associated with the confidence interval of microorganism enumeration (Linden and Darby, 1998). Higher dose–response observations can be obtained with the collimated beam apparatus than with a flow-through reactor. Only when all microorganisms receive the same dose (an ideal reactor) would a correct dose measurement result from biodosimetry. If a dose distribution occurs among the microorganisms, biodosimetry gave a volume average decimal reduction dose lower than the arithmetic mean of the dose distribution.

Although UV treatment has received less attention than other nonthermal processing methods, there is considerable evidence in the literature of the success of this method in reducing most types of microorganisms.

23.6 CONCLUSIONS

New high-technology approaches have a great potential for realizing a breakthrough in improving food safety and extending products shelf life without appreciable changes in quality and with excellent sensory and nutritional benefits. Recent advances in the science and engineering of microwave and radio-frequency heating, high-pressure treatment, and ionizing and ultraviolet light irradiation make them a feasible option for commercialization in the sterilization and pasteurization of foods, in addition to traditional thermal processing.

REFERENCES

Bengtsson NE, Green W, Vaue F (1970): Radio-frequency pasteurization of cured hams. *J Food Sci*. 35:681–687.

Bridgman PW (1931): The Physics of High Pressure. G. Bells & Sons, London.

Considine KM, Kelly AL, Fitzgerald GF, Hill C, Sleator RD (2008): High pressure processing: effects on microbial food safety and food quality. *FEMS Microbiol Lett*. 281:1–9.

Farber J (2000): Health Risk Assessment: Qualitative risk assessment unpasteurized fruit juice/cider. Food Directorate, Health Protection Branch, Health Canada, Ottawa, Ontario, Canada.

Forney LJ, Pierson JA, Ye Z (2004): Juice irradiation with Taylor–Couette flow: UV inactivation of *Escherichia coli*. *J Food Prot*. 67:2410–2415.

Gedye RN, Smith FE, Westaway KC (1988): The rapid synthesis of organic compounds in microwave ovens. *Can J Chem*. 66:17–26.

——— (1991): Microwaves in organic and organometallic synthesis. *Microwave Power Electromagn Energy*. 26:3–17.

Heldman D, Newsome R (2003): Kinetics models for microbial survival during processing. *Food Technol*. 57:40–48.

Houben J, van Roon P, Krol B (1994): Continuous radio-frequency pasteurization in sausage manufacturing lines. *Fleischewirtsch Int*. 2:35–36.

Knorr D, Heinz V (2001): Development of nonthermal methods for microbial control. In: Block SS (Ed.) *Disinfection, Sterilization, and Preservation,* 5th ed. Lippincott Williams & Wilkins, Philadephia, pp. 853–881.

Koutchma T, Parisi B (2004): Biodosimetry of *E. coli* UV inactivation in model juices with regard to dose distribution in annular UV reactor. *J Food Sci*. 69:14–22.

Koutchma T, Keller S, Chirtel S, Parisi B (2004): Ultraviolet disinfection of juice products in laminar and turbulent flow reactors. *Int Food Sci Emerg Technol*. 5:179–189.

Koutchma T, Guo B, Patazca E, Parisi B (2005a): High pressure–high temperature sterilization: from kinetic analysis to process verification. *J Food Process Eng*. 28:610–629.

Koutchma T, Parisi B, Patazca E (2005b): Validation of UV coiled tube reactor for fresh fruit juices. In *Proc. 3rd International UV World Congress*, Whistler, Canada, May 24–27.

Lin W, Sawyer C (1988): Bacterial survival and thermal responses of beef load after microwave processing. *Microwave Power Electromagn Energy*. 23:183–194.

Linden KG, Darby JL (1998): UV disinfection of marginal effluents: determining UV absorbance and subsequent estimation of UV intensity. *Water Environ Res*. 70:214–223.

Lopez-Fandino R, Villamiel M, Corzo N, Olano A (1996): Assessment of the thermal treatment of milk during continuous microwave and conventional heating. *J Food Prot*. 59:889–892.

Mechenova VA, Yakovlev VV (2004): Efficiency optimization for systems and components in microwave power engineering. *Microwave Power Electromagn Energy*. 39:15–29.

Nikdel S, Chen C, Parish M, MacKellar D, Friedrich L (1993): Pasteurization of citrus juice with microwave energy in a continuous-flow unit. *J Agric Food Chem*. 41:2116–2119.

O'Bryan CA, Crandall PG, Ricke SC, Olson DG (2008): Impact of irradiation on the safety and quality of poultry and meat products: a review. *Crit Rev Food Sci Nutr*. 48:442–457.

Patazca E, Koutchma T, Ramaswamy HS (2006): Inactivation kinetics of *Geobacillus stearothermophilus* spores in water using high-pressure processing at elevated temperatures. *J Food Sci*. 71:M110–M116.

Patazca E, Balasubramaniam VM, Ramaswamy HS, Koutchma T (2007): Quasi-adiabatic temperature increase during high pressure processing of selected foods. *J Food Eng*. 8:199–205.

Pflug IJ, Zeghman LG (1985): Microbial death kinetics in the heat processing of food: determining an *F*-value. In *Proc. Aseptic Processing and Packaging of Foods*, Tylosand, Sweden, September 9–12, pp. 211–220.

Pircon LJ, Loquercio P, Doty DM (1953): High-frequency heating as a unit operation in meat processing. *Agric Food Chem*. 1:844–847.

Piyasena P, Dussault C, Koutchma T, Ramaswamy HS, Awuah GB (2003): Radio frequency heating of foods: principles, applications and related properties—a review. *Crit Rev Food Sci Nutr*. 43:587–606.

Ramaswamy HS, Koutchma T, Tajchakavit S (2000): Enhanced thermal effects under microwave heating conditions. In *Proc. International Congress on Engineering and Food*, ICEF 8, Mexico DF, April 6–12.

Rasanayagam V, Balasubramaniam VM, Ting E, Sizer CE, Bush C, Anderson C (2003): Compression heating of selected fatty food materials during high-pressure processing. *J Food Sci*. 68:254–259.

Rehkopf A, Koutchma T (2005): Quality validation of a microwave-pasteurization process for shell-eggs. In *Proc. Institute of Food Technologists Annual Meeting*, New Orleans, LA, July 15–20.

Risman P (1996): Guest editorial. *Microwave Power Electromagn Energy*. 31:69–70.

Stuerga DAC, Gaillard P (1996): Microwave athermal effects in chemistry: a myth's autopsy. *Microwave Power Electromagn Energy*. 31:87–113.

Sugarman C (2004): Pasteurization redefined by USDA committee. *Food Chem News*. 46:21.

USFDA-CFSAN (U.S. Food and Drug Administration–Center for Food Safety and Applied Nutrition) (2000a): 21CFR179 Irradiation in the production, processing and handling of food. http://www.cfsan.fda.gov/~lrd/FCF179.html. Accessed June 2008.

——— (2000b): Kinetics of microbial inactivation for alternative food processing technologies: microwave and radio frequency processing. http://www.cfsan.fda.gov/~comm/ift-toc.html. Accessed June 2008.

Yakovlev VV (2001): Commercial EM codes suitable for modeling of microwave heating: a comparative review. In: van Reinen U, Günther M, Hecht D (Eds.). *Scientific Computing in Electrical Engineering*, Vol. 18. Springer-Verlag, Dordrecht, the Netherlands, pp. 87–96.

——— (2004): Examination of contemporary electromagnetic software capable of modeling problems of microwave heating. In: Willert-Porada M (Ed.). *Advances in Microwave and Radio Frequency Processing*. Springer-Verlag, Dordrecht, the Netherlands, pp. 178–190.

Yakovlev VV, Celuch M (2003): Computer modeling and microwave power industry. Short course, Industrial Microwave Modeling Group. http://www.wpi.edu/Academics/Depts/Math/CIMS/IMMG/seminar5.html. Accessed June 2008.

CHAPTER 24

FOOD PRESERVATION TECHNIQUES OTHER THAN HEAT AND IRRADIATION

RONALD LABBÉ and LINDA L. NOLAN

24.1 INTRODUCTION

Preservation of food is a centuries-old objective. In this chapter we discuss physical and chemical methods of food preservation and give examples of each. Also given are examples of the more recent use of biological preservatives as well as the growing application of hurdle technology, a concept that promises to reduce the use of chemical and physical treatments needed for food protection.

24.2 TRADITIONAL PHYSICAL METHODS OF FOOD PRESERVATION

24.2.1 Water Activity

Long ago, the need to preserve foods during nongrowing seasons led to preservation by drying. Although this presumably originated with vegetable crops, protein foods such as meat and fish were also dried for long-term preservation and later, in the case of fish, by the addition of salt.

Water activity (a_w) of a solution is defined as the ratio of the vapor pressure of the solution to the vapor pressure of pure water at the same temperature. The a_w value is adjusted by the addition of solutes or by dehydration. It is the relative unavailability of water (i.e,. a_w rather than moisture content) that is responsible for control of microbial growth as well as chemical reactions in foods. That water availability rather than water content is the more important parameter is shown by the example of *Staphylococcus aureus*, which has been shown to grow in dried meat and soup having water contents of 23% and 62%, respectively, but possessing water activities of 0.88 to 0.86 (Christian, 2000). Typical water activity levels of certain foods are given in Table 1. High-a_w foods (i.e., 0.95 to 0.99) are spoiled easily by

Microbiologically Safe Foods, Edited by Norma Heredia, Irene Wesley, and Santos García

TABLE 1 Value of Water Activity for Some Common Foods

Range	Food
1.00–0.95	Fresh foods (meats, fish, milk, fruits, vegetables)
0.95–0.90	Ham, salami, bacon, mayonnaise
0.90–0.85	Aged hard cheese, dry ham, fruit juice concentrates, maple syrup
0.85–0.75	Sweet condensed milk, fruit cake, salted fish, molasses, jams
0.75–0.65	Dates, figs, nuts
0.65–0.60	Honey
Below 0.60	Dry pasta, crackers, cereals, dry milk

both gram-positive and gram-negative bacteria. Spoilage of intermediate-moisture foods (a_w 0.60 to 0.90) is caused primarily by molds and osmophilic yeasts.

Solutes function to inhibit growth by removing intracellular water, leading to plasmolysis in which cell volume is reduced, resulting in dormancy or death. Under osmotic stress cells can accumulate solutes such as proline and glycine betaine in *S. aureus* (Jablonski and Bohach, 1999; Townsend and Wilkinson, 1992) to restore turgor, but the resulting environment may be inhibitory to enzyme activity (O'Bryne and Booth, 2000). As the a_w value falls below the optimum, the stationary population falls and the duration of the lag phase increases (Table 2). Osmoregulation, control of the influx and efflux of solutes, is reviewed in detail elsewhere (O'Bryne and Booth, 2000).

Whether by removing moisture or by binding moisture with solutes, the lowered a_w value of foods leads to the inhibition or death of toxigenic and spoilage molds as well as non-spore-forming bacterial cells, for most bacteria growth is limited to a_w levels above 0.9, with the exception of certain halophiles (Table 3).

Minimum a_w levels for growth of microbial groups and bacteria involved in foodborne illness are given in Table 4 using NaCl to control a_w. At the lower end is *Listeria monocytogenes*, which has a lower limit of 0.92 in sodium chloride. Because of its psychrotrophic nature, it is of particular concern in chilled foods. By far the most outstanding of the foodborne pathogens with regard to growth at low a_w is *S. aureus*. Most strains grow at a_w as low as 0.86 under aerobic conditions, with

TABLE 2 Effect of a_w on Growth of *S. aureus* in a Complex Laboratory Medium

a_w	Time (hr) Stationary Phase	$\log_{10}$ Plate Count at Stationary Phase
0.99	20	10
0.97	60	9.7
0.96	80	9.5
0.93	82	8.5
0.90	>100[a]	7.2[b]

Source: Modified from Troller (1971).
[a]40 hr lag phase.
[b]At 100 hr.

TABLE 3 Approximate Minimum a_w Levels for Various Groups of Microorganisms in Foods

	a_w
Most spoilage bacteria	0.90
Most spoilage yeast	0.88–0.90
Most spoilage molds	0.80
Halophilic bacteria	0.75
Xerophilic molds	0.61
Osmophillic yeasts	0.61

the production of *S. aureus* toxins A and D (Ewald and Notermans, 1988). On the other hand, a_w in the range 0.96 to 0.93 prevented synthesis of enterotoxins B and C (Notermans and Heuvelman, 1983; Troller, 1971). In general, gram-negative species have a higher a_w requirement, about 0.95, than gram-positive species.

The use of water-depressing solutes other than salt affects minimal a_w levels for growth. For example, *Clostridium perfringens* grows at an a_w value of between 0.97 and 0.95 in laboratory media in which sucrose or sodium chloride is used to adjust the a_w, but at 0.93 in media adjusted with glycerol (Kang et al., 1969). For *C. botulinum* as well, growth occurs at lower a_w values when controlled by glycerol instead of salt (Baird-Parker and Freame, 1967). In contrast to growth, bacterial spores germinate at an a_w value below that limiting growth (Sperber, 1983). For example, *C. botulinum* types A and B grow at a_w 0.96 (NaCl as solute), but their spores can germinate at 0.93 (Baird-Parker and Freame, 1967).

For both bacterial spores and vegetative cells, heat resistance increases with decreases in minimum a_w. Near ambient temperature, vegetative cells in milk survive longest at a_w 0.05 to 0.20 (Higginbottom, 1953). The increased heat resistance of *Salmonella* to low-a_w, high-fat foods such as peanut butter and chocolate is well established (Baird-Parker et al., 1970; Kirby and Davis, 1990; Mattick et al., 2000; Shachay and Yaron, 2006). Spores also increase heat resistance as the a_w decreases

TABLE 4 Minimum Water Activity Levels for Growth of Selected Bacteria in Laboratory Media

	Minimum a_w	Reference
Bacillus cereus	0.93	Marshall et al., 1971
Clostridium botulinum type A	0.94	Baird-Parker and Freame, 1967
C. botulinum type B	0.94	Ohye and Christian, 1967
C. botulinum type E	0.97	Ohye and Christian, 1967
C. perfringens	0.97	Kang et al., 1969
Escherichia coli	0.95	Marshall et al., 1971
Listeria monocytogenes	0.92	Tapia et al., 1991
Staphylococcus aureus	0.86	Scott, 1957
Vibrio parahemolyticus	0.95	Beuchat, 1974

from 1.0 to a maximum in the range 0.4 to 0.2 (Murrell and Scott, 1966). Even the relatively heat-sensitive spores of *C. botulinum* type E increase their heat resistance several thousand-fold at such low a_w levels, with obvious implications for the heat processing of low-acid foods. Because they grow more rapidly, bacteria are more competitive than yeasts and molds at high a_w. However, many yeasts have a_w abilities below those of bacteria, with osmophilic species such as *Zygosaccharomyces* able to grow in high-sugar-containing foods with a_w values between 0.60 and 0.65 (Corry, 1987). Only yeasts and certain fungi can grow in high concentrations of sugar. However, as with bacteria, yeasts and molds grow better at a_w levels higher than the minimum for growth.

Molds in particular are resistant to low a_w conditions and are responsible for spoilage of foods with lower a_w, and most microorganisms capable of growth below 0.90 are fungi. Fungistatic substances (e.g., sorbic acid, sulfur dioxide, smoke) are often used to inhibit them. Molds represent important spoilage flora of nuts, seeds, and grains. The aflatoxins of *Aspergillus* are of particular concern with such products. The minimum a_w value for growth of this genus is 0.82, with mycotoxin formation requiring an a_w value of 0.83 to 0.87 (Farkas, 2007; Pitt and Miscamble, 1995). Detailed data regarding limiting a_w levels for growth of a number of bacteria, molds, and yeasts are presented elsewhere (Corry, 1987; ICMSF, 1980).

Christian (2000) has reviewed in detail the role of a_w on microbial growth in a variety of plant and animal foods. It should be noted that at the minimum values given in the literature, growth of microorganisms is very slow, and the minima are for conditions in which other environmental factors are optimal. For example, as mentioned above, the published minimum a_w for *S. aureus* is 0.86, but as stated by Troller (1987), "the 'casual' observer would be hard-pressed to obtain growth of most strains much below 0.89 a_w and if determined in many foods the minimum a_w for growth of *S. aureus* might be as high as 0.90–0.91." In fact, the interdependence among extrinsic factors can be exploited by the use of hurdle technology (see below); that is, the slightly deleterious effects of lowered a_w, unfavorable pH, temperature, and so on, are combined so that none has a predominant role but together they function to inhibit microbial growth. The combination of a_w and pH is used to define the term *hazardous foods*. The U.S. Food and Drug Administration defines hazardous foods as having a pH above 4.6 and a_w above 0.85 (USFDA-CFSAN, 1998). Processing of such foods must result in a minimum of a 12-log-cycle kill of *C. botulinum*.

24.2.2 Low Temperature

In addition to moisture and nutrients, proper temperature is a prerequisite for microbial growth. Each microorganism has its minimum, maximum, and optimum temperature for growth. The latter is usually based on the rate of growth, and the maximum is usually only a few degrees above the optimum.

Traditionally, microorganisms are defined as psychrophilic, mesophilic, and thermophilic. There is disagreement on the specific temperature ranges of these groups, but generally the optimum for each group is 20°C or below, 25 to 40°C, and 45°C or above, respectively. The terms *obligate* and *facultative* confuse the categorization further.

Those microorganisms able to grow at low temperatures are of obvious importance to the low-temperature preservation of food and, again, there is some debate on the terms used to define them, in particular, use of the terms *psychrotrophic* and *psychrophilic*. Psychrophilic microorganisms are those that have an optimum growth temperature below 15°C, a maximum at 20°C, and a minimum at 0°C, while psychrotrophs have a temperature optimum above 15°C and an upper limit above 25°C but are still capable of growth at low temperatures (Morita, 1975). Psychrotrophs are more commonly associated with food, while psychrophiles are found in permanently cold environments. The result is that psychrotrophs have a broad temperature range approaching 40°C, in contrast to psychrophiles, which have a narrower range. For example, *Listeria* can grow in temperatures as low as 3°C and at 37°C, human body temperature, making this genus a significant public health concern. Psychrotrophs are found in nearly all raw foods. Stokes (1968) found that psychrophiles constituted 35 to 95% of the bacterial population on meats and 67% of the population on fresh chicken. Molds and yeast are more commonly associated with growth at low temperatures than are bacteria, especially in the range 0 to 5°C (Stokes, 1971).

The minimum, maximum, and optimum growth temperatures of selected bacterial foodborne pathogens given in Table 5 are for optimal growth conditions near

TABLE 5 Minimum, Maximum, and Optimum Temperatures for Growth of Certain Bacterial Foodborne Pathogens

	Temperature (°C)		
Organism	Min.	Opt.	Max.
B. cereus			
Psychrotrophic	4–5	28–35	30–35
Mesophilic	10–15	35–40	50–55
Campylobacter	32	42–45	45
C. botulinum			
Proteolytic	12.5	35	50
Nonproteolytic	3.0–3.3	30	45
C. perfringens	12	43–47	50
E. coli (0157:H7)	8	35–40	42–44
L. monocytogenes	0–4	30–37	45
P. shigelloides	8–10	30	45
Salmonella	5	35–37	45–47
Shigella sonnei	7	37	45–47
S. aureus[a]	7	35–40	48
V. cholerae	10	37	43
V. parahemolyticus	5	37	43
Y. enterocolitica	−1	28–30	42

Source: Adapted from Herbert and Sutherland (2000).

[a]For enterotoxin production, the range is 10–46°C and the optimum is 40–45°C.

neutrality, elevated a_w, and lack of preservatives. The ability for microbial growth can vary between laboratory media and food. *L. monocytogenes* grew in laboratory broth, pH 7.2, at 2°C after a lag of 40 h, but grew without lag on pork fat tissue at −0.3°C (Gill et al., 1997). Similar differences in growth in laboratory media versus food were observed for *Aeromonas hydrophila*, suggesting caution in applying to foods growth models obtained in commercial broths.

Growth at low temperature can induce cold shock proteins (CSPs), enabling an organism to grow at low temperature. For example, *L. monocytogenes*, cold-shocked from 37°C to 5°C, induces a dozen CSPs (Bayles et al., 1996). CSPs are involved in protein synthesis and mRNA folding (Abee and Wouters, 1999; Graumann and Marahiel, 1996). Many other bacteria, including *E. coli, B. cereus*, and *Salmonella* (Abee and Wouters, 1999), synthesize small (ca. 7 kDa) CSPs following a sudden decrease in temperature. CSPs are overexpressed in all bacteria studied to date. In addition, cold-adapted bacteria express an additional set of proteins, cold acclimation proteins (CAPs), which, unlike CSPs, are not present at milder temperatures. Such CAPs differentiate them from mesophiles (Berger et al., 1996; Hebraud and Potier, 2000).

The generation times are shortened considerably with only a slight increase in temperature. For example, in the case of *L. monocytogenes*, the generation time decreased more than threefold (ca. 17 min to ca. 5 min) as the temperature was increased from 5°C to 10°C. A similar situation exists not only with foodborne pathogens but with spoilage organisms as well; for example, in meat slices, psychrotrophic pseudomonad generation time fell from 8.2 min to 5.4 min as the temperature was increased from 2°C to 5°C (Gill and Newton, 1977).

It is generally recognized that the inhibition of microbial growth at low temperature is due to altered membrane structure. To maintain membrane fluidity at low temperatures, psychrotophs increase their proportion of unsaturated fatty acid levels at the expense of the corresponding saturated fatty acids. For example, up to a 50% increase in unsaturated bonds of fatty acids was found in *Candida* grown at 10°C compared to 25°C (Kates and Baxter, 1962). On the other hand, *C. perfringens* responds to low temperature by a reduction in fatty acid chain length rather than increasing unsaturated fatty acids (de Jong et al., 2004). At low temperatures there is also inhibition of microbial enzyme activity. The effect of low temperature on each is discussed elsewhere (Herbert and Sutherland, 2000; Russell, 2002).

A number of bacterial foodborne pathogens have been shown to grow in laboratory media and food products at temperatures below 10°C (summarized by Herbert and Sutherland, 2000). Nonproteolytic *C. botulinum* grows and produces toxin at 3 or 3.3°C (Graham et al., 1997) in laboratory media after a month or more. In the case of food (fish), 18 to 21 days was required to detect *C. botulinum* growth or toxin at 4°C (Graham et al., 1997; Post et al., 1985). Holding at 8°C reduced time to toxin detection in fish to 8 days. The concern here is the increasing availability of minimally processed foods, for which few hurdles exist other than low temperature.

Even if unable to grow, microbes, including foodborne pathogens, can survive at low temperatures. For example, no change in viability of *Campylobacter jejuni* held in ground beef occurred after 14 days at 4°C (Stern and Kotula, 1982).

24.2.3 Freezing

The preservation of frozen food, especially fish and meat, began in earnest at the beginning of the twentieth century, although as early as 1880, frozen meat had been transported from Australia to England. With the introduction of blanching, a preliminary heating step, frozen vegetables became widely available at the retail level. With minor exception (e.g., *Salmonella* in ice cream), frozen products have a good record of quality and safety. Lund (2000) has summarized foodborne outbreaks during recent decades due to the consumption of frozen food.

Water in foods starts to freeze at -1 to $-3°C$ and lowers the temperature of the food to $-18°C$. The a_w value also decreases. During freezing ice crystals are formed from the free water, resulting in the concentration of cellular solutes and denaturation of cellular proteins, among other events (Jay et al., 2005). During freezing, intracellular ice crystals can cause mechanical injury. In addition, the concentration of unfrozen liquid affects pH and ionic strength, in turn affecting cellular organelles. Death during frozen storage probably results from the concentrated, unfrozen remaining solutes from the freezing process. The extent of death, injury, or survival also depends on the freezing rate and temperature. Ice crystallization occurs extracellularly during slow freezing, resulting in the loss of intracellular water. The duration of such osmotic effects decreases with increase in freezing rate, resulting in an increase in survival rates. High freezing temperatures are usually more lethal than lower temperatures. For example, *Salmonella* survived better (60 to 83% after 126 days) at $-20°C$ than at $-5°C$ ($<6\%$ after 5 days). Unfortunately, the lower freezing temperatures that are harmful to microorganisms also affect the quality of many foods.

Microbes vary widely in their sensitivity to frozen storage. Gram-positive bacteria are generally more resistant than gram-negative bacteria. For example, in frozen ground beef held at $-30°C$, the proportion of gram-positive genera increased from 22% to 75%, while that of gram-negative fell from 78% to 23% (2% were yeast) (ICMSF, 1980). Similarly, the percentage of frozen vegetables containing enterococci remained at nearly 90% after 1 year at $-20°C$, while the percentage of such products with *E. coli* fell to 60% (Burton, 1949). In the case of certain strains of *E. coli* O157:H7, about 99% are freeze-injured following freezing at $-20°C$ (Hara-Kudo et al., 2000). Regardless of the organism, a nonselective medium must be employed if freeze-injured cells are to be resuscitated.

As in the case of chilling, cold shocking renders certain bacterial genera resistant to freezing. The viability after freezing of *E. coli* cultures cold-shocked at 10°C for 6 h was greater than that of cultures frozen without cold shock (Goldstein et al., 1990). Similarly, the survival of *L. monocytogenes* after freezing was 90% if they were cold-shocked beforehand at 10°C versus 50% without cold shock (Wemekamp-Kamphuis et al., 2002).

Bacterial spores are resistant to freezing, and indeed, freezing or freeze drying is an effective method of culture carriage. On the other hand, higher organisms (eukaryotes) such as protozoans, roundworms, and tapeworms, are more sensitive than prokaryotes. Freezing for specific times and temperatures are effective methods for inactivating such potential foodborne pathogens. For example, the U.S. Department of

Agriculture requires that ready-to-eat smoked sausage be held at −20°C for 20 days for meat <15 cm thick (lower temperatures require fewer days of holding) (Leighty, 1983).

Certain compounds, such as proteins and glycerol, have a cryprotective effect against freeze injury. Indeed, glycerol is used routinely for culture carriage of vegetative cells at −80°C. The extensive reduction of *C. jejuni*, 3 log cycles at −15°C after 3 days, could be reduced by about half in the presence of 10% glycerol versus 0.1% peptone (Stern and Kotula, 1982). Similar lethal effects during frozen storage of *C. perfringens* (Labbé and Juneja, 2006) led to the recommendation that in the case of this microorganism, for prolonged frozen storage or shipping under dry ice, suspected outbreak food samples should be mixed with a buffered glycerol–NaCl solution (Rhodehamel and Harmon, 2001). Nevertheless, freeze tolerance is genus- and species-specific, with certain psychrophilic bacteria susceptible to frozen storage even in the presence of 10% glycerol (Yamasato et al., 1973).

24.3 FOOD ANTIMICROBIALS

Food preservatives are defined as chemicals that prevent or retard deterioration of food but do not include, in the case of the FDA, salt, sugars, vinegars, oil from spices, spices, or wood smoke. Those that affect microbial growth are considered antimicrobial agents. Most have a broad-spectrum effect, with a select few used against specific pathogens. Traditionally used chemical food antimicrobials are listed in Table 6. A selected number are mentioned here. Davidson et al. (2005) have provided an excellent detailed description of each. Reviews of traditional and approved natural antimicrobials, such as lactoferrin, lysozyme, nisin, essential oils, and phenolic compounds, have also been published (Davidson and Zivanovic, 2003; Galvez et al., 2007; Naidu, 2000; Stopforth et al., 2005; Vigil et al., 2005).

TABLE 6 Traditionally Used Food Antimicrobials

Compound(s)	Target	Applications
Acetic acid, acetates, diacetates, dehydroacetic acid	Yeast, bacteria	Baked goods, condiments, confections, dairy products, fats/oils, meats, sauces
Benzoic acid, benzoates	Yeasts, molds	Beverages, fruit products
Dimethyl dicarbonate	Yeasts	Beverages
Lactic acid, lactates	Bacteria	Meats, fermented foods
Nitrite, nitrate	*Clostridium botulinum*	Cured meats
Parabens (alkyl esters(propyl, methyl, heptyl) of *p*-hydroxybenzoic acid)	Yeasts, molds, bacteria (gram-positive)	Beverages, baked goods, syrups, dry sausage
Propionic acid, propionates	Molds	Bakery products, dairy products
Sorbic acid, sorbates	Yeasts, molds, bacteria	Most foods, beverages, wines
Sulfites	Yeasts, molds	Fruits, fruit products, wines

Source: Adapted from Davidson et al. (2005).

24.3.1 Organic Acids

All organic acids used as antimicrobials have pK_a values below 5.0. Other organic acids are used primarily as flavorings (Table 6). The most effective antimicrobial form is the undisasociated acid. Therefore, their maximum activity is in high-acid foods (pH <5.5). The undissociated organic acid can penetrate the cell membrane's lipid bilayer and dissociate inside the cell, due to the higher pH of the cell interior. The ATP required to maintain neutral internal pH by removal of protons results in a depletion of cellular energy. The net effect is interference in maintaining membrane potential and metabolite transport (Davidson and Zivanovic, 2003). Although less effective, dissociated organic acids may also have antimicrobial action, at least in the case of sorbates (Stopforth et al., 2005). In any event, it is clear that the precise mode of action of organic acids remains to be determined.

Benzoic acid and sodium benzoate are used primarily against yeasts and molds which are inhibited by 0.05 to 0.10% of the undissociated acid. As with most antimicrobial agents, there is wide genus and species variation in susceptibility. An outbreak of *E.coli* 0157:H7 in apple cider has resulted in the commercial pasteurization of cider as well as the addition of benzoate and sorbate, which were shown to be effective in inactivating this organism in cider (Zhao et al., 1993).

Related to benzoic acid are the esters of *p*-hydroxybenzoic acid (parabens), and their use as antimicrobials is permitted in several countries. They differ from benzoate in being less sensitive to pH and are more effective against molds than against yeast. The effective concentration depends on the particular ester form as well as the target group (molds, yeast, bacteria). As the alkyl chain length increases, inhibitory activity generally increases. In the United States, the methyl and propyl forms are generally regarded as safe (GRAS) up to a concentration of 0.1%. Though historically not widely used, they may find future applications in antimicrobial packaging.

Closely related to benzoic acid are sorbic acid and especially, its potassium salt. With a pK_a of 4.8, activity is greatest at a pH below 6.0 and is more effective than sodium benzoate between pH 4.0 and 6.0. Sorbates are effective primarily against yeasts and molds and certain bacteria. The resistance of lactic acid bacteria to sorbate results in its use as a fungistat in lactic fermentations. A common application is in cheese spreads and on the surface of non-mold-ripened cheese, to prevent mold development. The sorbates are used in a wide variety of other products, including vegetable, fruit, and bakery products. The formation of carcinogenic nitrosamines during cooking of cooked, cured meat led to the proposed use of sorbates and reduced nitrite levels in such products while maintaining the latter's antibotulinal activity. Despite extensive evidence of the antimicrobial properties of sorbate in a variety of meat products, the proposal to reduce nitrite levels in bacon and add sorbate was not adopted because of an apparently single report that consumption of experimental bacon caused allergic-type reactions in certain persons. Nevertheless, because of their GRAS status and broad spectrum of activity, sorbic acid and sorbates remain one of the most widely used chemical food preservatives.

The three-carbon propionic acid and its calcium and sodium salts are used in breads and cakes primarily to inhibit molds present as a result of post-processing contamination. Since they have little or no effect on yeast, propionates can be added to bread dough. As with benzoates and sorbates, the undissociated molecule is necessary for its antimicrobial activity. Swiss cheese contains significant amounts of propionic acid because of the growth and metabolism of propionic bacteria associated with its manufacture.

A long list of other organic acids are used in foods. Many are added for their secondary effects rather than solely for their antimicrobial activities. These have been described elsewhere (Doores, 2005).

24.3.2 Nitrites

The use of nitrates for meat preservation is an old technology. A vast amount of literature has been published on its activity and safety. The realization in the mid-twentieth century that it is the nitrite formed by microbial reduction of nitrate that is the effective agent led to the current use of nitrite salts. Together with sodium chloride, these are commonly referred to as curing salts. In the United States, the use of nitrite is limited to meat, although in other countries it is used to prevent "late gasing" in cheese.

Nitrite plays two primary roles in meat preservation. The first is to maintain a desirable red color. The nitrous acid formed under acidic conditions decomposes to yield nitric oxide (NO), the important product for color fixation. Erythrobate or ascorbic acid also reduce nitrite to NO and are commonly included today in cured meats. The actual red pigment is nitrosomyoglobin, which forms when NO reacts with myoglobin.

A second primary use for nitrite is to inhibit *C. botulinum* growth and toxin formation, although not necessarily spore germination. Its effectiveness is affected by temperature and salt concentration. Although 50 ppm (mg/kg) initial nitrite levels are sufficient for the meat color desired, up to 200 ppm, depending on the country, is used for antibotulinal activity. The result has been the almost total absence of botulism in cured meat. Its effect on non-spore-formers is distinctly genus dependent. As with the organic acids, lower pH noticeably improves the antimicrobial activity of nitrite. Indeed, the pH of meat (ca. 6.0) is at the upper end of its effective range at permissible concentrations. Nitrite can react with secondary amines (e.g., from meat) under acidic conditions (as in the human stomach) to form nitroseamines. The discovery in the late 1960s that nitroseamines come from foods containing nitrite led to a reexamination of its use by regulatory agencies. Considerable resources of time and effort were devoted to determining its continued use in meats and, ipso facto, such products themselves. The result was that in the United States, for example, input levels of nitrite for bacon were reduced to 120 mg/kg as well as the addition of 550 mg/kg of ascorbate or isoascorbate. These reducing agents decrease nitrosamine formation. Nitrates are no longer permitted. Nitrite alternatives have been proposed, such as replacement with sorbic alone or together with reduced nitrite levels, or replacement with sorbate plus betalains (beet juice). The inhibiting effect of nitrite and NaCl against microbes other than *C. botulinum* varies with the bacterial genus. *Salmonellae* and S. *aureus*, for example, are able to grow in cured meat but not under proper refrigeration. Lactic acid bacteria are a major component of the spoilage flora of these products. Microbial spoilage of cured meat has been reviewed extensively by Gardner (1983).

24.3.3 Sulfur Compounds

The use of sulfur for sanitation purposes spans millennia, from the fumigation of homes in ancient Greece (Hammond and Carr, 1976) to its use as a larvicide during construction of the Panama Canal (McCullough, 1977). The primary applications of sulfur dioxide and its salts are in fruits and vegetables. For example, the gaseous form is used widely to prevent mold growth on dried fruits, and in the sulfite form in virtually all wines to inhibit molds, bacteria, and undesirable yeasts, although in the United States, wines with more than 10 mg/L sulfites must be labeled to indicate its presence, due to possible allergic reactions. The inhibitory effect of sulfites is greatest in the hydrate $SO_2{\cdot}H_2O$ form, which occurs at acidic pH values presumably because of the nonionized molecule's ability to pass across cell membranes. For example, a 10-fold increase in SO_2 occurs between pH 4.0 and 3.0.

In most countries, sulfites are not permitted in meat or foods recognized as sources of thiamin. In addition, due to potential hypersensitivity reactions, the FDA rescinded the GRAS status of sulfites used on raw fruits and vegetables, as had been commonplace in salad bars to maintain fresh appearance and prevent browning reactions.

Because sulfite can react with various critical cell components as well as the effect of pH on the molecular form, there is probably more than one mode of action by sulfur compounds. Summaries of possible targets of inhibition are given in the primary references listed above.

24.4 PRESERVATIVES FROM BIOLOGICAL SOURCES

As consumers become weary of chemical preservatives, the use of "natural" antimicrobials become attractive, and certain ones have been approved for use in foods. Compared to chemical preservatives, their use or proposed use in foods is relatively recent. Nisin and lysozyme will be given as examples. An even more recent proposal is the use of bacteriophages as a biopreservative tool. This is discussed as well.

24.4.1 Nisin

Bacteriocins are low-molecular-weight antimicrobial peptides which are inhibitory to closely related producer bacteria. The bacteriocin nisin is the prototype foodborne bacteriocin produced by the dairy starter culture *Lactococcus lactis*. It is widely used in many countries as a food preservative and achieved GRAS status in the United States in 1988 (Delves-Broughton, 2005).

A vast amount of literature on nisin has been published. Extensive research has been conducted on its mode of action. In effect, the antimicrobial activity of nisin is due to its pore-forming abilities on cell membranes, resulting in the efflux of ions, solutes, and cellular ATP. It is available commercially and is effective against gram-positive bacteria but not against fungi and gram-negatives. It is a 34-amino acid peptide with five internal rings, yielding a molecular weight of 3510. Because it is relatively heat stable, it is used in pasteurized or heat-treated foods. The spore-forming bacteria that might survive such processes are inhibited by nisin, which prevents spore outgrowth. *Listeria* is another susceptible target.

Levels of nisin remain stable during refrigerated storage and decline at higher temperatures in a temperature-dependent manner. Degradation of nisin may occur in minimally processed or unheated foods, due to proteolytic enzymes in the food. It is considered a natural preservative and can occur at low levels in cheese. A major application of nisin as a preservative is in processed cheese products in the form of slices and spreads to inhibit spoilage by *Clostridium* species. Its use in unheat-treated milk allows reduced heat treatment, avoiding the perceived burned flavor of such products (Wirjantoro et al., 2001).

Nisin has also been used as a preservative in low- and high-acid canned foods to prevent thermophilic spoilage by gram-positive, thermophilic spore-formers. Abee and Delves-Broughton (2003) have summarized the use of nisin to control spoilage in canned vegetables. In contrast to numerous other food systems, nisin is only variably effective in meat systems. In vitro–sensitive organisms are less sensitive to nisin when growing in meat. This is proposed to be due to binding by the sulfhydryl group of glutathione, a reducing tripeptide found in meat and poultry. Proteases from meat were presumed responsible for reduced antilisterial effectiveness of nisin on raw pork (Murray and Richard, 1997). On the other hand, nisin spray treatments did reduce levels of inoculated *Listeria* and spoilage organisms on beef carcasses (Cutter and Siragusa, 1995). Other examples of the uses of nisin and other bacteriocins in meat are summarized in the primary literature sources cited below.

Fish is another food in which nisin has shown effectiveness. For example, it prevented or delayed growth and toxin formation by *C. botulinum* in carbon dioxide–packaged fish (Taylor et al., 1990) and growth of *L. monocytogenes* in smoked salmon (Szabo and Cahill, 1999), products that are not heated before being consumed. The above involves the direct addition of nisin as a preservative. Other approaches to introducing nisin and other bacteriocins could include inoculation of food with lactic acid bacteria that produce bacteriocin or use of products containing bacteriocin by previous fermentation.

The limitations of nisin and other bacteriocins, such as narrow activity spectra, will probably see its use in conjunction with other agents. These could include the use of chelating agents to render nisin accessible to gram-negative cell membrane, the use of multiple bacteriocins, the combination of nisin with other antimicrobials, and the incorporation of nisin into packaging films (Ye et al., 2008). Recently, the acid-tolerant spore-forming bacterium *Alicyclobacillus acidoterrestris* was identified as a cause of spoilage of fruit juices. Nisin was shown to be very effective in its inhibition as well as reducing spore *D*-values (Yamazaki et al., 2000). In addition, nisin decreases spore resistance (Penna and Moraes, 2002) and is bacteriostatic against spores of several *Bacillus* species (Montville et al., 2006). Since it is unlikely that new chemical preservatives will be proposed for use in foods, this synergistic effect of existing natural antimicrobials together with existing GRAS substances is a likely approach. Certain of these, such as organic acids, essential oils, and chelating agents, are synergistic with nisin. Used together, often with physical methods of preservation, the concept is referred to as hurdle technology and is discussed in more detail below. Recent work has shown the enhanced effectiveness of nonthermal processing procedures such as pulsed electric field and high hydrostatic pressure (see Chapter 23) when used with nisin and other bacteriocins. In the case of nisin, for example, nisin and high pressure together resulted in a several-log reduction in *Lactobacillus plantarum* and *E. coli* (ter Steeg et al., 1999). Future work with nisin will probably involve further synergistic effects with ultrahigh-pressure processing and its incorporation into or coating of food packaging materials as well as incorporation into edible films. Detailed summaries of the mode of action of nisin and its use alone or with other additive and processing procedures are reviewed elsewhere (Abee and Delves-Broughton, 2003; Johnson and Larson, 2005; Montville and Chikindas, 2007; Roller and Board, 2003; Thomas and Delves-Broughton, 2005). With regard to antimicrobial packaging, Tewari (2002) has presented a summary of the antimicrobial compounds used in such packaging, although few are commercially available.

24.4.2 Bacteriophages

Bacterial viruses have presented problems for dairy and meat starter culture, leading to failed fermentations. As biocontrol agents, it has been known for decades that bacterial viruses are able to lyse bacteria from meat, fish, and dairy products. Phage prophylaxis is a known treatment for animal and human illness (Sulakvelidze et al., 2001). The use of bacteriophages has been shown to be effective as a preharvest control method against pathogens such as *E. coli* 0157:H7 and *Campylobacter* (Carrillo et al., 2005; Raya et al., 2006; Sheng et al., 2006).

The direct addition of bacteriophages to food for spoilage control is a more recent development. Unlike chemicals used as preservatives, bacteriophages are very host specific. They may specifically target *Salmonella*, for example, while not affecting native microflora, which are useful for competitive reasons. The limited host specificity of bacterial viruses will probably require a cocktail of phages for biocontrol purposes. Another reported limitation is their requirement for host replication for phage activity, a concern for refrigerated foods. Even so, phage adsorption can occur at low temperatures. When conditions permissible for growth are encountered, such as in the human gut, lysis of targeted pathogens can occur.

Although one report (Whitman and Marshall, 1971) indicated that half of retail food examined contained up to 38 phage-specific host systems, most of the phages were specific for pseudomonads. This reflects the large population levels (log 3 to 5 CFU/g) required for the recovery of phages from foods (i.e., coliforms and psychrotrophic spoilage organisms). This may limit the usefulness of phages as biocontrol agents in products such as produce, where relatively low pathogen loads may be encountered. By contrast, much more information has been published on their use in post-harvest bacterial control in dairy, poultry, and meats (summarized by Greer, 2005). Two bacteriophage products have been approved for use on food products in the United States (Bren, 2007). Both target *Listeria* and are for use on ready-to-eat meat and poultry products and for cheese. The myriad factors affecting the success of bacteriophages as biocontrol agents have been reviewed elsewhere (Greer, 2005; Hudson et al., 2005).

24.4.3 Lysozyme

Another naturally occuring antimicrobial agent receiving increasing attention in recent years is lysozyme. Lysozyme is one of a number of antimicrobial systems present in avian eggs designed to keep it free of infection during embryo development. It is obtained by extraction of egg whites, and its biochemical and physical properties are well known (Proctor and Cunningham, 1988). Its action results in hydrolysis of the 1,4 glycosidic bond between *N*-acetylglucosamine and *N*-acetylmuramic acid in the peptidoglycan layer of the bacterial cell wall. The lipopolysaccharide (LPS) layer of the outer layer of gram-negative bacteria limits its effectiveness to gram-positive bacteria, although a certain few, such as *C. perfringens* and *S. aureus,* are not inhibited. The chelating agent EDTA can increase the antimicrobial spectrum of lysozyme as well as nisin by destabilizing the LPS layer. The antimicrobial spectrum of lysozyme has been summarized by Johnson and Larson (2005).

Although present in milk from humans and other animals, only that from hen egg white is used in food preservation. Its high solubility, presence as a component of the human immune system, specificity for bacterial peptidoglycan, and relative resistance to heat and pH make it an ideal food preservative. Indeed, although an enzyme, it is remarkably stable, surviving refrigerated storage for several years. It can resist boiling for 1 to 2 min at low pH and is not affected by temperatures up to 55°C, although its activity can be affected significantly by nonthermal food-processing procedures (Johnson and Larson, 2005). Its activity remaining after pasteurization prevents late blowing of cheese by *Clostridium tyrobutyricum.*

As an enzyme with an optimum pH of 9.2, it is not surprising that high concentrations of acid (lactic, acetic) affect activity adversely. While low NaCl concentrations, below 10 mM, improves lysis of sensitive bacteria, activity is inhibited at concentrations greater than 0.05 to 0.1 M (Chang and Carr, 1971). Its use in foods is at concentrations in the range 20 to 400 ppm with an estimated 100 tons used annually (Gould, 2002). Despite its relative stability, lysozyme is an enzyme, and if considered for use in food systems, its stability should be evaluated under conditions of use. Nevertheless, certain specific applications of lysozyme in foods have been adopted over the years. As mentioned above, it is commonly used to prevent late blowing of cheese by its addition to milk at levels that do not affect the starter culture.

A novel application of lysozyme is its use on packaging films, allowing its direct contact with pathogens on the surface of foods and avoiding its inactivation during heat-processing procedures (see Chapter 25). A promising approach along these lines would be its use in combination with other antimicrobials. Activity of lysozyme is unaffected by certain other antimicrobial compounds, such as sodium nitrite, calcium propionate, and potassium sorbate, but is affected negatively by fatty acids and certain ions and proteins during processing, perhaps by the formation of mixed disulfides. Lysozyme–nisin combinations were more effective than either used alone to control the growth of gram-positive and meat spoilage bacteria (Nattress et al., 2001). In another example, lysozyme, EDTA, and nisin applied as a surface coating inhibited spoilage and pathogenic bacteria on ham and bologna (Gill and Holley, 2000). This concept of hurdle technology is described below.

24.5 HURDLE TECHNOLOGY

The trend toward minimally processed convenience foods, as well as foods with reduced sugar, salt, and preservatives, has led to challenges in maintaining the stability and safety of such products. It has long been known that interactions of temperature, a_w, preservatives, low pH, and so on, serve to preserve food. In the 1970s, the term *hurdle technology* was applied to this long-known phenomenon. If the antimicrobial targets vary (DNA, membrane, and enzyme system), the effect can be synergistic rather than additive. Some 60 potential hurdles for foods of animal or plant origin have been described (Leistner, 2000).

The concept of hurdle technology is elegantly simple. Simply put: Some of the microorganisms can overcome one or more hurdles, but none can jump over all the hurdles when used together. Historically, single hurdles have been commonly used, such as low pH (4.6), for inhibition of C. *botulinum* or high temperatures for canned foods. Some hurdles can be of greater intensity than others (e.g., low a_w but moderate pH). Other factors in the successful application of hurdle technology are microbial load (e.g., following poor hygienic conditions) and the nutrient content of the food. Important, well-known hurdles used in food preservatives are listed in Table 7. Some of these are interactive, such as low pH and weak organic acids (sorbic, propionic, and benzoic). Often-used traditional hurdles are physical hurdles and microbiological hurdles such as starter cultures and nisin.

To overcome adverse conditions imposed by preservatives, cells must induce repair mechanisms or maintain homeostasis (internal equilibrium), requiring the expenditure of energy stores (e.g., to maintain internal pH) a concept termed metabolic exhaustion (Leistner, 2000). If the stability of foods (e.g., holding temperature, presence of antimicrobials) is near the threshold of growth, vegetative cells that cannot grow will die. However, cells including *Salmonella* could survive if such foods are refrigerated

TABLE 7 Traditional Hurdles in Food Preservation

Parameter	Application
High temperature	Heating
Low temperature	Chilling, freezing
Reduced a_w	Drying, curing, conserving (e.g., fruits)
Increased acidity	Acid addition formations
Reduced redox potential	Removal of oxygen, addition of reducing agents
Preservatives	Sorbate, sulfite, nitrite, etc.
Competitive flora	Microbial fermentation

(Leistner, 1995), leading to conditions where refrigeration is not necessarily desirable for food safety and quality in, for example, developing countries.

The laboratory confirmation of the effectiveness of multiple hurdles can be a daunting task using traditional challenge testing. The need for obtaining data on microbial survival and death for various inhibitory parameters led to the development of modeling programs developed in the UK (Micromodel, Leatherhead Food Research Association) and the United States (Pathogen Modeling Program, U.S. Department of Agriculture) (see Chapter 30).

The concept of hurdle technology has also been adopted by regulatory agencies. For example, among the options for storage of meat products, the U.S. Department of Agriculture and Canadian Food Inspection Agency requirements are a pH of 4.6 or less or an a_w of 0.90 or less and 100 ppm or more of nitrite (Lemay et al., 2002).

Hurdle technology has also been used to reduce the initial load of microorganisms on raw materials so that few subsequent preservative hurdles mentioned above are necessary. An example is the sequential use of steam vacuuming, pre-eviseration carcass washing, and rinsing with organic acids (Bacon et al., 2000). Combinations of multiple treatments were more effective than single or double treatments in reducing pathogens.

Newer nonthermal technologies such as high pressure and pulsed electric fields (discussed in Chapter 23) can be combined with traditional techniques, avoiding the extreme use of any single treatment. Ross et al. (2003) have reviewed the combined effect of nonthermal processes with traditional preservation techniques. Such combined treatment will probably play a major role in food preservation in the future.

REFERENCES

Abee T, Delves-Broughton J (2003): Bacteriocins—nisin. In: Rusell NJ, Gould GW (Eds.). *Food Preservatives*, 2nd ed. Kluwer Academic/Plenum Publishing, New York.

Abee T, Wouters J (1999): Microbial stress response in minimal processing. *Int J Food Microbiol*. 50:65–91.

Bacon R, Belk K, Sofos J, Clayton R, Reagan J, Smith G (2000): Microbiol populations of animal hides and beef carcasses at different stages of slaughter in plants employing multiple sequential interventions for decontamination. *J Food Prot*. 63:1080–1086.

Baird-Parker A, Freame B (1967): Combined effects of water activity, pH, and temperature on the growth of *Clostridium botulinum* from spores and vegetative inocula. *J Appl Bacteriol*. 30:420–429.

Baird-Parker A, Boothroyd M, Jones E (1970): The effect of water activity on the heat-resistance of heat-sensitive and heat-resistant strains of *Salmonella*. *J Appl Bacteriol*. 33:515–522.

Bayles D, Annous B, Wilkinson B (1996): Cold stress proteins induced in *Listeria monocytogenes* in response to temperature downshock and growth at low temperatures. *Appl Environ Microbiol*. 62:1116–1119.

Berger F, Morellet N, Menu F, Potier P (1996): Cold shock and cold acclimation proteins in the psychrotrophic bacterium *Athrobacter globiformis* SI55. *J Bacteriol*. 178:2999–3007.

Beuchat L (1974): Combined effects of water activity, solute and temperature on the growth of *Vibro parahemolyticus*. *Appl Microbiol*. 27:1075–1080.

Bren L (2007): Bacteria-eating virus approved as food additive. *FDA Consumer Mag*. http://www.fda.gov/fdac/features/2007/107_virus.html. Accessed June 2008.

Burton M (1949): Comparison of coliform and enterococcus organisms as indices of pollution in frozen foods. *Food Res*. 14:434–438.

Carrillo C, Atterby R, El-Shibiny A, et al. (2005): Bacteriophage therapy to reduce *Campylobacter jejuni* colonization of broiler chickens. *Appl Environ Microbiol*. 71: 6554–6563.

Chang K, Carr C (1971): Studies on the structure and function of lysozyme. I: The effect of pH and cation concentration on lysozyme activity. *Biochim Biophys Acta*. 229:496–503.

Christian J (2000): Drying and reduction of water activity. In: Lund B, Baird-Parker T, Gould G (Eds.). *The Microbiological Safety and Quality of Foods*, Vol. 1. Aspen Publishers, Gaithersburg, MD, pp. 146–174.

Corry J (1987): Relationships of water activity to fungal growth. In: Beuchat L (Ed.): *Food and Beverage Mycology*, 2nd ed. Van Nostrand Reinhold, New York, pp. 51–100.

Cutter C, Siragusa G (1995): Population reductions of gram negative pathogens following treatments with vision and chelators under various conditions. *J Food Prot*. 58: 977–983.

Davidson M, Zivanovic S (2003): The use of natural antimicrobials. In: Zeuthen P, Bogh-Sorensen L (Eds.). *Food Preservation Techniques*. Woodhead Publishing, Cambridge, UK, pp. 5–30.

Davidson M, Sofos J, Branen A (Eds.) (2005): *Antimicrobials in Food*. CRC Press, Boca Raton, FL.

De Jong AEI, Rombouts F, Beumer R (2004): Behavior of *Clostridium perfringens* at low temperatures. *Int J Food Microbiol*. 97:71–81.

Delves-Broughton J (2005): Nisin as a food preservative. *Food Aust*. 57:525–527.

Doores S (2005): Organic acids. In: Davidson M, Sofos J, Branen A (Eds.). *Antimicrobials in Foods*, 3rd ed. CRC Press, Boca Raton, FL, pp. 91–142.

Ewald S, Notermans S (1988): Effect of water activity on growth and enterotoxin D production of *Staphylococcus aureus*. *Int J Food Microbiol*. 6:25–30.

Farkas J (2007): Physical methods of food preservation. In: Doyle M, Beuchat L, Montville T (Eds.). *Food Microbiology: Fundamentals and Frontiers*. 3rd ed. ASM Press, Washington, DC, pp. 685–712.

Galvez A, Abriouel H, Lopez RL, Ben Omar N (2007): Bacteriocin-based strategies for food biopreservation. *Int J Food Microbiol*. 120:51–70.

Gardner GA (1983): Microbial spoilage of cured meats. *Soc Appl Bacteriol Symp Ser*. 11:179–202.

Gill A, Holley R (2000): Surface application of lysozyme, nisin, and EDTA to inhibit spoilage and pathogenic bacteria on ham and bologna. *J Food Prot*. 63:1338–1346.

Gill C, Newton K (1977): Development of aerobic spoilage flora on meat stored at chill temperatures. *J Appl Bacteriol*. 43:189–195.

Gill C, Greer G, Dilts B (1997): The aerobic growth of *Aeromonas hydrophila* and *Listeria monocytogenes* in broths and on pork. *Int J Food Microbiol*. 35:67–74.

Goldstein J, Pollitt S, Inouye M (1990): Major cold shock protein of *Escherichia coli*. *Proc Natl Acad Sci*. 87:283–287.

Gould G (2002): Control with naturally occurring antimicrobial systems including bacteriolytic enzymes. In: Juneja V, Sofos J (Eds.). *Control of Foodborne Microorganisms*. Marcel Dekker, New York, pp. 281–302.

Graham A, Mason D, Maxwell F, Peck M (1997): Effect of pH and NaCl on growth from spores of non-proteolytic *Clostridium botulinum* at chill temperatures. *Lett Appl Microbiol*. 24:95–100.

Graumann P, Marahiel M (1996): Some like it cold: response of microorganisms to cold shock. *Arch Microbiol*. 166:293–300.

Greer G (2005): Bacteriophage control of foodborne bacteria. *J Food Prot*. 68:1102–1111.

Hammond S, Carr J (1976): The antimicrobial activity of SO_2^- with particular reference to fermented and non-fermented fruit juices. *Appl Bacteriol Symp Ser.* 5:89–110.

Hara-Kudo Y, Ifedo M, Kodaka H, et al. (2000): Selective enrichment with resuscitation step for isolation of *Escherichia coli* 0157:H7 from foods. *Appl Environ Microbiol*. 66: 2872.

Hebraud M, Potier P (2000): Cold acclimation and cold shock response in psychrotrophic bacteria. In: Inouye M, Yamanaka K (Eds.). *Cold Shock Response and Adaptation*. Horizon Press, Norfolk, UK, pp. 41–60.

Herbert R, Sutherland J (2000): Chill storage. In: Lund B, Baird-Parker T, Gould G (Eds.). *The Microbiological Safety and Quality of Foods*, Vol. 1. Aspen Publishers, Gaithersburg, MD, pp. 101–121.

Higginbottom C (1953): The effect of storage at different relative humidities on the survival of microorganism in milk powder in the intermediate moisture range. *J Dairy Res*. 20:65–75.

Hudson J, Billington C, Carey-Smith G, Greenina G (2005): Bacteriophages as biocontrol agents in food. *J Food Prot*. 68:426–437.

ICMSF (International Commission on Microbiological Specifications for Foods) (1980): Reduced water activity. In: *Microbial Ecology of Foods*, Vol. 1. Academic Press, New York, pp. 70–91.

Jablonski L, Bohach G (1999): *Staphylococcus aureus*. In: Doyle M, Beuchat L, Montville T (Eds.). *Food Microbiology: Fundamentals and Frontiers*. ASM Press, Washington, DC, pp. 411–434.

Jay J, Loessner M, Golden D (2005): Modern Food Microbiology, 7th ed. Springer, New York.

Johnson E, Larson E (2005): Lysozyme. In: Davidson M, Sofos J, Branen A (Eds.). *Antimicrobials in Foods*, 3rd ed. CRC Press, Boca Raton, FL, pp. 361–387.

Kang C, Woodburn M, Pagenkopf A, Cheney R (1969): Growth, sporulation and germination of *Clostridium perfringens* in media of controlled water activity. *Appl Microbiol*. 18: 798–805.

Kates M, Baxter R (1962): Lipid comparison of mesophilic and psychrotrophic yeasts (*Candida* species) as influenced by environmental temperatures. *Can J Biochem Physiol*. 40:1213–1227.

Kirby R, Davis R (1990): Survival of dehydrated cells of *Salmonella typhimurium* LT 2 at high temperatures. *J Appl Bacteriol*. 68:241–246.

Labbé R, Juneja V (2006): *Clostridium perfringens*. In: Rieman H, Cliver D (Eds.). *Foodborne Infections and Intoxications*, 3rd ed. Academic Press, San Diego, CA, pp. 137–184.

Leighty J (1983): Regulatory action to control *Trichinella spiralis*. *Food Technol*. 37:95–97.

Leistner L (1995): Principle and applications of hurdle technology. In: Gould G (Ed.): *New Methods of Food Preservation*. Blackie Academic and Professional, London, pp. 1–21.

——— (2000): Basic aspects of food preservation by hurdle technology. *Int J Food Microbiol*. 55:181–186.

Lemay M-J, Choquette J, Delaguis P, Gariepy C, Rodrique N, Saucier L (2002): Antimicrobial effect of natural preservative in a cooked and acidified meat model. *Int J Food Microbiol*. 78:217–226.

Lund B (2000): Freezing. In: Lund B, Baird-Parker T, Gould G (Eds.). *The Microbiological Safety and Quality of Foods*, Vol. 1. Aspen Publishers, Gaithersberg, MD, pp. 112–145.

Marshall B, Ohye D, Christian J (1971): Tolerance of bacteria to high concentration of NaCl and glycerol in the growth medium. *Appl Microbiol*. 21:363–364.

Mattick K, Jorgensen F, Legan J, Lappin-Scott H, Humphrey T (2000): Habituation of *Salmonella* at reduced water activity and its effect on heat tolerance. *Appl Environ Microbiol*. 66:4921–4925.

McCullough D (1977): *The Path Between the Seas: The Creation of the Panama Canal*. Simon and Schuster, New York.

Montville T, Chikindas M (2007): Biopreservation of foods. In: Doyle M, Beuchat L (Eds.). *Food Microbiology: Fundamentals and Frontiers*, 3rd ed. ASM Press, Washington, DC, pp. 747–766.

Montville TJ, De Siano T, Nock A, Padhi S, Wade D (2006): Inhibition of *Bacillus anthracis* and potential surrogate bacilli growth from spore inocula by nisin and other antimicrobial peptides. *J Food Prot*. 69:2529–2533.

Morita R (1975): Psychrophilic bacteria. *Bacteriol Rev*. 39:146–167.

Murray M, Richard JA (1997): Comparative study of the anlilisterial activity of nisin A and pediocin in AcH in fresh ground pork stored at 5°C. *J Food Prot*. 60:1534–1540.

Murrell W, Scott W (1966): The heat resistance of bacterial spores at various water activities. *J Gen Microbiol*. 43:411–425.

Naidu A (Ed.) (2000): *Natural Food Antimicrobial Systems*. CRC Press, Boca Raton, FL.

Nattress F, Yost C, Baker L (2001): Evaluation of the ability of lysozyme and nisin to control meat spoilage bacteria. *Int J Food Microbiol*. 70:111–119.

Notermans S, Heuvelman C (1983): Combined effect of water activity, pH and sub-optimal temperature on growth and enterotoxin production of *Staphylococcus aureus*. *J Food Sci*. 48:1832–1840.

O'Byrne C, Booth I (2002): Osmoregulation and its importance to foodborne microorganisms. *Int J Food Microbiol*. 74:203–216.

Ohye D, Christian J (1967): Combined effects of temperature, pH and water activity on growth and toxin production by *Clostridium botulinum* types A, B, and E. In: Ingram M, Roberts T (Eds.). *Clostridium botulinum*. Chapman & Hall, London, pp. 136–143.

Penna V, Moraes DA (2002): The effect of nisin on growth kinetics from activated *Bacillus cereus* spores in cooked rice and milk. *J Food Prot*. 65:419–422.

Pitt J, Miscamble B (1995): Water relations of *Aspergillus flavus* and closely related species. *J Food Prot*. 58:86–90.

Post L, Lee D, Solberg M, Furgang D, Specchio J, Graham C (1985): Development of botulinal toxin and sensory deterioration during storage of vacuum and modified atmosphere packaged fish fillets. *J Food Sci*. 50:990–996.

Proctor A, Cunningham F (1988): The chemistry of lysozyme and its use as a food preservative and pharmaceutical. *Crit Rev Food Sci Nutr*. 26:359–395.

Raya P, Varey P, Oot R, et al. (2006): Isolation and characterization of a new T-even bacteriophage, CEV1 and determination of its potential to reduce *Escherichia coli* 0157:H7 in sheep. *Appl Environ Microbiol*. 72:6405–7410.

Rhodehamel EJ, Harmon S (2001): *Clostridium perfringens*. In: *Bacteriological Analytical Manual* online. http://www.cfsan.fda.gov/;ebam/bam-toc.html. Accessed February 2007.

Roller S, Board R (2003): Naturally occurring antimicrobial systems. In: Russell N, Gould G (Eds.). *Food Preservation*, 2nd ed. Kluwer Academic/Plenum Press, New York, pp. 262–290.

Ross A, Griffiths M, Mittal G, Deeth H (2003): Combining non-thermal technologies to control foodborne microorganisms. *Int J Food Microbiol*. 39:125–138.

Russell N (2002): Bacterial membranes: the effects of chill storage and food processing. *Int J Food Microbiol*. 79:27–34.

Scott W (1957): Water relations of *Staphylococcus aureus* at 30°C. *Aust J Biol Sci*. 6:549–564.

Shachay D, Yaron S (2006): Heat tolerance of *Salmonella enterica*, and serovars Agona, Enterica, and Typhimurium in peanut butter. *J Food Prot*. 69:2687–2691.

Sheng H, Knecht H, Kudvra I, Horde C (2006): Application of bacteriophages to control intestinal *Escherichia coli* 0157:H7 levels in ruminants. *Appl Environ Microbiol*. 72:5359–5366.

Sperber W (1983): Influence of water activity on foodborne bacteria; a review. *J Food Prot*. 46:142–150.

Stern N, Kotula A (1982): Survival of *Campylobacter jejuni* inoculated into ground beef. *Appl Environ Microbiol*. 444:1150–1153.

Stokes J (1968): Nature of psychrophilic microorganisms. In: Hawthorne J (Ed.): *Low Temperature Biology of Foodstuffs*. Pergamon Press, Oxford, UK.

——— (1971): Influence of temperature on the growth and metabolism of yeasts. In: Rose AH, Harrison J (Eds). *The Yeasts*, Vol. 2, *Physiology and Biochemistry of Yeasts*. Academic Press, New York, pp. 119–134.

Stopforth J, Sofos J, Busta F (2005): Sorbic acid and sorbates.In: Davidson M, Sofos J, Branen A (Eds.). *Antimicrobials in Foods*. CRC Press, Boca Raton, FL, pp. 49–90.

Sulakvelidze Z, Alavidze Z, Morris J (2001): Bacteriophage therapy. *Antimicrob Agents Chemother*. 43:649–659.

Szabo EA, Cahill ME (1999): Nisin and ALTATM 2341 inhibit the growth of *Listeria monocytogenes* on smoked salmon packaged under vacuum or 100% CO_2. *Lett Appl Microbiol*. 28:373–377.

Tapia de Daza M, Villegas Y, Martinez A (1991): Minimal water activity for growth of *Listeria monocytogenes*. *Int J Food Microbiol*. 14:333–337.

Taylor LY, Cann DD, Welch BJ (1990): Antibotulinical properties of nisin in fresh fish packaged in an atmosphere of carbon dioxide. *J Food Prot*. 53:953–957.

ter Steeg PF, Hellemons JC, Kok AE (1999): Synergistic actions of nisin, sublethal ultrahigh pressure, and reduced temperature on bacteria and yeast. *Appl Environ Microbiol*. 65:4148–4154.

Tewari G (2002): Microbial control by packaging. In: Juneja V, Sofos J (Eds.). *Control of Foodborne Microorganisms*. Marcel Dekker, New York, pp. 191–233.

Thomas L, Delves-Broughton J (2005): Nisin. In: Davidson PM, Sofos JN, Branen A (Eds.). *Antimicrobials in Foods*, 3rd ed. CRC Press, Boca Raton, FL, pp. 239–275.

Townsend D, Wilkinson B (1992): Proline transport in *Staphylococcus aureus:* a high-affinity system and a low affinity system involved in osmoregulation. *J Bacteriol.* 174:2702–2710.

Troller J (1971): Effect of water activity on enterotoxin B production and growth of *Staphylococcus aureus*. *Appl Microbiol.* 21:435–439.

——— (1987): Adaptation and growth of microorganism environments with reduced water activity. In: Rockland L, Beuchat L (Eds.). *Water Activity: Theory and Applications*. Marcel Dekker, New York, pp. 101–117.

USFDA-CFSAN (U.S. Food and Drug Administration–Center for Food Safety and Applied Nutrition) (1998): 21CFR113. Thermal processed low acid foods packaged in hermetically-sealed contains. http://www.cfsan.fda.gov/~lrd/FCF113.html. Accessed February 2007.

Vigil A, Palou E, Alzamora S (2005): Naturally occurring compounds: plant sources. In: Davidson M, Sofos J, Branen A (Eds.). *Antimicrobials in Foods*. CRC Press, Boca Raton, FL, pp. 429–452.

Wemekamp-Kamphuis H, Karatzas A, Wouters J, Abee T (2002): Enhanced levels of cold-shocked proteins in *Listeria monocytogenes* LO28 upon exposure to low temperature and high pressure. *Appl Environ Microbiol.* 68:456–463.

Whitman P, Marshall RT (1971): Isolation of psychrophilic bacteriophage: host systems from refrigerated food products. *Appl Microbiol.* 22:220–223.

Wirjantoro TI, Lewis MJ, Grandison AS, Williams GC, Delves-Broughton J (2001): The effect of nisin on the keeping quality of reduced heat-treated milks. *J Food Prot.* 64:213–219.

Yamasato K, Okuno D, Ohtomo T (1973): Preservation of bacteria by freezing at moderately low temperatures. *Cryobiology.* 10:453–463.

Yamazaki K, Murakami M, Kawai Y, Inoue N, Matsuda T (2000): Use of nisin for inhibition of *Alicyclobacillus acidoterrestris* in acidic drinks. *Food Microbiol.* 17:315–320.

Ye M, Neetoo H, Chen H (2008): Control of *Listeria monocytogenes* on ham steaks by antimicrobials incorporated into chitosan-coated plastic films. *Food Microbiol.* 25:260–280.

Zhao T, Doyle MP, Besser RE (1993): Fate of enterohemorragic *Escherichia coli* O157:H7 in apple cider with and without preservatives. *Appl Environ Microbiol.* 59:2526–2530.

CHAPTER 25

FOOD SAFETY AND INNOVATIVE FOOD PACKAGING

JUNG (JOHN) H. HAN

25.1 INTRODUCTION

25.1.1 Food Safety

Food safety is of public concern and its definition is evolving due to its highly political nature and its global health importance (Nestle, 2003). Food safety is an integrated index of a degree of protection from hazards, of reliability, and of edibility of foods; therefore, safe foods are securely protected, reliably produced, and harmless edible and nutritious products. *Protection* means to secure the food products out of harm's way. *Reliability* implies dependable, trustworthy, and careful actions of the entire food stream, from producers to consumers. *Edibility* describes the nondangerous, harmless, or nontoxic nature of foods as well as their positive health benefits.

Hazards endangering food safety are of chemical, physical, or biological origin. Chemical hazards include pesticides, herbicides, insecticides, and other agrochemicals, and toxic compounds. Explosion, blade-cut, broken glass, stones, and other dangerous obstacles are physical hazards. Pathogens, virus, parasites, insects, rodents, and other unwanted organisms are biological hazards. Most of these hazards may inadvertently compromise the safety level of food products; however, intentional tampering of foods for any political reason and, more seriously, massive and destructive acts of terrorism represent another category (see Chapter 29). The unintended hazards may break out accidentally despite thorough quality and security assurance programs. However, malicious tampering and acts of bioterrorism are unpredictable, despite vigilant food inspection programs and regulations of oversight agencies, and not only jeopardize the level of public health but also destroy innocent human life and society.

Microbiologically Safe Foods, Edited by Norma Heredia, Irene Wesley, and Santos García

25.1.2 Food Security

Food security refers to the availability of food and one's access to it. Food security exists when all people at all times have access to sufficient, safe, and nutritious food to meet their dietary needs and food preferences for an active and healthy life (Nestle, 2003). Therefore, hunger or starvation is the consequence of a low level of food security. After September 11, 2001, the meaning of food security broadened to encompass reliable access to safe food (Andrews and Prell, 2001). Thus, the common meaning of food security changed to protection of the food system against bioterrorism (Nestle, 2003). Basic approaches to antiterrorism and food safety actions involve (1) multiple layered defense lines (protecting systems), which is a great example of hurdle technology to enhance the level of newly defined security; (2) a reliable and prompt tracing system of data involved; and (3) precise assessments of risk and benefit (i.e., toxicity vs. health benefit in the case of food safety). The effectiveness of antiterrorism and food safety programs is balanced with the convenience and quality of public services. In the case of food systems, the more convenient foods, such as ready-to-eat case products or minimally processed foods, are more likely to be contaminated with undesirable hazards than are fully cooked foods, canned foods, or military rations. For example, unpasteurized cheese may satisfy the consumer's preference, but it is more likely to have pathogenic bacteria in the final products than is fully pasteurized processed cheese.

25.1.3 Food Packaging

Functions of Food Packaging Hurdle technology is an application of combined preservation factors (i.e., hurdles) to improve total quality, including safety, by utilizing an intelligent mix of hurdles (Leistner, 2000). Is packaging another hurdle to enhance the protection level, liability, and edibility of food products? Before answering the question, basic functions of food packaging should be reviewed. Most food packaging systems have five common functions: containment, protection/preservation, handling, information, and sale promotion (Table 1). There is no function to increase the safety of foods. To have an extra functional hurdle enhancing food safety, the packaging should be designed to possess new and effective

TABLE 1 Functions of Food Packaging

Technical functions
• Containment
• Protection/preservation
• Handling
Marketing functions
• Information
• Sale promotion
Newly determined functions
• Securing safety

TABLE 2 Applications of Active and Intelligent Packaging

Active Packaging	Intelligent Packaging
Oxygen-scavenging packaging	Time–temperature integrator
Antimicrobial packaging[a]	Freshness indicator[a]
Moisture-scavenging packaging	Gas permeation control packaging
Ethylene-scavenging packaging	Radio-frequency identification[a]
Ethanol-emitting packaging	Shock/vibration abuse indicator
Carbon dioxide control packaging	
Self-heating/self-cooling packaging	
Edible/biodegradable packaging	

[a]Related directly to food safety.

functions related to food safety with an intelligent concept involving a combination of other conventional hurdles. By changing the design or material of a common packaging system, it is possible to give the system an extra function that has not existed in the most common packaging systems. An extra food safety function can be added to the conventional functions of food packaging to increase the level of safety. If the new packaging system incorporates a proactive function, the new system could be identified as another hurdle.

Active and Intelligent Packaging Active packaging is defined as a packaging system that possesses attributes beyond basic barrier properties. Intelligent packaging is characterized by the extra functions of monitoring internal changes in packages, responding to changes, or containing electronic information technology devices (Rodrigues and Han, 2003). In Table 2 we list some examples of applications of active packaging and intelligent packaging. The extra functions oriented to food safety enhancement might include antimicrobial packaging, tamper-resistant packaging, a freshness indicator, or a radio-frequency identification tag, among many other practical extra functions not related directly to food safety.

25.2 INNOVATIVE PACKAGING TO ENHANCE FOOD SAFETY

25.2.1 Antimicrobial Packaging

Antimicrobial packaging, including packaging materials and design architecture, incorporates antimicrobial agents to kill or inhibit spoilage and pathogenic microorganisms during storage and distribution (Han, 2000, 2003). This function can be achieved by adding antimicrobial agents in the packaging system and/or by using antimicrobial polymers. Antimicrobial packaging is one of very promising applications of active food packaging. Since antimicrobial packaging is designed for foods, it should satisfy entire basic requirements and functions of regular food packaging (Han, 2003).

Antimicrobial packaging systems can be designed in the form of films, pouches, paper, sachets, or edible coatings (Han, 2002, 2003). These common antimicrobial packaging designs enable the food industry to adapt the new packaging materials and systems for their products without significant modification of their current packaging lines. For the commercialization of antimicrobial packaging systems, various marketing factors (e.g., logistics, cost, and consumer acceptance) should be considered (Meroni, 2000). The adaptation of antimicrobial packaging systems should not conflict with current logistic systems in the food industry or with consumers' lifestyles (Han, 2003).

Purpose and Functions of Antimicrobial Packaging The primary goal of the use of antimicrobial system is to reduce the risk caused by any hazardous microorganisms that may break into food streams from contaminated raw materials or unintentional contamination of products during the manufacturing and distribution process. In addition to this primary goal, antimicrobial packaging can decrease any intentional contamination of foods by health-related pathogens which have possibly been injected into the food for the reason of sabotage or bioterrorism. Antimicrobial packaging can also create secondary benefits besides enhanced food safety, such as shelf-life extension resulting from the elimination of spoilage microorganisms. This secondary benefit is very attractive to perishable-food manufacturers, as that could expand their market geographically. As an example, air-chilled fresh chicken meats have 2 or 3 weeks at most of shelf life at refrigeration temperatures. The poultry industry has immediate interest in the control of *Pseudomonas*, which is a major spoilage bacterium of fresh poultry meats. Control of *Pseudomonas* using an antimicrobial packaging system could extend the shelf life of air-chilled fresh chicken meats an extra 1 or 2 weeks. Bacterial foodborne pathogens such as *Salmonella*, *Listeria*, and *Campylobacter* may also exist in fresh poultry, and antimicrobial packaging should also control their growth at refrigeration temperatures as well as at 10 to 12°C in the event of possible temperature abuse during processing and distribution. Poultry companies located in the midwestern region of the United States could open their markets to all of North America with the extended shelf life provided by antimicrobial packaging and a highly controlled cold-chain system. Antimicrobial packaging augments the level of food safety by controlling pathogens and increases the degree of food quality through controlling spoilage microorganisms. Unlike the case with antimicrobial packaging, most common packaging systems can maintain only a limited level of food safety and quality because at the end of processing they do not possess any active functions to increase the degree of food safety and quality during distribution.

Antimicrobial packaging systems can be designed to help the packaging structure to release antimicrobial agents to foods or to absorb essential elements of microbial growth from foods (Fig. 1). For the release system, common antimicrobial agents incorporated into packaging system were mostly food-grade preservatives with Generally Regarded as Safe (GRAS) status, such as organic acids, enzymes, bacteriocins, natural plant extracts, or antimicrobial polymers (Table 3). For example, polyethylene cheese films containing potassium sorbate inactivated yeast and molds that grow on cheese surfaces (Han and Floros, 1997). The second mode of antimicrobial action is to remove essential growth requirements, such as oxygen or moisture, from food and packaging systems. An oxygen-absorbing system can remove oxygen inside

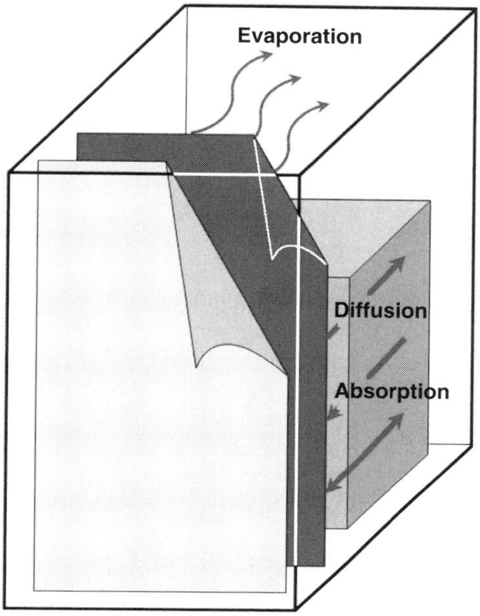

FIG. 1 Design of an antimicrobial packaging system.

packages and inhibit the growth of aerobic microorganisms such as molds. A dehydrating system reduces water activity inside packages and inhibits microbial growth. No matter which action mode (i.e., release or absorption) is used, antimicrobial packaging systems should be designed for maximum effectiveness. This is totally dependent on the antimicrobial mechanisms, physical and chemical nature of antimicrobial agents, physiology of target microorganisms, and such characteristics of foods as nutritional content, moisture content, pH, storage temperature, and shelf life.

Three Important Factors: Antimicrobial Agent, Food Composition, and Microorganism It is very important to evaluate the efficiency of antimicrobial agents before selecting any agent and constructing an antimicrobial packaging system. Antimicrobial activity can be determined by various methods. Common and basic methods are an agar diffusion test and a viable microbial count in broth culture. The clear zone of inhibition in the agar diffusion test is very simple to measure and is used most widely to determine the antimicrobial activity of water-soluble agents (Fig. 2). This method determines the effectiveness of antimicrobial agents. The microorganisms, which are either spread-plated onto the surface of the agar or incorporated (pour plated) in the agar, cannot grow with the diffused antimicrobial agents. The zone of inhibition is the area measured to evaluate antimicrobial activity. However, this method cannot be used for nontransferring antimicrobial agents, which are not soluble in water. Hydrophobic agents cannot migrate into agar media rich in water, and therefore no clear zone will be observed. For hydrophobic agents, the viable

TABLE 3 Examples of Food-Grade Antimicrobial Agents That Can Be Used for Antimicrobial Food Packaging Systems

Classification	Antimicrobial Agents
Organic acids and their derivatives	Acetic acid, benzoic acid, lactic acid, citric acid, malic acid, propionic acid, sorbic acid, succinic acid, tartaric acid, mixture of organic acids, potassium sorbate, sodium benzoate, sorbic anhydride, benzoic anhydride, propyl paraben, methyl paraben, ethyl paraben
Alcohol	Ethanol
Bacteriophages	Phages A511 and P100 for *L. monocytogenes*
Bacteriocins	Nisin, pediocin, subtilin, lacticin
Fatty acids and fatty acid esters	Lauric acid, palmitoleic acid, glycerol monolaurate
Chelating agents	EDTA, citrate, lactoferrin
Enzymes	Lysozyme, glucose oxidase, lactoperoxidase
Metals	Silver, copper, zirconium, titanium oxide
Antioxidants	BHA, BHT, TBHQ, iron salts
Antibiotics	Natamycin
Fungicides	Benomyl, imazalil, surfur dioxide
Sanitizing gas	Ozone, chlorine dioxide, carbon monoxide, carbon dioxide
Sanitizers	Cetylpyridinium chloride, acidified NaCl, triclosan, trisodium phosphate, cresol
Polysaccharide	Chitosan
Phenolics	Catechin, hydroquinone
Plant volatiles	Allyl isothiocyanate, cinnamaldehyde, eugenol, isoeuginol, linalool, terpineol, thymol, carvacrol, pinene
Plant/spice extracts	Grape seed extract, grapefruit seed extract, hop beta acid, *Brassica erucic* acid oil, rosemary oil, oregano oil, basil oil, clove oil, cinnamon oil, other herb/spice extracts and their oils
Probiotics	Lactic acid bacteria

Source: Modified from Han (2000, 2003), Suppakul et al. (2003a).

cell count in liquid broth media estimates the antimicrobial activity. However, these antimicrobial activities measured with culture media in vitro may not predict their efficacy in real food matrices. Compared to defined culture media, foods have more complex ingredients. The agar diffusion test or viable cell count is a good screen for potential antimicrobial agents. But when the antimicrobial packaging system is utilized commercially, the antimicrobial activity should be reevaluated by the viable cell counting test with real foods. Overall, there is no standard method to quantify antimicrobial activity. Based on the nature of antimicrobial agents and media ingredients, researchers should develop suitable determination procedures for antimicrobial activity. Each antimicrobial agent has its own chemical and physical characteristics, such as polarity, volatility, dissociation–association of ions depending on pH, and boiling temperature. These characteristics should be considered carefully in selecting

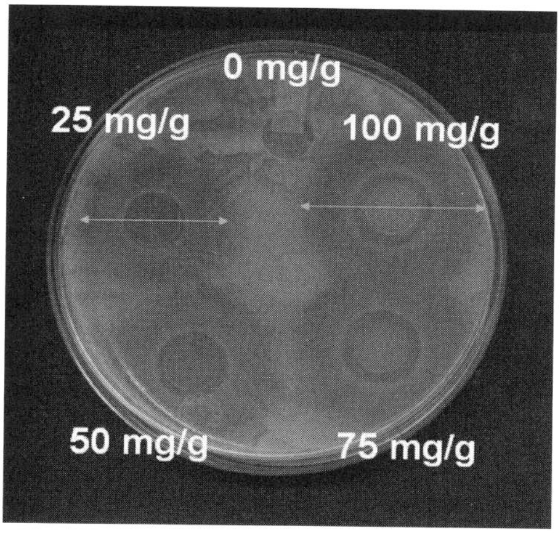

FIG. 2 Agar diffusion test. Disk-shaped films contain various concentration of lysozyme. Clear zone indicates no growth of *Brochthorix thermosphacta*.

effective antimicrobial agents with respect to such conditions as packaging material fabrication, incorporation methods of the agent into the packaging material, residual antimicrobial activity, and antimicrobial mechanisms. However, the most important aspect of the use of antimicrobial agents is to satisfy all regulations of authorized governmental agencies or associations. The antimicrobial agents should be food ingredients, food-grade additives, or food-contact substances. They must satisfy all regulations related to constituents to be used in an antimicrobial packaging system. The use of natural antimicrobial agents such as organic acids, herb extracts, or other plant volatile oils, which are generally regarded as safe (GRAS), are very promising approaches (Nadarajah et al., 2005b; Suppakul et al., 2003b). Research on natural antimicrobial agents and the development of the packaging systems incorporating natural agents are growing in popularity because these agents are found in food ingredients, have GRAS status, and are partially or wholy free of food regulations.

Foods are complex systems with multiple ingredients representing various chemical and physical characteristics. In addition to these food characteristics, food products have optimal storage conditions, including storage temperature, time period, and in-package atmosphere. Among this complexity of foods and storage conditions, the most important variables related to food quality and safety are water activity, pH, nutrients (sugar and nitrogen contents), other compositions, and storage temperature. These food characteristics and storage conditions dictate the balance of the microbial world in the food: the microflora. Therefore, these characteristic food compositions and storage temperatures provide optimal environments to only a small number of different microorganisms, which may be spoilage, pathogenic, or fermentative. Because of these typical microbial characteristics of foods, we can predict the microflora and assign specific target hazardous microbes for food products (Fig. 3).

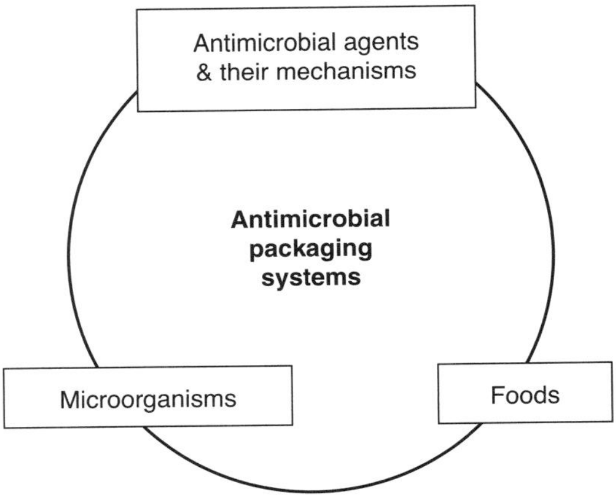

FIG. 3 Antimicrobial packaging systems with three important factors related to research and development.

Every microorganism has its own physiological characteristics and responds to specific environmental conditions for its survival. Based on oxygen requirements, microorganisms are broadly divided into aerobes, microaerobes, anaerobes, and facultative anaerobes. The oxygen requirement is a very important factor in the design of a food packaging system with regard to the prevention of spoilage and pathogenic microorganisms. Cheeses are packaged in gas-impermeable thick films with vacuum treatments. This oxygen-free packaging system inhibits the growth of the molds that reduce the shelf life, quality, and chemical safety of cheeses. However, not only for cheese but also for fresh meats, such a vacuum packaging system could provide a favorable atmosphere for anaerobic microorganisms which have never before been of concern. Storage temperature is also an important factor in determining potential microbial growth. Based on the optimal growth temperature, microbes are classified as: thermophiles, mesophiles, and psychrotrophs. As an example, a cold-chain system maintains low storage and distribution temperatures and prevents the growth of thermophiles and mesophiles. A cold-chain system could protect foods from the activation of most pathogens, which are generally mesophiles. But this refrigeration may create a temperature condition favorable to psychrotrophs. Therefore, we could predict the growth of certain microorganisms in a specific food item and select the most suitable antimicrobial agent to inactivate the potential target microorganisms. Properly designed antimicrobial packaging system could therefore eliminate the risk of foodborne illness by inhibiting the predicted growth of potential pathogens under the specific conditions of food composition and storage and distribution systems.

Example of Studies on Antimicrobial Food Packaging Antimicrobial packaging systems could be constructed in various ways, the first being to use antimicrobial packaging films. Antimicrobial packaging films can be fabricated by direct incorporation of agents into plastic or paper raw materials and by casting a film or sheet with the raw materials. Han and Floros (1997) blended potassium sorbate into low-density polyethylene and produced antifungal cheese packaging films. Potassium sorbate is released from the plastic film into cheeses at the specific mass transfer rate. Besides the blending of agents into packaging materials, antimicrobial film can also be produced by a coating method. This process mixes antimicrobial agents into a solvent of binder polymers applied to one side of packaging films, which when dried forms a coated film. Another way to produce antimicrobial films is to utilize antimicrobial polymers. Natural polymers have inherent antimicrobial functionality which can be used as a food packaging material. For example, medium-molecular-weight chitosan (i.e., acetaldehyde-removed chitin) has effective antimicrobial activity. Chitosan can form a brittle film, and this film can be used for food packaging that exhibits an inhibitory effect on the growth of microorganisms (Hong et al., 2000; Sebti et al., 2005).

In the case of most packaged solid or semisolid foods, microorganisms grow primarily at the surface of foods (Brody et al., 2001). Therefore, the contact antimicrobial films with the surface of packaged foods is critical unless the antimicrobial agents are volatile. Antimicrobial packaging containing volatile agents does not require the surface contact of packaging materials with the food. They can vaporize into headspace and control the microbes at any surface of the food.

The second method of constructing antimicrobial packaging systems is to insert an antimicrobial sheet, sachet, tray, or other form of object into common barrier packages with foods. In one investigation, butcher's paper containing volatile horseradish oil, of which allyl isothiocyanate is a major compound, was inserted into a plastic pouch with ground beef (Fig. 4). This paper insert effectively controlled the growth of *E. coli*

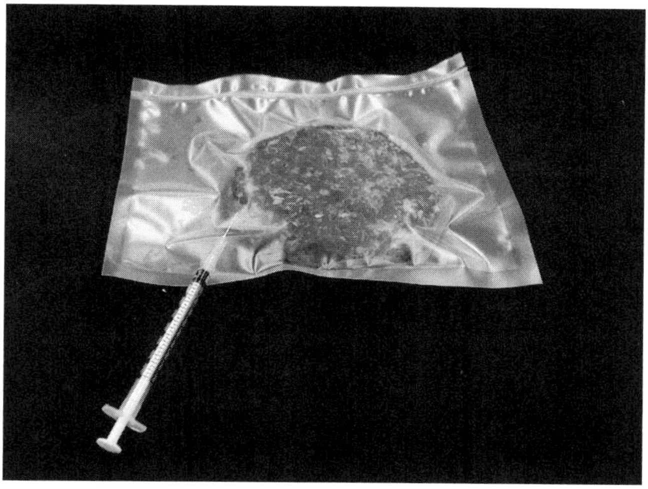

FIG. 4 Antimicrobial packaging of ground beef. The plastic pouch contains antimicrobial paper under the ground meat, which releases volatile antimicrobial agent (allyl isothiocyanate). The syringe takes headspace gas samples to monitor the effective concentration of the volatile antimicrobial agent inside the pouch to inactivate *Escherichia coil* O157:H7. (From Nadarajah et al., 2005b.)

O157:H7 in the ground beef (Nadarajah et al., 2005b). Nadarajah et al. (2005a) also investigated the use of mustard powder to inactivate the pathogen in the ground beef. Their antimicrobial packaging system completely killed inoculated *E. coli* O157:H7 during storage in the refrigerator. In addition to the inserts, sachets are also very convenient carriers of volatile antimicrobial agents. An ethanol-emitting sachet is commercially available for controlling molds and alcohol-sensitive bacteria (Smith et al., 1987). This sachet releases ethanol into the headspace of a package and increases the ethanol vapor above the critical inhibitory concentration for microbial growth.

The third way to create an antimicrobial packaging system is to apply antimicrobial edible coatings directly on foods before conventional packaging. Min and Krochta (2005) incorporated lactoferrin (natural antimicrobial peptide existing in milk) into whey protein isolate coating solutions and demonstrated antimicrobial activity against mold. Common edible coating materials are whey protein, corn zein, soy protein, wheat gluten, cornstarch, modified starch, beeswax, and shellac (Krochta and De Mulder-Johnston, 1997). Recently, the U.S. Food and Drug Administration approved the use of a surface spray consisting of six bacteriophages to be used on ready-to-eat meats and poultry (hot dogs and luncheon meat) to kill *Listeria monocytogenses* (USFDA-CFSAN, 2006).

An antimicrobial packaging system strives for safety very actively by inactivating potential hazardous pathogens. Through this reactive antimicrobial action, the level of safety of packaged food can be upgraded during storage and distribution. Antimicrobial packaging could enhance food safety through the concept of hurdle technology with other progressive actions and systems of safety management.

25.2.2 Tamper-Resistant Packaging

Goals and Advantages of Tamper-Resistant Packaging Tamper-resistant packaging is very different from tamper-evident packaging. However, the two functions are related and it is practically meaningless to separate them. Because a tampered package with damaged seals is easy to spot and remove from the food stream, tamper-evident packaging reduces the possibility of successful tampering attempts, whereas tamper-resistant packaging also decreases the chance of tampering. Of course, many tamper-evident packages lack the tamper-resistant function. However, the resistance is not perfectly effective in preventing or proving tampering. Commercially, there is no tamper-proof packaging.

Tamper-resistant packaging can be used to prevent counterfeit generation. Counterfeit of genuine products or tax payment seals could easily be identified by tamper-resistant packaging. The counterfeit-evident function of tamper-resistant packaging can be used effectively not only for food products but also for more expensive commodities such as tobacco, pharmaceutical and medical products, software (e.g., programs, games, audio CD), portable electronic devices, and other items.

Designs and Materials of Tamper-Resistant Packaging The tamper-resistant function of a package can be achieved by exploiting new structural designs or new sealing materials. The child-resistant caps used on pharmaceuticals exemplifies the tamper-resistant function obtained by design innovation. Materials for tamper-resistant packaging include tapes, shrinkwraps, wires, metal taps, imprinted waxy sealants, and holographic seals. They are designed to prohibit counterfeit generation and to break upon any attempt at tampering.

As illustrated by the example of safety (or security) seals, the role of the safety seal is very important to shield pre-inspected sites visually. This security seal does not improve the safety level at the site; however, it maintains the degree of safety. By analogy, tamper-resistant packaging does not improve the level of quality or safety of packaged foods, but it verifies the security of safe packages and can therefore maintain the safety level of packaged foods assured visually. Tamper-resistant packaging is a practical but passive or defensive method of safety action, as it is not responsive or reactive.

25.2.3 Freshness Indicator

Mechanisms of Freshness Indication A freshness indicator is designed to detect a specific target chemical inside a package. The target chemical could be a metabolite of undesired microbial growth or unwanted chemical reaction. A freshness indicator functions at different checkpoints in the safety deterioration process as noted by a time–temperature integrator (TTI) (Fig. 5). A TTI is a device that records the time–temperature profile of a product. It may use any chemical reaction or compounds changing in physical properties in response to time and temperature. Its changing mechanism should be studied thoroughly for the kinetics of the changes. Therefore, a TTI indicates the temperature and time history of the products. A TTI may be used to identify preexisting temperature abuse because temperature abuse can cause the growth of unexpected microorganisms or any physicochemical changes in food products. A TTI does not identify the growth of pathogens or their metabolites; instead, it warns that the food product has been treated improperly at an abnormal temperature that may provide favorable atmospheric conditions to pathogens,

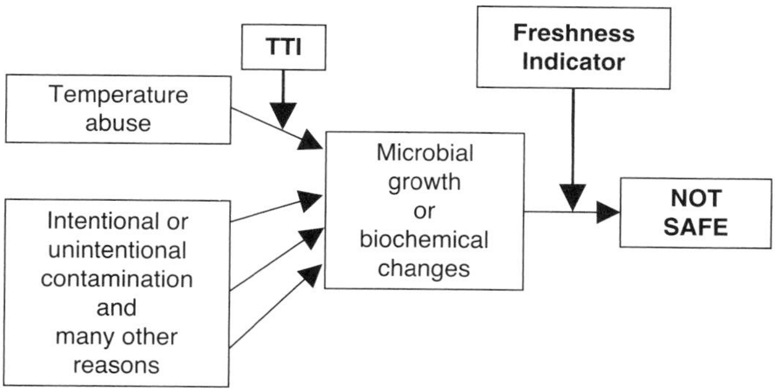

FIG. 5 Working position of a time–temperature integrator (TTI) and a freshness indicator in a cause-and-effect diagram of safety degradation.

TABLE 4 Common or Potential Mechanisms of Freshness Indicators

Detecting Compounds	Causes of the Changes
pH changes	Organic acids, alkali chemicals, oxidizing enzymes
Nitrogen compounds	Ammonia from protein degradation, biogenic amines
Sulfuric compounds	H_2S from the degradation of sulfur-containing biocompounds
Biochemical metabolites	Diacetyl, aldehydes, and alcohol produced by fermentative microbes
Energy sources	Glucose depletion, ATP reduction

Source: Adapted from Brody et al. (2001), Smolander (2003).

regardless of the microbial growth. In contrast, the freshness indicator detects the specific biochemical compound formed during the growth of target microorganisms or target metabolisms. Both TTI and freshness indicators are good applications of active packaging to ensure the quality of the packaged products.

Benefits and Concerns of Freshness Indication A freshness indicator generally uses the changes in color due to the reaction of target chemical agents to indicator dye compounds. Various mechanisms to indicate the target chemicals exist. Table 4 shows the general categories of the freshness-indicating mechanisms. All freshness indicators are designed to sense target chemical compounds. Therefore, it is a sensing-target-oriented technology regardless of the main causes of target compound generation, which could initiate a false alarm. In the case of a pH indicator, the pH of packaged food could be changed for many reasons. If the pH changes through different reactions—for example, the growth of lactic acid bacteria rather than by a sensing target chemical compound such as pathogen metabolites—the freshness indicator registers a false alarm. Or, the packaged food could be spoiled or contaminated by hazardous chemicals or unexpected pathogens other than the target compounds, in which case the freshness indicator will show "Safe."

No matter which specific mechanisms or principles of freshness indication are applied, the reaction indicated should be irreversible, so that the unsafe notification of the indicator remains after the specific target compounds are diminished. A freshness indicator neither improves nor maintains the degree of safety or security. However, this technology can also be used effectively to screen unsafe products and remove them from food streams.

25.2.4 Radio-Frequency Identification

Electronic Product Code An electronic product code (EPC) is a compact license plate identifying each product, case, box, or pallet in a supply chain (Michel, 2005). Manufacturers and retailers have more accurate management, inspection, and information control through wireless reading of the electronic tag. A radio-frequency identification (RFID) system (Fig. 6) is an application of EPC systems currently utilized by large-scale chain stores and distribution channels. Although there are

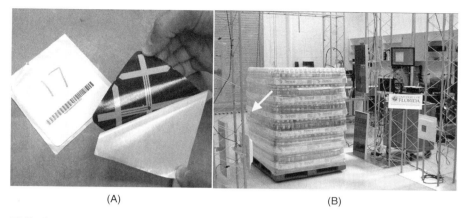

(A) (B)

FIG. 6 (A) RFID tag and a tag on a pallet (B, arrow) at a receiving dock door equipped with an RF antenna. (Courtesy of Bruce Welt at the University of Florida, and published with permission.)

different designs, all RFID tags are transducers emitting radio-frequency signals. Each RFID has its own coded signal of identification. The overall RFID system requires RFID tags, a receiving antenna, readers connected to the antenna, and a computer system for data storage or communication. In the production supply chain of food products, RFID tags could be used on four different levels: individual packages, display cartons, shipping boxes, and/or pallets. If products had tags attached on all four-levels, one scan of a pallet could read not only the information regarding the pallet, but also of all cases on the pallet, all display cartons in the cases, and all individual packages without contacting the tags to the antenna or opening the packaging materials to reveal the tags.

Advantages of RFID for Food Safety Enhancement The RFID benefits the food industry in shipping and receiving, averting product theft, preventing counterfeiting, and minimizing the time to mobilize a product recall (Michel, 2005). RFID facilitates accurate delivery of the exact amounts of the correct food products. Since an RFID system creates a record of the chain of custody for each product, it prevents item loss or theft. The identical signal for each RFID can determine the authenticity of a shipment, resulting in prevention of counterfeiting. Above all, by enabling more accurate identification, the RFID system allows immediate access to the exact location of recalled products in the distribution channel. Therefore, an RFID system enhances the traceability of food products as a consequence of safety assurance. ISO 8402 defines traceability as the ability to trace the history, application, or location of an entity through recorded identifications. More traceable food products are considered safer. Therefore, an RFID system can enhance the level of safety by providing more accurate, precise, and immediate tracking of food products and by improving the traceability of the foods.

25.3 CONCLUSIONS

Food packaging is constructed to protect packaged foods from quality deterioration. Conventional food packaging is essentially required to maintain the initial quality of foods but cannot increase the level of food safety. However, active and intelligent packaging systems are good means to improve the level of food safety. Promising applications of active and intelligent packaging to enhance the safety level of foods include antimicrobial packaging, tamper-resistant packaging, freshness indication, and radio-frequency identification.

REFERENCES

Andrews MS, Prell MA (2001): *Second Food Security Measurement and Research Conference*, Vol. 2. USDA/ERS, Washington DC.

Brody AL, Strupinsky ER, Kline LR (2001): *Active Packaging for Food Applications*. Technomic Publishing, Lancaster, PA, pp. 131–196.

——— (2000): Antimicrobial food packaging. *Food Technol*. 54:56–65.

——— (2002): Protein-based edible films and coatings carrying antimicrobial agents. In: Gennadios A (Ed.): *Protein-Based Films and Coatings*. CRC Press, Boca Raton, FL, pp. 485–499.

——— (2003): Antimicrobial food packaging. In: Ahvenainen R (Ed.). *Novel Food Packaging Techniques*. Woodhead Publishing, Cambridge, UK, pp. 50–70.

Han JH, Floros JD (1997): Casting antimicrobial packaging films and measuring their physical properties and antimicrobial activity. *J Plastic Film Sheeting*. 13:287–298.

Hong SI, Park JD, Kim DM (2000): Antimicrobial and physical properties of food packaging films incorporated with some natural compounds. *Food Sci Biotechnol*. 9:38–42.

Krochta JM, De Mulder-Johnston C (1997): Edible and biodegradable polymer films: challenges and opportunities. *Food Technol*. 51:61–74.

Leistner L (2000): Basic aspects of food preservation by hurdle technology. *Int J Food Microbiol*. 55:181–186.

Meroni A (2000): Active packaging as an opportunity to create packaging design that reflects the communicational, functional and logistical requirements of food products. *Packag Technol Sci*. 13:243–248.

Michel R (2005): Reality meets radio-frequency identification. *Manuf Bus Technol*. 23:20–22.

Min S, Krochta JM (2005): Inhibition of *Penicillium commune* by edible whey protein films incorporating lactoferrin, lacto-ferrin hydrolysate, and lactoperoxidase systems. *J Food Sci*. 70:M87–M94.

Nadarajah D, Han JH, Holley RA (2005a): Inactivation of *Escherichia coli* O157:H7 in packaged ground beef by allyl isothiocyanate. *Int J Food Microbiol*. 99:269–279.

——— (2005b): Use of mustard flour to inactivate *E. coli* O157:H7 in refrigerated ground beef under nitrogen flushed packaging. *Int J Food Microbiol*. 99:257–267.

Nestle M (2003): *Safe Food: Bacteria, Biotechnology, and Bioterrorism*. University of California Press, Berkeley, CA.

Rodrigues ET, Han JH (2003): Intelligent packaging. In: Heldman DR (Ed.). *Encyclopedia of Agricultural and Food Engineering*. Marcel Dekker, New York, pp. 528–535.

Sebti I, Martial-Gros A, Carnet-Pantiez A, Grelier S, Coma V (2005): Chitosan polymer as bioactive coating and film against *Aspergillus niger* contamination. *J Food Sci*. 70:M100–M104.

Smith JP, Ooraikul B, Koersen WJ, van de Voort FR, Jackson ED, Lawrence RA (1987): Shelf life extension of a bakery product using ethanol vapor. *Food Microbiol*. 4:329–337.

Smolander M (2003): The use of freshness indicators in packaging. In: Ahvenainen R (Ed.). *Novel Food Packaging Techniques*. Woodhead Publishing, Cambridge, UK, pp. 127–143.

Suppakul P, Miltz J, Sonneveld K, Bigger SW(2003a): Active packaging technologies with an emphasis on antimicrobial packaging and its applications. *J Food Sci*. 68:408–420.

——— (2003b): Antimicrobial properties of basil and its possible application in food packaging. *J Agric Food Chem*. 51:3197–3207.

USFDA-CFSAN (U.S. Food and Drug Administration–Center for Food Safety and Applied Nutrition) (2006): FDA approved of *Listeria*-specific bacteriophage preparation on ready-to-eat (RTE) meat and poultry products. http:www.cfsan.fda.gov/~dms/opabacqa.html. Accessed June 2008.

PART V

DETECTION OF FOODBORNE PATHOGENS

CHAPTER 26

TRADITIONAL METHODS FOR DETECTION OF FOODBORNE PATHOGENS

LUISA SOLÍS, EDUARDO SÁNCHEZ, SANTOS GARCÍA, and NORMA HEREDIA

26.1 INTRODUCTION

Microbiological examination of foods and food ingredients helps to assess safety to consumers, stability or shelf life under normal storage conditions, and the level of sanitation used during processing. Thus, routine examination of foods to detect selected pathogens is necessary. Most analyses look for indicator organisms, which are more rapidly enumerated and whose presence in foods indicates exposure to conditions that might introduce hazardous organisms and/or the probable proliferation of infectious or toxigenic species. Precautions should be taken by laboratory personnel handling foods for examination, since one or more pathogenic microorganisms or toxins can be present.

The three basic categories of tests in microbiology include presence–absence tests, enumeration tests, and identification or characterization tests. Pioneers of microbiology developed the fundamental methods traditionally used for many of these tests. In this chapter we describe briefly the most commonly used techniques in this area.

26.2 GENERAL QUANTIFICATION METHODS

26.2.1 Conventional Plate Count

The most important information used to assess the quality, spoilage, and safety of foods and to determine potential implications of foodborne pathogens is determination of total viable cell counts in food, water, food–contact surfaces, and air in food plants. The aerobic plate count (APC), also known as the aerobic colony count

Microbiologically Safe Foods, Edited by Norma Heredia, Irene Wesley, and Santos García

(ACC), heterotrophic plate count (HPC), total plate count (TPC), or standard plate count, estimates the number of total viable aerobic bacteria per gram or milliliter of product. Detailed procedures for determining the APC of foods have been developed by the Association of Official Analytical Chemists (AOAC) and the American Public Health Association (APHA) (Maturin and Peeler, 2001).

In the APC method, a portion of the sample is mixed with a specified agar medium and incubated under specific conditions of time and temperature. It is assumed that each viable aerobic bacterium will multiply under these conditions and give rise to a visible colony that can be counted. Bacteria that can be enumerated include psychrophiles, which grow optimally at or below 15°C; mesophiles, whose optimum growth temperature is between 20 and 45°C; and thermophiles, which grow optimally at temperatures above 45°C (Health Canada, 2001a).

A very important aspect of APC analysis requires that a truly representative analytical sample be taken by mixing liquid or free-flowing material until the contents are homogeneous. In solid samples, portions should be taken from several locations within the sample unit.

Samples received in the laboratory must be analyzed as soon as possible. Shellfish must be analyzed within 24 h of collection. However, frozen samples can be softened by storing up to 18 h at 2 to 5°C, or under time and temperature conditions that prevent microbial growth or death. The procedure for analysis of frozen, chilled, precooked, or prepared foods is usually similar. Dilutions of 1 : 10 are usually prepared to a concentration of 25 g or 25 mL per 225 mL of the required diluents [commonly 0.1% peptone water (PW)]. According to the APHA, at least 10 g or 10 mL of sample is homogenized with exactly nine times the weight or volume of diluent. After homogenizing by blending or shaking, decimal dilutions (10^{-2}, 10^{-3}, 10^{-4}, and others as appropriate) are prepared (Health Canada, 2001a). One milliliter of each dilution is dispensed into petri dishes and 12 to 15 mL of plate count agar (45 ± 1°C) is added. This procedure should not take more than 15 min after the initial dilution (Maturin and Peeler, 2001). Petri dishes are then rotated and tilted to homogenize the content. After the agar solidifies, plates are inverted and incubated for 48 ± 4 h, or up to 5 days, for psychrophilic and thermophilic organisms. The incubation temperature will depend on the growth temperature requirements of target organisms. Psychrophilic bacteria should be cultured between 15 and 20°C, mesophilic bacteria between 30 and 35°C, and thermophilic bacteria at 55°C.

After the incubation period, colonies are enumerated on plates with 20 to 200 or 25 to 250 colonies, including pinpoint colonies. When plates have less than 25 or more than 250 colonies, the results should be reported as "estimated aerobic plate counts (EAPC)." When no colonies are detected in any plate dilution, APC is reported as less than 1 times the corresponding lowest dilution used (Maturin and Peeler, 2001).

In some samples such as meat and milk powder, food particles could interfere with colony enumeration. In these cases it is recommended that one extra plate of each dilution be made and held under refrigeration as a control for comparison during counting. Alternatively, after incubation, plates can be flooded with 2 mL of 0.1% 2,3,5-triphenyltetrazolium chloride. After gently rotating the plates to ensure that the solution is distributed homogeneously, the plates are allowed to stand at room temperature for 3 h in an inverted position. The bacteria will reduce the indicator to a formazan, which results in red colonies and aids in enumeration (Health Canada, 2001a).

26.2.2 Enumeration of Yeast and Molds

Fungi are ubiquitous organisms that often are associated with the spoilage and biodeterioration of a large variety of foods and feedstuffs. Because of the importance of fungi in assessing food quality, quick and accurate procedures to detect and enumerate these contaminants in food commodities are essential (Bleve et al., 2003).

Prior to analysis, it should be assumed that xerophilic molds and osmophilic yeast are organisms that prefer reduced water for growth. With the exception of shelf-stable products, samples should be refrigerated (0 to 5°C) during storage and transport. Frozen products should be kept frozen until analysis. Frozen samples should be thawed in a refrigerator or under time and temperature conditions that prevent microbial growth or death (Douey and Wilson, 2004).

Traditionally, a 25- to 50-g sample is diluted 1 : 10 in 0.1% PW as diluent (Tournas et al., 2000). After homogenization, decimal dilutions are prepared. Two different procedures can be followed for plating and incubation of sample. In the spread-plate method, 0.1 mL of each dilution is aseptically added to pre-poured, solidified dichloran rose bengal chloramphenicol (DRBC) agar plates and spread with a sterile bent glass rod. Dichloran 18% glycerol (DG18) agar is preferred when the water content of the sample being analyzed is lower than 0.95. In the pour-plate method, 1 mL of each dilution is added to plates and 20 to 25 mL of tempered DG18 agar is added over the sample. The contents are mixed by gently swirling plates clockwise and then counterclockwise. It is important to note that no more than 20 min should elapse from preparation of sample dilutions and pouring or surface plating. Spread plating is considered superior to the pour-plate method, since surface plating results in more uniform growth and makes colony isolation easier (Tournas et al., 2000).

Molds that have been stressed should be enumerated by a surface spread plate technique, which provides maximal exposure of the cells to atmospheric oxygen and avoids heat stress from molten agar. Pour plates may be used when yeast or nonstressed mold cells are being detected (Douey and Wilson, 2004).

Ideally, the media chosen for enumeration of xerophiles or osmophiles should reflect the characteristics of the food to be analyzed. Glucose-, sucrose- or glycerol-supplemented agars and diluents should be used for analysis of high-sugar products, whereas for high-salt foods, media containing sodium chloride, perhaps in combination with a sugar, is more suitable. Also, for high-fat foods such as cheese, utilization of 2% sodium citrate solution prewarmed to 45°C as diluent is recommended (Douey and Wilson, 2004).

Plates are incubated in the dark for 3 to 5 days at 25°C and should not be inverted. If no growth is observed after 5 days, reincubation for another 48 h is recommended (Tournas et al., 2000). Osmophilic yeast may be incubated for up to 7 days. Plates are examined on the third day of incubation, and if mold or yeast colonies are numerous, these are counted and then counted again on the fifth day, if possible (Douey and Wilson, 2004).

In all cases, plates containing 10 to 150 colonies are enumerated, distinguishing, if required, yeast from mold colonies, according to their colonial morphology. Microscopic examination after staining with crystal violet may be necessary to distinguish yeast colonies from some bacterial colonies that may resemble yeast. Microscopically, yeast cells are significantly larger than bacteria and some cells may be budding (Douey and Wilson, 2004). Results are reported as colony-forming units (CFU)/g or CFU/mL. When no colonies are observed in any of the plates, the count is reported as less than 1 times the corresponding lowest dilution used (Tournas et al., 2000).

26.2.3 Most Probable Number: Presumptive Test for Coliforms, Fecal Coliforms, and *E. coli*

The coliform group includes aerobic and facultative anaerobic, gram-negative, non-spore-forming rods that ferment lactose and form acid and gas within 48 h at 35°C. The most probable number (MPN) technique is a widely used quantification method. An MPN is estimated from responses where results are reported as positive or negative in one or more decimal dilutions of the sample (Peeler et al., 1992). Thus, unlike the aerobic plate count, the MPN does not provide a direct measure of the bacterial count.

Frequently, the composition of many food products makes it difficult to use standard plate procedures, particularly when the microbial concentration of the sample is less than 10 CFU/g. At these low concentrations, the MPN technique gives more accurate counts than the plate count method for bacterial populations.

Fifty grams or milliliters of sample are mixed with 450 mL of Butterfield's phosphate-buffered water to make a 1 : 10 dilution. A 0.5% PW solution is recommended as diluent for shellfish. Water samples should be used undiluted. After blending for 2 min, decimal dilutions of the sample are made and 1-mL aliquots from each dilution are transferred to each of three lauryl tryptose (LST) tubes with a fermentation vial. A five-tube MPN is recommended for analysis of shellfish and shellfish harvest waters. At least three consecutive dilutions should be analyzed and tubes labeled according to the dilution inoculated (Christensen et al., 2002; Feng et al., 2002).

Inoculated LST broth tubes are incubated at 35°C for 24 ± 2 h and then examined for gas formation, which may be either a gas bubble in the fermentation vial or effervescence. Gas-negative tubes should be reincubated (except raw shellfish and fish products) for an additional 24 ± 2 h. Following incubation, the number of additional gas-positive tubes are recorded and confirmation tests for coliforms, fecal coliform, and *E. coli* tests are initiated, as required. The absence of gas in all the tubes at the end of 48 ± 4 h (24 ± 2 h for raw shellfish and fish products) of incubation constitutes a negative presumptive test (Christensen et al., 2002).

MPN Confirmative Test for Coliforms One loop of culture from each positive LST tube is transferred to a tube of brilliant green lactose bile (BGLB) broth with a fermentation vial. Avoid transferring the pellicle (Christensen et al., 2002). Incubate BGLB tubes at 35°C and examine for gas production at 48 ± 2 h. Calculate MPN of coliforms based on proportion of confirmed gas-positive LST tubes for three consecutive dilutions (Feng et al., 2002).

MPN Confirmative Test for Fecal Coliforms and E. coli A loop of culture from each gas-positive LST tube from the presumptive test is transferred to a tube of *E. coli* broth (EC broth) with or without 4-methylumbelliferyl-β-D-glucuronide (MUG), incubated for 24 ± 2 h at 45.5°C and then examined for gas production. Water, shellfish, and shellfish harvest water analysis should use an incubation temperature of 44.5 ± 0.2°C. If negative, the culture is reincubated and examined again at 48 ± 2 h. Results of this test are used to calculate fecal coliform MPN. The MUG assay is based on the enzymatic activity of β-glucuronidase (GUD), which cleaves the substrate MUG, to release 4-methylumbelliferone (MU). When exposed to long-wave (365-nm) UV light, MU exhibits a bluish fluorescence. The tubes containing EC-MUG broth should also be examined under UV light (366 nm) for glucuronidase activity, where blue–green fluorescence indicates a positive presumptive *E. coli* test (Christensen et al., 2002).

Confirmative Tests for E. coli Gently shake each gas-positive EC broth tube or fluorescing EC-MUG broth tube and streak a loopful of the culture onto an L-EMB or Endo agar plate. Plates are incubated at 35°C for 18 to 24 h. Nonmucoid, nucleated, dark-center colonies with or without a metallic sheen are indicative of *E. coli* (Christensen et al., 2002). Gram-negative isolates with lactose fermentation and gas production within 48 h at 35°C, with IMViC (indole, methyl red, Vog–Proskauer, citrate) patterns of + + - - for biotype 1, or - + - - for biotype 2, are considered to be *E. coli* (Feng et al., 2002).

Calculation of MPN Compute the MPN of coliform, fecal coliform, and *E. coli* per g (mL) of food (per 100 g of shellfish and fish products or per 100 mL of water) using MPN tables (Christensen et al., 2002).

26.2.4 Coliforms: Plate Method

A 1 : 10 dilution of sample dilution is prepared by aseptically blending or stomaching 25 g or mL into 225 mL (or 50 in 450 mL) of the required diluents. Decimal dilutions may be prepared as required, after obtaining a homogeneous suspension. One-milliliter aliquots of each dilution are transferred to petri dishes, and either of the following two pour-plating methods is used, depending on whether injured or stressed cells are suspected to be present:

1. Pour 10 mL of violet red bile agar (VRBA) warmed to 48°C into plates, swirl the plates to mix, and let the agar solidify. To prevent surface growth and spreading of colonies, overlay using 5 mL of VRBA, and let the agar solidify (Feng et al., 2002).
2. When resuscitation is necessary, for example in refrigerated, frozen, and processed foods, pour approximately 10 mL of tryptic soy agar (TSA) into each plate. After mixing by gentle rotation, allow the agar to solidify on a level surface. Plates are incubated at room temperature for 2 ± 0.5 h. Overlay with 5 mL of agar or an amount necessary to give a thin, even layer of double-strength VRBA (Feng et al., 2002; Wilson, 2001).

For both pour-plate methods, inverted plates are incubated for 24 ± 2 h at 35°C (Wilson, 2001). The incubation is carried out at 32°C for analysis of dairy products (Feng et al., 2002). Plates containing 25 to 250 purple-red colonies that are 0.5 mm or larger in diameter and surrounded by a zone of precipitated bile acids are counted.

To confirm coliforms, pick a representative number of colonies of each morphological type and transfer to a tube containing BGLB broth (Wilson, 2001), incubate at 35°C, and examine at 24 and 48 h for gas production. If a gas-positive BGLB tube shows a pellicle, perform a gram stain to ensure that gas production was not due to gram-positive, lactose-fermenting bacilli. The number of coliforms per gram is determined by multiplying the number of suspected colonies in percent confirmed in BGLB by the dilution factor (Feng et al., 2002).

Alternatively, *E. coli* colonies can be distinguished from coliform colonies on VRBA by adding 100 μg/mL of MUG in the VRBA overlay. After incubation, observe for bluish fluorescence around colonies under long-wave UV light (Feng et al., 2002). MacConkey agar may also be used for generic *E. coli* when incubated at 44°C for 24 h.

26.3 QUANTIFICATION AND DETECTION METHODS FOR SPECIFIC MICROORGANISMS

26.3.1 *Aeromonas*

Aeromonas species are oxidase and catalase positive, ferment glucose, and measure 1.0 to 4.4 μm by 0.4 to 1 μm. *A. hydrophila* is motile by a single polar flagellum. These organisms do not grow in 6% sodium chloride and are resistant to the vibriostatic compound O/129.

The *Aeromonas* medium base (Ryan's XLD Medium) is a commercial selective diagnostic medium available from Oxoid for the isolation of *Aeromonas* from clinical and environmental specimens when used with an ampicillin-selective supplement. It is useful for detecting *Aeromonas* spp. in tap water, bottled water, and foods, including meat, poultry, fish, and seafood. The API 20 NE is useful for identification of the isolates.

26.3.2 *Arcobacter*

The original methods for isolation of *Arcobacter* spp. were based on those developed for *Campylobacter* spp., where the protocols usually involved aerobic growth at 30°C. A commercial enrichment broth [Arcobacter broth (AB)] has been developed, and when supplemented with either CAT (cefoperazone, amphotericin, teicoplanin) or mCCDA (modified cefoperazone, charcoal, deoxycholate), may be used for the isolation of *Arcobacter* spp. or *A. butzleri*, respectively. Although both CAT and mCCDA agars support growth of *Arcobacter* spp., *Arcobacter* grows better in CAT, which also tends to support a wider range of *Arcobacter* (*A. butzleri*, *A. cryaerophilus*, and *A. skirrowii*, although *A. nitrofigilis* grows poorly) and *Campylobacter* species.

Another advantage of AB is that *Arcobacter* can reach higher population densities than when using biphasic growth methods such as a solid phase of 10% bovine blood agar and a liquid-phase overlay of brain heart infusion broth in tissue culture vessels (Phillips, 2001).

A combination of new enrichment and solid media has been developed by Johnson and Murano (JM formulation), allowing optimal aerobic growth of these bacteria at 30°C. In the solid medium, the addition of 0.05% thioglycolic acid, 0.05% sodium pyruvate, 5% sheep's blood, and cefoperazone (pH 6.9) results in a growth medium that supports *A. butzleri*, *A. cryaerophilus*, and *A. nitrofigilis*. In this medium, a deep red color develops around the *Arcobacter* colonies, making presumptive positives easier to recognize.

CIN (cefsulodin–irgasan–novobiocin) agar, which is a *Yersinia* spp.–selective media, has been used for recovery of *Arcobacter* from pork meat samples and from human cases of enteritis.

For analysis of meat samples, enrichment in *Arcobacter* selective broth (ASB) is widely used, followed by plating onto semisolid *Arcobacter* selective medium using cefoperazone, trimethoprim, piperacillin, and cycloheximide as inhibitors of accompanying flora. Cultures are incubated at 24°C (Phillips, 2001).

To recover this organism from raw poultry, *Arcobacter* enrichment broth (AEB) containing cefoperazone as the selective agent and a microaerobic incubation at 30°C, or a filter method onto mCCDA or CAT agar followed by aerobic incubation at 30°C, is recommended (Phillips, 2001).

Although species and strain identification may not always be required in clinical or food-monitoring situations, it is necessary to identify strains and clones further to determine the source(s) of infection in epidemiological studies. *Arcobacter* species are described as gram-negative, curved rods, oxidase positive, and display a corkscrew or darting motility by means of a single unsheathed polar flagellum. The main phenotypic tests used for species identification are catalase activity, nitrate reduction, cadmium chloride susceptibility, microaerobic growth at 20°C, and growth on MacConkey agar and in the presence of 3.5% sodium chloride and 1% glycine. Swarming may occur after aerobic incubation at 30°C on fresh blood agar (Phillips, 2001).

Several studies comparing protocols for isolation and identification of *Arcobacter* spp. have been published and use a combination of PCR and culturing techniques. These methods allow detection of several nonculturable and culturable forms of *A. butzleri*. DNA-based assays have also been established for rapid and specific identification of *Arcobacter* spp. and *Campylobacter* spp. (Snelling et al., 2006).

26.3.3 *Bacillus cereus*

Several methods for isolation and identification of *B. cereus* in foods have been described. In food samples where *B. cereus* may be present in spore form, non-spore-forming contaminants may be removed by treating the sample with 50% sterile ethanol for 60 min, or by heating the sample with an equal volume of deionized water at 62.5°C for 15 min before plating onto selective medium (Drobniewski, 1993).

Enumeration of *B. cereus* may be performed by the MPN method when fewer than 1000 organisms per gram of material are expected, or by a surface plating technique when expecting highly contaminated samples. The plate technique is usually performed as follows: 50 g of sample is mixed with 450 mL of Butterfield's phosphate-buffered dilution water (1 : 10 dilution), and after homogenization, serial dilutions are made. Then 0.1 mL of 10^{-2} to 10^{-6} dilutions are inoculated onto the surface of mannitol–egg yolk–polymyxin (MYP) agar plates using a sterile glass spreading rod. Other alternative media include Kim and Goepfert medium and polymyxin–pyruvate–egg yolk–mannitol plus bromothymol blue or bromocresol purple. The latter media use polymyxin B as the selective agent. Unlike many *Bacillus* species, *B. cereus* does not ferment mannitol, but does produce phospholipase C (lecithinase). Incubation for 24 to 48 h at 30°C is optimal with or without prior enrichment in media, including brain heart infusion or trypticase–soy–polymyxin broth.

After incubation at 30°C for 24 h, suspect colonies in MPY media are pink and surrounded by a precipitate zone, which indicates that lecithinase is produced. If cultures are not positive or suspicious colonies appear, it is recommended that the plates be reincubated for an additional 24 h. Pick five or more presumptive positive colonies and transfer them to nutrient agar slants for confirmation as *B. cereus* (see below).

The MPN method usually involves a three-tube MPN series using trypticase–soy–polymyxin broth (TSP). The tubes are inoculated with 1 mL of sample dilutions 10^{-1} to 10^{-3}. After incubation for 48 h, at 30°C, the presence of dense growth typical of *B. cereus* is determined. An aliquot from the tubes is streaked onto MYP agar plates and incubated for 24 to 48 h at 30°C. Transfer one or more characteristic colonies that are eosin pink, lecithinase-positive, to nutrient agar slants for confirmation as *B. cereus*. Calculation of MPN of *B. cereus* cells/g of sample is made using appropriate tables (Rhodehamel and Harmon, 2001).

B. cereus identification generally includes morphological characteristics such as colonies 5 to 6 mm in diameter with a ground-glass or matte appearance, and edges that range from circular and entire to irregular and fimbriate. Microscopically, *B. cereus* will appear as large gram-positive bacilli in short or long chains. The spores are ellipsoidal or cylindrical, central to subterminal and do not swell the sporangia.

Confirmation of *B. cereus* involves conventional biochemical tests such as production of lecithinase and lack of fermentation of mannitol on MYP agar, growth and production of acid from glucose anaerobically, reduction of nitrate to nitrite, production of acetylmethylcarbinol, decomposition of L-tyrosine and growth in the presence of 0.001% lysozyme (Drobniewski, 1993; Rhodehamel and Harmon, 2001). Serotyping and phage typing methods are available if necessary (Drobniewski, 1993; Schoeni and Lee Wong, 2005).

26.3.4 *Campylobacter*

Enrichment is required for *Campylobacter* isolation from foods and environmental samples because these bacteria are usually present in these samples in low numbers with a high level of competing microflora. In addition to enrichment, isolation media should contain oxygen quenchers and antibiotics (Trachoo, 2003).

According to the FDA methods, preparation of samples will depend on the type of food. For lobster tail or crab claws, weigh 50 to 100 g into a filter-lined bag and rinse with 100 mL of enrichment Bolton broth. For a whole meat carcass or samples that cannot be reduced to 25 g, 200 mL of 0.1% PW is added to the sample in a sterile bag and the contents are swirled for 2 to 3 min to rinse, and the rinse is poured through a sterile cheesecloth-lined funnel. The sample is centrifuged at 16,000 × *g* for 15 min, the supernatant is discarded, and the pellet is suspended in 10 mL of 0.1% PW. An aliquot (3 mL) of pellet mixture is then transferred to 100 mL of enrichment broth.

For a liquid egg yolk or whole egg mixture, weigh 25 g into 125 mL of Bolton broth to result in a dilution of 1 : 6. After mixing, 25 mL is transferred to another 100 mL of Bolton broth (1 : 48). For shellfish, a minimum of 12 shellfish should be taken to obtain a representative sample. After blending for 60 s, 25 g of shellfish homogenate is placed into a bag and 225 mL of enrichment broth is added. Make a second dilution, analyzing both the 1 : 10 and 1 : 100 enrichments. For water samples, collect 2 to 4 L of chlorinated water and mix with 5 mL of 1.0 M sodium thiosulfate per liter of sample. The sample is then filtered through 45-μm, 47-mm-diameter Zetapor filters, and the filter is immediately placed into enrichment broth. Place a swab into flask with 10 mL of enrichment broth (Hunt et al., 2001).

In the case of raw milk, other milk types, and ice cream, the pH of sample is adjusted to 7.5 with sterile 1 to 2 N NaOH, and 50 g is centrifuged for 40 min at 20,000 × *g*. The supernatant is discarded and the pellet suspended in 10 mL of enrichment broth, and then added to 90 mL of enrichment broth. For cheese, weigh 50 g of the sample into a filter bag and add 50 mL of 0.1% PW. After homogenization, the filtrate is centrifuged and the pellet suspended in 10 mL of enrichment broth, and then added to 90 mL of enrichment broth (Hunt et al., 2001). For other samples, weigh 25 g (50 g if fruit or vegetables) into a filter bag and add 100 mL of enrichment broth. After shaking gently for 5 min, the sample is held for 5 min and the filter lining is removed and allowed to drain for a few seconds.

A pre-enrichment of samples, including dairy products, is performed under microaerobic conditions (anaerobe jars with a modified atmosphere using Gas Pack, or gas tanks with a mixture of 5% O_2, 10% CO_2, and 85% nitrogen) and shaking at 37°C for 4 h. For water or shellfish samples, and samples that have been refrigerated for ≥10 days, incubate at 30°C for 3 h followed by incubation for 2 h at 37°C. Then for enrichment, incubate the samples at 42°C under microaerobic conditions for 23 to 24 h. Shellfish samples should be incubated an extra 4 h. Dairy samples are incubated for 48 h total (Hunt et al., 2001; Trachoo, 2003).

A great variety of selective media for the isolation of campylobacters have been reported. Since species differ in their resistance to antibiotics and other selective agents, no single medium is satisfactory for the isolation of all *Campylobacter* spp.

According to FDA procedures, after 24 and 48 h of incubation in enrichment broth, streak an aliquot onto either Abeyta–Hunt–Bark agar or modified Campy blood-free agar (mCCDA) and incubate at 37 to 42°C. A variety of other selective agars for isolation of campylobacters from human and animal feces have been developed, including the Skirrow agar, which is based on blood agar supplemented with trimethroprim, polymyxin B, and vancomycin; the blood-containing media Butzler agar and Campy-BAP; the Campy Line agar, based on *Brucella* agar supplemented with reducted agents and seven antibiotics; the charcoal-based media mCCDA agar; and the Preston agar, which was developed for *Campylobacter* isolation from feces and environmental samples (Höök, 2005; Hunt et al., 2001; Potturi-Venkata et al., 2007).

Several phenotypic tests are used to differentiate between *Campylobacter* species and include growth at 25°C and 42 to 43°C; catalase production; nitrate and nitrite reduction; H_2 requirement for microaerophilic growth; indoxyl acetate hydrolysis; growth in the presence of 3.5% NaCl, 1% glycine; and susceptibility to specific antibiotics such as nalidixic acid and cephalothin. *C. jejuni* is the only *Campylobacter* species that hydrolyzes hippurate. *C. jejuni* subsp. *doylei* may vary in this reaction. Therefore, hippurate hydrolysis has become the most widely used test to identify *C. jejuni*, and especially to differentiate it from the phenotypically and genotypically similar *C. coli*. However, some strains of *C. jejuni* have been shown to be hippurase negative. This indicates the need for alternative or additional tests (Höök, 2005).

A simple alternative method for *Campylobacter* isolation was proposed by the UK Health Protection Agency. Weigh a representative 25-g sample and homogenate with nine times that weight or volume of *Campylobacter* enrichment broth. Transfer the suspension to a sterile screw-capped container, leaving very little headspace (ca. 16%), and close the top tightly. If the amount of sample available is less than 25 g, add sufficient medium to ensure minimal headspace. Incubate at 37°C for 22 ± 2 h and then at 41.5°C for a further 22 ± 2 h. An aliquot is then streaked onto *Campylobacter* selective agar (CCDA) and incubated microaerobically at 37°C for 48 ± 2 h. *C. jejuni* and *C. lari appear as* flat, glossy, effuse colonies with a tendency to spread along the inoculation track, which resemble droplets of fluid. *C. coli* are less effuse, often convex colonies with the surface usually remaining shiny. Biochemical identification is recommended for typical colonies (Health Protection Agency, 2005).

26.3.5 *Clostridium botulinum*

For a complete analysis, it is recommended one portion of a food sample be used for detection of viable *C. botulinum* and another portion for toxicity testing. Detection of viable *C. botulinum* from foods involves inoculation with 1 to 2 g or mL of the food into two tubes of reduced cooked meat medium and two tubes of trypticase–peptone–glucose–yeast extract (TPGY) medium. Tubes are then incubated at 35°C and 28°C, respectively, for 5 days (Solomon and Lilly, 2001).

When honey or syrup is analyzed, take 25 g of sample into a sterile foil-covered beaker and add 100 mL of sterile distilled water containing 1.0% Tween-80 and stir the solution until homogeneous. The sample is then centrifuged and the supernatant filtered through a 0.45-μm membrane filter. Transfer the membrane and the sediment into 110 mL of trypticase–glucose–peptone–yeast extract–beef extract medium (TPYGB) and incubate at 35°C for 7 days. For cereals, 25 g of sample is mixed with 600 mL of TPGYB medium heated to 65°C, and this mixture is kept at 65°C for 30 min. Incubation is then carried out anaerobically at 35°C for 7 days (Austin, 1998).

In all cases it is recommended the inoculum be introduced slowly beneath the surface of the broth to the bottom of tube. After 5 to 7 days of incubation at 35°C, turbidity, gas production, and digestion of meat particles in the enrichment cultures (cooked meat medium, TPYG, and TPYGB) are determined (Austin, 1998; Solomon and Lilly, 2001). Look for typical clostridial cells, which resemble a tennis racket under the microscope (Solomon and Lilly, 2001).

Toxin Testing The supernatant fluid from centrifuged food samples is used for the toxin assay. Liquid foods should be tested directly (Solomon et al., 2001). Supernatant fluid from cultures of *C. botulinum* also can be used for toxin examination (Austin, 1998). Toxins of nonproteolytic types may need trypsin activation to be detected. Thus, parallel tests should be conducted using both trypsin-treated supernatants and heat-treated supernatants (10 min at 100°C) that would inactivate the toxin if present. For trypsin-treated supernatants, add 0.2 mL of aqueous trypsin solution to 1.8 mL of each supernatant fluid and incubate at 37°C for 1 h. The trypsin solution is prepared by dissolving 0.5 g of Difco trypsin (1 : 250) in 10 mL of warmed distilled water.

A bioassay using mice is the traditional test for *C. botulinum*. Pairs of mice are injected intraperitoneally with 0.5 mL of heat-treated, undiluted, and diluted (1 : 5, 1 : 10, and 1 : 100 in gel–phosphate buffer) samples of untreated and trypsin-treated supernatant fluids. To avoid or minimize nonspecific death of mice, supernatant fluids are filtered through 0.45-μm Millipore filters prior to injection (Austin, 1998; Solomon et al., 2001). After injection, the mice are observed for symptoms of botulism each hour for 48 h (Solomon et al., 2001) to 4 days (Austin, 1998). Mice injected with a positive supernatant should die. Death should not occur in mice injected with heat-treated supernatant. However, death without clinical symptoms of botulism is not sufficient evidence. If after 48 h of observation, all mice except those injected with heat-treated and trypsin-treated preparations have died, the toxicity test is repeated, using higher dilutions of supernatant fluids in order to establish an endpoint or the minimum lethal dose (MLD) as an estimate of the amount of toxin present (Solomon et al., 2001).

Toxin Typing Inject pairs of mice previously protected by specific monovalent antitoxin injection (Solomon et al., 2001) intraperitoneally with each dilution of the toxin preparation. Inject a pair of unprotected mice (without antitoxin injection) with each toxin dilution as a control. Observe mice for 48 h for symptoms of botulism and record the number of deaths. If the mortality results indicate that the toxin was not neutralized, the test is repeated using polyvalent antitoxin pool (Solomon et al., 2001).

26.3.6 *Clostridium perfringens*

Enumeration of *C. perfringens* in foods may be performed as follows: A 1 : 10 dilution of the food is prepared by aseptically shaking, stomaching, or blending 25 g or mL of food into 225 mL of peptone dilution fluid (Health Canada, 2001b; Rhodehamel and Harmon, 1998). The 1 : 10 sample/dilution ratio is maintained when the sample size is other than 25 g or m (Health Canada, 2001b). After homogenization, decimal serial dilutions are prepared, usually 10^{-1} to 10^{-6}. One milliliter of the appropriate dilution is dispensed into duplicate sterile dishes previously filled with 6 to 7 mL of TSC agar without egg yolk. After the inoculum is absorbed, 15 mL of TSC agar without egg yolk at 45°C is added. An alternative plating method consists of spreading 0.1 mL of sample or dilution over plates previously filled with TSC agar containing egg yolk emulsion. Once the inoculum has been absorbed, plates are overlaid with 10 mL of TSC agar without egg yolk emulsion (Rhodehamel and Harmon, 1998). A one-layer system has also been reported using 20 mL of sulfite cycloserine (SC) agar that is poured into each plate and then mixed by gentle rotation with the sample dilution (Health Canada, 2001b).

After agar solidification, plates are incubated under anaerobic conditions at 35°C for 20 to 24 h (Health Canada, 2001b; Rhodehamel and Harmon, 1998). Five (maximum 10) presumptive colonies (black and 1 to 2.5 mm in diameter) are randomly selected (Health Canada, 2001b; Rhodehamel and Harmon, 1998); and tested by gram stain. *C. perfringens* is a short, thick, gram-positive bacillus, and presumptive confirmation includes growth in recently prepared fluid thioglycollate broth and the iron–milk presumptive test. The latter test verifies rapid coagulation of milk followed by fracturing of curd into spongy mass (stormy fermentation). Cultures that fail to exhibit stormy fermentation within 5 h are unlikely to be *C. perfringens* (Rhodehamel and Harmon, 1998).

Complete confirmation is achieved by biochemical tests, which include nitrate-motility agar, lactose fermentation, and gelatin liquefaction. *C. perfringens* is nonmotile, reduces nitrates to nitrites, produces acid and gas from lactose, and liquefies gelatin within 48 h. Isolates can be tested for sporulation and enterotoxin production (Health Canada, 2001b; Rhodehamel and Harmon, 1998).

26.3.7 *Listeria monocytogenes*

Several methods for isolation and identification of *Listeria* spp. and *Listeria monocytogenes* from foods have been proposed. Among the most widely used protocols are those developed by the USDA, FSIS (for meat products), and FDA (for dairy products, fruits, vegetables, and seafood) (Donnelly, 2001). The conventional methodology is described below.

Twenty-five-gram samples from food are pre-enriched in 225 mL of enrichment broth [the most widely used is *Listeria* enrichment broth [(LEB base or FDA medium 52) containing sodium pyruvate]. After 4 h of incubation at 30°C, selective agents (sodium nalidixate, acriflavine, and cycloheximide) with the capacity of suppress other microbial contaminants present in foods are added.

Samples are incubated for 48 h at 30°C. An aliquot of the culture is then streaked onto selective agar [Oxford (FDA medium 118), or LPM fortified with esculin and Fe^{3+} (FDA medium 82)] and incubated for 24 to 48 h at 35°C for Oxford agar or 30°C for LMP agar (Farber and Peterkin, 1991; Hitchins, 2002). The suspect *Listeria* colonies appear in both media as black with a black halo. Confirmation is made by transferring five or more colonies to trypticase soy agar with 0.6% yeast extract (TSAye, FDA medium 153) and incubating at 30°C for 24 to 48 h (Hitchins, 2002). This culture can be used for further identification. Members of *Listeria* genus are identified by tests, including (1) examination of a TSAye colony under phase-contrast microscopy, where *Listeria* spp. appear as short rods with slight rotating or tumbling motility; (2) catalase-positive; (3) gram-positive rods in younger cultures; (4) nitrate reduction test, where only *L. grayi* sp. *murrayi* is able to reduce nitrates; (5) motility test in SIM or MTM media incubated for 7 days at room temperature, where the *Listeria* spp. are motile, giving a typical umbrella-like growth pattern (Hitchins, 2002).

The CAMP reaction is useful for identifing *Listeria* species. This test uses horse blood agar and streaks of β-hemolytic *Staphylococcus aureus* and *Rodococcus equi* in combination with *Listeria* isolates. The *L. monocytogenes* and *L. seeligeri* hemolytic reactions are enhanced in the zone influenced by the *S. aureus* streak, while the other species remain nonhemolytic in this zone. In contrast, the hemolytic reaction of *L. ivanovii* is enhanced in the zone influenced by *R. equi*.

Further characterization is obtained by inoculating purple carbohydrate broth supplemented (0.5%) with different carbohydrates, such as dextrose, maltose, rhamnose, mannitol, and xylose. After incubation for 7 days at 35°C, all species should be positive for dextrose and maltose. All *Listeria* spp. except *L. grayi* should be mannitol negative. *L. monocytogenes*, *L. innocua*, and *L. grayi* are xylose negative, and *L. monocytogenes* is rhamnose positive (Hitchins, 2002). *L. monocytogenes* and *L. ivanovii* can also be distinguished using commercial confirmatory methods (see Chapter 27).

26.3.8 *Salmonella*

Isolation of *Salmonella* spp. depends in large part on the composition of food analyzed. It is suggested that readers review Chapter 9 for more information about *Salmonella*. For pre-enrichment, a 25-g sample is transferred into an appropriate sterile container (wide-mouth flask or Whirl-Pak bag), and 225 mL of sterile lactose broth (Andrews and Hammack, 2000), nutrient broth (NB), or buffered peptone water (BPW) (D'Aoust and Purvis, 1998) is added (1 : 9 sample/broth ratio). After mixing well by swirling, the pH is adjusted if necessary to 6.8 ± 0.2 by addition of sterile 1 N NaOH or 1 N HCl, followed by incubation for 24 ± 2 h at 35°C.

In some cases, the pre-enrichment broth could differ depending on the food tested. For dried yeast, spices, and hard-boiled eggs, trypticase soy broth is recommended. For eggs, trypticase soy broth supplemented with ferrous sulfate is the best option (Andrews and Hammack, 2000). Brilliant green water is used for milk powders and nonfat dry milk (Andrews and Hammack, 2000; D'Aoust and Purvis, 1998). The universal pre-enrichment broth is recommended for analysis of lactic casein, orange juice, cantaloupes, and tomatoes. For candies and candy coating, including chocolate, reconstituted nonfat dry milk is used. Tetrathionate broth is used for food dyes and food coloring substances, and buffered PW is used for mangoes (Andrews and Jammack, 2000).

The enrichment is performed by transferring 0.1 mL into a tube with 10 mL of Rappaport–Vassiliadis (RV) medium and 1 mL into 10 mL of tetrathionate (TT) broth (Andrews and Hammack, 2000). Selenite cystine (SC) and tetrathionate brilliant green (TBG) broths also can be used as enrichment media, transferring 1.0 mL of the pre-enrichment culture (D'Aoust and Purvis, 1998). Incubation is carried out at $42 \pm 0.2°C$ for 24 ± 2 h in the case of the RV and TBG media. For TT and SC broths, the incubation is at $35 \pm 2.0°C$ for 24 ± 2 h (Andrews and Hammack, 2000; D'Aoust and Purvis, 1998). Streak replicates using a 3-mm loop of selective enrichment cultures onto plates of xylose lysine desoxicolate agar (XLD), Hektoen enteric agar (HE), and bismuth sulfite agar (BS) (Andrews and Hammack, 2000), or brilliant green sulfa (BGS, D'Aoust and Purvis, 1998). Plates are incubated for 24 ± 2 h at 35°C. If colonies suggestive of *Salmonella* have not developed on BS plates (brown, gray, or black colonies), incubate for an additional 24 ± 2 h (D'Aoust and Purvis, 1998). Typically, *Salmonella* colony morphology in HE agar is blue–green to blue colonies with or without black centers. In XLD agar, colonies are pink with or without black centers; colonies in BS agar are brown, gray, or black, and sometimes display a metallic sheen. In BGS agar, colonies are pink to fuchsia, surrounded by red medium (D'Aoust and Purvis, 1998). XLT-4 is an improved medium recommended for the isolation of this microorganism; typical colonies in this medium appear black or black-centered with a yellow periphery after 18 to 24 h of incubation.

Pick two or more isolated typical colonies with a sterile inoculating needle and inoculate TSI and LIA slants (Andrews and Hammack, 2000) and Christensen's urea agar (D'Aoust and Purvis, 1998). Incubate at 35°C for 24 ± 2 h. Store selective agar plates at 5 to 8°C (Andrews and Hammack, 2000; D'Aoust and Purvis, 1998). *Salmonella* typically produce alkaline (red) slant and acid (yellow) butt, with or without production of H_2S (blackening of agar) in TSI. In Christensen's urea agar, the urea test is negative (D'Aoust and Purvis, 1998), whereas in LIA, it produces alkaline (purple) reaction in the butt of the tube (Andrews and Hammack, 2000). Most *Salmonella* cultures produce H_2S in LIA. All cultures that give an alkaline butt in LIA, regardless of TSI reactivity, should be retained as potential *Salmonella* isolates. Cultures that give an acid butt in LIA and alkaline slant/acid butt in TSI also should be considered potential *Salmonella* isolates and should be analyzed with more biochemical tests [urease (−), lysine decarboxylase broth (+), phenol red dulcitol broth (+), KCN broth (−), malonate broth (−), indole (−), phenol red lactose broth (−), phenol red sucrose broth (−), Voges–Proskauer (−), methyl red (+), and Simmons citrate tests (+/variable)]. Serotyping using polyvalent and single-grouping somatic and flagellar antisera is also recommended. Cultures that have typical reaction patterns are reported as *Salmonella* (Andrews and Hammack, 2000).

26.3.9 *Shigella*

For the recovery of *Shigella*, a 25-g or 25-mL sample is added to 225 mL of *Shigella* broth containing 0.5 μg/mL (or 3 μg/mL for other than *S. sonnei*) of novobiocin and stomach (Andrews and Jacobson, 2000; Kingombe et al., 2006). Suspension is held for 10 min, shaking periodically at room temperature (Kingombe et al., 2006). Pour the supernatant into a sterile flask or new stomacher bag and incubate at 42°C for 20 ± 2 h in a CO_2 incubator (Kingombe et al., 2006) or into anaerobic jars containing CO_2 generator bags (GasPak; in this case incubate at 44°C) (Andrews and Jacobson, 2000).

After incubation, streak a loop of culture onto at least two selective media, such as MacConkey agar (low selectivity) (Andrews and Jacobson, 2000), xylose lysine desoxycholate (XLD, high selectivity) or Hektoen enteric (HE, moderate to high selectivity) agars and incubate for 20 to 24 h at 35°C (Andrews and Jacobson, 2000; Kingombe et al., 2006). Examine the plates for characteristic *Shigella* colonies. In MacConkey agar, colonies are slightly pink and translucent, with or without rough edges (Andrews and Jacobson, 2000). In XLD agar, colonies are red or colorless, and in HE, colonies are green (Kingombe et al., 2006).

Suspect colonies are inoculated into TSI and LIA and subjected to motility tests. Incubate at 35°C for 24 to 48 h. Typical *Shigella* spp. are positive for methyl red and negative for motility, H_2S, lysine, and gas from glucose. They are also negative for urease, sucrose, adonitol, inositol, lactose (2 days), KCN, malonate, citrate, and salicin (Andrews and Jacobson, 2000; Kingombe et al., 2006). However, some *Shigella* species may produce some gas (Kingombe et al., 2006). Reactivity with specific antiserum is recommended for identification of serotype. For serotyping, colony growth from 24 h is suspended in 3 mL of 0.85% saline. Two drops of this suspension are mixed with antiserum, and the extent of agglutination is recorded (Andrews and Jacobson, 2000).

26.3.10 *Staphylococcus aureus*

The traditional technique for isolation and enumeration of *Staphylococcus aureus* generally includes direct plate count, especially in cases when high contamination is expected (over 100 *S. aureus* cells/g). The MPN method is recommended for samples with low levels of contamination and those suspected to contain a large population of competing species.

The direct plate count method usually involves 50 g of sample (solid or liquid), which is mixed with 450 mL of Butterfield's phosphate-buffered dilution water (Bennett and Lancette, 1998). However, there are methodologies that prepare a 1 : 10 dilution of food by aseptically adding 11 or 10 g or mL to 99 or 90 mL, respectively, of PW diluent (Szabo, 2005). After shaking each dilution for 2 min, 1 mL of sample suspension is distributed among three plates of Baird–Parker agar. Then 0.4 mL is added to one plate and 0.3 mL to the others (Bennett and Lancette, 1998) and spread. In some cases, in accordance with the laboratory in-house specifications (Szabo, 2005), lower amounts of sample can be spread (e.g., 0.2 or 0.4 mL).

After the inoculum has absorbed, plates are inverted and incubated for 45 to 48 h at 35°C (Bennett and Lancette, 1998; Szabo, 2005). Presumptive *S. aureus* colonies are circular, smooth, convex, moist, 2 to 3 mm in diameter on uncrowded plates, gray to jet black, shiny black without well-defined clear zones or frequently with a light-colored (off-white) margin, surrounded by an opaque zone and frequently with an outer clear zone. When touched with an inoculating needle, colonies have a buttery to gummy consistency (Bennett and Lancette, 1998; Szabo, 2005).

For MPN determination, a three-tube series of TSB (trypticase soy broth) containing 10% NaCl and 1% sodium pyruvate are inoculated with 1-mL aliquots of decimal dilutions of each sample. The highest dilution must give a negative endpoint. After incubation for 48 ± 2 h at 35°C, a loop (10 μL) from each tube showing growth is transferred to Baird–Parker plates with a properly dried surface, incubated for 48 h at 35°C (Bennett and Lancette, 1998), and then examined for presumptive *S. aureus*. Continue with the procedure for identification and confirmation of *S. aureus* and report *S. aureus* per gram as MPN/g, according to the appropriate tables.

The coagulase test is considered the initial step for confirmation of *S. aureus*. In this test, suspect colonies are transferred into small tubes containing 0.2 to 0.3 mL of BHI broth (BD Difco United States) and incubated for 18 to 24 h at 35°C. Then 0.5 mL of reconstituted certified coagulase plasma with EDTA is added to the culture and mixed thoroughly. Tubes are incubated at 35°C and then examined periodically for 6 h, observing for clot formation (Bennett and Lancette, 1998). Negative tubes should be incubated overnight at room temperature and reexamined (Bennett and Lancette, 1998; Szabo, 2005). Other confirmatory tests include catalase, glucose, and mannitol fermentation, lysostaphin (25 μg/mL) sensitivity, and thermostable nuclease production. All of the tests above are positive for *S. aureus*. Positive and negative control cultures as well as media controls should be run simultaneously when performing all confirmation tests (Bennett and Lancette, 1998; Szabo, 2005).

26.3.11 *Vibrio*

Vibrio species are anaerobic facultative organisms that grow best under alkaline conditions and are able to grow in the presence of high levels of bile salts. These characteristics are very useful during the isolation and identification process.

V. cholerae The conventional method to detect this pathogen in food or environmental samples is usually as follows. Enrichment is made by preparing a 1 : 10 (v/v or w/v) sample dilution using alkaline peptone water (APW, pH 8.4 to 9.2) as diluent. Less common are APW with tellurite, Monsur's tellurite–taurocholate broth, and sodium–gelatin phosphate broth (Kaper et al., 1995). All the enrichment broths are incubated at 35 to 37°C for 6 to 8 h for products such as seafood or vegetables. If the product was subjected to a processing step such as heating, freezing, drying, or when low population density is expected, or to resuscitate injured cells, the incubation period should be extended to 18 to 24 h. If the sample is raw oysters, the enrichment is made in APW (1 : 100 w/v) followed by incubation at 42°C for 18 to 21 h (Kaysner and DePaola, 2004).

After enrichment, a loopful of surface growth is plated onto selective agar, the most common of which is thiosulfate–citrate–bile salts–sucrose (TCBS) agar, and incubated for 18 to 24 h at 35 to 37°C. The sucrose-fermenting *V. cholerae* characteristic colonies are detected as large, yellow, and smooth. Other less common selective agars include Monsur's tellurite–taurocholate gelatin agar, vibrio agar, and polymyxin–mannose–tellurite agar (Kaper et al., 1995).

Suspected *V. cholerae* isolates can be subcultured in nonselective agar, and standard series of biochemical tests used for identification of members of the Enterobacteriaceae and Vibrionaceae families are recommended (Kaper et al., 1995). These include (1) the arginine glucose slant, where *V. cholerae* and *V. mimicus* cultures will have an alkaline (purple) slant and an acid (yellow) butt (arginine is not hydrolyzed); (2) salt tolerance, where *V. cholerae* and *V. mimicus* cultures grow without NaCl; and (3) oxidase reaction, which is positive for *V. cholerae* (Kaysner and DePaola, 2004). However, the key confirmation test for *V. cholerae* serogroup is the agglutination test using polyvalent antisera against different antigens (Kaper et al., 1995; Kaysner and DePaola, 2004).

V. parahaemolyticus and V. vulnificus A MPN procedure is commonly used to identify these species. Weigh 50 g of seafood sample. Normally, 12 animals are pooled and blended for 90 s. Fifty grams of homogenate are used for analysis. Add 450 mL of phospate-buffered saline (PBS) to result in a 1 : 10 dilution, and homogenize. For molluscan shellfish, pool 12 animals, blend for 90 s with an equal volume of PBS, and then prepare a 1 : 10 dilution. Prepare decimal dilutions in PBS. For product that has been processed (heated, dried, or frozen) inoculate 3 × 10 mL portions of the 1 : 10 dilution into three tubes containing 10 mL of 2X APW. This represents the 1-g portion. Inoculate 3 × 1 mL portions of the 1 : 10, 1 : 100, 1 : 1000, and 1 : 10,000 dilutions into 10 mL of single-strength APW. Incubate overnight at 35 ± 2°C. Streak a loopful of culture onto TCBS agar for *V. parahaemolyticus* and onto mCPC or CC agar for V. *vulnificus*, and incubate overnight at 35 ± 2°C and 39 to 40°C, respectively. Generally, *V. parahaemolyticus* appear as round, opaque, green or bluish colonies, 2 to 3 mm in diameter on TCBS agar. Most strains of *V. parahaemolyticus* will not grow on mCPC or CC agar. If growth occurs, colonies will be green–purple in color due to lack of cellobiose fermentation. *V. vulnificus* will grow on mCPC or CC agar as round, flat, opaque, yellow colonies 1 to 2 mm in diameter.

Confirm isolates by biochemical tests (Table 1). Refer to the original positive dilutions in the enrichment broth and apply the three-tube-MPN tables for final enumeration of the organism.

26.3.12 *Yersinia*

When suspect *Yersinia* is present in food, water, or environmental samples, samples should be rapidly analyzed or stored at 4°C until analysis. Then 25 g of sample is homogenized with 225 mL of either peptone sorbitol bile broth (PSBB) or phosphate-buffered saline (PBS) and incubated for 10 days at 10°C. After incubation, the enrichment broth is mixed well and 0.1 mL of enrichment culture is transferred to a tube containing 1 mL of 0.5% KOH in 0.5% saline solution and mixed. This treatment reduces the background flora, making selection of *Yersinia* colonies less laborious (Fredriksson-Ahomaa and Korkeala, 2003; Weagant et al., 1998). After KOH treatment, one loopful is streaked onto selective agar plates. Different selective agar plating media are available. The most widely used is MacConkey (MAC) agar and cefsulodin–irgasan–novobiocin (CIN) agar. S*almonella–Shigella* deoxycholate

TABLE 1 Biochemical Characteristics of Frequently Isolated Pathogenic *Vibrio*[a]

	V. cholerae	*V. parahaemolyticus*	*V. vulnificus*
TCBS agar	Yellow	Green	Green
mCPC agar	Purple	No growth	Yellow
CC agar	Purple	No growth	Yellow
Arginine–glucose slant	Slant alkaline/ butt slightly acid	Slant alkaline /butt acidic	Slant alkaline /butt acidic
Oxidase	+	+	+
Arginine dihydrolase	−	−	−
Ornithine decarboxylase	+	+	+
Lysine decarboxylase	+	+	+
Growth (w/v):			
0% NaCl	+	−	−
3% NaCl	+	+	+
6% NaCl	−	+	+
8% NaCl	−	+	−
10% NaCl	−	−	−
Growth at 42°C	+	+	+
Acid from:			
Sucrose	+	−	−
D-Cellobiose	−	V	+
Lactose	−	−	+
Arabinose	−	+	−
D-Mannose	+	+	+
D-Mannitol	+	+	V
ONPG	+	−	+
Voges–Proskauer	V	−	−
Sensitivity to:			
10 μg O/129	S	R	S
150 μg O/129	S	S	S
Gelatinase	+	+	+
Urease	−	V	−

Source: Adapted from Kaysner and DePaola (2004).
[a]S, susceptible; V, variable among strains; R, resistant.

calcium chloride (SSDC) agar can also be used. After incubation at 30°C for 24 h, *Yersinia* spp. colonies in MAC agar are small (1 to 2 mm in diameter), flat, colorless, or pale pink. Red or mucoid colonies should be rejected. CIN plates show small colonies 1 to 2 mm in diameter with deep red centers and sharp borders surrounded by a clear colorless zone with an entire edge. Suspect colonies are inoculated into lysine arginine iron agar (LAIA) slant, anaerobic egg yolk (AEY) agar, and Christensen's urea agar plate or slant. Incubation is carried out at room temperature for 48 h. Presumptive *Yersinia* isolates give alkaline slant and acid butt, no gas, and no H_2S (KA–) reaction in LAIA, and are urease-positive. *Yersinia* in AEY agar is lipase-positive.

When high levels of *Yersinia* are suspected, the following methodologies are recommended: (1) Spread 0.1 mL of sample onto MAC agar and 0.1 mL onto CIN agar before inoculation into enrichment broth; (2) transfer 1 mL of the sample or homogenate to 9 mL of 0.5% KOH in 0.5% saline solution, and after homogenization for several seconds, spread-plate 0.1 mL on MAC and CIN agars. Plates are incubated at 30°C for 24 h. Suspect colonies may be transferred to sterile Whatman 541 filter paper and examined for a *Yersinia* virulence gene by DNA colony hybridization (Weagant et al., 1998).

Biochemical identification of the isolates is recommended (Bottone, 1997; Fredriksson-Ahomaa and Korkeala, 2003). *Y. enterocolitica* (or even *Y. pseudotuberculosis*) produces anaerogenic fermentation of glucose and other carbohydrates, it is motile at 25°C but not 37°C, and is negative for oxidase, phenylalanine deaminase, lysine decarboxylase, and arginine dihydrolase tests (Bottone, 1997).

Virulent and avirulent *Y. enterocolitica* strains can be differentiated by growth in Congo Red agar. Virulent *Y. enterocolitica* strains take up Congo Red (CR1), which correlates with the presence of the 60- to 75-kb virulence plasmid. Colonies that do not take up Congo Red (CR2) are lacking this plasmid and are designated negative in this assay (Bottone, 1997).

REFERENCES

Andrews WH, Hammack TS (2000): *Salmonella*. In: Bacteriological Analytical Manual online, 8th ed., Rev. A, Chap. 5. http://www.cfsan.fda.gov/~ebam/bam-5.html. Accessed January 18, 2007.

Andrews WH, Jacobson A (2000): *Shigella*. In: Bacteriological Analytical Manual online, 8th ed., Rev. A, Chap. 6. http://www.cfsan.fda.gov/~ebam/bam-6.html. Accessed January 26, 2007.

Austin JW (1998): Health Protection Branch: detection of *Clostridium botulinum* in honey and syrups. MFLP-50. Bureau of Microbial Hazards, Health Canada, Ottawa, Ontario, Canada. Published on the Food Directorate's (Health Canada's) website, http://www.hc-sc.gc.ca/fn-an/res-rech/analy-meth/microbio/index_e.html. Accessed February 9, 2007.

Bennett RW, Lancette GA (1998): *Staphylococcus aureus*. In: Bacteriological Analytical Manual online, 8th ed., Rev. A, Chap. 12. http://www.cfsan.fda.gov/~ebam/bam-12.html. Accessed January 18, 2007.

Bleve G, Rizzotti L, Dellaglio F, Torriani S (2003): Development of reverse transcription (RT)-PCR and real-time RT-PCR assays for rapid detection and quantification of viable yeasts and molds contaminating yogurts and pasteurized food products. *Appl Environ Microbiol*. 69:4116–4122.

Bottone EJ (1997): *Yersinia enterocolitica*: the charisma continues. *Clin Microbiol Rev*. 10:257–276.

Christensen D, Crawford C, Szabo R (2002): Enumeration of coliforms, faecal coliforms and of *E. coli* in foods using the MPN method. Health Products and Food Branch, MFHPB-19. Microbiology Evaluation Division, Bureau of Microbial Hazards, Health Canada, Ottawa, Ontario, Canada. http://www.hc-sc.gc.ca/fn-an/res-rech/analy-meth/microbio/volume2/mfhpb19-01_e.html Accessed March 1, 2007.

D'Aoust JY, Purvis U (1998): Isolation and identification of *Salmonella* from foods. MFHPB-20. Health Protection Branch, Health Canada, Ottawa, Ontario, Canada. http://www.hc-sc.gc.ca/fn-an/res-rech/analy-meth/microbio/volume2/mfhpb20-01_e.html. Accessed January 25, 2007.

Donelly C (2001): *Listeria monocytogenes*. In: Labbé RG, García S (Eds.). *Guide to Foodborne Pathogens*. Wiley, New York, pp. 99–132.

Douey D, Wilson P (2004): Enumeration of yeasts and moulds. In: *Foods*. Health Products and Food Branch, Microbiology Evaluation Division, Bureau of Microbial Hazards, Health Canada, Ottawa, Ontario, Canada. http://www.hc-sc.gc.ca/food-aliment. Accessed January 15, 2007.

Drobniewski FA (1993): *Bacillus cereus* and related species. *Clin Microbiol Rev.* 6:324–338.

Farber JM, Peterkin PI (1991): *Listeria monocytogenes*, a food-borne pathogen. *Microbiol Rev.* 55:476–511.

Feng P, Weagant SD, Grant MA (2002): Enumeration of *Escherichia coli* and the coliform bacteria. In: Bacteriological Analytical Manual online, 8th ed. http://www.cfsan.fda.gov/;ebam/bam-tic.html. Accessed February 15, 2007.

Fredriksson-Ahomaa M, Korkeala H (2003): Low occurrence of pathogenic *Yersinia enterocolitica* in clinical, food, and environmental samples: a methodological problem. *Clin Microbiol Rev.* 16:220–229.

Health Canada (2001a): Determination of the aerobic colony count in foods. MFHPB-18. Microbiology Evaluation Division, Bureau of Microbial Hazards, Health Products and Food Branch, Health Canada, Ottawa, Ontario, Canada. Published on the Food Directorate's (Health Canada's) website, http://www.hc-sc.gc.ca/fn-an/alt_formats/hpfb-dgpsa/pdf/res-rech/mfhpb18_e.pdf. Accessed May 2008.

——— (2001b). Enumeration of *Clostridium perfringens* in foods. MFHPB-23. Microbiology Evaluation Division, Bureau of Microbial Hazards, Health Canada, Ottawa, Ontario, Canada. Published on the Food Directorate's (Health Canada's) website, http://www.hc-sc.gc.ca/fn-an/res-rech/analy-meth/microbio/volume2/mfhpb23-01_e.html. Accessed May 2008.

Health Protection Agency (2005): Standard operating procedure: Detection of Campylobacter species. F21. Issued by Standards Unit, Evaluations and Standards Laboratory Specialist and Reference Microbiology Division, pp. 1–10. http://www.hpa-standardmethods.org.uk/documents/food/pdf/f21.pdf. Accessed May 2008.

Hitchins AD (2002). Detection and enumeration of *Listeria monocytogenes* in foods. In: Bacteriological Analytical Manual online. 8th ed. http://www.cfsan.fda.gov/;ebam/bam-toc.html. Accessed February 20, 2007.

Höök H (2005): *Campylobacter* epidemiology: insights from subtyping by pulsed-field gel electrophoresis. Doctoral dissertation Swedish University of Agricultural Sciences, Uppsala.

Hunt JM, Abeyta C, Tran T (2001): *Campylobacter*. In: Bacteriological Analytical Manual online, 8th ed. http://www.cfsan.fda.gov/˜ebam/bam-7.html. Accessed May 2008.

Kaper JB, Glenn Morris J, Levine MM (1995): Cholera. *Clin Microbiol Rev.* 8:48–86.

Kaysner CA, DePaola A (2004): *Vibrio*. In: Bacteriological Analytical Manual online, 8th ed. http://www.cfsan.fda.gov/~ebam/bam-9.html. Accessed May 2007.

Kingombe CB, Cerqueira-Campos ML, Trottier YL, Houle J (2006): Health products and food branch: isolation and identification of *Shigella* spp. from foods. MFLP-25. Research Division, Health Canada, Ottawa, Ontario, Canada. Published on the Food Directorate's (Health

Canada's) website, http://www.hc-sc.gc.ca/fn-an/res-rech/analy-meth/microbio/volume3/mflp25_e.html. Accessed May 2008.

Maturin L, Peeler JT (2001): Aerobic plate count. In: Bacteriological Analytical Manual online. 8th ed. http://www.cfsan.fda.gov/~ebam/bam-3.html. Accessed May 2008.

Peeler JT, Houghtby GA, Rainosek AP (1992): The most probable number technique. In: Vanderzant C, Splittstoesser DF (Eds.): *Compendium of Methods for the Microbiological Examination of Foods*. 3rd ed. American Public Health Association, Washington, DC, pp. 105–120.

Phillips CA (2001): *Arcobacter spp* in food: isolation, identification and control. *Trends Food Sci Technol*. 12:263–275.

Potturi-Venkata LP, Backert S, Lastoviaca AJ, et al. (2007): Evolution of different plate media for direct cultivation of *Campylobacter* species from live broilers. *Poult Sci*. 86:1304–1311.

Rhodehamel EJ, Harmon SM (1998): *Clostridium perfringens*. In: Bacteriological Analytical Manual online, 8th ed. http://www.cfsan.fda.gov/~ebam/bam-16.html. Accessed May 2008.

——— (2001): *Bacillus cereus*. In: Bacteriological Analytical Manual online, 8th ed. http://www.cfsan.fda.gov/~ebam/bam-14.html. Accessed May 2008.

Schoeni JL, Lee Wong AC (2005): *Bacillus cereus* food poisoning and its toxins. *J Food Prot*. 68:636–648.

Snelling WJ, Matsuda M, Moore JE, Dooley JSG (2006): Review: under the microscope—*Arcobacter*. *Lett Appl Microbiol*. 42:7–14.

Solomon HM, Lilly T (2001): *Clostridium botulinum*. In: Bacteriological Analytical Manual online, 8th ed. http://www.cfsan.fda.gov/~ebam/bam-17.html. Accessed May 2008.

Szabo RA (2005): Enumeration of *Staphylococcus aureus* in foods. MFHPB-21. Microbiological Methods Committee, Health Products and Food Branch, Microbiology Evaluation Division, Bureau of Microbial Hazards, Health Canada, Ottawa, Ontario, Canada. Published on the Food Directorate's (Health Canada's) website, http://www.hc-sc.gc.ca/fn-an/res-rech/analy-meth/microbio/volume2/mfhpb21-01_e.html. Accessed May 2008.

Tournas, Stack ME, Mislivec PB, Koch HA, Bandler R (2000): Yeasts, molds and mycotoxins. In: Bacteriological Analytical Manual online, 8th ed. http://www.cfsan.fda.gov/~ebam/bam-18.html. Accessed May 2008.

Trachoo N (2003): *Campylobacter jejuni*: an emerging pathogen. *Songklanakarin J Sci Technol*. 25:141–157.

Weagant SD, Feng P, Stanfield JT (1998): *Yersinia enterocolitica*. In: Bacteriological Analytical Manual online, 8th ed. http://www.cfsan.fda.gov/~ebam/bam-8.html. Accessed May 2008.

Wilson P (2001): Determination of coliforms in foods using violet red bile agar. MFHPB-31. Health Products and Food Branch, Microbiology Evaluation Division Bureau of Microbial Hazards, Health Canada, Ottawa, Ontario, Canada. Published on the Food Directorate's (Health Canada's) website, http://www.hc-sc.gc.ca/fn-an/alt_formats/hpfb-dgpsa/pdf/res-rech/mfhpb31_e.pdf. Accessed May 2008.

CHAPTER 27

RAPID METHODS FOR FOODBORNE BACTERIAL ENUMERATION AND PATHOGEN DETECTION

PETER FENG and NORMA HEREDIA

27.1 INTRODUCTION

Foods are routinely tested with the objectives of establishing the absence of specific pathogens or toxins, to ensure food safety, and to test for total microbial load or for indicators to monitor the sanitary quality of foods. These fundamental objectives have long been achieved with traditional microbiological methods, which are labor-, time-, and material-intensive. Hence, rapid methods have had a major impact, as evidenced by the vast numbers of papers that describe the use of rapid methods in food testing. Many of these papers have, however, focused on pathogen testing, which is expected, due to the health risk of pathogen presence in foods, and accordingly, numerous pathogen test kits are available (Feng, 2007). But a large percentage of food testing is for the enumeration of total counts and indicators, yet rapid enumeration assays are covered sparsely in the literature. In this chapter we provide a brief overview of pathogen testing, focusing instead on the technologies and advancements made in rapid enumeration methods.

Initially, rapid methods were simple, manual devices that shortened test time. However, with scientific advancements, rapid method technologies continue to change and are increasingly being automated using highly sophisticated instruments. Although convenient, these assays are costly and not easily accessible worldwide, due to limited resources, import regulations and tariffs, reagent availability, and short shelf life, nor may they be as cost-effective, due to the local economy and cheap labor costs. Hence, we also examine the practical and logistical issues of the application of rapid methods in food testing.

Microbiologically Safe Foods, Edited by Norma Heredia, Irene Wesley, and Santos García

27.2 LOGISTICS OF FOOD TESTING

Testing for pathogens or toxins in foods is usually done on a present–absent basis to conform to the "zero tolerance" or "absence" regulations for these agents in foods. However, enumeration assays for total bacteria or indicators yield actual or estimated counts that are used to assess food quality, shelf-life stability, effectiveness of HACCP (hazard analysis of critical control points) during processing, as well as indirectly indicating pathogen presence or compliance with microbial limits, if any, specified for those foods. Because of these distinct testing objectives, the logistics and approaches used in analysis are also very different.

27.2.1 Pathogen Detection

Conventional methods used to establish the absence of a pathogen in foods seems fairly straightforward, where food homogenates are plated on selective/differential media to screen for presumptive pathogens, which are then isolated and identified. But food matrices are extremely complex (Feng, 2007; Stevens and Jaykus, 2004), and pathogens, if present, may be found in low levels and not distributed uniformly in foods. In addition, the presence of normal flora bacteria, especially in raw foods, the presence of ingredients that can interfere with assays, bacterial stress injury that may result from food processing, and limitations in assay sensitivity all pose formidable challenges to pathogen testing (Feng, 2001). As a result, it is essential to subject the samples to a series of enrichments to dilute the effects of inhibitors, resuscitate cell injury, suppress normal flora, and to growth-amplify target pathogens, to improve the odds of detecting the pathogens that may be present. Although effective, enrichment is very time consuming, and as a result, analysis takes several days to complete.

27.2.2 Enumeration

Enumeration methods can be divided into direct methods that give a count of colony-forming units (CFU) of the bacteria present or indirect methods that use various parameters to estimate the bacterial count. In contrast to pathogen testing, enrichment is not used and is actually detrimental to enumeration methods, as it will amplify the cells and thus overestimate the actual number of organisms present. As a result, enumeration methods are simpler than pathogen testing methods. However, the microbial levels in foods can vary greatly, ranging from low in processed foods to very high in raw foods. Thus, it is essential to serially dilute the food homogenate and test each dilution in order to obtain an accurate count. Enumeration methods are therefore media- and labor-intensive.

The most common direct method is the aerobic plate count (APC), also known as heterotrophic plate count (HPC) or total plate count (TPC), where food homogenates are serially diluted and plated directly onto agar medium. The numbers of colonies that grow are counted and by multiplying with the dilution factor, a total microbial count is obtained. Enumeration for indicator bacteria such as coliforms and generic *E. coli* often uses the most probable number (MPN), which is an indirect method, where sample dilutions are inoculated into multiple tubes of lactose media. Tubes that show lactose fermentation are confirmed with a more selective lactose medium, and by using the combinations of confirmed positive tubes, a statistical estimation of indicator bacteria level is obtained from the MPN table. A common, direct enumeration method for indicators is the membrane filtration (MF) test, where a defined volume of liquid is vacuum-passed through a filter to trap the bacteria present. The filter is then incubated on specific agar media, and the numbers of colonies that grow are counted. MF is most often used in water testing and may be used on liquid foods, but those containing particulates will clog the filter. Also, the filter has a limited counting range that is easily exceeded in contaminated samples, so dilutions of the samples may need to be tested to obtain an accurate count.

Many procedures generate bioaerosols, which can be complex and may contain bacteria, filth, and even toxins. Hence, bacterial enumerations are also done on production environments to monitor cleanliness of air and food contact surfaces. In some countries, there are no legislations regarding air quality, but some food processors will conduct environmental testing as part of internal quality control. A common method for air sampling is to expose an open agar plate for a specified time, then incubate and count the numbers of bacterial colonies that have fallen onto the plate. Unsanitary food-contact surfaces are well-known sources of food contamination. Surface sampling is often done by using a sterile swab to sample an area, rinse the swab to release bacteria, and do APC for the levels of bacteria present. All of these are media- and labor-intensive procedures.

27.3 RAPID PATHOGEN TESTING METHODS

Rapid pathogen testing methods have been covered elsewhere (Feng, 2001, 2007), hence only an overview is presented. Rapid pathogen testing may be divided into identification and detection methods, but in both instances the term *rapid* should be interpreted with caution, as identification assays require the isolation of a pure culture prior to testing, and rapid detection methods that are intended for testing food homogenates continue to need some culture enrichment to deal with the problems associated with food testing and matrix complexity. As a result, the rapid assays may take only minutes or a few hours to complete, but the overall food analysis time is much longer, due to the dependence on conventional methods for isolation and enrichment.

Bacteria may be identified by many attributes, including fatty acid and carbon oxidation profiles, but most still rely on biochemical analyses, which are labor- and media-intensive procedures. Miniaturized biochemical identification kits, which have been in use for years, have greatly simplified this process, but identification assays are becoming even more user-friendly, as many are now automated. These assays continue to change and some have undergone modifications to accommodate larger and more accurate databases and have been expanded to identify other microorganisms. The use of specialized substrates or media for presumptive identification of bacteria is another area that has seen a lot of changes. The use of special substrates became popular with the fluorogenic substrate 4-methylumbelliferone-β-D-glucuronide (MUG) for identifying *E. coli* based on β-glucuronidase activity (Feng and Hartman, 1982), but has now expanded to include many more substrates or media that target unique enzyme or metabolic traits in various pathogens (Feng, 2007). These fluorogenic and chromogenic substrates, however, continue to be used in rapid enumeration tests for indicators (see Section 27.4).

Antibody-based assays comprise the majority of rapid pathogen detection kits and they use various assay formats. Simple latex agglutination tests that use antibody-bound colored latex beads to serotype pure bacterial cultures have become very popular. Used initially for serotyping *E. coli* O157:H7 isolates from foods, latex assays are now available for many pathogens, including other enterohemorrhagic *E. coli* serotypes that are increasingly causing foodborne illness worldwide (Brooks et al., 2005). Immunomagnetic separation (IMS) is another antibody-based format that has undergone major advancements, as many are realizing that the selective antibody capture of target by IMS can often improve the sensitivity of other assays (Benoit and Donahue, 2003). Hence, the diversity of antibodies coupled to beads has increased, and automated IMS assays have also become available. Similarly, lateral flow or immunoprecipitation format is used increasingly in assays for many pathogens. These disposable, single-use devices offer the advantages of simplicity, flexibility, virtual hands-off assay, and stability, as some can be stored or transported at ambient temperatures. Pathogen detection using the antibody enzyme–linked immunosorbent assay (ELISA) format continues to exist, but few manual tests are being introduced. Several manual ELISA tests that were the gold standards of pathogen testing have also been phased out, as many are being modified to become automated tests. Antibodies are also being used increasingly in biosensors, which have biological components (antibodies and ligands) that are coupled with sensitive physicochemical transducer to measure specific biological interactions. Biosensors can simultaneously detect multiple targets (Taitt et al., 2004) and are very fast and sensitive in the detection of bacterial cultures in solutions, but their efficiency in food testing can be variable and is still being explored (Alocilja and Radke, 2003).

DNA-based pathogen detection assay formats consist of DNA probes (Olson, 2002), cloned phages (Favrin et al., 2001), and polymerase chain reaction (PCR). Until recently, most PCR assays, however, used manual gel-based detection that was labor-intensive, hence not very popular. As a result, DNA-based rapid pathogen methods formed only a small percentage of commercially available kits. Advances in genomics (Abee et al., 2004), however, introduced such technologies as real-time PCR (RT-PCR) (Exner, 2005) and DNA chips (microarrays) (Call, 2005), which caused a resurgence in DNA-based assays. As a result, RT-PCR has surpassed other DNA formats, and many new assays for pathogens have been introduced. These assays use fast amplification and a variety of detection technologies (Kubista and Zoric, 2005) for real-time data monitoring that will give results in an hour. But the complexity of foods continues to pose problems, so that most RT-PCR still require proper sample preparation procedures (Stevens and Jaykus, 2004), including some culture enrichment steps, to minimize the effects of PCR inhibitors that may be present in foods (Vaneechoute and Van Eldere, 1997).

27.4 RAPID ENUMERATION METHODS

Both direct and indirect enumeration methods are used extensively in food testing; hence, rapid enumeration assays have been developed in both formats to meet these testing needs. In some cases these rapid enumeration assays are simple miniaturization of existing methods to reduce material costs and time (Walser, 2000), but there are also assays that use novel technologies. We have divided rapid enumeration methods into those that are used for environmental (Table 1) and food testing (Table 2), but as evident by the table listings, some assays can be used in many situations—hence there are overlaps.

27.4.1 Rapid Enumeration Methods for Air, Environmental, and Surface Samples

With the emphasis on food safety from "farm to fork," there is an increasing trend to do testing on production areas that are often remote, creating problems in logistics, transport, and sample integrity. To simplify field testing of water sources, some devices have been developed for sampling, incubation, and direct count enumeration

TABLE 1 Rapid Enumeration Methods for Air, Environmental, and Surface Samples

Type	Assay	Principle/Description	Applications
Air	Biotest's Hycon System SAS Super 100 Air Ideal Oxoid MAQS II MicroBio MB2 Burkhard Microflow M Air T System Sartorius MD8	RCS centrifugal sampling and impaction Impaction	Pharmaceutical, automotive, indoor air quality, health care, food, and cosmetic industry
Surface and environmental	RODAC plates (direct method)	Surface contact plates with specific media	Surfaces and personnel
	Petrifilm (direct method)	Dual-layer film coated with dehydrated media and gelling agents soluble in cold water	
	Biotest Hycon contact slides (direct method)	Contact slides filled with specific media	
	Enliten ATP Assay System Lightning MVP Zygiene 100 Rapid Hygiene System	ATP biolumniscence	Dairy products, meat, poultry, beer, fruits and vegetables

TABLE 2 Rapid Enumeration Assays for Food Samples

Type	Assay	Principle/Description	Applications
Manual	Petrifilm Sanitakun	Dual-layer film coated with nutrients and gelling agents soluble in cold water	Food, water, environmental
	Iso-Grid	Membrane filtration using hydrophobic grid membranes that are placed on selective agar for enumeration by MPN	Wide range of foods, beverages, ingredients, water
	Easygel	Special petri dish coated with gelling agents and nutrients	Wide range of foods, beverages
	Simplate Quanti-Disc	Multienzyme technology Correlate enzyme activity with the presence and number of viable organisms in foods	Wide variety of foods (Simplate), water (Quanti-Disc)
	ColiTrak, ColiTrak Plus (fecal coliform)	MPN assay utilizing LST and MUG (fecal coliform)	Food, water, environmental
	Millipore's Samplers	Ready-to-use plastic paddle with nutrients, membrane filter for sampling and incubation	Water
Automated	Spiral, Wasp II Spiral Plater	Precise delivery of 1 : 1 to 1 : 10,000 sample dilution in a spiral pattern on each plate	Food, water, environmental
	Tempo	Automated MPN: coliforms, *E. coli*, and Enterobacteriaceae	Poultry, egg, meat, meat products
	Bactometer, Rabbit Impedance Detection System, Bac Trac	Impedance	Food, water, environmental
	Malthus	Conductance	Food, water, environmental
	BacT/Alert Automated Microbial Detection System	Colorimetric sensor and reflected light to monitor cell presence by production of CO_2	Food, beverages
	ChemScan RDI System	Flow cytometry (fluorescent cell labeling and laser scan)	Pharmaceutical, personal care, food, beverages
	D-Count	Flow cytometry (fluorescent cell labeling, laser excitation, and digital processing)	Pharmaceutical, personal care, food, beverages
	Milliflex Rapid Microbiology Detection System	ATP bioluminescence	Water and filterable samples

in situ. The HPC and total count samplers (Millipore, United States), consist of a plastic paddle with a 0.45-μm filter backed with a pad with dehydrated medium. A sample (1 mL) is drawn through the filter by capillary action to trap the bacteria present and to rehydrate the medium. After incubation, the number of colonies on the grid-marked filter is counted. These disposable, ready-to-use devices are self-contained, sterilized, and individually packaged, and have been used to test water sources in the pharmaceutical, food, and beverage industries.

The microbiological quality of air in production areas can be a critical factor in manufacturing. Traditional air-sampling methods simply exposed open agar plates in the area to be tested, but several rapid air-sampling devices have been developed. The RCS Microbial Air Sampler (Biotest, Germany) is a handheld, battery-powered air sampler, which can be coupled with the Hycon (hygiene control) system for air analysis. It is based on the impaction principle, where viable airborne bacteria are collected onto a semisoft agar strip, which is inserted into the instrument's sampling head for counting. Impaction is also used in other air samplers, which come with variable features such as size, weight, power, battery life, program options, and special collectors for difficult-to-access areas. These include the SAS Super 100 (Bioscience International, United States), Air Ideal 3P air sampler (bioMerieux, United States), MAQS II Microbiological Air Sampler (Oxoid, UK), Microflow (Geneq, Inc, Canada), M Air T System (Millipore, United States), MD8 Microbiological Air Sampler (Sartorius, Germany), and MicroBio MB2 Portable Air Sampler and the Burkhard Portable Air Sampler (both from Spiral Biotechnology, United States) (Table 1). Many such devices are used to monitor indoor air quality, but also in pharmaceutical, automotive, food, and cosmetic manufacturing industries (Mehta et al., 2000).

Although not a new test, the replicate organism detection and counting (RODAC) plate (Hall and Hartnett, 1964) is a simple, direct method that uses agar media to contact any surface directly (e.g., tabletops, walls, benches, floors, garments, gowned personnel) to pick up any bacteria present. The media may be formulated to contain a neutralizer to inactivate cleaning and disinfection agents that may inhibit bacterial growth, as do the Hycon contact slides (Biotest, Germany).

The APC portion of the swab surface sampling enumeration method can be simplified with devices like Petrifilm (3M, United States) plates. These consist of disposable cardboard with a gridded, defined area containing dehydrated media and a gelling agent, both of which are rehydrated by 1 mL of sample inoculum to allow colony growth. These tests can be used for enumeration of total counts but are also available with different selective or differential media for counting indicators such as coliforms and *E. coli*, yeast, and molds, and some are also used for specific pathogens (Table 1).

The microbial quality of surfaces may also be monitored with indirect methods using bioluminescence to measure bacterial adenosine triphosphate (ATP). This assay is based on the ATP-dependent luciferase activity, which oxidizes luciferin to oxyluciferin with photon emissions that are measured with a luminometer (Poulis et al., 1993). Most ATP assays have sensitivity in the range of 10^3 to 10^4 CFU/mL, but by using a standard curve, the intensity of light may be correlated to cell density. This, however, is only an estimation of bacterial levels present. Also, since all living cells have ATP, the assays will not differentiate the types of bacteria present. There are many ATP-based rapid enumeration methods and many are handheld, portable devices that give results in 5 min. A few examples are the Enliten ATP assay system (Promega, United States), Lightning MVP (Idexx BioControl, United States), Zygiene 100 Rapid Hygiene (Biotest Diagnostics Corp., United States), and Profile 1 (New Horizon Diagnostics, United States). Some ATP assays are also used for testing total microbial load in dairy products, meats, and other foods (Table 2).

27.4.2 Rapid Enumeration Methods for Foods

A wide range of both direct and indirect rapid enumeration methods have been developed for testing for total and indicator bacteria in foods. Several of these were introduced many years ago, but are worthy of mention. Also, for ease of discussion, we have divided these systems into manual and automated tests.

Manual Techniques APC uses many dilution blanks and agar plates. The Easygel (Micrology Labs, United States) has simplified the pour-plate APC method by precoating petri dishes with a gelling agent and using pre-measure media containing pectin, which solidifies when it contacts the gelling agent to allow the formation of bacterial colonies. Similarly, the Petrifilm and Sanita-kun (Chisso Co., Japan) plates are devices that simplify the APC enumeration method. These are disposable, convenient, space-saving tests that are well suited for quality control labs that test large numbers of samples. These assays have been tested on a wide range of food and environmental samples, but their sensitivities may vary depending on foods, and the presence of injured cells may cause false-negative results (Gracias and McKillip, 2004). These tests are also available for lactic acid bacteria, coliforms, *E. coli*, Enterobacteriaceae, *S. aureus, Listeria,* and yeast and molds.

The MPN and MF are most often used to enumerate indicators. The Iso-Grid (QA Labs, Canada) is a MF assay that uses a larger hydrophobic grid filter to confine colony growth within gridded cells. This prevents overlapping colony growth and also has a larger counting capacity, thereby reducing the need to dilute the sample. By placing the filter on a specific media, the numbers of colony squares indicative of the target organism are counted and converted to MPN. This method has been used in the analysis of pathogens and indicators in foods, beverages, and water samples.

Many assays use special enzymatic substrates for enumeration. The ColiTrak (BioControl, United States) is a simple, disposable, self-contained, ready-to-use, miniaturized MPN that uses a coliform-specific chromogenic substrate to detect lactose fermentation or MUG for *E. coli* (ColiTrak Plus). These have been used for indirect enumeration of indicators in food, water, and environment samples. The SimPlate (BioControl, United States) developed by Idexx uses a special 84-well plate containing dehydrated medium and chromogenic substrates. The sample inoculum hydrates the wells, and the specific enzyme activity causes color changes in the wells. The numbers of positive wells are counted, multiplied by the dilution factor, and the bacterial load is estimated from a chart. Another SimPlate incorporates a fluorogenic substrate in addition to the chromogen for the enumeration of *E. coli*. These assays have been used to test a variety of foods (Beuchat et al., 1998) for total counts, coliforms, *Campylobacter*, and yeast and molds. The Quanti-Disc (BioControl, United States), also developed by Idexx, is an enzymatic assay for total counts in water. The assay uses multienzyme technology and a special disk with 50 channels that lead to individual wells. The wells are filled with the sample through capillary action, and after incubation are checked for fluorescence either manually or with a reader. The number of fluorescence-positive wells is converted to MPN using a chart. It has a counting range of less than 1.8 to greater than 391 cells per milliliter.

Automated Technologies The first automated total count assay was the spiral plater that used a single plate per sample, thus realizing great saving in time and materials (Campbell and Gilchrist, 1973; Gilchrist et al., 1973). The system, developed over 30 years ago, delivered precisely 35 μL of sample on a rotating plate in an Archimedes spiral pattern with gradually decreasing volumes equivalent to sample dilutions from 1 : 1 to 1 : 10,000. The colonies are counted visually or with an automated laser colony counter (Donnelly et al., 1976). Different versions of the spiral plater are now commercially available (Table 2).

The Tempo EB (bioMerieux, France) is an automated MPN for enumeration of total counts, coliforms, *E. coli,* and Enterobacteriaceae. The assay uses a disposable plastic card with three levels of 16 wells each that are of different sizes at each level, representing different dilutions. The wells contain a selective medium with a fluorogenic substrate. Once inoculated, the system is automated and it incubates and calculates the MPN based on a combination of fluorescence positive wells. It can provide MPN data in 22 h, including confirmation, as compared to the 3 to 4 days needed for traditional MPN.

The impedance and/or conductance technology measures changes in electrical conductivity in the media caused by metabolic growth of the organism. Hence, by using substrates that can be utilized only by certain bacterial species, the presence of those organisms can be monitored continuously by electrical changes in the medium, and the degree of change in conductance is directly (impedance is inversely) proportional to the number of cells initially present. Rapid enumeration assay that use impedance include the Bactometer (bioMerieux), BacTrac (SY-Lab), Rabbit Impedance (Microbiology International), and Microbial Detection (Malthus) (Moldenhauer, 2003).

Metabolic products from microbial growth can also be measured to determine cell density. The BactT/ALERT Microbial Detection (bioMerieux) developed by Organon Teknika uses a colorimetric sensor to monitor CO_2 and other metabolic by-products of microbial growth that are dissolved in the medium. The presence or level of CO_2 changes the color of the gas-permeable sensor at the bottom of each culture bottle to yellow, which is detected and analyzed by the instruments' decision-making software (Thorpe et al., 1990).

The ATP bioluminescence assay has also been developed into automated, rapid enumeration assays. The Milliflex Rapid Microbiology Detection (Millipore, United States) for testing water or liquid foods uses filtration to trap bacterial cells. The filter is then sprayed with permeabilizing reagent to release ATP, followed by bioluminescence reagents. The numbers of live (luminescent) cells are counted with a CCD camera, and the results are available in hours as compared to the days required for a typical MF assay.

Advances in instrumentation and microfluidics have produced some very sophisticated instruments for enumerating bacteria. The ChemScan RDI (Chemunex, France) is a flow cytometry assay for filterable samples using fluorescent cell labeling and laser scanning. The assay uses a nonfluorescent substrate (fluorassure) which is cleaved enzymatically by metabolically active cells to release a fluorochrome that is detected by a laser. By using target-specific substrates, labeled antibodies, or nucleic acid probes, the assay can be formatted to detect specific bacteria. The Chemunex D-Count uses the same technology but is an automated assay for the analysis of nonfilterable samples. These assays, which can provide results within hours and potentially capable of detecting one cell, are being explored for cell enumeration in the pharmaceutical, cosmetics, personal care, food, and beverage industries (Reynolds and Fricker, 1999). It will be interesting to see their detection efficiencies in complex food matrices.

27.5 LOGISTICS, RESOURCES, AND APPLICABILITY

The rapid methods industry is constantly evolving in response to scientific and technological advances, so there are vast numbers and varieties of rapid methods, ranging from simple devices that shorten test time to assays that use sophisticated instruments. Understandably, there are tendencies for assay developers to become enamored with technologies and try to develop assays or apply instruments designed for research to applications that are not very practical or cost-effective to the user. Hence, despite the fact that analysts would like to use rapid methods to simplify and speed up food testing, there are many factors to consider, as these methods also have their limitations. In addition, there are problems in logistics and resources that are associated with the actual implementation of these methods in food testing.

One of the primary applications of rapid methods is for rapid screening of large quantities of foods, where negative results are accepted, but positives are only considered as presumptive and need to be confirmed, often by traditional microbiological methods. The need to confirm presumptive positives may not pose great inconveniences to some segments of the food industry, such as processed or ready-to-eat food manufacturers, as most of these foods would be expected to have low counts and test negative for the presence of pathogens. However, in other manufacturing segments, where higher numbers of presumptive positives are expected, the need to confirm presumptive positive rapid method results by conventional assays may be perceived as redundant testing and not very labor- and cost-effective.

Once a user has gone through the difficult task of selecting a rapid method from the vast numbers that are available, the actual implementation is also not very straightforward, especially in countries worldwide. Most countries have regulations regarding the importation and transportation of biological agents, including test kits, and some of these regulations have become even more stringent, due to increasing concerns with bioterrorism. As a result, documentations, certifications, and import permits are often needed prior to the importation of test kits. The application process for these documents can in itself be very complex and requires local knowledge to navigate through the various authorities, procedures, and overlapping jurisdictions, which can be different from country to country. In addition, import taxes are often levied on test kits, which can drive up the cost of the assay, and some countries may even levy a tax on a specific component, such as the plasticware contained in the kits. Having proper documentations will facilitate the transit of test kits through customs, which is critical, as most biological reagents require refrigeration. However, bureaucratic procedures may sometime cause unexpected delays, which raise user's concerns about shelf-life stability and effectiveness of the kits due to time and temperature abuse. As a result, some manufacturers will subject their kits to ruggedness testing to ensure that they will perform according to specification even after passages through harsh holding conditions.

In developed countries, the analyst's time is often the most costly expense of testing; hence, the use of a rapid method may be an attractive alternative for reducing costs. This, however, does not apply in other countries, where labor costs are not as big a concern as the cost and availability of test reagents. Manufacturers will often use local distributors to resolve availability issues and will take into consideration differences in currency exchange to try to adjust the cost of their assays in accordance with local economy. But even with such efforts, by the time the additional costs are added, such as distributor markup, permits, taxes levied, and exchange rates, sometimes even the most inexpensive rapid methods can be costly in other countries, making it difficult for them to be competitive with cheap labor cost.

The user's knowledge, needs, and testing situations are also factors that can have an impact in the implementation of rapid methods worldwide. In some instances, users may be reluctant to try new assays, due to lack of familiarity with the new technology or, perhaps, due to the cost or the inconvenience of having to modify their existing procedures to adapt to new testing methods or even their facilities to accommodate the requirements of the new instrument. On the contrary, the lack of knowledge may also compel some users to be too eager to embrace new methods. For example, a testing lab may get requests from customers insisting that molecular biology methods be used, on the assumption that these methods are better. But the customer may not be fully cognizant of the method's validation status, the significance of validation, or realize that these methods also have their limitations. Rapid methods are available in all formats and configurations, ranging from manual, single-use, disposable devices to multitest kits that are often automated and intended for large-volume testing. Understandably, small labs that do not routinely test large numbers of samples tend to prefer single-use devices to minimize the waste of having to discard unused assays and reagents that have expired. Nor is it cost-effective for small labs to invest in an instrument with the added cost of maintenance contracts for upkeep if the instrument will not be used extensively. On the other hand, larger testing labs and food manufacturers tend to prefer automated, multitest kits in order to maximize cost reduction benefits. Many of the automated assays also offer the advantage in being configured with state-of-the-art information technologies to facilitate the fast and broad dissemination of test data as well as to provide test kit and data traceability, such as kit production lot and expiration date and time, and the date and name of the analyst who performed the assay. Ideally, a test would be available in multiple formats to suit the various users, needs, but often it is not economically feasible to produce an assay in multiple formats, and it may actually increase the cost of the assays. There is, however, an abundance of rapid assays for pathogen testing, and in ample formats to suit the user's needs and testing situations.

Several logistical issues on the application of rapid methods have been discussed above. However, the largest hindrance to the widespread use of rapid methods worldwide seems to be the lack of harmonized standard methods. Many countries have their own food safety regulations, microbial limits, and specification of the methods to be used for food testing. Hence, even if a rapid method has been approved and is considered a standard method in one country, it is often validated versus the other country's official method prior to acceptance and implementation in that country. From the assay standpoint, this seems logical since the local food types, varieties, microbial flora/load, and processing practices may be different, so it is essential to verify the effectiveness of the assay for their particular testing situations. But these requirements can be bureaucratic, lengthy, and discouraging to implement. In some countries, rapid methods are used mostly to screen food products destined for export, in which case it is critical that the rapid method used is an official method or a method accepted by the importing country. One of the consequences of the lack of method harmonization is that the exporter may need to test the same food by various methods, depending on destination requirements, thereby increasing labor and cost expenditures. Sometimes, the importer may even specify the methods to be used, which leaves the user with no alternative or the flexibility to explore other rapid assays that may be better suited for their particular testing situation.

Finally, the logistical issues of using rapid methods may be getting more complex with the increasing food safety emphasis from "farm to fork." As a result, testing may be expanding from foods to include analysis of the production environment for sanitation or certification purposes. This shift in testing practices will present new challenges to rapid methods in having to deal with whole new sets of complex sample matrices.

Acknowledgments

The authors would like to express their sincere gratitude to their friends and colleagues from various countries around the world for their helpful comments, opinions, and contributions to the discussion of logistical issues regarding the use of rapid methods.

REFERENCES

Abee T, van Schaik W, Siezen RJ (2004): Impact of genomics on microbial food safety. *Trends Biotechnol.* 22:653–660.

Alocilja EC, Radke SM (2003): Market analysis of biosensors for food safety. *Biosens Bioelectron.* 18:841–846.

Benoit PW, Donahue DW (2003): Methods for rapid separation and concentration of bacteria in food that bypass time-consuming cultural enrichment. *J Food Prot.* 66:1935–1948.

Beuchat LR, Copeland F, Curiale MS, et al. (1998): Comparison of the SimPlate total count method with Petrifilm, Redigel and conventional pour plate method for enumerating aerobic microorganism in food. *J Food Prot.* 61:14–18.

Brooks JT, Sowers EG, Wells JG, et al. (2005): Non-O157 Shiga toxin–producing *Escherichia coli* infections in the United States, 1983–2002. *J Infect Dis.* 192:1422–1429.

Call DR (2005): Challenges and opportunities for pathogen detection using DNA microarrays. *Crit Rev Microbiol.* 31:91–99.

Campbell JE, Gilchrist JE (1973): Spiral plate technique for counting bacteria in milk and other foods. *Dev Ind Microbiol.* 14:95–102.

Donnelly CB, Gilchrist JE, Peeler JT, Campbell JE (1976): Spiral plate count method for the examination of raw and pasteurized milk. *Appl Environ Microbiol.* 32:21–27.

Exner MM (2005): Multiplex real-time PCR. In: Fuchs J, Podda M (Eds.). *Encyclopedia of Diagnostics, Genomics, and Proteomics.* Marcel Dekker, New York, pp. 855–859.

Favrin SJ, Sabah AJ, Griffiths MW (2001): Development and optimization of a novel immunomagnetic separation-bacteriophage assay for detection of *Salmonella enterica* serovar Enteritidis in broth. *Appl Environ Microbiol.* 67:217–224.

Feng P (2001): Development and impact of rapid methods for detection of food borne pathogen. In: Doyle M, Beuchat L, Montville T (Eds.). *Food Microbiology Fundamental and Frontiers*, 2nd ed. ASM Press, Washington, DC, pp. 775–796.

——— (2007): Rapid methods for the detection of food borne pathogens: current and next generation technologies. In: Doyle M, Beuchat L (Eds.). *Food Microbiology Fundamental and Frontiers*, 3rd ed. ASM Press, Washington, DC, pp. 911–934.

Feng P, Hartman PA (1982): Fluorogenic assays for immediate confirmation of *Escherichia coli*. *Appl Environ Microbiol.* 43:1320–1329.

Gilchrist JE, Campbell JE, Donnelly CB, Peeler JT, Delaney JM (1973): Spiral plate method for bacteria determination. *Appl Microbiol.* 25:244–252.

Gracias KS, McKillip JL (2004): A review of conventional detection and enumeration methods for pathogenic bacteria in foods. *Can J Microbiol.* 50:883–890.

Hall LB, Hartnett MJ (1964): Measurement of the bacteria contamination on surfaces. *Public Health Rep.* 79:1021–1024.

Kubista M, Zoric N (2005): Real-time PCR platforms. In: Fuchs J, Podda M (Eds). *Encyclopedia of Diagnostics, Genomics, and Proteomics.* Marcel Dekker, New York, pp. 1126–1130.

Mehta SK, Bell-Robinson DM, Groves TO, Stetzenbach L, Pierson DL (2000): Evaluation of portable air samplers for monitoring airborne culturable bacteria. *Am Ind Hyg Assoc J.* 61:850–854.

Moldenhauer J (2003): Industry perceptions regarding rapid microbiology cripple the industry. *Rapid Microbiol Newsl.* 1:1–7.

Olson WP (2002): DNA probes for the identification of microbes. In: *Encyclopedia of Pharmaceutical Technology.* Marcel Dekker, New York, pp. 729–738.

Poulis JA, de Pijper M, Mossel DAA (1993): Assessment of cleaning and disinfection in the food industry with the rapid ATP-bioluminiscence technique combined with the tissue fluid contamination test and a conventional microbiological method. *Int J Food Microbiol.* 20: 109–116.

Reynolds DT, Fricker CR (1999): Applications of laser scanning for the rapid and automated detection of bacteria in water samples. *J Appl Microbiol.* 86:785–795.

Stevens KA, Jaykus LA (2004): Bacterial separation and concentration from complex sample matrices: a review. *Crit Rev Microbiol.* 30:7–24.

Taitt CR, Golden JP, Shubin YS, et al. (2004): A portable array biosensor for detecting multiple analytes in complex samples. *Microbial Ecol.* 47:175–185.

Thorpe TC, Wilson ML, Turner JE, et al. (1990): BacT/Alert: an automated colorimetric microbial detection system. *J Clin Microbiol.* 28:1608–1612.

Vaneechoute M, Van Eldere J (1997): The possibilities and limitations of nucleic acid amplification technology in diagnostic microbiology. *J Med Microbiol.* 46:188–194.

Walser PE (2000): Using conventional microtiter plate technology for the automation of microbiology testing of drinking water. *J Rapid Methods Automat Microbiol* 8:193–208.

CHAPTER 28

LABORATORY ACCREDITATION AND PROFICIENCY TESTING

DEANN L. BENESH

28.1 INTRODUCTION

Laboratory accreditation and proficiency testing play an important role in today's food industry. The food on our tables may come from several regions of the globe and experienced various levels of processing (or not) before arriving on our plates. As consumers, we want to have confidence that the products we purchase have been properly inspected and tested by laboratories certified to conduct these tests. Today, all regions of the globe are actively involved in the globalization of requirements and certification of food-testing laboratories.

Verification that laboratories and their personnel can demonstrate that they are capable of performing their laboratory operations correctly and produce valid results is the job of recognized accreditation bodies. Accreditation bodies within each country work together with accreditation bodies in other regions to provide mutual recognition and acceptance of practices and assessment schemes throughout the globe. Ultimately, the goal for laboratory accreditation is to improve consistency of auditing, assessment, and performance of testing and calibration laboratories worldwide, and to provide assurance in the quality of laboratory results.

28.2 LABORATORY ACCREDITATION

Every country has its own regulations, recognized scientific organizations, and politics that have contributed to the approaches that have been taken regarding accreditation in their various industries. Accreditation of laboratories today is based on an international standard that was developed as a result of many years of experience using the International Standards Organization /International European Cooperative (ISO/IEC) Guide 25 (ISO, 1990) and the European Norm (EN) 45001 (CEN, 1989).

Microbiologically Safe Foods, Edited by Norma Heredia, Irene Wesley, and Santos García

The International Laboratory Accreditation Cooperation (ILAC) first issued the ISO/IEC Guide 25 in 1978. ISO/IEC Guide 25 and EN 45001 both defined general good laboratory practices (GLPs) and quality procedures for testing laboratories. For many years, these were used as guides for assessment and accreditation of laboratories in industries throughout the globe.

In December 1999, ISO/IEC Guide 25 and EN 45001 were integrated and became a unified ISO document—ISO/IEC standard 17025: General Requirements for the Competence of Testing and Calibration of Laboratories (ISO/IEC, 2005). This standard details the requirements that calibration and testing laboratories should meet to demonstrate that they operate a high-quality system based on recognized criteria, that they are technically competent, and that they can therefore produce valid results. Accreditation of testing laboratories provides a means of determining the competence of laboratories to perform specific types of testing, measurement, and calibration. This standard is meant for use in all industries, including the food and beverage industries.

ISO/IEC Guide 25 was focused on the general technical competency of the laboratory, whereas ISO/IEC 17025 places more emphasis on the quality system of the laboratory as a whole, with specifics regarding the role of management of laboratory operation and ongoing efforts toward improvements. Because many testing laboratories are a part of larger quality and manufacturing organizations that follow ISO 9001:2002 systems, it was important for ISO/IEC 17025 to incorporate the requirements of these systems. Laboratories that fully comply with ISO/IEC 17025 will therefore also operate in accordance with ISO 9001:2002 systems. A simple statement of what these ISO standards have in common is that laboratories will now have defined, written procedures that document what they *say* they do, and verify that they *do* what they say.

Two important clauses of ISO/IEC 17025 that highlight the key areas of focus in the standard are clauses 4 and 5 (ISO/IEC, 2005). Clause 4 specifies requirements for sound management of the laboratory. Clause 5 specifies technical requirements for demonstration of competency of the methods and calibration used within the laboratory. These requirements, listed in Tables 1 and 2, when linked together, form a laboratory's operational quality system.

From these tables one can see that laboratory accreditation encompasses the entire laboratory. It requires defining and documenting all quality management systems, technical requirements for operations, and then initiating a third-party assessment

TABLE 1 Clause 4: Requirements for Sound Management of a Laboratory

Organization	Quality System
Document control	Review of requests, tenders, and contracts
Subcontracting of tests and calibrations	Purchasing services and supplies
Service to the client	Complaints
Control of nonconforming work	Corrective action
Preventive action	Control of records
Internal audits	Management reviews

TABLE 2 Clause 5: Technical Requirements for the Demonstration of Competency in the Methods and Calibration Used Within a Laboratory

General	Personnel
Accommodation and environmental conditions	Test and calibration methods
Method validation	Uncertainty of measurement
Control of data	Equipment
Measurement traceability	Reference standards and materials
Sampling	Handling test and calibration items
Assuring quality of test and calibration results	Reporting results

of technical competence. Accreditation bodies located in each region of the globe conduct these third-party assessments.

ILAC is an international organization that represents a cooperation of these third-party global accreditation schemes. Key responsibilities of the ILAC organization are:

1. To act as a forum for the development of lab accreditation practices
2. To promote lab accreditation as a trade facilitation tool
3. To provide assistance to develop accreditation systems
4. To recognize competent global test facilities

In 1996, 44 national bodies signed a memorandum of understanding (MOU) in Amsterdam to formalize ILAC cooperation. The MOU provides the basis for the development of cooperation and for the continual establishment of multilateral recognition agreements between ILAC member bodies.

Each participating country generally has its own accreditation body, or a small region may choose to share an accreditation body. Each accreditation body may choose to sign mutual recognition partnerships with individual accreditation bodies in the other countries. In addition, within major global regions (e.g., Europe, Asia-Pacific), there are joint agreements signed with collections of individual country accreditation bodies to form larger, regional accreditation cooperatives, such as the European cooperation for Accreditation (EA) or the Asia Pacific Laboratory Accreditation Cooperation (APLAC). In turn, these regional accreditation cooperatives may then sign multilateral agreements between their respective regions, agreeing to accept each other's accreditation cooperatives.

Some examples of the layers of agreements that may occur between the many accreditation cooperatives around the globe are shown in Table 3. These agreements between cooperatives recognize and promote the equivalence of each other's systems, certifications, and reports. It means they agree on equivalency and that they will assess each other for compliance to the standards. This resulting effort could potentially have an impact on international trade, because it could mean that the results from an accredited laboratory in one global region may be accepted at face value, without

TABLE 3 Examples of the Layers of Agreements That May Occur Between the Many Accreditation Cooperatives Around the Globe

Description	Examples
Individual accreditation body (per *country)*	EMA (Mexican Accreditation Entity)
Mutual recognition agreement partners (between *individual accreditation bodies*)	UKAS (United Kingdom Accreditation Services), COFRAC (French Committee of Accreditation), NATA (National Association of Testing Authorities)
Accreditation cooperatives (between *countries within a region*)	EA (European Cooperation for Accreditation), APLAC (Asian Pacific Laboratory Accreditation Cooperation)
International forum (between *regional accreditation groups*)	ILAC (International Laboratory Accreditation Cooperation)

additional testing, by another laboratory in another region. As an example, a shipment of frozen fish tested at an accredited laboratory in Chile may only need to provide one product certificate from their accredited laboratory to satisfy all governments to which the fish is exported (provided that those governments are members of one of the international cooperatives operating under a multilateral agreement). This could be a very real competitive advantage for companies and for customers!

Accreditation of microbiology laboratories can provide benefits for both a laboratory and its clients. Many laboratories already have numerous quality practices in place, and the effort to bring their laboratories into compliance to meet ISO/IEC 17025 requirements has in the end brought all of these practices into one overall system. Using one quality system has brought improvement in the overall process throughout laboratories. By gaining more control over testing protocols and providing and documenting ongoing training, laboratories have improved confidence in their own results due to increased control measures and fewer repeat analyses.

Benefits for the customer can mean greater confidence in the reliability of test data and greater acceptance of these results by government departments. There is also the assurance that calibration standards used in test procedures are traceable to national standards and that these national standards are measured against international standards, making it easier for results to be accepted both nationally and abroad.

Some of the realities of accreditation are the costs incurred by the laboratory in the process of achieving accreditation. These costs will need to be absorbed by the laboratory, and some costs will be passed on to the customer (as the price to be paid for increased reliability in results). Most likely, at least in the early stages of the changeover to improved quality systems, there will be a slower sample throughput, due to increased control measures that are now in place.

The costs associated with accreditation are not insignificant. There are fees to initiate the laboratory assessment, costs to follow through on any recommended laboratory improvements observed during the initial assessment, costs for the hiring of consultants to help formalize the quality system and prepare standard operating

TABLE 4 Estimated Costs of Laboratory Accreditation

Accreditation Step	Cost
Training	$20,000
Supplies	10,000
Consultants	6,000
Technical writer	65,000
Contract employee	75,000
Certifying auditor	15,000
Total variable costs	191,000
Total fixed costs	153,000
Total cost	344,000

procedures (SOPs), and an ongoing assessment fee for periodic audits that help maintain the laboratory's accreditation status.

The general variable and fixed costs associated with efforts of installation and maintenance of a quality system in a contract laboratory in the United States during the process of gaining laboratory accreditation are listed in Table 4. The variable costs represent additional personnel and time needed to complete all phases of installation of the quality system. Fixed costs represent the hours incurred by the current laboratory staff to complete the process of installing the quality system. "The total variable and fixed costs amounted to approximately 10% of the laboratory's total revenue. This level of expense was anticipated before the project began and it was determined that the long-term benefits would significantly outweigh the up-front costs" (Arnold, 1999).

Despite all the work and costs to ensure that quality systems and measures are in place and that a laboratory has demonstrated competence to perform certified tests, there are some limitations to accreditation. Accreditation can provide increased assurance that the methods, measures, competence, and quality systems have been assessed. But accreditation is still not a *guarantee* of results. Remember, only small sample volumes of very large batch quantities of foods are tested to represent the entire batch, so it is possible that proper testing in an accredited laboratory may still miss potential food spoilage or potential food poisoning.

Gaining accreditation can be expensive and time consuming, but without accreditation, some laboratories may lose their competitive edge over other laboratories that have made the effort to become accredited.

28.3 PROFICIENCY TESTING

Proficiency tests are external controls that are used to measure a laboratory's accuracy and competency in performing methods. These controls are made up of samples that have known levels of the analyte(s) that are being routinely tested and measured in the laboratory. There are numerous suppliers of proficiency test schemes. Many of these proficiency test providers' laboratories are also accredited to, or working toward, accreditation to ISO/IEC 17025. In addition, many are also accredited to be proficiency test providers per ILAC-G13:2000: ILAC Guidelines for the Requirements for the Competence of the Providers of Proficiency Testing Schemes (ILAC, 2000), and EA-2/09 (2000): EA Policy on the Accreditation of Providers of Proficiency Testing Schemes.

Participation in a proficiency test scheme is considered to be an important control used to verify that a laboratory and its technicians are competent. Different schemes may use different matrices as carriers of the target organisms, such as dried powders, lyophilized pellets, liquids, wet product, and other inert carriers.

Samples with known levels of target organisms are shipped periodically (several times per year) to laboratories participating in the scheme. Each participating laboratory is expected to treat the proficiency sample the same as they would a food sample in their laboratory. The tendency of many laboratories is to treat proficiency samples as "special" or to have only the best technician test all the proficiency test samples, because they want to be sure to get the "right answer." This runs absolutely conter to the real purpose of participating in a proficiency test sample program. Participation should be rotated between all technicians in the laboratory who routinely conduct testing, using the methods they are accredited to perform. All methods should be conducted as they are performed routinely each day. Results of the proficiency samples are reported back to the proficiency test provider according to the methods used to obtain the results. For each method used, results reported from each laboratory participating in the test scheme are compared to results reported by every other participating laboratory and to the results generated on each sample by the proficiency test provider. How close the laboratory's results are to the true value is a measure of the competence of the technician and the competence of the laboratory to conduct the test methods for which the laboratory is certified.

Participation in a proficiency test scheme can also provide a competitive edge over other laboratories and may be used as a tool to qualify vendors. To ensure that the certificate of analysis supplied by a supplier is meaningful, often a company may ask a vendor to verify its participation in a proficiency test program. It can be one way for the laboratory to demonstrate it is competent to perform the tests used to certify their product for sale to another company.

28.4 GLOBAL PERSPECTIVES

ISO/IEC 17025 states key requirements for testing and calibration laboratories; however, the details of some of these requirements are written broadly because the use of the standard is intended for many different types of testing laboratories and procedures. In many cases, being too specific could be too restrictive or nonapplicable for some types of testing laboratories.

However, this vagueness leaves many points subject to interpretation—and interpretation of these key points may be very different between laboratories, assessors, and accreditation bodies. Additionally, each assessor's level of experience or comfort can play a key role in interpretation of the standard. The openness in the writing of the standard's requirements allows for some individuality within accreditation schemes and can also result in extreme differences.

An area of note in the standard is the validation of methods in Section 5.4.5. Note 2 under this section states,

> The techniques used for the determination of the performance of a method should be one of, or a combination of, the following:
>
> - calibration using reference standards or reference materials;
> - comparison of results achieved with other methods;
> - interlaboratory comparisons;
> - systematic assessment of the factors influencing the result;
> - assessment of the uncertainty of the results based on scientific understanding of the theoretical principles of the method and practical experience.

This particular note is interpreted quite differently by various accreditation agencies around the globe. Examples of differences observed are listed in Table 5. As a result, there can be quite a variation in interpretation of this section between accreditation bodies regarding the use of method validation. No accreditation body is more right or wrong than others. It is therefore up to each laboratory, in each country, to speak with their specific accreditation body and seek clarification and mutual understanding as to the definition and interpretation of the standard's requirements.

TABLE 5 Variation in Interpretation of Validation of Methods in Section 5.4.5, Note 2, Between Accreditation Bodies

Accreditation Body	Interpretation
COFRAC (France)	Any ANFOR method may be used. No additional testing is required within the lab to validate the use of these ANFOR-validated methods.
NATA (Australia)	For all methods other than Australian Standard Methods, data points should be generated in compliance with ANZ 4659 series qualitative or quantitative equivalence methods and analyzed in comparison to the standard method used for that food. This is usually equivalent to 5 to 10 samples of each food matrix, depending on whether the food matrix includes natural contamination or requires artificial contamination. This is necessary to verify both the methods used within the laboratory, and the food matrices.
UKAS (United Kingdom)	The laboratory, through comparative study, must validate every method and have the analysis of data verified by the accreditation body before the lab can be accredited to use the new method.

Due to the costs and benefits of laboratory accreditation, currently the majority of laboratories around the globe that seek to become accredited fall into three categories: (1) contract laboratories, (2) corporate laboratories, and (3) government laboratories. The costs necessary to achieve accreditation at this time are too steep for most average food plant laboratories to absorb and demonstrate a return on the investment. However, these three groups of laboratories may find it necessary to make this investment in order to stay competitive. Contract laboratories may need it to demonstrate that their laboratory provides reliable testing services. Corporate laboratories may use it to enhance testing methods for use in their regional plant laboratories. And all of these laboratory groups may find it necessary to be accredited in order to compete in international trade and assure the acceptance of their product for import and/or export.

In some regions, all food-testing laboratories are required to have some form of accreditation. In Australia, nearly all food-testing laboratories are accredited by the National Association of Testing Authorities (NATA). The concept of laboratory accreditation initiated in Australia, so it has been in wide use in some form for many years prior to the issue of ISO/IEC 17025. In the United Kingdom (UK), approximately 95% of all food-testing laboratories are also accredited. There are three recognized accreditation groups in the UK: United Kingdom Accreditation Scheme (UKAS), Campden Laboratory Accreditation Scheme (CLAS), and LabCred (developed and operated by Bodycote Lawlabs). UKAS is the accreditation scheme formally recognized by other international accreditation bodies; however, the majority of food laboratories are accredited to CLAS and LabCred. These two schemes service a key role in assessing the level of quality in routine food and beverage laboratories in the UK. They are based on ISO/IEC 17025, but were developed to provide a more affordable, "practical," independent assessment and monitoring of laboratories in the UK food industry.

As with all ISO standards, documentation is required. This means that laboratories must gather and keep on file all necessary method references, method regulatory approvals, certificates of analysis of the media and reagents used, package inserts (or the legal document of the product's use) of any product used, and document the measurement of uncertainty for the methods for which the laboratory is certified. The accreditation assessor will use these documents to verify that the laboratory is following their written procedures to the letter.

The measurement of uncertainty of a method has been the subject of an ongoing discussion between laboratories and accreditation bodies as they try to put a simple definition to a complex concept. Uncertainty of measurement is meant to measure the variability or uncertainty that the result is repeatable and reproducible. To measure this, one must determine the precision of each step throughout each procedure, and make assumptions about the analyte and the food matrix.

In a chemical measurement, the measurement of uncertainty can be determined fairly easily. When mixed into a solution a chemical analyte can generally be found in an even distribution throughout the sample. The analyte is stable—not increasing or decreasing. The analyte either is or is not present, and the variables of the method can be tabulated.

The measurement of uncertainty is much more difficult for microbiological analysis. The analyte in microbiological analysis is *Alive*, and changing. Distribution of the analyte throughout the sample is not even. Microorganisms may grow in clumps and perhaps may only be found in "pockets" of the food matrix where key ingredients are providing the "right" nutrients for their growth. Thus, it can only be assumed, for the sake of analysis, that the analyte is evenly distributed. Because the analyte is a living organism, measurement of the organism is very method dependent, making it difficult to define and add up the variables.

But determining the measurement of uncertainly for methods is important. The following commentary appear in the current draft of the ILAC document [ILAC/LLC (00)006]: Guidance for accreditation to ISO/IEC 17025 and what evidence to look for:

> There are going to be instances where the client does not care or even want an estimation of the measurement of uncertainty. I have heard where clients have become angry at a laboratory when they reported the uncertainty of a test. They were upset that the laboratory was not "certain" about their results. They were going to look for a new testing laboratory, one that was certain whether the product met the specification or not. It is important to note that the laboratory should have a procedure for estimating the uncertainty of these tests, even if the client does not want or need them. They need to be able to provide this information to the client should they ever need it, but I would not go to all the trouble of establishing the estimate of uncertainty for a test if no one wants it. Finally, the most important factor is educating your clients about what an appropriate estimate of uncertainty is and how it should be used. (Fox, 2000)

Because such a wide variance in the definition of the measurement of uncertainty has been observed, based on different accreditation bodies, it is recommended that laboratories seek counsel and agreement from their local accreditation body to help define the measurement that will be used. There are also local courses offered on this topic. Locations for these and related accreditation courses can be found on the ILAC website at www.ilac.org.

The bottom line for those who work in the food industry is that everyone wants to ensure that we provide, or are provided with, products and services that support food safety worldwide. Laboratory accreditation and proficiency testing are two measures that can help support this global effort.

REFERENCES

Arnold EA (1999): Case study: accreditation of a microbiological laboratory. Land O'Lakes/R-Tech Analytical Laboratory. Laboratory Accreditation and Proficiency Testing. *Bull Int Dairy Fed*. 344:19–21.

Comite Europeen de Normalisation (CEN) (1989): *General Criteria for the Operation of Testing Laboratories*. EN 45001. January.

EA (European co-operation for Accreditation) (2000): *EA Policy on the Accreditation of Providers of Proficiency Testing Schemes*. EA-2/09. September 2000.

Fox A (2000): What's new in ISO 17025? Identification of client needs: inside laboratory management. *AOAC Int*. September:15.

ILAC (International Laboratory Accreditation Cooperation) (2000): *ILAC Guidelines for the Requirements for the Competence of the Providers of Proficiency Testing Schemes*. G13:2000. International Organization for Standardization, Geneva, Switzerland.

ISO (International Organization of Standardization) (1990): *General Requirements for the Competence of Calibration and Testing Laboratories*, 3rd ed. Guide 25., ISO, Geneva, Switzerland.

ISO/IEC (International Organization for Standardization/International Electrotechnical Commission) (2005): *General Requirements for the Competence of Testing and Calibration of Laboratories*, 2nd ed. ISO/IEC 17025:2005(E), 2005-05-15. ISO/IEC, Geneva, Switzerland.

PART VI

CURRENT AND FUTURE ISSUES IN FOOD SAFETY

CHAPTER 29

BIOTERRORISM AND FOOD SAFETY

BARBARA A. RASCO and GLEYN E. BLEDSOE

> The way we produce things makes it somewhat easy for a terrorist to infiltrate our food supply, whether it is live animals or the manufacturing process. So this is a real issue. This is not a hypothetical situation.
>
> —Lawrence Dyckman, Head of the Natural Resources and Environment Section of the U.S. General Accounting Office (GAO, 2004a)

29.1 INTRODUCTION

The potential for intentional contamination must be incorporated as an integral part of current food safety considerations, and measures to prevent sabotage should augment, but not replace, other food safety activities (WHO, 2002). Proactive risk analysis and preventive measures can be developed using familiar food safety models.

29.2 THE NEED FOR PROTECTIVE FOOD SECURITY PROGRAMS

Malicious contamination of food for terrorist purposes is a real and current threat, with the deliberate contamination of food at a single location potentially having a global public health impact (GAO, 2004a; WHO, 2002). Biological weapons of mass destruction remain a possible threat and have been the focus of numerous preparedness and response strategies; however, such weapons are not the most likely risk to food systems or to the public at large because these agents are relatively difficult to stabilize, transport, and effectively disseminate on a large scale within the food system.

The most likely venue for an attack on food would involve foodborne pathogens or chemicals that are relatively easy to grow or obtain. An attack could employ pathogens or toxicants developed specifically for biological warfare, however, the use of readily available toxic chemicals such as pesticides, heavy metals and industrial chemicals,

Microbiologically Safe Foods, Edited by Norma Heredia, Irene Wesley, and Santos García

and naturally occurring microbiological pathogens are more likely (Rasco and Bledsoe, 2004; WHO, 2002). The impact of an attack would depend on the potential public health impact of the agent, the food used for dissemination, and the point of introduction into the food chain. Those agents causing rapid acute effects, death, paralysis, incapacitating symptoms, or long-term consequences would be most effective.

Attacks could be targeted at a specific commercial entity, industry segment, or a specific country's exports involving the real or threatened introduction of an animal or plant pathogen (or its genetic material) at a production, distribution, or retail facility (Crutchley et al., 2007; Miller et al., 2008). Agents could be disseminated in a somewhat crude form and in a number of what initially appear to be isolated incidents. Deliberate attacks on food, compared to air or water, would be easier to control, making food a relatively reliable vehicle for a terrorist attack (WHO, 2002). Fortunately, there are measures that we can take to reduce the likeliness of an occurrence of, and/or the public health impact of, an attack on our food supply. For example, having better traceability and safety controls in the production and distribution of food would reduce opportunities to contaminate a product intentionally. Also, dietary diversity and multiple food choices make it unlikely that every person in an area would be affected, thus diluting the overall public health impact of an attack. However, food remains highly vulnerable because of the diversity of sources of food, the distribution system of food in global markets, and the complexity of the supply chain, which make prevention of an intentional contamination incident difficult, if not impossible, to prevent. Furthermore, many developing countries still lack a basic food safety infrastructure, making their food supply even more vulnerable (WHO, 2002).

Just the threat of a food-tampering incident involving harmless materials (or no materials) can be as effective as a real attack. Simply claiming that a product has been purposely contaminated with a dangerous material is sufficient to precipitate an extensive product recall, with the associated adverse publicity, short-term economic loss, and longer-term loss of market share (Bledsoe and Rasco, 2001a,b, 2003).

Perpetrators of a terrorist activity targeting the food industry will probably have a variety of motivations. The most common will be to cause economic damage to a specific company, type of product, a particular country's exports, or to the industry at large. Food can be used to make a political statement (e.g., animal right activists) or to influence a political outcome (e.g., the 1984 Rajneshee activities in northern Oregon) (Bledsoe and Rasco, 2003; Miller et al., 2001). Malicious mischief, copy cat crimes, or personal revenge are other possible motives. The type of attack and desire for publicity will depend on the motive (Bledsoe and Rasco, 2002, 2003; Hollingsworth, 2001; Washington State, 2001).

29.3 VULNERABILITY ASSESSMENT

Specific threats and vulnerability assessments have been difficult to obtain and many have been classified by governmental agencies, making development of effective food security planning by the private sector even more difficult. This unfortunate situation deprives people who have the greatest need to know—those involved in the production and distribution of safe food—from having the information needed to reduce these risks in their operations. Failure to provide critical information to the private sector also dilutes the efforts of both business and the government to protect the food supply and means that the most reasonable and effective preventive measures that could be developed to protect food safety may not be undertaken.

For nations with weak food safety and public health infrastructure, any vulnerability assessment is not likely to be complete, since it will be difficult to conduct the necessary studies to ascertain the actual risks to the food supply. Often, there is little reliable information regarding food production and distribution. For companies operating in situations such as this, or for those importing products from countries with a poorly developed public health and food safety infrastructure, response planning will have relatively greater importance, since the development of effective preventive measures will be difficult, diffuse, and sporadic.

Unfortunately, as security tightens up in other sectors and away from "spectacular high casualty, high profile attacks, the focus of terrorist strikes will shift to softer, primarily economic targets" (Drees, 2004). An intentional introduction of a devastating plant or animal disease is one of the risks with the greatest potential impact, and the gaps in security and inherent weakness of the farm sector make it fairly easy to introduce disease. Cost estimates of a foot-and-mouth disease incident could exceed $24 billion dollars (GAO, 2003, 2004b,2004c). A large-scale incident involving human foodborne illness would have a greater psychological impact, along with a significant economic impact on food markets.

29.4 EMERGENCY RESPONSE AND PRODUCT RECOVERY

Emergency response and product recovery involve a coordinated effort of governmental responders (www.fernlab.org). Response to a terrorist attack, a major disease outbreak, or a natural disaster would have many similarities. The degree of private-sector participation in these activities will depend on the jurisdiction. Regardless, businesses are encouraged to develop their own emergency plans and response programs to protect personnel and assets and to mitigate damages from a disaster. In the United States, catastrophic loss from any cause is increasingly self-insured, as liability policies restrict covered losses and/or add exclusions for terrorist activity, damage caused by environmental agents (e.g., environmental mold), and etiologic agents (e.g., food- or waterborne bacteria) (GAO, 2004b,c; Rasco, 2001).

29.5 PREVENTION AS THE FIRST LINE OF DEFENSE

Prevention is the first line of defense. Key to preventing food terrorism is establishing and enhancing existing food safety management programs and implementing reasonable food security measures (WHO, 2002). Preparation of a food security preparedness plan can be based on concepts familiar to food safety professionals such as hazard analysis of critical control points (HACCP; see Chapter 22). The strategies and models presented here are applicable to production agriculture, food processing, food distribution, or food service. [These are designed to be compatible with current U.S. regulations on HACCP (e.g., for fishery products: 21 *Code of Federal Regulations* (CFR) Part 123; meat and poultry products: 9 CFR 301 et seq. and 381 et seq.), good manufacturing practices (GMPs): 21 CFR 110; and recall programs: 21 CFR 7; and provisions under the Bioterrorism Act: 21 CFR 1 (CFR, 2007).]

A related strategy, organization risk management (ORM), is another option. However, in the opinion of these authors, while ORM provides an excellent tool in the hazard and risk analysis phase of a HACCP-based system, the introduction of a new and independent system provides an unnecessary burden on those responsible for administering and executing a food security program.

WHO outlines cooperative efforts between industry and government that can be effective in countries where the government or governmental employees have a vested interest in the successful operation of a business. Such arrangements are quite commonplace. This cooperative approach is less likely to work in countries where the relationship between government and the private sector is adversarial, or where the role of government agencies is focused on the exercise of police power to protect the public health by forcing compliance with food safety regulations (reasonable or not).

Regardless of the governmental structure in place, the WHO guidance focus on strengthening national response systems for food terrorism is applicable as well to private-sector planning activities. WHO also emphasizes the need to integrate food security programs, including foodborne illness surveillance and communicable disease control systems, with emergency preparedness and response systems. The WHO-proposed models and strategies are based on those already in place for terrorist attacks involving chemical, biological, or radiological agents (such as dirty bombs).

HACCP-based food safety and security programs are already in effect in the European Union and throughout North America. Such programs have a greater likelihood of successful adoption in the private sector than do other models and are promoted by WHO and the National Academies of Sciences in the United States as the most feasible approach for food security planning (GAO, 2003; NAS, 2002; WHO, 2002).

Although personal safety, preventing the kidnapping or assault of employees and/or their families, and defenses against armed attacks are important parts of a security program, these are not discussed here. Rather, the focus is directed toward protecting the integrity of the food produced, the systems and facilities used in its production, and employee safety as affected by food-related pathogens while at work.

29.6 DEVELOPMENT OF A FOOD SECURITY PLAN BASED ON HACCP PRINCIPLES

Each organization is unique and should develop a sensible and individualized security plan. Because different units and locations will probably have different vulnerabilities and be at different levels of risk, each location should be evaluated separately and the overall food security program be modified locally as required. Critical factors in a plan include evaluating specific hazards, determining their relative risk, and evaluating the public health and economic realities associated with managing these risks. Further, these factors may change seasonally or from year to year.

As mentioned above, there is a strong parallel between developing a preventive strategy for a terrorist attack and the development of preventive measures under HACCP plans (see, e.g., 21 CFR 123; CFR, 2007). The emphasis here, as with HACCP, is placed on preventive, and not on reactive measures, recognizing that HACCP is a systematic approach to the identification, evaluation, and control of food safety hazards. An outline of suggested steps in a HACCP-based plan is provided in Table 1.

An effective security plan must be built on a foundation that includes and integrates an effective HACCP plan with the existing security and food safety aspects of good manufacturing practices, sanitation standard operating procedures, and recall programs. [From U.S. regulations, the following apply: good manufacturing practices (GMPs) (21 CFR 110), workable and effective sanitation standard operating procedures (21 CFR 110; 21 CFR 123.11), and current product recall program (21 CFR 7) (CFR, 2007).] The security plan should be a written, confidential document that is reviewed and updated periodically to ensure that it is current and workable. Whereas dissemination of the relevant portions of the plan should be throughout the organization, certain elements therein should be confidential, and access to such information should be based on a bona fide need for that information. Vigilance in maintaining current food safety programs coupled with increased employee awareness are vital if a rapid determination of product contamination has to be made. Rapid communication regarding an incident to those with responsibility to manage it, recover and handle the affected product, and ensure employee and public safety is critical.

Similarly, a threat evaluation assessment and management (TEAM) approach can be used. This may be a variant of a company's total quality management (TQM) or operational risk management (ORM) program. The objective should be to provide a systematic approach to identifying and focusing on food security efforts on addressing the most critical risks. Operational risk management includes the following:

1. Accept no unnecessary risk; there must be a commensurate return in terms of real benefits or opportunities.
2. Make risk decisions at the appropriate level, as this establishes clear accountability. Include those accountable in the risk decision process.
3. Accept risk when the benefits outweigh the cost. HACCP requires hazards that are reasonably likely to occur to be controlled; however, latitude is provided regarding the means selected for controlling a particular hazard, and lower-cost options can be selected.
4. Integrate ORM into planning at all levels. HACCP programs are also integrated into facilities operations. Regulatory HACCP has focused only on food safety, limiting its scope.

The six steps in an ORM program (USFDA-CFSAN, 2001) are essentially identical to those of the HACCP-based model described above and include: (1) identifying

TABLE 1 Suggested Steps for Developing a Food Security Plan Based on an HACCP Model

Develop comprehensive flowchart(s).	Depict the operation from primary production or receiving through to consumption by the end user. This may incorporate steps outside your operation; however, this will be useful for determining suitable traceability measures to institute.
Determine possible food security hazards and evaluate the risk that these hazards may occur.[a]	Examine each operation in the flowchart to determine whether a significant food security hazard exists or could be introduced at this point.
	Consider possible risks posed by the food ingredients, packaging, and other materials that could come into contact with the food.
	Determine which of these hazards are most likely to occur and which ones, if they did occur, would cause the greatest harm.
Develop and institute risk control measures.	These risk control measures are similar to preventive measures under HACCP. The objective is to control an identified food security hazard.
	Product tracking programs or traceability features can be included within this category since the ability to conduct rapid inventory control and locate product in the marketplace can reduce risk.
	Information management factors can be included here.
Determine *points* in the operation that are *critical* for managing particular food security risks.	A critical point is a point, step, or procedure at which a control can be applied that will prevent, eliminate, or reduce a hazard to an acceptable level. A critical control point in this context could be a location inside the facility or a particular process, function, or time when the operation is at greatest risk.
Where appropriate, establish *critical limits* that are not to be violated or breached without a resulting corrective action being taken and completed.	A critical limit is a maximum or minimum value placed on a parameter at a critical control point to ensure that a particular hazard can be prevented, eliminated, or reduced to an acceptable level.
Develop *monitoring* procedures for critical control points.	Monitoring is a systematic periodic activity to ensure that critical controls are in place and have not been breached in any way.
	The monitoring program should be in writing and can include checklists or other forms of monitoring records.
	Test the monitoring program to make sure that it works and is workable for your operation.
	Review monitoring records.

TABLE 1 (*Continued*)

Develop a procedure to *fix security problems* or failures that occur if a critical control has been breached or compromised.	This is similar to corrective actions under HACCP. Ensure that problems are fixed. The objective is to reduce the likelihood that a similar breach would happen again. First and foremost, ensure that any affected product has been located, segregated (either under this program or under HACCP), and evaluated for safety. Then evaluate the current food security program and determine if the critical control points and limits are appropriate. Revise the security plan to include any changes to the critical control points and/or monitoring procedures that might be necessary so that this security breach does not reoccur. Then rigorously retest the system and its risk monitoring procedures. Corrective actions may also include prompt notification of appropriate law enforcement or emergency response authorities, or execution of ancillary procedures such as an evacuation, lockdown, or similar activity.
Initially *verify* and then periodically re-verify the security program to make sure it is suitable, current and workable.	Examine the security plan and revise written protocols (if necessary) when the operation or any of its key features change. Reexamine your security plan, starting at the flowchart step, if suppliers, ingredients, product form, distribution systems, or end users change, as these could introduce or remove hazards and require that the plan be revised. Reexamine security programs if there is credible information that the food supply in general, or your particular product type or operation, is at heightened risk. If necessary, take stricter precautions. Verification programs should be in writing and maintained as confidential files. The supervisory personnel tasked with implementing the food security program should systematically review food security monitoring and corrective action records. A weekly review may be appropriate. The purpose of this review is to ensure that the program is being implemented and remains effective for addressing current food security risk within an operation. Inclusion of superfluous and unnecessary documentation should be avoided.

(*Continued*)

TABLE 1 (*Continued*)

	Updating other important company programs can be tied in with periodic verification activities to make sure that all programs are integrated, implementable, not conflicting or redundant, and are up to date. These additional programs can include: • Employee training program in food security with training records • Review of recall programs and any associated press releases • Emergency preparedness and response plan and response team information and roles • Emergency contact information for key employees, law enforcement, and public safety officials • Media relations plan, contacts, and press releases Conduct exercises periodically to verify the ability to successfully execute the overall and/or the individual elements of the plan.
Maintain *records* for the security program	Adequate, comprehensive, and confidential records need to be developed. These records include the plan objectives, flowcharts, plant and site layout, risk analysis and preventive measures, justification and establishment of critical control points and critical limits, monitoring, corrective action plan and deviations, and verification activities. Incorporated within the plan should be current contact information for law enforcement, food safety and public health agencies, and employees. Also, consider developing a family notification plan. Wherever possible, utilize existing records modified as necessary. Avoid generating an overburdening system of unnecessary and/or redundant records.

[a]Under HACCP, only two assessments are made relating to risk assessment: (1) whether a hazard may cause food to be unsafe for human consumption (see e.g., 21 CFR Sec. 123.3.f), and (2) whether a hazard is reasonably likely to occur (see e.g., 21 CFR Sec. 123.6a). A hazard that is reasonably likely to occur is one for which a prudent processor would establish controls.

threats, (2) assessing the risk, (3) analyzing risk control measures, (4) making control decisions, (5) implementing risk controls, and (6) supervising and reviewing.

ORM is more complicated. We have modified the classic matrix to more closely reflect the situation facing food businesses (Table 2), including the important category of "unknown," commonly incorporated into the risk assessment matrices of intelligence professionals. Frankly, in most instances the likelihood and severity of many food-associated risks are not known, and recognizing this fact will help to focus efforts on filling knowledge gaps.

TABLE 2 An Operational Risk Assessment Matrix

	Probability[b]					
Severity[a]	Frequent	Likely	Occasional	Seldom	Unlikely	Unknown
Catastrophic	Extremely high	Extremely high	High	High	Medium	Unknown
Critical	Extremely high	High	High	Medium	Low	Unknown
Moderate	High	Medium	Medium	Low	Low	Unknown
Negligible	Medium	Low	Low	Low	Low	Unknown
Unknown	Unknown	Unknown	Unknown	Unknown	Unknown	Unknown

[a]Severity:

- *Catastrophic*: food contamination incident that causes total business failure. Fatalities and numerous serious illnesses or injuries.
- *Critical*: food contamination incident that has caused a major loss of business. Serious illnesses or injuries.
- *Moderate*: food contamination incident that causes some loss of business. No serious illnesses or injuries.
- *Negligible*: food contamination incident that causes minor loss of business. No serious illnesses or injuries.
- *Unknown*: food contamination with a severity that is difficult or not possible to predict.

[b]Probability:

- *Frequent*: food contamination incident that occurs often. Specific individuals or the general population is continuously exposed.
- *Likely*: food contamination incident that has occurred several times. Specific individuals or the general population is regularly exposed.
- *Occasional*: food contamination incident that occurs. Exposure is sporadic.
- *Seldom*: food contamination incident that may occur. Exposure is low.
- *Unlikely*: food contamination incident that is not likely to occur. Exposure is rare.
- *Unknown*: food contamination incident that may or may not occur. Probability of occurrence is difficult or not possible to predict. Exposure of targeted individuals or the population at large is difficult to predict.

Our experience implementing ORM risk assessment in food operations is that people get "hung up" with the hazard analysis and have difficulty getting past this and on to the development of a workable food security plan. Companies often have limited concrete information on which to make risk assessments, and this fact must be recognized. Because of the unnecessary complexity of ORM and the tendency for most companies, and their employees, to be familiar with HACCP, we recommend, initially at least, that a company employ the HACCP-based model. The added level of sophistication in ORM can be incorporated into the initial planning or into later versions of a food security plan as additional risk assessment data becomes available. Further, one of the weaknesses of ORM as promulgated for food security planning is that it assumes that "severity" and "probability" of occurrence are known, which is often not true. Often the hardest decision to make is to determine that any element is unknown. Such goes against our very nature. Therefore, we have modified the matrix to add "unknown" to each axis, and Table 2 portrays the ORM risk assessment matrix as we have modified it.

TABLE 3 Analysis of Risk Control Measures

Action	Justification
Reject	Refuse to take the risk if the overall costs of the risk exceed its benefits to the business or operation. *Example*: Placing a new employee on night shift with minimal or no supervision when the person has not been properly cleared or vetted. Another example is providing lockers to which only the employee has access.
Avoid	Avoiding a risk altogether requires canceling or delaying a job or operation, and is rarely used. *Example*: Removing a salad bar from a restaurant to avoid intentional contamination of its contents with pathogenic bacteria.
Delay	Is it possible to forestall the risk? If time is not critical, a risk could be delayed. During the delay, the risk may go away. *Example*: A business could decide to retain a salad bar in a restaurant while threat levels are low. However, if threat levels increase, or public health or law enforcement officials notify a business or class of businesses regarding a particular threat, the business could decide to switch to providing individual servings of salad instead.
Transfer	Risk transfer does not change the probability or severity of a hazard, but it may decrease the probability or severity of the risk actually experienced. Risk transfer could also be accomplished by forming a cooperative to ensure against a terrorist loss experienced by a member of the cooperative. *Example*: Have a professional society or trade association provide an audited certification program for members of a particular industry segment. Such a program would reduce risk by increasing overall awareness and preparedness. For example, the National Restaurant Association has prepared guidelines and training materials to address the needs of restaurants.
Spread	Distribute the risk either by increasing the exposure distance or by lengthening the time between exposure events. *Example*: Spread deliveries in time and between different suppliers and carriers.
Compensate	Create a redundant capacity. This includes backup systems for critical equipment, staff, materials, information systems, and logistics.
Reduce	Plan operations and design systems that do not contain hazards by minimizing risk, instituting preventive measures, adding safety and warning devices, exercising programs, and providing training.

Source: Modified from USFDA-CFSAN (2001).

ORM includes an analysis of risk control measures that involve cost considerations that can be incorporated into evaluations of possible preventive measures in HACCP-based plans (Table 3). The overall objective is not to reach the least level of risk, but instead, to reach the best level of risk for overall food safety and security (USFDA-CFSAN, 2001). A possible deficiency with the ORM approach is a failure to specifically include provisions to verify the effectiveness of the program, to develop a series of control decisions for possible breaches of security in advance, and to maintain adequate and systematic records.

Regardless of the model used, to the extent possible, keep details of any food security plan confidential, to limit the possibility of information falling into the wrong hands. Although food security plans are not yet mandated by governmental agencies, guidance has been issued, and it will not be long before food security issues start to creep into food safety inspections. There is a legitimate fear that security guidance will morph into de facto regulations as we have seen happen with HACCP over the past eight years in the United States. Food security programs are and should be at the company level and be market driven. Many aspects of food security are beyond the scope of the expertise of individual food safety inspectors, and there are several necessary components outside their jurisdiction. Many companies had food security programs in place for the years prior to governmental concern over these matters. Further, their plans are evolving as they gain a better understanding of food security risks, as the sources of the risks increase or evolve, as new knowledge is gained on how to control these risks, and as technologies develop in support of managing risks.

29.7 EVALUATING SECURITY RISKS AND IDENTIFYING HAZARDS

Initially, a company or organization should complete an analysis of its facilities and operations to identify significant hazards and the potential exposure to a particular hazard, and to evaluate the risks of an occurrence. The scope of this effort should include relevant physical, human, and technical factors. This analysis, sometimes called a vulnerability assessment, incorporates scientific, economic, political, and social circumstances and measures the extent of the threat when possible. Further vulnerability assessment should consider external factors such as first responders, activities of regulating agencies, and the protection of evidence, and set priorities for resource utilization (WHO, 2002). Priorities must be set so that any action taken to deal with a security threat is commensurate with its severity and impact. This assessment will provide the company, if nothing else, with an idea of how the emergency response from the public health sector may proceed. Obviously, any incident will have major market impact, regardless of the agent used, the terrorist motivation or the level of preparedness, and effectiveness in executing a governmental emergency response preparedness program. Vulnerability assessments should include evaluation of the following factors:

1. The public health impact, severity of illness, or risk of death of deliberate exposure to the agent to the general public and susceptible subpopulations.
2. Potential for delivery of the agent to large populations.
3. Possibility of mass production or distribution of the agent.
4. Potential for person-to-person transmission.
5. Public perception of the agent, fear, and potential for civil disruption.
6. Special needs for public health preparedness, including stockpiles of drugs, vaccines, etc.

7. Need for enhanced surveillance or diagnosis capabilities.
8. Possibility of obtaining necessary quantities of agent.
9. Means to do harm and opportunity to carry out a terrorist act.
10. Identification of potential terrorists and willingness to do harm.
11. Availability of effective preparedness plans and capacity for effective response; means to avert harm.

A risk analysis should not be limited to the production facility or to times of peak operations. The evaluation should cover the entire scope of operations, including:

1. Agricultural production methods and harvest methods of ingredients.
2. Storage and transport of raw materials.
3. Receiving operations.
4. Materials and goods-in-process holding.
5. Security risk presented by other materials used within the facility (process or sanitizer chemicals, pesticides, pressurized gases, water and boiler treatments).
6. Suppliers of various components, their potential vulnerabilities, and their degree of preparedness planning.
7. Type of processing used for the manufacture of particular food items and risks associated with this.
8. Processing lines and their configuration.
9. Subcontracting facilities, packaging, warehousing, rolling stock, distribution of processed goods, physical plant, wholesale and retail distribution, retail and consumer use. Evaluation of the risks presented by neighboring facilities is also important (WHO, 2002) and includes power plants, fuel or chemical manufacture, storage or distribution, military, law enforcement or government facilities, transportation and communication operations, and infrastructure.
10. Factors not normally associated with conventional HACCP planning, such as security fencing, perimeter lighting, restrictive access, and facility monitoring, should be included.

Any point in the food chain where product changes hands or may not be monitored directly is vulnerable. Access to any critical areas should be controlled with additional and sometimes unique factors applicable to research centers, farms, and/or ancillary sites that may need to be taken into consideration. Any evaluation of risk requires an examination of the raw materials and distribution methods, as well as the handling practices of common carriers and other third parties. Water sources and supplies may be of specific concern, particularly if water is used as an ingredient or comes into direct contact with consumable products. In effect, the "chain of custody" for the product and its components should be monitored from farm to table.

As with HACCP, a team should be used to develop the plan and conduct a vulnerability assessment. This evaluation should include personnel from human resources, marketing, distribution, and sales as well as those involved with quality control, production, and security functions. In larger organizations, this team may actually consist of a series of smaller groups formed within identifiable units. Regardless of the structure of an organization, good leadership and a comprehensive integration of the team recommendations into corporate programs are critical factors, as is the buy-in to the resulting program by both management and employees at all levels.

29.8 MANAGING RISK: PREVENTIVE MEASURES

Since it will probably be impossible to eliminate all hazards, a reasonable procedure must be instituted to manage them. Probably the best strategy is to develop preventive or risk control measures that would reduce or eliminate the most significant hazards, then work down the list to control less likely or less serious hazards. As part of this risk management program, points in an operation identified as critical for controlling the security risks determined may require specific attention and developmental emphasis. These points may change or fluctuate during the course of a day, seasonally, with changes in ingredient sourcing, suppliers (e.g., domestic or imported product), product type or form, processing and packaging methods, distribution, and end user.

Following this evaluation, establish a monitoring procedure for these risk control points (similar to the program already be in place for monitoring critical control points in a HACCP plan). Along with these monitoring protocols should be corrective actions (again, similar to those in a HACCP program) in case of a breach of security or a security failure. A plan for verifying the effectiveness of the preventive and risk controls measures in a food security plan should be included (the use of forms such as the HACCP Hazard Analysis Worksheet or the HACCP Plan Form (see, e.g., USFDA-CFSAN, 2001) may be of benefit in some cases and are the forms used in the example at the end of the chapter). An example of a food security plan with forms is presented as an appendix to this chapter.

29.9 SECURITY STRATEGIES

Specific recommendations for the detailed development of a food security plan are available and are only summarized here (Table 4) (Bledsoe and Rasco, 2003; USFDA, 2007a,b; USFDA-FSIS, 2002; WHO, 2002). The key to a successful program is vigilance by management and all employees. Training is critical. Clear standard operating procedures must be developed and followed for day-to-day operations, in handling suspicious incidents or persons, and for actual attacks. The problems arising from an actual attack may be similar to the outcome already included within an existing crisis management plan for natural disasters, loss of power or communications, and so on. If product safety is an issue, recall procedures would need to be followed. As with recall programs, individual farms, companies, or research institutions should use periodic exercises and drills to test whether a security plan is current, workable, and effective. Unfortunately, cost will often be the controlling factor in the

TABLE 4 Suggestions for a Food Security Plan

Security Issue	Suggestions
Site survey	Include construction plans or blueprints for facility, floor plan, aerial photos. Have an up-to-date floor plan accessible from a secure location near the site. Identify copies on file at local police, fire, building, and planning departments as confidential. Request that these recipients place appropriate restrictions on access to these files.
Farming operations	Implement an animal traceability system. Improve lot traceability for fungible items such as grain. Restrict commingling of lots. Institute tracking systems for supplies and shipments. Provide bin locks, tamper-evident devices, or other control devices on feed bins and water delivery systems. Closely monitor stocks of fuel, ammonia, ammonia-containing fertilizers, agricultural chemicals, and applicator equipment. Avoid stockpiling hazardous materials, and keep materials secure. Evaluate supplier guarantee and third-party audit programs to ensure that shipments of feed, seed, and chemicals are to specification and are not contaminated. Restrict access to cropland and livestock to the extent practical. Consider compartmentalizing livestock operations, reducing opportunities for cross-contamination, and improving sanitation to reduce risk of spreading a disease.
Manufacturing or food preparation operations	Evaluate physical security of a building: screens, closable and lockable doors, windows, window wells, roof entry, and ventilation inlet/outlet. Control access to site (buildings, outbuildings, chemical storage, boiler, water and waste handling) and to processing and storage areas. Keep traffic in food preparation areas to a minimum. Remove hiding places in facility, particularly in food preparation and storage areas. Have surveillance programs for the exterior and interior of the facility. Inspect the facility at least daily for compliance with sanitary, safety, and security programs. Maintain records. Maintain an accurate inventory of product, ingredients, tools, utensils, knives, etc. Inspect incoming raw materials for integrity, cleanliness, temperature, etc. Train employees on how to recognize, segregate, and handle suspicious ingredients, components, and products. Ensure that there is enough information for adequate traceability (supplier, production lot, location) on incoming materials. Compare delivery slips or load manifests with orders for both content and quantity.

TABLE 4 (*Continued*)

Security Issue	Suggestions
	Have current contact information for key personnel, emergency response, law enforcement, and public health posted in the facility.
	Know and mark the location of equipment and utilities controls and safety switches, escape routes, and emergency exits. Make sure that escape routes, are clearly marked and accessible.
Facilities configuration	Construct or modify the facility to control product flow in a rational way.
	Compartmentalize functions, such as physical segregation of raw and cooked product.
	Install good interior and exterior lighting.
	Provide adequate and functional sprinklers and alarm systems.
	Evaluate plant ventilation, filtration, and air cleaning systems to protect building environments.
	Reduce points of access to a facility.
	Have an appropriate number of accessible and alarmed emergency exits.
	Consider stricter control of parking and vehicle access to the site, including the use of parking permits and vehicle registration.
	Enclosing the parking area, increasing physical security, installing no parking safe-zones, and/or instituting a vehicle inspection program are possible options.
Water and air supplies	Evaluate the security of on-site and municipal wells, hydrants, and water storage and water handling facilities.
	Secure access to wells, standpipes, reservoirs, and pumping stations.
	Consider checking water quality more frequently, regardless of its source.
	Locate an alternative source of potable water and provide additional on-site storage in case of an emergency, or consider a backup water purification system.
	Take precautions to ensure that air entering the operation is not contaminated. Examine air intake points for physical integrity and access.
Suppliers	Request letters of guarantee from suppliers and require a showing of protected transportation of components.
	Consider a preferred supplier programs for companies that can comply with your quality specifications, and safety and security standards. This will include periodic inspections of vendors and an examination of their distribution systems.
	Require tamper-proof packaging or shipping containers as well as numbered seals that can be independently verified with the vendor.
	Do not accept unordered ingredients/shipments or product received in opened or damaged containers.
	As part of your recall program, ensure that any specific lot of an ingredient can be tracked from its source through production to final product and distribution.

(*Continued*)

TABLE 4 ***(Continued)***

Security Issue	Suggestions
	Have sufficient air circulation in the plant to maintain a slight overpressure.
Distribution and transit	Require carrier to secure loads during transit, and if the product or container is to be held, that fencing, locks, etc. to prevent unauthorized access to food contents secure the container.
	Tamper-evident and tamper-resistant seals unique to any given bulk container should be used. If possible, communicate seal information electronically, separate from the shipment, to the receiver and sender; verify numbers and seal integrity prior to opening the container.
	Consider a more sophisticated tracking program for shipments.
	Conduct-off-loading under controlled conditions, with periodic testing of off-loading security.
	Use temperature recorders on loads where appropriate and analyze the data for indications of unauthorized access to the load (e.g., a temperature spike or other unusual fluctuation).
Wholesale and retail distribution	Control access and monitor activities. Employee vigilance is even more critical in retail that it may be in manufacturing.
	Camera systems set up to deter robbery should be reevaluated to improve their effectiveness as part of a food security program.
	Have self-service sections (delis, produce, bakery, bulk foods, automatic dispensers of beverages and sauces) positioned in the store where they can be closely monitored (high-traffic area, greater employee control) to reduce the likelihood of intentional contamination.
	Exclude nonemployees from food preparation and storage areas. Improve the physical barriers between public and restricted areas in the facility.
Research and quality control labs	Control access to laboratories, test plots, and their supporting infrastructure.
	Increase security of hazardous materials. Consider locked access to dangerous biological or chemical materials. Maintain an accurate inventory and investigate shortages immediately.
	Make sure that hazardous materials are properly labeled, stored, and handled properly to avoid contamination of food and food-contact surfaces.
	Avoid taking hazardous materials into food processing or storage areas.
	Conduct random product and environmental testing as a preventive measure against contamination within the processing environment.
	Develop a good working relationship with local or regional food testing and forensic laboratories, as their services may be critical if an issue of product or facilities contamination arises.

TABLE 4 (*Continued*)

Security Issue	Suggestions
Employee and contractor screening	Check references and background on employees and contractors (construction, pest control, truckers, security, cleaning crew, etc.) looking for signs of dishonesty.
Employees and contractors	A "two person" rule should be in effect for both safety and food security reasons. No one should be left alone during food preparation or handling.
	Employee and sub/contractor rosters, job, and shift assignments should be current, reviewed on a daily basis, and updated as needed. No one should be on the site who is not scheduled to be there.
	ID should be provided.
	No personal items such as lunches, purses, etc. should be permitted into a food-processing area. You may wish to extend this procedure to restrict certain personal objects entirely from the facility.
	A condition of employment can be that the employer may inspect the personal property of any employee at any time.
	Job functions within a facility should be compartmentalized to the extent practicable. This would mean restricting access to specific areas in a facility only to people who need to be there.
	Unusual behavior on the part of employees or contractors, such as staying unusually late, or arriving early, reviewing or removing documents or materials not necessary for their assigned work, removing materials or documents from the facility, or seeking information about sensitive subjects should cause suspicion.
	Discharged employees/contractors should immediately surrender keys, badges, etc. They should be promptly escorted from the facility and not be permitted to return except as an (escorted) visitor. Computer and electronic access codes should be terminated when employment ends.
	Ensure that all keys can be accounted for and that each key has discreet identification numbers. Keys should be marked "do not duplicate." Better yet, consider the use of card-swipe electronic locks that eliminate the need for metal keys. Most key card systems allow for improved control over access and maintain a record when a person gains entry. Individual access can also be controlled on a timely basis, thus permitting entry only during scheduled hours.
	Employees should be made aware of their responsibilities to stay alert for and report suspicious activities, objects, and persons at their workplace or at home. The responsibility for specific security functions should be assigned to qualified persons and included within job descriptions.
Visitors and inspectors	Inspectors should provide appropriate identification and be vetted by backup procedures.

(*Continued*)

TABLE 4 ***(Continued)***

Security Issue	Suggestions
	Consider a "no photography" policy.
	Escort visitors at all times.
	Limit access to processing areas, lockers, and break rooms by visitors (truckers, delivery people, supplier representatives, customers, applicants for employment, or other visitors).
	Have a check-in procedure and issue visitor badges in a reception area or another location that is not adjacent to the processing area or accessible to the processing area without proceeding through physical barriers. All visitor badges should be accounted for on a daily basis.
Emergency evacuation plan	Have an emergency evacuation plan. Review for appropriateness at least annually.
	File a copy with the local municipal planning department and with emergency response agencies. Require these governmental entities to safeguard the documents and *prohibit their release to any party without your knowledge and written consent*. Another option is to have the evacuation plan along with the facility layout placed into a locked and sealed container outside the facility in case access to the facility is limited in an emergency.
	Conduct unannounced tests of evacuation plans.
	Train employees how to respond to certain types of emergencies (flood, fire, earthquake, chemical spill) and include this training as part of new employee orientation.
	Train as many people as possible in CPR and basic first aid.
	Make certain that contractors and visitors know company evacuation procedures and the special hazards at the operation (e.g., high-voltage electricity, steam, toxic and corrosive chemical storage and use).
	Ensure that visitors are escorted through the facility, can understand instructions of their escort in case of an emergency, and that exits are clearly marked.
	Make sure that contact information with emergency responders is up to date.
Other issues	*Data security*. Ensure that operational, mandatory records, and business confidential materials (including product formulations, analytical results, and operational parameters) are backed up with electronic and/or hard copies stored at a separate location.
	Restrict access to computer systems and remove access immediately for persons no longer employed or contracted by the firm. Test and update firewalls and virus detection and cleaning systems. Evaluate computer systems on a regular basis for security.
	Mail handling. Ensure that packages received within your facility do not have suspicious labeling or appearance. Establish procedures to handle suspicious mail.

development of a food security program, since it is impossible physically and financially to guard against every eventuality. Further, not all of the recommendations included here will be appropriate, practical, and cost-effective for every individual entity. As with HACCP, food security programs will often be market driven, and each company will have to make managerial and policy decisions based on their own unique circumstances.

APPENDIX: AN EXAMPLE

Production and Retail Distribution of Ready-to-Eat Potato Salad

In this example, food security issues surrounding the receipt, processing, storage, and distribution of a ready-to-eat deli-style potato salad are addressed (Fig. A1).

Product Description Ready-to-eat potato salad, refrigerated, packaged in plastic tubs with tamper-evident seals, for sale to the general public at retail outlets.

1. *Raw material acquisition*. Fresh potatoes and onions are obtained in 50-lb bags; and fresh celery in 10-lb boxes. These produce items are obtained from a local fresh food distributor. They are from local sources when in season, and from Mexico or California out of season. Product can be traced to individual farms or cooperatives (domestic production) and to a specific distributor (for imported product).

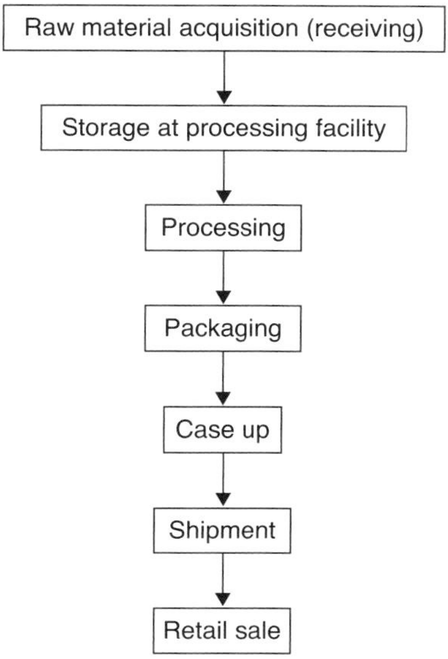

FIG. A1 Flowchart: ready-to-eat potato salad.

Salad dressing, salt, and pepper are obtained from a local food service distributor. Salad dressing is in 5-gallon plastic containers, salt in 50-lb sacks, and pepper and spices in 1-lb plastic containers. Manufacturer contact information, including lot codes, is required on individual containers. Packaging (8-oz plastic tubs with plastic snap-top closures) is obtained from a regional manufacturer and is received in cardboard boxes.

The packaging of the ingredient components is tamper-evident only to the extent that it should be clear that the package had been opened and resealed (torn tape or stitching).

All materials arrive by common carrier. Shipments are scheduled in advance.

Product is received at the processing facility within 24 hours after the order has been placed (Monday through Friday delivery only). Product type, container size, quantity, and lot number are checked against order sheets.

2. *Storage at processing facility*. Products are held in a cool, dry, walk-in food storage area until needed. This area is separate from, but adjacent to, the processing room. Product flow is first in, first out.
3. *Processing*. The amount of each ingredient required for a single 50-lb batch of product is removed from storage immediately prior to production. Lot numbers from each lot are recorded on production sheets. Commingling ingredients from different lots into a single batch of salad is avoided. Potatoes are peeled by an automatic peeler. Potatoes are chopped and then cooked in boiling salted water in a steam-jacketed kettle until soft (about 15 min). Onions are peeled and then chopped in a food processor, transferred to a sealed plastic container, and held in a walk-in refrigerator until used. Celery is chopped in a food processor and then held similarly. Dry ingredients are blended together in the appropriate ratio and held in a sealed plastic container. Ingredients, with the exception of the cooked potatoes, are folded together in a mixer until uniformly blended. Product temperature is not permitted to exceed 50°F for more than 1 h from the time of initiating blending. The final processing step is the combination of the blended ingredients with the cooked potatoes.
4. *Packaging*. Eight ounces (net weight) of the potato salad is filled by hand into plastic tubs. A plastic closure is placed on the container. A preprinted label is applied to the top of each closure. A "best if used by date" is stamped on the bottom along with a lot code, which is a combination of time and Julian date. Then a plastic tamper-evident heat-shrinkable band is applied to each container. Containers are placed onto metal racks and placed in a cooler (40°F). Specifications are for the product to reach 60°F within 1 h and 42°F within an additional hour. The label includes the product name, manufacturer name, location and contact information, net weight, an ingredient statement, nutrition facts, prominently displayed instructions to keep the product refrigerated until use, and a bar code.
5. *Case up*. After the product has reached 42°F, 24 tubs are packed into a master case. The master case is sealed with a specially designed tape with the company logo. A label is generated that has product identification and content, lot code,

bar code, and company contact information. Both the tape and the box are prominently marked "keep refrigerated".

6. *Shipment*. Since product is made to order, it is shipped within 24 h to regional customers by common carrier. Retailers receive only full cases of product. Quantity and lot code are tied to each customer shipment. Trucks are inspected before each shipment is loaded to ensure that the vehicle is clean, the refrigeration system is working, and the identity of the driver and the expected time of delivery are verified. The customer is notified electronically or by phone when the order has been shipped and is given a tracking number (contains product ID, quantity, and lot codes) and estimated time of arrival.
7. *Retail sale*. Personnel at the retail store inspect the product for package integrity and take the product temperature. Delivery is checked against vendor information. Personnel from the deli department replace stock on the sales shelves as necessary: first in, first out. The consumer removes the product from the deli case.

A key to ensuring that shipment integrity has been maintained is inspection at receiving (Figs. A2 and A3). It is entirely practical and possible for the receiving company to match the data output from even the simplest of the aforementioned devices against schedule profiles. Product that does not meet the critical limits established by the purchasing firm should be rejected, isolated, and the vendor notified immediately. The receiving records and supporting documents should be reviewed in a timely manner by a qualified supervisor for every shipment. Where practical, this review should be backed up by comparative automated data analysis.

At receiving, vendor certification and lot numbers should be matched against that provided by the vendor, normally through the purchasing department of the purchasing company. Volumes and weights should also be compared and matched against purchasing documents. In a similar manner, receiving as well as other personnel at all stages of production should inspect packaging integrity. A copy of the critical receiving information should be transmitted independently to the producer and shipper for comparative verification.

Part of this step would be assurance that the receiving department has the appropriate seal numbers available to them. The driver or other delivery agent should have this data and use it periodically for inspection while transporting the materials. However, for security reasons, the driver should not provide seal data to the receiver. This information should be provided directly from the supplier to the receiver electronically or by fax. The integrity of seals and locks should be verified by the company's receiving personnel both as to identification code and integrity and not removed until immediately prior to unloading. Inspecting agencies that remove the seals enroute should replace the seals with new units and then independently transmit the new seal numbers to the intended receiver.

The printout from the truck recorder (often this will be provided electronically by the common carrier from remotely downloaded data) should be examined for indications of unauthorized deviations.

Firm Name: **Address:**	Fresh Salad Co. 16 Penn Ave. Columbia, WA 98765		**Product line/description**: Ready-to-eat potato salad, packed (8 oz plastic tubs) for retail sale **Intended use/consumer**: Retail sale, general public	
Item, Step or Function	***Identify Potential Hazards Introduced, Controlled, Or Enhanced at this Step***	***Are Any Hazards Significant?***	***What Control Measure(s) Can be Applied to Prevent the Significant Hazard***	***Is this Control Measure Critical?***
Raw material acquisition	Purposeful Contamination	YES	Certification of lot by vendor/Supplier guarantee for packaging materials.	YES
			Ensure product secure and access limited to authorized individuals only.	YES
			Verifying paperwork at receipt, check lot, product type, quantity, number of units, origin.	YES
			All openings, vents, doors etc. on truck or conveyance locked and sealed.	YES
			Verify seal numbers and integrity	YES
			Check product and packaging integrity.	YES
			Tamper evident packaging.	YES
			Transit vehicles held in secured facility when unattended	YES
			Vehicle secured when driver absent	YES
Storage at processing facility	Purposeful contamination	YES	Product remains in original packaging, storage is for a short period and poses little risk.	NO
			Ensure product secure and access limited to authorized individuals only.	YES
			Product properly inventoried	NO
Processing	Purposeful contamination	YES	Contamination of final product with hazardous materials would not be evident to retailer or retail customer	YES
Packaging	Purposeful contamination	YES	Contamination of final product with hazardous materials would not be evident to retailer or retail customer	YES
			Product properly inventoried	YES
			Tamper evident features applies to individual containers	YES
			Traceability features incorporated into individual units	YES
Case-up	Purposeful Contamination	YES	Product Properly Inventoried	NO
			Tamper evident seals present and intact on unitized packaging	YES
			Traceability features incorporated into unitized product	YES
Shipment	Purposeful Contamination	YES	All openings, vents, doors, etc. on truck or conveyance locked and sealed. Seals recorded.	YES
			Data and temperature logger included in load	YES
Retail	Purposeful Contamination	YES	Control receipt and storage of inventory	YES
			Control stock rotation, first in first out	YES
			Ensure that all food is properly labeled and has suitable traceability features	YES
			Do not resell perishable food items found in other store locations or returned by customers	YES
			Check package integrity of product on shelves	YES
			Be alert for suspicious activities	YES
Prepared by:	T. Thompson	Date:	19 October 2004	

FIG. A2 Hazard analysis workseet.

Firm Name: **Address:**	Fresh Salad Co. 16 Penn Ave. Columbia, WA 98765	**Product line/description**: Ready-to-eat potato salad, packed (8 oz plastic tubs) for retail sale	**Intended use/consumer**: Retail sale, general public						
Critical Control Point	***Significant Hazard(s)***	***Critical Limits for each Critical Control Measure***	***Monitoring***				***Corrective Actions***	***Verification***	***Records***
			What	***How***	***Frequency***	***Who***			
Raw material acquisition	Purposeful Contamination	Vendor certification received with shipment	Certification received	Check against shipping docs	Each lot	Receiving QC	Isolate and investigate. If required records verification is possible, accept. If not, reject.	Daily record review	Receiving record
		Lot ID#s	Lot identification	Check product ID against shipping docs	Each lot		Isolate and investigate. If can't adequately ID lots, then reject.		
		All units have functional tamper evident packaging. Packaging is intact.	Package integrity	Visual	Each unit		Reject and isolate. Retain product if criminal activity is suspected and contact law enforcement.		
		Vehicle secured when driver absent	Vehicle security	Trip report	Each shipment		Examine carrier practices and discontinue use of carriers that cannot comply with security program		
Processing	Purposeful Contamination	No introduction of hazardous materials into food	Restrict opportunity to contaminate product by monitoring worker activities	Two workers at all times	Each lot	Process foreman, other workers	Isolate product and evaluate safety. Investigate and report any suspicious activity. If tampering is possible, reject and destroy. If criminal activity is suspected, isolate and retain product and contact law enforcement	Daily records review	Scheduling roster

FIG. A3 Food security plan form.

		Ingredient lot(s) in each batch. Proper quantities measured and recorded.	Ingredient lot numbers, ingredient amount	Visual inspection for lot numbers, volume or weight for quantity	Each lot		Properly record lots for each batch of product. Do not ship product that cannot be traced back to specific ingredients		Production log
Packaging	Purposeful Contamination	Product integrity	Product handled by trusted individuals only	Two person rule. Employee vigilance for suspicious activity	Each lot	Packaging lead	Isolate suspicious product and evaluate. If tampering is possible, reject and destroy. If criminal activity is suspected, isolate and retain product and contact law enforcement	Daily records review	Packaging log
		Package integrity and tamper evident features in each unit	Package properly sealed	Visual	Each unit	Line worker	Reject, then isolate damaged product		
		Each package can be traced back	Proper package labeling	Visual	Each unit	Line worker	Isolate, and relabel uncoded product. If this is not possible, reject and destroy product.		
		Product properly inventoried	Accurate count of containers from each lot	Calculate yield	Each lot	Packaging lead	Check calculations to determine proper number of units per log. Account for all units. Do not ship any units from a production lot until yield can be confirmed.		
Case-Up		Tamper evident features present on cases	Package properly sealed	Visual	Each unit	Packaging lead	Isolate improperly labeled product and relabel.	Daily records review	Packaging log
		Traceability features present on master cases	Features present	Visual	Each unit				
Shipment	Purposeful Contamination	All openings, vents, doors, etc., on truck or conveyance are locked and sealed prior to shipment	Seals present and numbers recorded.	Check numbers against vendor docs	Each shipment	Receiving QC at retailer	If seal, lot and quantity documentation not reliable, do not accept shipment until adequate confirmation can be obtained	Daily review of shipping records	Shipping records

FIG. A3 *(Continued)*

		Data and temperature recorder device(s) included in shipment	Data logger and temperature recorder present and functional	Check for any unexplained deviations			Reject shipments with unexplained deviations		
		Automated trip recorder/report	Trip recorder set	Recover and review report			Isolate shipments for which there is questionable information. Reject if suspicious activity is possible. If criminal activity is suspected retain product and contact law enforcement		
Retail Sale	Purposeful Contamination	Receipt and storage of product controlled	Product delivered to secure area and unloaded under supervision of retailer	Offload monitored by retail personnel	Each shipment	Receiving QC	Isolate shipment. Do not offload into retail facility until security issues have been adequately addressed. Reject if security cannot be assured. Isolate and retain product if criminal activity is suspected.	Daily review of shipping & receiving records and security inspection reports	Shipping and receiving records. Reports of security inspections
		All food is properly labeled and has traceability features	Examine master cases at unload for labeling and traceability features	Visual	Each shipment	Receiving QC	Isolate any food not properly labeled and note defect. Reject. If criminal activity is suspected, retain product and contact law enforcement	Daily review of inventory control and product reports	Inventory reports
			Examine retail units when stocking	Visual	Each unit	Inventory control staff	Isolate unit and note defect if labeling is not clear and traceability or tamper evident features are damaged or absent. If criminal activity is suspected, retain product and contact law enforcement.	Daily review of inventory control report	Inventory control reports
		Perishable foods are not restocked; returned perishable food items are not resold	Restocked or returned perishable food items	Product recovery location and sale history	Any affected unit	Any employee	Isolate and discard	Review of inventory control and departmental	Inventory control and security inspection

FIG. A3 *(Continued)*

								shift reports	reports
		Package integrity for product on shelf	Examine products on shelf during shift and when stocking shelves	Visual	Any affected unit	Department manager	Isolate, report defect, and discard. Retain product if criminal activity is suspected.	Review of inventory control and departmental shift reports	Inventory control and security inspection reports
		No suspicious activity that could jeopardize food safety	Monitor customers and employee behavior	Visual or via surveillance system	Any individual	All employees	Question suspicious individual. If criminal activity is suspected, retain and contact law enforcement	Daily review security report	Security inspection report

Prepared by: *T. Thompson* Date: October 19, 2004 Reviewed by: R Cheney Date: 21 Oct 04

FIG. A3 *(Continued)*

Although measures such as those described in this example may appear onerous at first glance, many of the steps are current accounting, quality control, and production records commonly in use. Many of these recommendations are just good business practices that should be employed regardless of a perceived bioterrorist threat.

Note: A company might also employ the following practices to improve employee monitoring:

1. Enhance external and internal security control measures by instituting a system of identity tags that all employees must display when working. The identity tag is left at the entrance control point when the employee is not at work and is picked up when the employee checks in. One common method for compartmentalizing job functions uses employee uniforms of different styles or colors. This is a common practice in both large and small food-processing companies in many countries. For example, employees working in the immediate processing area wear white uniforms or smocks, while those in the receiving area wear blue and in the shipping area, red. Maintenance personnel could wear blue uniforms with red panels on the shoulders.
2. To improve site security, the entire plant might be surrounded by an 8-foot wire fence with a personnel gate through which visitors and employees pass. The shipping and receiving areas are within an interior fence, and access is through a locked gate that is staffed any time it is opened. Personal vehicles are not permitted in this interior area.
3. Perimeter lighting should be installed on posts away from the building but illuminating all portions of the building, grounds, and employee parking areas. Security cameras, with recorders, should be installed in strategic locations. The cameras are monitored by the company security personnel and reviewed by the security lead.

Although these steps may seem like overkill to many small businesses, they are becoming quite common throughout the food industry at home and abroad, particularly with small businesses.

REFERENCES

Bledsoe GE, Rasco BA (2001a): Taking the terror out of bioterrorism. *Food Qual.* November–December: 33–37.

——— (2001b): Terrorists at the table. II: Developing an anti-terrorism plan. *Agrichem Environ News*. 187; 5–8.

——— (2003): Effective food security plans for production agriculture and food processing. *Food Prot Trends*. 23:130–141.

CFR (Code of Federal Regulations) (2007): Code of Federal Regulations (CFR) homepage. http://www.gpoaccess.gov/CFR/INDEX.HTML. Accessed May 2008.

Crutchley TM, Rodgers JB, Whiteside HP Jr, Vanier M, Terndrup TE (2007): Agroterrorism: where are we in the ongoing war on terrorism? *J Food Prot*. 70 (3):791–804.

Drees C (2004): US food sector may be vulnerable to attack. Feb. 25, 2004. Citing Combating Terrorism: Evaluation of Selected Characteristics of National Strategies Related to Terrorism, GAO-04-408T. http://www.gao.gov/new.items/d04408t.pdf. Accessed September 2004.

GAO (General Accounting Office) (2003): Food processing security: voluntary efforts are underway, but federal agencies cannot fully assess their implementation. GAO-03-342. Report to Senators Richard J. Durbin and Tom Harkin, Washington, DC.

——— (2004a): Combating terrorism. Evaluation of selected characteristics in national strategies related to terrorism. GAO-04-408T. Subcommittee on National Security, Emerging Threats, and International Relations, Committee on Government Reform, House of Representatives, Washington, DC.

——— (2004b): Terrorism insurance. Implementation of the terrorism risk insurance act of 2002. USGAO Report GAO-04-307. Report to the chairman, Committee on Financial Services, House of Representatives. Washington, DC.

——— (2004c): Terrorism insurance: effects of the terrorism risk insurance act of 2002. USGAO Report GAO-04-806T, testimony before the Committee on Banking, Housing and Urban Affairs, May 2004.

Hollingsworth P (2001): Know a crisis when you see one. *Food Technol.* 54:24.

Miller J, Engelberg S, Broad W (2001): *The Attack, Germs: Biological Weapons and America's Secret War.* Simon & Schuster, New York, pp. 15–24.

Miller RL, Israelsen C, Jensen J (2008): Agroterrorism: a mixed methods study examining the attitudes and perceptions of Utah producers. *J Agric Safety Health.* 14 (3):273–282.

NAS (National Academy of Sciences) (2002): Human and agricultural health systems. In: *Making the Nation Safer: The Role of Science and Technology in Countering Terrorism.* National Research Council, National Academies Press, Washington, DC, Chapter 3.

Rasco BA (2001): It's the water: legal issues and rural H_2O. *Agrichem Environ News.* 186:18–21.

Rasco BA, Bledsoe GE (2004): *Bioterrorism and Food Safety.* CRC Press, Boca Raton, FL.

USDA-FSIS (U.S. Department of Agriculture–Food Safety and Inspection Service) (2002): FSIS security guidelines for food processors. http://www.fsis.usda.gov/OA/topics/SecurityGuide.pdf. Accessed May 2008.

USFDA (U.S. Food and Drug Administration) (2007a): Guidance for industry. Food producers, processors, and transporters: food security preventive measures guidance. http://www.cfsan.fda.gov/~dms/secgui14.html. Accessed May 2008.

——— (2007b): Guidance for industry. Importers and filers: food security preventive measures guidance. http://www.cfsan.fda.gov/~dms/secgui15.html. Accessed May 2008.

USFDA-CFSAN (U.S. Food and Drug Administration–Center for Food Safety and Applied Nutrition) (2001): Food safety and security: operational risk management systems approach. November 29. http://foodsafety.cas.psu.edu/Food_Safety_and_Security.pdf. Accessed May 2008.

Washington State (2001): Eco-terrorism. Public hearing, June 11, Washington State Senate, Senate Judiciary Committee, Olympia, WA.

WHO (World Health Organization) (2002): Food safety issues: terrorist threats to food. *Guidance for Establishing and Strengthening Prevention and Response Systems.* Food Safety Department, WHO, Geneva, Switzerland.

CHAPTER 30

PREDICTIVE MICROBIOLOGY: GROWTH *IN SILICO*

MARK L. TAMPLIN

30.1 INTRODUCTION

Early reports in the field of microbiology were based on morphological descriptions of microbes, with a particular focus on classification and on species of clinical importance. Over time, there was a gradual movement away from morphological characterization to descriptions of biochemical and molecular traits, and an understanding of how the environment influences microbial viability. In time, food microbiology evolved as a subspecialty that described bacterial applications in food production, and the influence of food composition, food storage, and thermal processing.

Approximately 25 years ago, the field of predictive microbiology formally emerged as a new discipline that sought to describe microbial viability in quantitative terms and to express it with mathematical expressions that predict microbial responses under environmental conditions not experimentally tested (Roberts et al., 1981; Roberts and Jarvis, 1983). Today, the products (tools) of predictive microbiology are widely used in food safety systems that manage human health risk and food quality in global commerce.

30.2 APPLICATIONS OF PREDICTIVE MICROBIOLOGY IN THE FOOD INDUSTRY

In the formative years of predictive microbiology, there were obvious extensions of research in food production and management systems. However, early studies focused on describing the effects of environment factors on the behavior of microorganisms and translating this information into models, both empirical and mechanistic. Only after vast quantities of data were produced (by a very few laboratories with large

Microbiologically Safe Foods, Edited by Norma Heredia, Irene Wesley, and Santos García

resource investments) did software interfaces evolve into the user-friendly risk management tools in use today.

The promulgation of U.S. federal regulations mandating implementation of HACCP plans in food-processing systems was responsible for "pulling" predictive microbiology into the food industry (USDA-FSIS, 1996). The coincidental availability of predictive models and an emerging industry requirement for tools to identify critical control points (CCPs) and critical limits (CLs) resulted in the development of user-friendly model interfaces such as the U.S. Department of Agriculture (USDA) Pathogen Modeling Program and the UK Food MicroModel.

As a consequence of industry use of predictive models, research programs began to address microbial behavior in raw and processed foods, instead of only bacteriological broths, and in mixed culture and nonsterile systems. These changes in research direction resulted in predictive models with greater relevance to and adoption by food companies as well as by public health and food regulatory organizations.

Indirectly, predictive models also affect the food industry, in that they are used to develop risk assessment that informs risk management practices, which then influence the development of regulations and trade and public health policies. As greater reliance is placed on models, attention has turned to ways to standardize experimental and model designs and to properly verify and validate models. Such advances will ultimately reduce uncertainties and costs associated with the design and management of food operations, accelerate the development of more accurate risk assessment, and lead to greater uniformity in national and international food safety regulations.

Predictive models with the greatest value to the food industry are those that have been validated under commercial food operations and that are recognized by regulatory bodies as valid tools for making food safety decisions (USDA-FSIS, 2005). Such tools reduce reliance on microbiological tests that, considering reasonable sampling plans, are expensive, slow, and destructive.

Additional benefits of predictive microbiology tools not commonly reported are those realized by regulatory agencies and the public. Predictive models inform the development of new guidelines and regulatory policies (personal communication, food safety, and inspection service) and increase public confidence in the safety of food when consumers understand that both industry practices and government regulations are based on solid and defendable science.

Of all models in the current public domain, two exemplify the positive attributes described in the preceding paragraphs. The Refrigeration Index (RI), produced through research funded by Meat & Livestock Australia (MLA), is used routinely by Australian beef exporters to predict the growth of *Escherichia coli* on chilled meat products.

As a result of rigorous evaluation of the science behind the development and evaluation of the RI, the Australian Quarantine Inspection Service (AQIS) revised the Export Control (Meat and Meat Products) Orders in *AQIS Meat Notice: 2001/19—Assessment of Deterioration of Refrigerated Meat Affected by Refrigeration Breakdown, Incidents and Accidents* (AQIS, 2001) and adopted the model to evaluate the hygienic quality of red meat. This has allowed industry greater flexibility in operations and more innovative approaches to chilling meat products.

The 2007 MLA publication *Food Safety: Predictive Microbiology, the Industry Impact* (MLA, 2007) states that the RI underpins the science behind new risk-based meat export regulations that have been accepted by numerous trading partners. The Centre for International Economics (CIE) undertook an evaluation of the benefits of MLA's investment in predictive microbiology (CIE, 2006) within their market access science and technology program. The CIE evaluated the impact of the RI on the basis of cost in the absence of predictive microbiology, including those for a variety of processing operations, such as cooling of meats, hot boning, refrigeration breakdowns, fabrication room temperature, refrigeration costs, product wastage, training, labor costs, work accidents, and microbiological testing.

Based on these assessments, the CIE determined that over a 30-year period, predictive microbiology would increase the value of the Australian meat industry by \$44 million, add \$162 million to Australia's gross domestic product, and produce \$71 million in benefits to consumers through improvements in quality and decreases in the cost of meat products. These impacts are based on a \$3.8 million investment in research, yielding \$11 in benefits for each dollar spent on research and development.

In another example, the U.S. Department of Agriculture's (USDA) *Pathogen Modeling Program* (PMP) (USDA-ARS, 2008) version 6.1 contains a suite of approximately 40 models. Models for *Clostridium botulinum* and *C. perfringens* are widely used by industry and are endorsed by the USDA Food Safety and Inspection Service (FSIS) for determining the disposition of cooked meat products during cooling operations (USDA-FSIS, 2005). Although benefit–cost analyses have not been published as for the RI described above, food companies state that these predictive tools markedly reduce the high costs of product testing and the destruction of otherwise safe food when cooling deviations occur. It is recognized that other models in the PMP suite are also used by industry to aid in designing product challenge tests, to identify CCPs and CLs in HACCP systems, and to inform food safety decisions when process deviations occur.

Other well-known modeling packages used by food companies include the ComBase Predictor and Perfringens Predictor developed by the UK Institute of Food Research (Anonymous, 2008). ComBase Predictor is a modified Web-based version of Growth Predictor and contains 20 growth models, seven thermal death models, and two nonthermal survival models. The Danish Institute of Fisheries Research produces the *Seafood Spoilage and Safety Predictor*, which predicts microbial spoilage of various fishery products under fixed and changing temperatures, and the growth of *Listeria monocytogenes* in smoked fish (DIFR, 2005).

30.3 MODELS

Predictive microbiology translates the primary patterns of microbial behavior (growth, survival, and inactivation) into mathematical algorithms which can then be used to predict microbial behavior under different environmental conditions. This is possible because parameters of microbial growth and inactivation display smooth curves as a function of change in environmental conditions. Consequently, predictions can be made over interpolative regions that have not been tested.

Predictive models are mathematical expressions of the effects of environmental conditions on bacterial viability. In the first step of model development, primary models are produced that describe microbial levels as a function of time. From these models, parameters are obtained for lag time, growth/inactivation rate, and maximum population density. These parameters are then translated into secondary models that predict change in primary parameters as a function of environmental condition. A tertiary model is the translation of primary and secondary models into a user interface which can then be accessed to predict the level and/or probability of growth in static and dynamic environments.

Predictive models can be kinetic or stochastic. Kinetic models dominate the literature and describe changes in microbial numbers as a function of time. In contrast, stochastic (probabilistic) models have received more recent attention and predict the probability that an event such as growth and death will occur (McKellar and Xu, 2004; Membre et al., 2006; Ross and Dalgaard, 2004). Stochastic models are used increasingly by food companies to optimize the costs of product formulations and processing operations while providing an acceptable level of risk.

The dynamic growth model of Baranyi and Roberts (1994) has gained widespread use in predictive microbiology by virtue of a mechanistically based parameter for lag time, its ability to predict microbial growth under dynamic conditions and superior performance (Juneja et al., 2007). The model expression is

$$\frac{dx}{dt} = \frac{q(t)}{q(t)+1}\mu_{\max}\left[1-\left(\frac{x(t)}{x_{\max}}\right)^{m}\right]x(t)$$

where x is the cell number at time t, $q(t)$ is the concentration of limiting substrate, and $x_{\max}$ is the maximum population density. Other primary growth models are discussed by McKellar and Xu (2004).

Secondary models predict changes in primary model parameters as a function of the environment. For example, growth rate can be estimated as a function of temperature, water activity, and pH. The literature describes square-root, gamma, cardinal, and various model forms for LPD (lag phase duration) and growth rate (Ross and Dalgaard, 2004).

30.4 TOOLS IN PREDICTIVE MICROBIOLOGY

Publishing a predictive model in the scientific literature subjects it to peer review, which is the first step in acceptance by regulatory authorities and policymakers. However, for implementation by the food industry, complicated algorithms must be translated into model interfaces that are intuitive and user friendly. Among the many models that have been published, those bundled within software packages are the most commonly used. Examples include the Growth Predictor, ComBase Predictor, Refrigeration Index, Pathogen Modeling Program (PMP), and Seafood Spoilage and Safety Predictor.

Growth Predictor is a package of models for microbial growth as a function of environmental conditions, such as temperature, pH, and water activity (IFR, 2008). Some models include a fourth environmental factor, such as carbon dioxide or acetic acid. An advantage of Growth Predictor is that the user controls the predicted lag time, based on the anticipated physiological state of the microorganism. Separate from Growth Predictor, within the Institute of Food Research's modeling toolbox, is Perfringens Predictor. This model uses an Excel-based interface and functions similar to the PMP *C. perfringens* model for the cooling of cooked meats. That is, both models recommend that less than 0.3 $\log_{10}$ predicted growth of *C. perfringens* is acceptable for human consumption. ComBase Predictor, located within the ComBase (www.combase.cc) modeling toolbox, is a modified Web-based form of Growth Predictor.

The Refrigeration Index (RI) predicts the growth of "generic" *E. coli* in raw meat products under dynamic cooling conditions (Fig. 1). The user inputs the product temperature profile, such as from a data logger, selects the temperature measurement time interval, the form of meat product, and other parameters. The RI predicts the level of *E. coli* growth, where less than a 1.0-$\log_{10}$ increase is considered acceptable.

The Pathogen Modeling Program (PMP) is a suite of models describing microbial growth, survival, and inactivation, as well as *Clostridium botulinum* neurotoxin

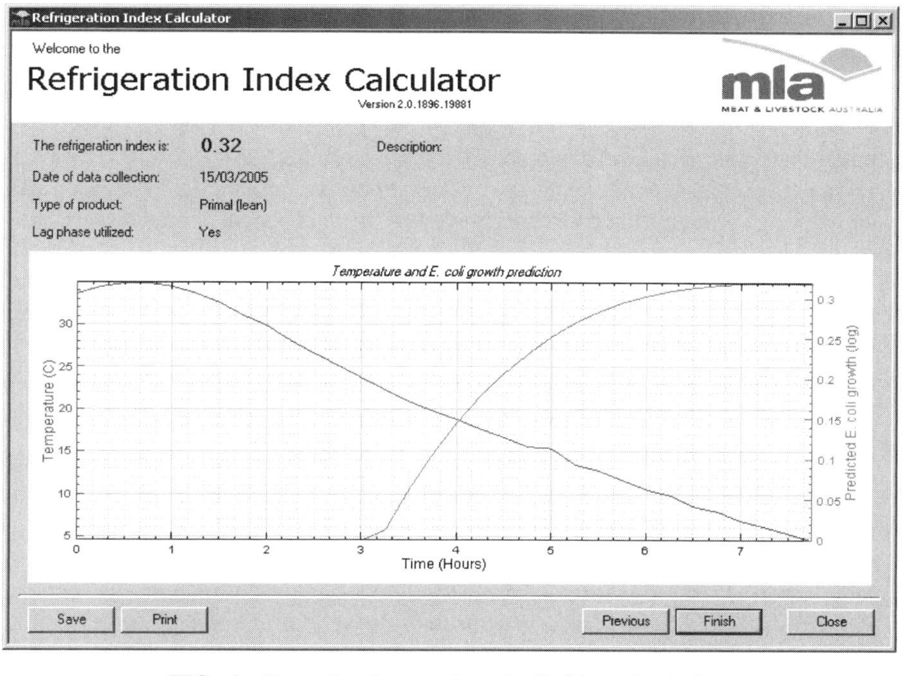

FIG. 1 Example of output from the Refrigeration Index.

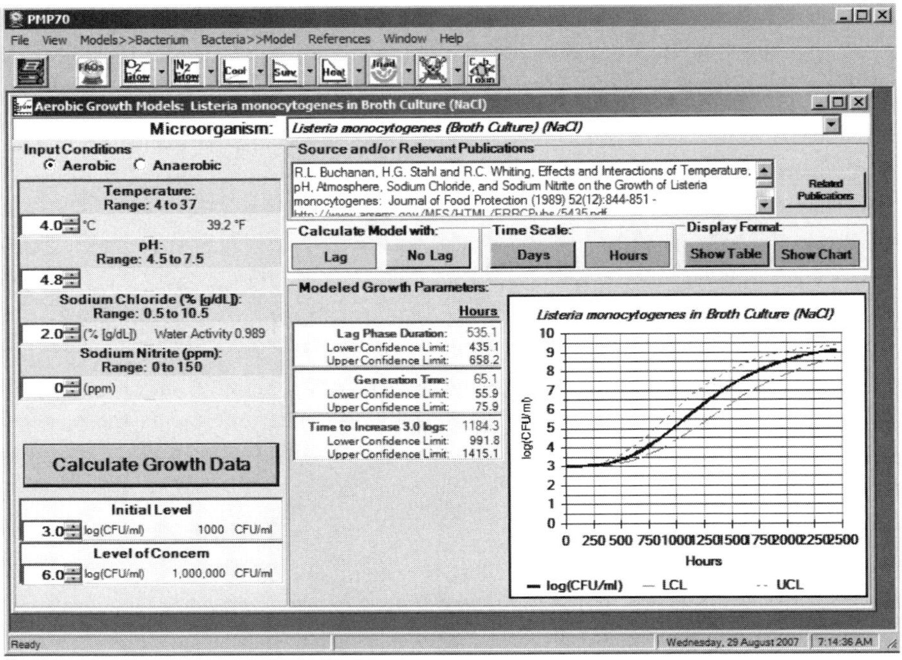

FIG. 2 Model interface for the Pathogen Modeling Program. This example displays a graphical output for the growth of *L. monocytogenes* in broth culture at 4°C, pH 4.8, 2.0% NaCl, with a lag phase.

production, under various environmental conditions (USDA-ARS, 2008). The PMP version 6.1 contains models for 10 species of pathogens, for a total of 37 models. As with ComBase Predictor and Growth Predictor, the user specifies product temperature, pH, and water activity (Fig. 2). Other environmental variables, depending on the model, include ionizing radiation, lactic acid, nitrite, and sodium pyrophosphate. The user can select "no lag time" for a more fail-safe prediction or a default lag time, but not the degree of flexibility offered by ComBase Predictor and Growth Predictor. Model outputs are displayed in both graphic and table form, and include 95% confidence intervals. For many PMP models, PDF versions of associated journal publications can be downloaded.

The Seafood Spoilage and Safety Predictor (SSSP) was developed by the Danish Institute of Fisheries Research and contains a suite of models for the spoilage of fish products and for the growth of *L. monocytogenes* in smoked salmon (DIFR, 2005). The SSSP predicts food spoilage for both fixed and fluctuating temperatures and is highly suited for predicting changes in product quality throughout cold chains. The SSSP has two model forms: one for the relative rate of spoilage (organoleptic changes) and the other for microbial spoilage.

30.5 DATABASES TO SUPPORT PREDICTIVE MICROBIOLOGY

Predictive models are based on large quantities of data that are translated into mathematical expressions. New data sets permit new models to be developed. With continued expansion, data sets can be organized into robust databases that permit new modeling techniques to be tested. As such, the discipline of predictive microbiology will depend increasingly on databases to allow models to be built, verified, and validated. In addition, databases allow the end users of predictive microbiology open access (transparency) to test and critique models, including the underlying assumptions.

In 2003, a public database of microbial responses to food environments was introduced at the Fourth Predictive Microbiology in Foods Conference in Quimper, France (Baranyi and Tamplin, 2004). Since that time, ComBase (www.combase.cc) has grown to over 45,000 records that describe microbial growth, survival, and inactivation under static and dynamic environmental conditions (Fig. 3).

The utility of ComBase has been advanced through the addition of various add-on tools that allow kinetic data to be compared with model predictions. Also, the user can customize model fits to ComBase data and can up-load and model data located outside ComBase.

In an effort to increase the rate of data submission, the ComBase consortium partnered with the International Association for Food Protection's *Journal of Food*

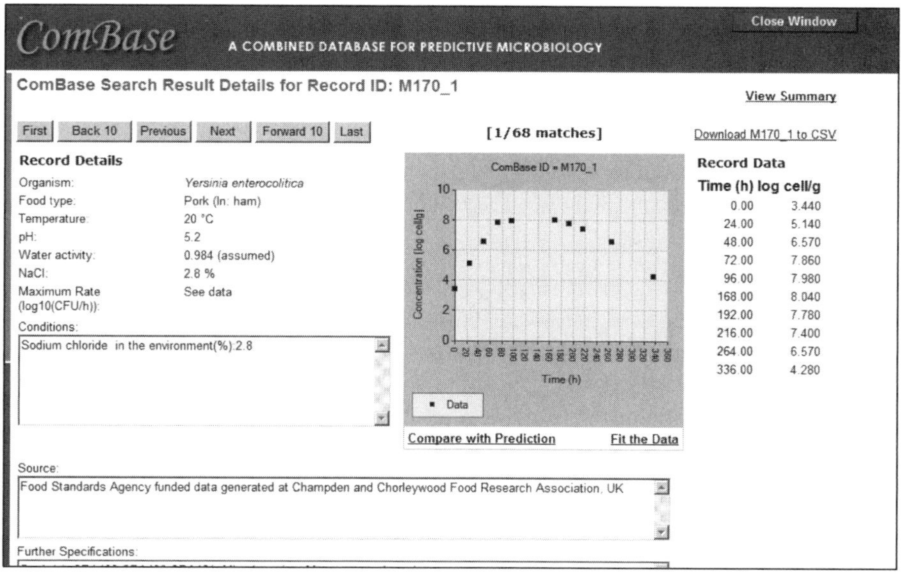

FIG. 3 Individual data record in ComBase showing experimental detail, table, and plot of time versus $\log_{10}$ CFU/g.

Protection to encourage authors to submit relevant data to ComBase. In an optimistic outlook, ComBase could one day serve a role similar to that of GenBank, which organizes nucleic acid sequence information into a database, and function as a central repository of food microbiology data.

30.6 CONCLUSIONS

In this chapter we have provided an overview of predictive microbiology, exploring applications of predictive models in the food industry, model development, software tools, and databases. For further information on general concepts and applications of predictive models, the reader is directed to publications by Burnham et al. (2008), McKellar and Xu (2004), McMeekin et al. (1993), Peleg (2006), and Ross and McMeekin (1994).

Undoubtedly, countries and economies depend on safe food supplies. Although we understand much about factors that control foodborne pathogens and spoilage organisms, we have yet to elucidate specific molecular and biochemical events that control microbial behavior, and more important, how to exploit this knowledge to improve food safety and quality. Recent advances in the relatively new fields of systems biology and network sciences are linking molecular events with microbial behavior. A yet-to-come "map" of cellular processes that control microbial behavior should result in penultimate models to manage the safety and quality of the food supply.

REFERENCES

Anonymous (2008): ComBase modelling toolbox. http://ifrsvwwwdev.ifrn.bbsrc.ac.uk/CombasePMP/GP/Login.aspx?ReturnUrl=%2fCombasePMP%2fGP%2fDefault.aspx. Accessed March 2008.

AQIS (Australian Quarantine Inspection Service). (2001): Export control (meat and meat products) orders assessment of deterioration of refrigerated meat affected by refrigeration breakdown, incidents and accidents. AQIS Meat Notice 2001/19.

Baranyi J, Roberts TA (1994): A dynamic approach to predicting bacterial growth in food. *Int J Food Microbiol*. 23:277–294.

Baranyi J, Tamplin ML (2004): ComBase: a combined database on microbial responses to food environments. *J Food Prot*. 67:1967–1971.

Burnham GM, Schaaffner DW, Ingham SC (2008): Predict safety. *Food Qual*. 15:14–22.

CIE (Centre for International Economics) (2006): MLA and predictive microbiology: an evaluation of the industry wide impacts. Report prepared for Meat and Livestock Australia, North Sydney, Australia.

DIFR (Danish Institute of Fisheries Research) (2005): Seafood spoilage and safety predictor, Version 2.0. http://www.dfu.min.dk/micro/sssp/Home/Home.aspx. Accessed January 2008.

IFR (Institute of Food Research) (2008): Growth predictor and *Perfringens* predictor. http://www.ifr.ac.uk/Safety/GrowthPredictor/. Accessed March 2008.

Juneja VK, Valenzuela MM, Huang L, Gumudavelli V, Subbiah J, Thippareddi H (2007): Modeling the effect of temperature on growth of *Salmonella* in chicken. *Food Microbiol.* 24:328–335.

McKellar RC, Xu X (2004): Primary models. In: McKellar RC, Lu X (Eds.). *Modeling Microbial Responses in Food.* CRC Press, Boca Raton, FL, pp. 21–62.

McMeekin TA, Olley JN, Ross T, Ratkowsky DA (1993): *Predictive Microbiology: Theory and Application.* Wiley, New York.

Membre J-M, Amezquita A, Bassett J, Giavedoni P, Blackburn CdeW, Gorris LGM. (2006): A probabilistic modeling approach in thermal inactivation: estimation of postprocess *Bacillus cereus* spore prevalence and concentration. *J Food Prot.* 69:118–129.

MLA (Meat and Livestock Australia) (2007): *Food Safety: Predictive Microbiology, The Industry Impact.* MLA, North Sydney, Australia.

Peleg M (2006): *Advanced Quantitative Microbiology for Foods and Biosystems.* CRC Press, Boca Raton, FL.

Roberts TA, Jarvis B (1983): Predictive modelling of food safety with particular reference to *Clostridium botulinum* in model cured meat systems. In: Roberts TA, Skinner FA (Eds.). *Food Microbiology: Advances and Prospects.* Academic Press, New York, pp. 89–95.

Roberts TA, Gibson AM, Robinson A (1981): Prediction of toxin production by *Clostridium botulinum* in pasteurised pork slurry. *J Food Tech.* 16:337–355.

Ross T, Dalgaard P (2004): Secondary models. In: McKellar RC, Lu X (EdS.). *Modeling Microbial Responses in Food.* CRC Press, Boca Raton, FL, pp. 63–150.

Ross T, McMeekin TA (1994): Predictive microbiology. *Int J Food Microbiol.* 23:241–264.

USDA-ARS (U.S. Department of Agriculture–Agriculture Research Service) (2008): PMP models. http://ars.usda.gov/Services/docs.htm?docid=6786. Accessed March 2008.

USDA-FSIS (U.S. Department of Agriculture–Food Safety and Inspection Service) (1996): Pathogen reduction; hazard analysis and critical control point (HACCP) systems; final rule. *Fed Reg.* 61:38806–38989.

——— (2005): Use of microbial pathogen computer modeling in HACCP plans. FSIS Notice 25–05. http://www.fsis.usda.gov/regulations_&policies/Notice_25-05/index.asp. Accessed March 2008.

CHAPTER 31

ROLE OF GENETICALLY MODIFIED ORGANISMS IN FOOD SAFETY

FIDEL GUEVARA-LARA

31.1 INTRODUCTION

Genetically modified organisms (GMOs) may be defined as organisms whose genetic material (DNA) has been altered in an artificial manner in order to confer upon them novel useful characteristics. This technology is generally known as modern biotechnology or genetic technology, sometimes also called recombinant DNA technology or genetic engineering. This technology appeared for the first time in 1973, as a result of the pioneering work of Cohen and co-workers in the United States, and allows for the introduction of a single selected gene (DNA sequence) from one organism to another, including transference between unrelated species, in a form that results in the integration of the transferred sequence into the chromosomes of the recipient organism, and its inheritance and expression in a specific fashion. Such methods are used to generate, for example, GM plants, which are then utilized to develop genetically modified (GM) food crops. Because gene transfer is involved in their production, GM organisms and foods are also referred to as transgenic or (more recently) bioengineered organisms and foods (Glick and Pasternak, 1998; Rowlands, 2002; Shewry et al., 2001; WHO, 2002).

The DNA sequence (gene) usually includes two parts: (1) a central coding region, which is transcribed to make a functional protein, and (2) adjacent regulatory sequences, which control the mechanics and specificity (i.e., level, cell and tissue type, timing) of expression. In the generation of GM crops, modern biotechnology provides three major advantages over classical plant breeding:

1. The coding region can be derived from any source, ranging from the recipient plant through related genotypes and species, to unrelated microbes and animals, thus bypassing fertility barriers that limit conventional plant breeding. It is also possible to mutate the coding sequence to alter the properties of the encoded

Microbiologically Safe Foods, Edited by Norma Heredia, Irene Wesley, and Santos García

characteristic (biological activity, nutritional quality, functional properties) or even to synthesize genes encoding characteristics of completely novel design.

2. Only single defined genes are transferred, or small numbers of genes, which can readily be identified and monitored in the progeny. This contrasts with conventional or mutation breeding, in which it is not possible to identify or precisely quantify the existence of gene transfer or mutation.
3. It is possible to control the level and pattern of transgene expression precisely and to decrease the expression of endogenous genes (Shewry et al., 2001).

There are two main aspects involving food safety and GMOs and genetically modified (GM) foods: (1) public concern with the safety of GMOs and GM foods, and (2) the use of modern biotechnology to generate GMOs and GM foods with enhanced safety in terms of a positive impact on human, animal, and environmental health. The first topic has been thoroughly addressed and reviewed (Chassy, 2002; EFSA-GMO Panel Working Group, 2008; FAO/WHO, 2000; Kaeppler, 2000; Kok and Kuiper, 2003; König et al., 2004; Kuiper et al., 2001, 2003; Kuiper and Kleter, 2003; Rowlands, 2002). Our main objective in this chapter is to present an overview of recent and potential future developments of GMOs and GM foods with promise to yield safer foods and food products, thus directly and indirectly benefitting human and animal health and the environment.

31.2 GENETICALLY MODIFIED FOODS IN THE WORLD MARKET

Most GM foods currently in the market are of microbial and plant origin. The first GM product that was granted approval for a food application and then entered the food market was the enzyme chymosin. On March 23, 1990, the U.S. Food and Drug Administration (FDA) granted the GRAS (generally recognized as safe) status to that Pfizer-developed enzyme (IFT, 1990). Chymosin causes hydrolysis and clotting of κ-casein, a major protein in milk, thus resulting in curd which is then processed into cheese. Chymosin is a key component of rennet, which was traditionally obtained from the fourth stomach of calves. Recombinant chymosin was obtained through expression of one of the calf's genes in the gut bacterium *Escherichia coli* K12 (Glick and Pasternak, 1998).

Recombinant DNA technology for plant genetic transformation was developed between 1982 and 1984. The first transgenic plant product to reach the market was the FlavrSavr, a slow-ripening tomato developed by Calgene, Inc. On May 18, 1994, the U.S. Food and Drug Administration (FDA) granted GRAS status, thus determining that FlavrSavr was as safe for human consumption as tomatoes developed through traditional plant breeding techniques, after which it could reach the market without the need for special food labeling (IFT, 1994). Other transgenic crops, such as squash, potatoes, soybeans, and maize, obtained GRAS status from the FDA and reached the market between 1994 and 1997. Since then, a large number of organisms of food importance, primarily plants, but also many microorganisms and animals,

TABLE 1 Global Area of Transgenic Crops Distributed by Country, 2005

Rank	Country	Area[a] (million hectares)	Transgenic Crops
1	United States[b]	49.8	Soybean, maize,cotton, canola, squash, papaya
2	Argentina[b]	17.1	Soybean, maize, cotton
3	Brazil[b]	9.4	Soybean
4	Canada[b]	5.8	Canola, maize, soybean
5	China[b]	3.3	Cotton
6	Paraguay[b]	1.8	Soybean
7	India[b]	1.3	Cotton
8	South Africa[b]	0.5	Maize, soybean, cotton
9	Uruguay[b]	0.3	Soybean, maize
10	Australia[b]	0.3	Cotton
11	Mexico[b]	0.1	Cotton, soybean
12	Romania[b]	0.1	Soybean
13	Philippines[b]	0.1	Maize
14	Spain[b]	0.1	Maize
15	Colombia	<0.1	Cotton
16	Iran	<0.1	Rice
17	Honduras	<0.1	Maize
18	Portugal	<0.1	Maize
19	Germany	<0.1	Maize
20	France	<0.1	Maize
21	Czech Republic	<0.1	Maize

Source: Adapted from James (2005).
[a]All data are rounded off to the nearest 100,000 hectares.
[b]Countries growing 50,000 hectares, or more, of transgenic crops.

have been transformed genetically (Table 1). Several plants and a few animals and their derivatives have been granted GRAS status by FDA and are currently in the market (Rowland, 2002). On the other hand, apparently no GM microorganisms are used commercially in food fermentations, although their many products and derivatives have been utilized routinely in the food industry since recombinant chymosin was granted GRAS status in 1990 (von Wright and Bruce, 2003).

In regard to GM crops, 2005 marked the tenth anniversary of their commercialization. The global area of approved GM crops in 2005 was 90 million hectares, an increase of 11% relative to the area planted in 2004. In fact, over the last decade, farmers have consistently increased their plantings of GM crops by double-digit growth rates every year since GM crops were first commercialized in 1996 (Fig. 1), with the number of biotech countries increasing from 6 to 21 in the same period (James, 2005). In the first decade, the accumulated global GM crop area was 475 million hectares, equivalent to almost half of the total land area of the United States or China, or 20 times the total land area of the United Kingdom. An historic milestone was reached in 2005 when 21 countries grew GM crops (Table 2), up significantly from 17 countries in the preceding year. Notably, of the four new

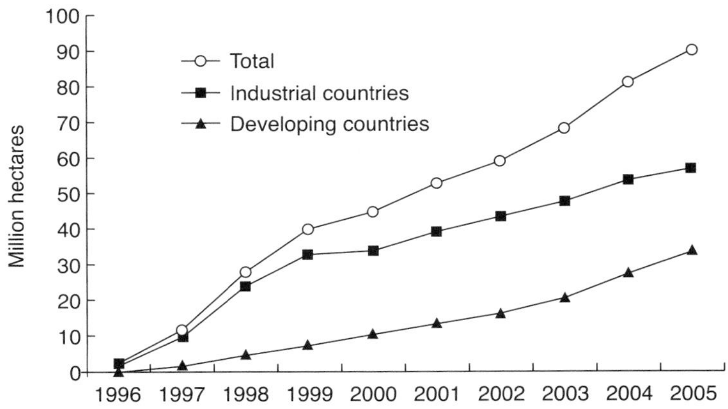

FIG. 1 Global areas cultivated with transgenic crops. (Adapted from James, 2005.)

countries that grew GM crops in 2005, three were EU countries (Portugal, France and the Czech Republic); the fourth was Iran. In 2005, the United States, followed by Argentina, Brazil, Canada, and China, continued to be the main adopters of GM crops in the world, with 49.8 million hectares planted in the United States (55% of the global GM crop area) (James, 2005). Mexico occupied eleventh place in the rank, with about 100,000 hectares of mostly GM cotton and soybean.

GM soybean continued to be the principal GM crop in 2005, occupying 54.4 million hectares (60% of the total), followed by GM maize, cotton, and canola (Fig. 2). During 1996–2005, herbicide tolerance has consistently been the dominant trait present in GM crops (71%) (Fig. 2), followed by insect resistance and stacked genes for the two traits. Also, in 2005 the first triple-gene GM crop (maize) was planted in the United States.

In 2005, the global market value of GM crops was estimated at $5.25 billion, representing 18% of the approximately $30 billion global commercial seed market. The accumulated global value for 1996–2005 is estimated at $29.3 billion. The global value of the GM crop market is projected at over $5.5 billion for 2006 (James, 2005). In 2006, a total of 252 million acres of transgenic crops were planted in 22 countries by 10.3 million farmers. In that year, countries that grew 97% of the global transgenic crops were the United States (53%), Argentina (17%), Brazil (11%), Canada (6%), India (4%), China (3%), Paraguay (2%) and South Africa (1%).

Despite ongoing public concern as to the safety of GM foods, the continuing rapid adoption of GM crops reflects consistent and substantial improvements in productivity, the environment, economics, and social benefits realized by both large and small farmers, consumers, and society in both industrial and developing countries. It is expected that the rapid growth in GM crop adoption will continue and probably be surpassed in the second decade, 2006–2015. Also, the number of countries adopting the four current major GM crops (soybean, maize, cotton, and canola) is expected to grow, and their global hectarage and number of farmers planting GM crops are

TABLE 2 Organisms of Food Importance That Have Been Genetically Modified

	PLANTS		
Alfalfa	Cranberry	Oat	Sorghum
Apple	Cucumber	Papaya	Soybean
Asparagus	Eggplant	Pea	Strawberry
Banana	Flax	Peanut	Sugar beet
Barley	Grape	Pear	Sugarcane
Bean	Kiwi	Pearl millet	Sunflower
Cabbage	Lettuce	Plantain	Sweet potato
Canola	Licorice	Potato	Tomato
Carrot	Maize	Rice	Wheat
Cauliflower	Melon	Rye	
	MICROORGANISMS		
Aspergillus oryzae	*Candida* spp.	*Kluyveromyces lactis*	*Saccharomyces* spp.
Bacillus licheniformis	*Corynebacterium* spp.	*Lactobacillus* spp.	*Streptococcus* spp.
Bacillus subtilis	*Escherichia coli*	*Lactococcus* spp.	*Streptomyces*
Brevibacterium spp.	*Fusarium venenatum*	*Leuconostoc* spp.	*Trichoderma reesei*
	ANIMALS		
Carp	Chicken	Quail	Sheep
Catfish	Goat	Rabbit	Shrimp
Cattle	Pig	Salmon	Tilapia

Source: According to Glick and Pasternak (1998), Maclean (2003), Rowlands (2002), Rowland (2002), Sang (2003), von Wright and Bruce (2003).

expected to increase as the first generation of GM crops is more widely adopted and the second generation of applications becomes available. Beyond the traditional agricultural products of food, feed, and fiber, entirely novel products to agriculture are expected to emerge, including the production of pharmaceutical products, oral vaccines, specialty and fine chemicals, and the use of renewable crop resources to replace nonrenewable, polluting, and increasingly expensive fossil fuels. In the near term, the use of multiple stacked traits is expected to grow, thus creating value and meeting the needs of both consumers and producers, who seek more nutritional and healthier food and feed at affordable prices (James, 2005).

31.3 POTENTIAL OF GMOs TO INCREASE FOOD SAFETY

31.3.1 Foods with Reduced Allergenicity

One of the main growing concerns over GM foods is the introduction of allergens as a result of the genetic modification. Actually, genetic engineering has the potential both to introduce new allergenic proteins into foods and to remove established allergens

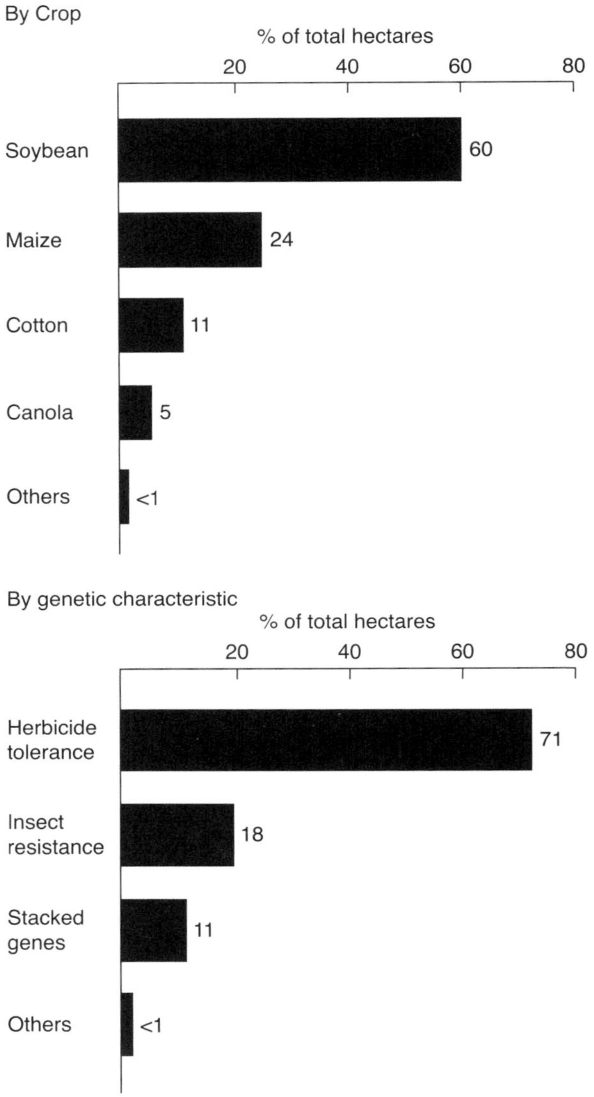

FIG. 2 Main transgenic crops grown in the world. Stacked genes generally refers to herbicide tolerance plus insect resistance. (Adapted from James, 2005.)

(Shewry et al., 2001). Many transgenic products will ultimately be consumed by humans, whether they have been introduced to improve food quality (e.g., aspects of nutritional quality, processing quality, flavor enhancements, nutraceuticals, post-harvest storage) or to improve agronomic performance, such as plant resistance to herbicides or insects. The possibility that some of the proteins responsible for these characteristics will prove to be allergenic is of great concern to consumers and regulatory authorities. This concern is not entirely unfounded. Many proteins with potential antimicrobial or antifungal properties, and hence biotechnological applications, are known allergens. The biotechnology industry will have to be careful in choosing safe proteins to use. Some examples of potentially allergenic proteins are:

1. 2S albumins, important storage proteins in seeds of many dicotyledonous plants, including legumes, composites, crucifers, and many nuts (Shewry and Pandya, 1999), are rich in cysteine or methionine and thus are attractive sources for expression in GM plants to improve sulfur-deficient species such as legumes. However, at least one of these, the Brazil nut albumin, is known to be a major allergen to humans (Nordlee et al., 1996).
2. Some lipid transfer proteins (LTPs), a family of small proteins present in seeds and other plant organs, show antifungal activity, although they are also allergens in the fruits of the family Rosaceae (e.g., peach, apple) (Osborn and Broekaert, 1999).
3. Pathogenesis-related (PR) proteins are synthesized by plants in response to microbial pathogens or chemical elicitors. They are a complex of proteins with various biological activities and may combine to provide a broad spectrum of resistance to pathogens. A number of plant allergens in chestnut, avocado, apples, cherries, celery, and carrots are known to be related to members of the PR protein complex (Shewry et al., 2001).
4. Low-molecular-weight enzyme inhibitors present in wheat, rye, and barley grain are active against α-amylases and proteinases from various organisms, including digestive α-amylases of some insect pests. However, these inhibitors are thought to be the most important allergens responsible for bakers' asthma, which is associated with the inhalation of wheat flour and is a major respiratory allergy in workers in the flour milling and baking industries. Some of these inhibitors are also thought to be associated with dietary allergy to wheat and rice, for which their use in transgenic crops and food would not be acceptable to consumers, regulatory authorities, or the industry (Carbonero and García-Olmedo, 1999).

These examples emphasize the importance of considering allergenic potential when identifying novel proteins to improve the resistance or quality of crop plants. This has also been highlighted by the well-publicized problems experienced with the Brazil nut 2S albumin. Expression of this methionine-rich protein in a number of plants, including *Arabidopsis*, tobacco, oilseed rape, narbon bean, and soybean, resulted in increased methionine levels by 20 to 300%. However, the commercial use of this gene was halted when it was demonstrated that the Brazil nut albumin is strongly allergenic to humans (Nordlee et al., 1996).

Although the experience with the Brazil nut protein exemplifies the potential problems of introducing allergens in GM plants, it also demonstrates that the plant biotechnology industry is well aware of such potential hazards, the problem being detected by testing procedures already in place. One of such systems proposed by FAO/WHO (2001) (Fig. 3) is aimed at ensuring that potential allergenic proteins

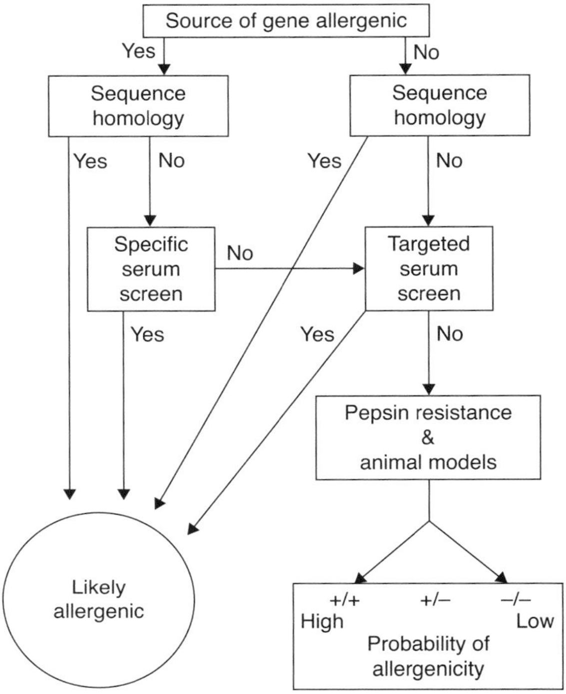

FIG. 3 FAO/WHO 2001 decision tree for the assessment of the allergenic potential of foods derived from biotechnology. (Adapted from FAO/WHO, 2001; Taylor, 2002.)

are identified and the work discontinued before material reaches the food chain, and preferably before GM plants are even produced. The routine use of internationally harmonized criteria and systems should ensure that GM foods have low added allergenicity, certainly when compared with new varieties and types of crops produced by conventional procedures, for which no testing for allergenicity is required.

In addition to the debate about the potential risk of increased allergenicity in GM food, there are several reports on the utilization of GM technology for the reduction or removal of allergenic proteins in plants, thus resulting in the generation of safer foods. For this purpose, two methods of silencing endogenous genes in plants have been used: the antisense and the co-suppression approaches. Both require the identification and cloning of the target gene and the reintroduction of all or part of it into the plant. Both have been applied to produce GM plants in which the trait is stably inherited. The ability to down-regulate gene expression using antisense and co-suppression techniques led to the proposal that genetic engineering could be utilized to remove allergens and toxic substances from plants. Both techniques can give almost complete gene inactivation. This has been attempted with one allergen present in rice grains, one of the world's most widely consumed foods. The major dietary allergens in rice grain have molecular weights of 14 to 16 kDa and belong to a family of α-amylase inhibitors.

Tada et al. (1996) showed that antisense expression of a single sequence resulted in substantial decreases in the total allergen content of transgenic rice seed. This work shows great potential toward the development of hypoallergenic rice, which would represent a major health benefit to many people (Nakamura and Matsuda, 1996).

An attractive alternative to removing whole allergenic proteins is to remove only the epitopes responsible for the allergenicity. For example, the allergenic sequences in the major allergens of peanuts have been identified (Shin et al., 1998). It should now be possible to design homologous, nonallergenic proteins with similar structures, stability, and biological and functional properties. This approach has been used successfully to remove conformational epitopes from the major allergens of apple (Son et al., 1999) and cherry (Scheurer et al., 1999). The next stage will be to use genes encoding such proteins to replace the endogenous allergen genes. Although more research needs to be done and the technology has to be refined, these studies, and the use of antisense and co-suppression of gene expression in other systems, demonstrate the feasibility of reducing or eliminating allergens by genetic engineering, which could result in safer foods.

31.3.2 Microbiologically Safer Foods

Infectious disease has major negative effects on poultry and livestock production, both in terms of economics and on animal welfare. Application of genetic modifications to livestock and poultry to improve resistance to disease is therefore a very attractive idea, although the implementation of such systems is still experimental. A major goal of the genomics programs in livestock and poultry is the identification of natural resistance genes or genes that enhance the immune response (Muller and Brem, 1998; Sang, 2003). Eventually, it may be possible to transfer resistance genes between breeds (intraspecies), between species, or to modify those genes and enhance their function.

A main focus of research in chicken genomics is the mapping of genes that confer resistance to major pathogens (Burt et al., 1995). For example, the chicken genome is being screened for genes that confer resistance to *Salmonella*, and this has led to mapping of a novel gene, not previously identified in other species, as conferring increased *Salmonella* resistance (Mariani et al., 2001). The function of such a gene may be investigated by classical breeding methods or by gene transfer. Similarly, major programs are under way to investigate the genetics of disease tolerance and disease resistance in livestock species.

There are several reports on the introduction of novel genes to confer resistance or to target expression of such genes in novel tissues. Transgenic sheep have been produced that express the visna virus envelope gene, normally expressed on the surface of the virus and not encoded by the host. These sheep provide a model to study whether expression of a viral envelope glycoprotein will prevent infection by the virus (Clements et al., 1994). Mammals provide passive immunity to their young by secretion of antibodies in their milk. It has been suggested that expression of specific antibodies in the mammary gland can be produced by using transgenic methods to direct expression of antibody sequences in the mammary gland. Expression of a single neutralizing antibody in the milk of transgenic mice has been shown to confer complete protection to suckling offspring against the strain of hepatitis virus that the antibody recognizes (Kolb et al., 1999). This approach could be developed further in livestock species, either in development of small herds for focused application in disease outbreaks or as production herds.

Relatively few single genes have been identified that have a major effect on disease resistance. One such gene is the *Mx* gene in mice, which mediates resistance to influenza virus. This gene confers resistance to influenza infection when expressed in chick embryo fibroblasts in culture, suggesting that its introduction via transgenesis could be protective (Garber et al., 1991). Another example of the possibility of transgenic expression of a gene from a different species, providing protection from a specific disease, has been modeled in mice. The directed expression of a modified lysostaphin gene from *Staphylococcus simulans*, which has an antistaphylococcal function, in the mammary gland has been reported (Kerr et al., 2001). The aim is to provide protection against *Staphylococcus aureus* infection, a major mastitis pathogen in dairy cattle. The transgenic mice show substantial resistance to experimental infection by *S. aureus*, but the milk protein content and profile are not affected. A demonstration of the possible application of antisense technology has been achieved in rabbits. Expression of an antisense RNA transgene to bovine leukemia virus (BLV) conferred a measurable level of resistance to infection by BLV (Korizeva et al., 1996).

There could be benefits to the environment from the introduction of specific GM livestock and poultry, in terms of supporting developments in sustainable agriculture. These include decreased environmental pollution and benefits from increasing disease resistance. Increased disease resistance will have benefits in terms of reduction in use of drugs, greater longevity, and animal welfare. Benefits to human health would also be the result of the use of GM animal food products. For example, overexpression of lysostaphin in cow's milk could protect cows against mastitis and also reduce the risk of *S. aureus* infection to humans. *Salmonella*-resistant chickens would also bring a reduced presence of this important pathogen in poultry products in the human food chain.

Expression of human lactoferrin, a natural antibiotic present in human milk, may protect infants against bacterial proliferation in the intestinal tract (Pintado and Gutierrez-Adan, 1999). Transmissible spongiform encephalopathies (TSE) are a threat to human health through consumption of meat products from infected animals. It has been shown that if the *prp* gene has been inactivated in mice, they are no longer susceptible to TSE infection, and there is no major phenotypic effect from the mutation. It has been suggested that it may be possible to inactivate the equivalent gene in livestock species, via gene targeting in somatic cells and nuclear transfer (Denning et al., 2001), although the long-term phenotypic effects of such a modification will require close monitoring.

All these aspects make the use of genetic modification to improve disease resistance particularly attractive, but this is probably the hardest area in which to develop effective systems. A possible issue that must be considered in these developments is that novel resistance mechanisms may introduce new selective pressures on pathogens harbored by resistant GM animals, resulting in changes to the pathogens to which non-GM animals are vulnerable.

31.3.3 Foods with Reduced Toxicity

A very recent subject of major concern and debate regarding GM organisms is that of nontarget (or unintended) effects that may be caused by genetic modification. Several cases have been reported of unexpected metabolic or biochemical changes arising in GM crops after the genetic modification. Unintended effects, however, are not all deleterious. One of the fortunate cases involves GM maize showing insect resistance through transformation with *Bacillus thuringiensis* δ-endotoxin (Bt corn). It has been reported that Bt transformation of maize hybrids can actually enhance their safety as food products because those hybrids are significantly less likely to contain harmful mycotoxins than are their non-Bt counterparts.

When insects attack maize plants, one possible result is an increase in microbial diseases. This occurs because insect pests carry pathogenic fungi, bacteria, and viruses and predispose plants to disease development. These diseases include ear and stalk rots that can reduce maize yield and quality. Some of the diseases are caused by fungi that produce mycotoxins in the maize crop. Mycotoxins, which are toxic compounds produced by fungi, pose a significant problem worldwide, affecting an estimated 25% of grain crops. The main mycotoxins in maize include aflatoxins, produced by fungi in the genus *Aspergillus*, and fumonisins, produced by several species of *Fusarium* fungi. Both aflatoxins and fumonisins can be fatal to livestock and are probable human carcinogens. The importance of fumonisins in human health is still a subject of debate, but they are carcinogenic to laboratory animals and there is evidence that they contribute to human cancer in some parts of the world. Fumonisin concentrations in maize are or will be under regulatory scrutiny in several nations. The economic impact of aflatoxins has been greater than that of fumonisins; thus many nations already regulate allowable aflatoxin concentrations in crops.

Symptoms of *Fusarium* and *Aspergillus* ear rots are often highly correlated with insect damage (Munkvold and Hellmich, 1999). Since 1994, several workers have studied the influence of Bt toxin expression on *Fusarium* ear rot and fumonisins in maize. In these studies, differences among types of Bt genes (also called Bt events) have become evident. These events differ in the specific Bt protein they express and in the tissue-specific expression of the proteins. Kernel expression of Bt proteins appears to be an important factor determining the amount of kernel feeding by European corn borer larvae and subsequently the intensity of *Fusarium* infection.

These studies have consistently demonstrated that hybrids containing two of the Bt events (MON810 and BT11) experience significantly less *Fusarium* ear rot and yield maize with lower fumonisin concentrations than that of their non-Bt counterparts (Dowd and Munkvold, 1999; ILSI, 1999; Munkvold, 2003; Munkvold and Hellmich, 1999, Munkvold et al., 1999).

When conventional hybrids were subjected to high populations of European corn borers, *Fusarium* ear rot severity and fumonisin levels became elevated, often to levels considered unsafe for swine and horses. Levels considered safe for horses and swine are less than 5 ppm and less than 10 ppm, respectively. Safe fumonisin levels for humans are unknown (Munkvold and Desjardins, 1997). *Fusarium* ear rot and fumonisin levels in MON810, CBH351, and BT11 hybrids were uniformly low (usually less than 10% of the concentrations in the non-Bt hybrids) and were unaffected by

European corn borer populations. More recent reports have analyzed the occurrence of maize stalk rot in Bt hybrids and their near-isogenic non-Bt counterparts, as well as the fungal species composition in maize stalks in relation to European corn borer injury and transgenic insect protection (Gatch et al., 2002; Gatch and Munkvold, 2002). Results indicate that although specific Bt events in some years may cause reductions in stalk rot, the overall effect of Bt transformation on stalk rot occurrence is highly variable. Also, it was found that the species composition of fungi infecting stalks of Bt hybrids differed from that of non-Bt hybrids, but the implications of this result are not yet clear.

Other studies also have shown reduced kernel infection by *A. flavus* and lower aflatoxin concentrations in BT11 and MON810 hybrids compared with their non-Bt counterparts. However, these reductions have been less dramatic than those seen for fumonisins (Windham et al., 1999). More recent evidence indicates that Bt maize hybrids should be effective in reducing aflatoxin contamination in areas where high southwestern corn borer infestations occur. Also, it was proposed that the reduced levels of aflatoxin accumulation associated with Bt hybrids are probably a consequence of reduced insect damage rather than resistance to *A. flavus* infection or aflatoxin accumulation per se (Williams et al., 2002, 2005).

The examples described above support the utility of Bt hybrids for management of *Fusarium* and *Aspergillus* ear rots and stalk rots of maize. New Bt hybrids now under development promise to exhibit more complete control of other kernel-feeding insects, so they should provide even better protection from insect-associated fungi, and there could be further contributions toward mycotoxin management. Transgenic control of insects and diseases offers an alternative that is much more effective, consistent, economical, and environmentally sound than foliar insecticides (Munkvold and Hellmich, 1999).

Debate surrounding the use of GM crops should be based on an assessment of all risks and benefits that can be measured, including environmental impacts, livestock impacts, and potential human health threats. Available data show that Bt transformation of maize hybrids enhances the food and feed safety of the grain by reducing its vulnerability to mycotoxin-producing fungi. A common criticism of currently available GM crops is a lack of apparent benefits to consumers. But lower mycotoxin concentrations represent a clear benefit to consumers of Bt grain, whether the intended use is for livestock or human food products. Consumers and regulatory agencies should consider these factors in decisions regarding Bt maize use (Munkvold and Hellmich, 1999).

Other very promising recent developments toward the production of less toxic foods through GM organisms include the generation of a model transgenic cereal plant (rice) with detoxification activity for the estrogenic mycotoxin zearalenone (Higa-Nishiyama et al., 2005), and the identification of a maize kernel pathogenesis-related protein and the gathering of evidence for its involvement in resistance to *Aspergillus flavus* infection and aflatoxin production (Chen et al., 2006). Proteins involved could later be transferred to other grain crops for enhanced protection, lower mycotoxin production, and the generation of safer food products.

31.4 INCREASED SAFETY OF GMOs FOR THE ENVIRONMENT AND HUMAN HEALTH

Recent reports provide the first evidence of a direct link between the adoption of GM crops and a positive impact on the environment and human health. Data from a 1999–2001 survey of cotton farmers in northern China showed that Bt cotton adoption reduced pesticide use and concomitant reductions in the risk and incidence of poisonings among those farmers (Hossain et al., 2004). Also, a report comparing the environmental and human health impacts of conventional sugar beet–growing regimes in the UK and Germany with those that might be expected from GM herbicide–tolerant (to glyphosate) sugar beet suggest that growing the GM crop would be less harmful to the environment and human health than would growing the conventional crop. This would be largely due to lower emissions from herbicide manufacture, transport, and field operations. Emissions contributing to negative environmental impacts, such as global warming, ozone depletion, and ecotoxicity of water and soil, were much lower for the herbicide-tolerant crop. Emissions contributing to summer smog, toxic particulate matter, and carcinogenicity, which have negative human health impacts, were also substantially lower for the GM crop (Bennett et al., 2004). These studies concur with recent reports of an accumulative reduction in pesticides for the period 1996–2004, estimated at 172 million kilograms of active ingredient, which is equivalent to a 14% reduction in the associated environmental impact of pesticide use on these crops (James, 2005).

On another vein, animal production has a major impact on the environment, and it is possible that specific genetic modifications may be designed to reduce negative environmental effects. Some genetic modifications may have a beneficial effect as a secondary advantage, and others may be designed specifically to tackle an environmental issue. The use of genetic modification to increase disease resistance may reduce the requirement for treatment with antibiotics and as a consequence also reduce the level of antibiotics in animal products and spread of antibiotic resistance. Phosphorus pollution from manure of monogastric animals, including pigs and poultry, is a major environmental issue. These animals are unable to digest plant phytate, which contains approximately 80% of phosphorus in common plant-derived feedstuffs. Excess phosphate in manure used as fertilizer results in eutrophication in rivers and lakes. Transgenic addition of phytase to the digestive enzymes of monogastric animals and poultry has been suggested as a route to reducing this problem, by enabling animals to utilize phosphorus in high-phytate diets. This approach was first modeled in mice and has now been demonstrated in pigs. Recently, the production and characterization of pigs carrying a transgene designed to express an *E. coli* phytase in saliva was described (Golovan et al., 2001). These pigs require almost no inorganic phosphate supplementation to their diet and excrete up to 75% less phosphorus than do nontransgenic pigs.

GM animals can contribute directly in various ways to increased food safety, which could translate to a positive impact on human health. The first dramatic demonstration of the potential power of transgenic manipulation was the production of mice carrying the human growth hormone gene that was expressed at high levels, which resulted in development of mice that were much larger than normal (Sang, 2003). Subsequent studies resulted in GM pigs containing a transgene with the zinc-inducible metallothionein promoter driving ovine growth hormone expression; these animals showed significant decrease in fat and increase in muscle tissue. Similarly, pigs have been produced that express human insulin-like growth factor 1 in skeletal muscle, using a transgene driven by the regulatory sequences of chicken skeletal α-actin. Female transgenic pigs showed significantly less fat and were leaner than nontransgenic pigs, whereas males were not significantly affected (Pursel et al., 1996, 1997). The growth factor myostatin has been shown to be a negative regulator of muscle growth and is highly conserved in mammals and birds. Mice in which the myostatin gene has been inactivated have a major increase in muscle mass and a significant reduction in fat accumulation with age (McPherron and Lee, 2002; McPherron et al., 1997). This suggests that myostatin manipulation via transgenesis in livestock and poultry may have a beneficial phenotypic effect in terms of increase in lean meat yield. This could be beneficial to human health in terms of reduction in animal fat consumption. Recently, Lai et al. (2006) have generated cloned transgenic piglets that express a *Caenorhabditis elegans* omega-3 fatty acid desaturase. The piglets' tissues are enriched in omega-3 fatty acids, a type of fat that is beneficial to human health.

Many possible modifications to milk via transgenesis have been proposed. These include alteration of endogenous proteins and addition of new proteins, with the aim of altering milk quality for specific food products or with benefits for human health. Modification of cow's milk to alter the composition and protein components is focused on making the milk more digestible and reducing the risk of allergic responses, called "humanization." The protein β-lactoglobulin is present in cow's milk but not in human milk, and approximately 10% of consumers develop an allergic response to the protein. Transgenic removal of the protein would benefit these consumers. Modifications to milk aimed at making it more suitable for use in production of infant formula, to make its composition more similar to that of human milk, would be an advantage, particularly for premature infants. Lactose intolerance limits the consumption of dairy products by many people; about 50 million Americans malabsorb lactose. Transgenic mice that produced a biologically active lactase in their milk were produced by targeting expression of an enzyme normally present in the small intestine to the mammary gland. The lactose content of the milk from the transgenic mice was reduced to one-half and the milk protein levels were not affected (Jost et al., 1999). A number of modifications to cow's milk have focused on modifying milk so that it is more suitable for humans, particularly for premature babies. Expression of bile salt stimulated lipase in the mammary gland, an enzyme normally expressed in the digestive tract, would be beneficial to cystic fibrosis patients and premature infants who do not express the enzyme. Another proposed modification is the reduction of phenylalanine content of milk by modifying the α-lactalbumin protein to replace phenylalanine in the coding sequence. Milk from animals modified in this way would be suitable for patients with phenylketonuria, who cannot tolerate dairy products (Karatzas and Turner, 1997; Lonnerdal, 1996). None of these modified milk products are currently close to market. It is important to note that the EU has instigated a zero-tolerance policy on GMOs.

31.5 FOOD SAFETY ISSUES AND PUBLIC CONCERNS REGARDING GMOs

Guidance provided by government regulators indicates that the main issues that pre-market food safety evaluation of GMOs should consider are (Chassy, 2002):

1. Safety of the source organism and gene(s)
   a. Safety of the inserted DNA
   b. Safety of DNA ingestion
   c. Safety of the antibiotic resistance marker (if present)
2. Food safety issues of the newly introduced product(s)
   a. Potential for toxicity (protein product)
   b. Potential for allergenicity (protein product)
   c. Safety of any unintended effects
3. Equivalence of composition
4. Retention of nutritional value
5. The human dietary exposure

Soon after the first successful transformation experiments in plants (tobacco) in 1988, several organizations and institutions began efforts toward the definition of internationally harmonized strategies for the safety evaluation of foods derived from GMOs. The International Food Biotechnology Council (IFBC) published the first report on the issue of safety assessment of the new varieties (IFBC, 1990). This laid the foundation for later safety evaluation strategies. Other international instances, such as the Organization for Economic Cooperation and Development (OECD), the Food and Agriculture Organization of the United Nations (FAO), the World Health Organization (WHO), and the International Life Sciences Institute (ILSI), have developed further guidelines for safety assessment which have obtained broad international consensus among experts on food safety evaluation (FAO/WHO, 2000, 2001; Kuiper et al., 2001). These internationally recognized guidelines and reports from expert consultation panels have been extremely useful for governmental commissions in both industrial and developing countries for the implementation of specific regulations and legislation during the last 15 years. As an example, the Law on Biosafety of Genetically Modified Organisms issued in Mexico on March 18, 2005 (CIBIOGEM, 2005) regulates the activities of confined utilization, experimental release, pilot-program release, commercial release, commercialization, and import and export of genetically modified organisms, in order to prevent, avoid, or reduce the possible risks that these activities could bring to human health, or to the environment and biological diversity, or to animal health, plant health, or water sanitation. Further refinements in the guidelines for the assessment of safety of GM foods are currently under way and are addressing major public concerns, such as the transfer and removal of selectable and reporter genes (antibiotic resistance, herbicide resistance, among others) and modern profiling (or "omics") approaches to study unintended (nontarget, unexpected) effects caused by genetic transformation (Cellini et al., 2004; Kok and Kuiper, 2003; König et al., 2004; Kuiper and Kleter, 2003; Kuiper et al., 2003; van den Eede et al., 2004).

In the view that the exchange of genetic information through horizontal (lateral) gene transfer (HGT) might play a more important role than hitherto imagined, a working group of experts dealing with HGT in the context of food and feed safety has been established in Europe (van den Eede et al., 2004). Attention has focused on the transfer of antibiotic and herbicide resistance genes and other selectable markers and reporter genes (Table 3) to soil- and plant-related microorganisms. This is particularly important since HGT has been shown to occur in bacteria in the food chain. However, the working European group concludes that the phenomenon of HGT is at the origin of the genetic diversity of life itself, and there is little reason to assume that consumption of transgenic food or feed adds any particular generalized risk. Also, at present, it is not necessarily the case that the use of systems that eliminate marker genes (Goldstein et al., 2005; Iamtham and Day, 2000; Yoder and Goldsbrough, 1994), or the use of markers alternative to antibiotic resistance markers, is safer than the use of certain antibiotic resistance marker genes themselves. Finally, whereas uptake of ingested DNA by mammalian somatic cells has been demonstrated, there is so far no evidence that such DNA may end up in germline cells as a consequence of the consumption of GM food (van den Eede et al., 2004).

Recently, a promising new technology has appeared that offers the possibility of making targeted gene mutations using hybrid molecules (chimeras) of DNA and RNA (Zhu et al., 2000). This system could be used to switch off gene expression by mutation of regulatory sequences or to replace individual amino acids involved in the active sites of enzymes or in allergenic epitopes. Although this technology is still under development, it could have a major impact on plant genetic engineering in the future, as a means of generating GM organisms without transgenesis.

Unintended effects of GM crops and products are those that go beyond that of the original modification and that might affect health primarily (Cellini et al., 2004). However, unintended effects do not automatically imply health hazards. The significance of unintended effects on consumer health must be evaluated in the risk assessment process, and must take into account the intended use of the food. A combination of targeted and nontargeted methods of analysis (to be decided on a case-by-case basis) is likely to be the best way to evaluate the safety of GM and conventionally bred crops. There is no indication that unintended effects are more likely to occur in GM crops than in conventionally bred crops. In fact, unintended effects occur in both GM and non-GM crops; however, GM crops are better characterized, because this is a legal requirement for GM crops. It has been suggested that non-GM crops should also be required to be analyzed for unintended effects (Cellini et al., 2004).

31.6 CONCLUSIONS

GMOs and GM foods are currently still a matter of intense public debate and scientific development. Although the list of cases presented above is far from being exhaustive,

TABLE 3 Examples of Marker Genes used in the Genetic Transformation of Organisms of Food Importance

Trait Conferred and Enzyme Activity	Gene	Substrate or Selective Agent or Trait
Antibiotic resistance		
Aminoglycoside-3′-phosphotransferase	*nptII, nptIII*	Kanamycin, neomycin, geneticin
Hygromycin phosphotransferase	*hpt*	Hygromycin B
β-Lactamase	*bla*	Ampicillin, penicillin G, amoxicillin
Chloramphenicol acetyltransferase	*cat*	Chloramphenicol
Aminoglycoside-3′-adenyltransferase	*aadA*	Streptomycin, spectinomycin
Herbicide resistance		
Acetolactate synthase	*als* and others	Sulfonylureas, imidazolines, and others
Bromoxynil nitrilase	*bxn*	Bromoxynil
5-enol-pyruvyl-shikimate-3-phosphate synthase	*epsps, epsps5*	Glyphosate
Glyphosate oxidoreductase	*gox*	Glyphosate
Phosphinothricine acetyltransferase	*bar, pat*	Phosphinothricine, bialaphos, glufosinate
Reporter genes		
β-Galactosidase	*lacZ*	Galactosides
β-Glucuronidase	*uidA (gus)*	β-Glucuronides, blue indicator product
Green fluorescent protein	*gfp*	Fluorescence, oxygen
Firefly luciferase	*luc*	Luciferin, ATP, oxygen
Metabolic traits		
6-Phosphomannose isomerase	*manA*	Mannose
Tryptophane decarboxylase	*tdc*	4-Methyltryptophane
Xylose isomerase	*xylA*	Xylose
Isopentenyl transferase	*ipt*	Shoot development

Source: Adapted from Glick and Pasternak (1998), Van den Eede (2004).

it does highlight the enormous potential that GMOs have for the generation of foods and food ingredients, with increased safety in terms of reduced allergenicity and toxicity, lower microbial loads, a greater applicability for particular age and health groups, and indirect benefits for a healthier environment with a direct impact on human and animal health. It is highly likely that as regulatory and risk assessment guidelines are implemented and refined in developed and developing nations, and specific legislation is put in place, many of the novel GMO and GM food developments aimed at conveying direct benefits to consumers will reach the market and have substantial impacts on human health and the environment.

REFERENCES

Bennett R, Phipps R, Strange A, Grey P (2004): Environmental and human health impacts of growing genetically modified herbicide-tolerant sugar beet: a life-cycle assessment. *Plant Biotechnol J.* 2:273–278.

Burt DW, Burnstead N, Bitgood JJ, Ponce de León FA, Crittenden L (1995): Chicken genome mapping: a new era in avian genetics. *Trends Genet.* 11:190–194.

Carbonero P, García-Olmedo F (1999): A multigene family of trypsin/α-amylase inhibitors from cereals. In: Shewry PR, Casey R (Eds.). *Seed Proteins*. Kluwer Academic, Dordrecht, The Netherlands, pp. 617–633.

Cellini F, Chesson A, Colquhoun I, et al. (2004): Unintended effects and their detection in genetically modified crops. *Food Chem Toxicol.* 42:1089–1125.

Chassy BM (2002): Food safety evaluation of crops produced through biotechnology. *J Am Coll Nutr.* 21:166S–173S.

Chen ZY, Brown RL, Rajasekaran K, Damann KE, Cleveland TE (2006): Identification of a maize kernel pathogenesis-related protein and evidence for its involvement in resistance to *Aspergillus flavus* infection and aflatoxin production. *Phytopathology.* 96:87–95.

CIBIOGEM (Comisión Intersecretarial de Bioseguridad de los Organismos Genéticamente Modificados) (2005): Ley de Bioseguridad de Organismos Genéticamente Modificados. http://www.cibiogem.gob.mx. Accessed May 2008.

Clements JE, Wall RJ, Narayan O, et al. (1994): Developments of transgenic sheep that express the visna virus envelope gene. *Virology.* 200:370–380.

Denning C, Burl S, Ainslie A, et al. (2001): Deletion of the α(1,3) galactosyl transferase (*GGTA1*) gene and the prion protein (*PrP*) gene in sheep. *Nat Biotechnol.* 19:562–571.

Dowd PF, Munkvold GP (1999): Associations between insect damage and fumonisin derived from field-based insect control strategies. In *Proc. 40th Annual Corn Dry Milling Conference,* Peoria, IL, June 3–4.

EFSA GMO Panel Working Group on Animal Feeding Trials (2008): Safety and nutritional aspects of GM plants and derived food and feed. *Food Chem Toxicol.* 46:S2–S70.

FAO/WHO (Food and Agriculture Organization/World Health Organization) (2000): Safety aspects of genetically modified foods of plant origin. Report of a joint FAO/WHO expert consultation on foods derived from biotechnology. Geneva, Switzerland, May 29–June 2.

——— (2001): Evaluation of allergenicity of genetically modified foods. Report of a joint FAO/WHO expert consultation on allergenicity of foods derived from biotechnology, Rome, January 22–25. http://www.fao.org/es/esn/gm/biotec-e.htm.

Garber E, Chute HT, Condra JH, Gotlib L, Colonno RJ, Smith RG (1991): Avian cells expressing murine Mx1 protein are resistant to influenza virus infection. *Virology.* 180:754–762.

Gatch EW, Munkvold GP (2002): Fungal species composition in maize stalks in relation to European corn borer injury and transgenic insect protection. *Plant Dis.* 86:1156–1162.

Gatch EW, Hellmich RL, Munkvold GP (2002): A comparison of maize stalk rot occurrence in Bt and non-Bt hybrids. *Plant Dis.* 86:1149–1155.

Glick BR, Pasternak JJ (1998): *Molecular Biotechnology: Principles and Applications of Recombinant DNA*, 2nd ed. ASM Press, Washington, DC.

Goldstein DA, Tinland B, Gilbertson LA, et al. (2005): Human safety and genetically modified plants: a review of antibiotic resistance markers and future transformation selection technologies. *J Appl Microbiol.* 99:7–23.

Golovan SP, Meidiner RG, Ajakaiye A, et al. (2001): Pigs expressing salivary phytase produce low phosphorus manure. *Nat Biotechnol.* 19:741–745.

Higa-Nishiyama A, Takahashi-Ando N, Shimizu T, Kudo T, Yamaguchi I, Kimura M (2005): A model transgenic cereal plant with detoxification activity for the estrogenic mycotoxin zearalenone. *Transgen Res.* 14:713–717.

Hossain F, Pray CE, Lu YM, Huang JK, Fan CH (2004): Genetically modified cotton and farmers' health in China. *Int J Occup Environ Health.* 10:296–303.

Iamtham S, Day A (2000): Removal of antibiotic resistance genes from transgenic tobacco plastids. *Nat Biotechnol.* 18:1172–1176.

IFBC (International Food Biotechnology Council) (1990): Biotechnologies and food: assuring the safety of foods produced by genetic modification. *Reg Toxicol Pharmacol.* 12:S1–S196.

IFT (Institute of Food Technologists) (1990): Washington news. *Food Technol.* 44:46.

——— (1994): Washington news. *Food Technol.* 48:46.

ILSI (Health and Environmental Sciences Institute) (1999): *An Evaluation of Insect Resistance Management in Bt Field Corn: A Science-Based Framework for Risk Assessment and Risk Management.* ILSI Press, Washington, DC.

James C (2005): *Executive Summary of Global Status of Commercialized Biotech/GM Crops: 2005. ISAAA Brief* 34. International Service for the Acquisition of Agri-biotech Applications, Cornell University, Ithaca, NY.

Jost B, Vilotte JL, Duluc I, Rodeau JL, Freund JN (1999): Production of low-lactose milk by ectopic expression of intestinal lactase in the mouse mammary gland. *Nat Biotechnol.* 17:135–136.

Kaeppler HF (2000): Food safety assessment of genetically modified crops. *Agron J.* 92:793–797.

Karatzas CN, Turner JD (1997): Toward altering milk composition by genetic manipulation: current status and challenges. *J Dairy Sci.* 80:2225–2232.

Kerr DE, Plaut K, Bramley AJ, et al. (2001): Lysostaphin expression in mammary glands confers protection against staphylococcal infection in transgenic mice. *Nat Biotechnol.* 19:66–70.

Kok EJ, Kuiper HA (2003): Comparative safety assessment for biotech crops. *Trends Biotechnol.* 21:439–444.

Kolb AF, Ansell R, McWhir J, Siddell SG (1999): Insertion of a foreign gene into the β-casein locus by Cre-mediated site specific recombination. *Gene.* 227:21–31.

König A, Cockburn A, Crevel RWR, et al. (2004): Assessment of the safety of foods derived from genetically modified (GM) crops. *Food Chem Toxicol.* 42:1047–1088.

Korizeva S, Konicheva V, Murovska M, et al. (1996): Investigation of an antisense RNA gene effect on the reproduction of the bovine leukaemia virus in vivo. *Transgenics.* 2:99–109.

Kuiper HA, Kleter GA (2003): The scientific basis for risk assessment and regulation of genetically modified foods. *Trends Food Sci Technol.* 14:277–293.

Kuiper HA, Kleter GA, Noteborn HPJM, Kok EJ (2001): Assessment of the food safety issues related to genetically modified foods. *Plant J.* 27:503–528.

Kuiper HA, Kok EJ, Engel K-H (2003): Exploitation of molecular profiling techniques for GM food safety assessment. *Curr Opin Biotechnol.* 14:238–243.

Lai L, Kang JX, Li R, et al. (2006): Generation of cloned transgenic pigs rich in omega-3 fatty acids. *Nat Biotechnol Adv Online Publ.* March 26.

Lonnerdal B (1996): Recombinant human milk proteins: an opportunity and a challenge. *Am J Clin Nutr.* 63:622S–626S.

Maclean N (2003): Genetically modified fish and their effects on food quality and human health and nutrition. *Trends Food Safety Technol.* 14 (5/8):242–252.

Mariani P, Barrow PA, Cheng HH, Groenen MM, Negrini R, Burnstead N (2001): Localization to chicken chromosome 5 of a novel locus determining salmonellosis resistance. *Immunogenetics.* 53:786–791.

McPherron AC, Lee SJ (2002): Suppression of body fat accumulation in myostatin-deficient mice. *J Clin Invest.* 109:595–601.

McPherron AC, Lawer AM, Lee SJ (1997): Regulation of muscle mass in mice by a new TGF-β superfamily member. *Nature.* 387:83–90.

Muller M, Brem G (1998): Transgenic approaches to the increase of disease resistance in farm animals. *Rev Sci Tech OIE.* 17:365–378.

Munkvold GP (2003): Cultural and genetic approaches to managing mycotoxins in maize. *Annu Rev Phytopathol.* 41:99–116.

Munkvold GP, Desjardins AE (1997): Fumonisins in maize: Can we reduce their occurrence? *Plant Dis.* 81:556–565.

Munkvold GP, Hellmich RL (1999): The good news about Bt corn. *ISB News Rep.* December, pp. 5–6. http://www.isb.vt.edu.

Munkvold GP, Hellmich RL, Rice LG (1999): Comparison of fumonisin concentrations in kernels of transgenic Bt maize hybrids and non-transgenic hybrids. *Plant Dis.* 83:130–138.

Nakamura R, Matsuda T (1996): Rice allergenic protein and molecular–genetic approach for hypoallergenic rice. *Biosci Biotechnol Biochem.* 60:1215–1221.

Nordlee JA, Taylor SL, Townsend JA, Thomas LA, Bush RK (1996): Identification of Brazil-nut allergen in transgenic soybeans. *N Engl J Med.* 334:688–692.

Osborn RP, Broekaert WF (1999): Antifungal proteins. In: Shewry PR, Casey R (Eds.). *Seed Proteins.* Kluwer Academic, Dordrecht, The Netherlands, pp. 727–752.

Pintado B, Gutierrez-Adan A (1999): Transgenesis in large domestic species: future development for milk modification. *Reprod Nutr Dev.* 39:535–544.

Pursel VG, Coleman ME, Wall RJ (1996): Regulatory avian skeletal α-actin directs expression of insulin-like growth factor-1 to skeletal muscle of transgenic pigs. *Theriogenology.* 35:348.

Pursel VG, Wall RJ, Soloman MB, Bolt DJ, Murray JD, Ward KA (1997): Transfer of an ovine metallothionein–oveine growth hormone fusion gene into swine. *J Anim Sci.* 75:2208–2214.

Rowland IR (2002): Genetically modified foods, science, consumers and the media. *Proc Nutr Soc.* 61:25–29.

Rowlands JC (2002): Determining the safety of bioengineered microorganisms. *Food Technol.* 56:28–31.

Sang H (2003): Genetically modified livestock and poultry and their potential effects on human health and nutrition. *Trends Food Sci Technol.* 14:253–263.

Scheurer S, Son DY, Boehm M, et al. (1999): Cross-reactivity and epitope analysis of Pru a 1, the major cherry allergen. *Mol Immunol.* 36:155–167.

Shewry PR, Pandya MJ (1999): The 2S albumin storage proteins. In: Shewry PR, Casey R (Eds.). *Seed Proteins.* Kluwer Academic, Dordrecht, The Netherlands, pp. 563–586.

Shewry PR, Tatham AS, Halford NG (2001): Genetic modification and plant food allergens: risks and benefits. *J Chromatogr B*. 756:327–335.

Shin DS, Compadre CM, Maleki SJ, et al. (1998): Biochemical and structural analysis of the IgE binding sites on Ara h1, an abundant and highly allergenic peanut protein. *J Biol Chem*. 273:13753–13759.

Son DY, Scheurer S, Hoffmann A, Haustein D, Vieths S (1999): Pollen-related food allergy: cloning and immunological analysis of isoforms and mutants of Mal d 1, the major apple allergen, and Bet v 1, the major birch pollen allergen. *Eur J Nutr*. 38:201–215.

Tada Y, Nakase M, Adachi T, et al. (1996): Reduction of 14–16 kDa allergenic proteins in transgenic rice plants by antisense gene. *FEBS Lett*. 391:341–345.

Taylor SL (2002): Protein allergenicity assessment of foods produced through agricultural biotechnology. *Ann Rev Pharmacol Toxicol*. 41:99–112.

Van Den Eede G, Aarts H, Buhk H-J, et al. (2004): The relevance of gene transfer to the safety of food and feed derived from genetically modified (GM) plants. *Food Chem Toxicol*. 42:1127–1156.

von Wright A, Bruce A (2003): Genetically modified microorganisms and their potential effects on human health and nutrition. *Trends Food Sci Technol*. 14:264–276.

WHO (World Health Organization) (2002): 20 Questions on genetically modified (GM) foods. http://www.who.int/foodsafety/publications/biotech/en/20questions_en.pdf. Accessed April 2007.

Williams WP, Windham GL, Buckley PM, Daves CA (2002): Aflatoxin accumulation in conventional and transgenic corn hybrids infested with southwestern corn borer (Lepidoptera: Crambidae). *J Agric Urban Entomol*. 19:227–236.

Williams WP, Windham GL, Buckley PM, Perkins JM (2005): Southwestern corn borer damage and aflatoxin accumulation in conventional and transgenic corn hybrids. *Field Crop Res*. 91:329–336.

Windham GL, Williams WP, Davis FM (1999): Effects of the southwestern corn borer on *Aspergillus flavus* kernel infection and aflatoxin accumulation in maize hybrids. *Plant Dis*. 83:535–540.

Yoder JI, Goldsbrough AP (1994): Transformation systems for generating marker-free transgenic plants. *Biotechnology*. 12:263–267.

Zhu T, Mettenburg K, Peterson DJ, Tagliani L, Baszczynski CL (2000): Engineering herbicide-resistant maize using chimeric RNA/DNA oligonucleotides. *Nat Biotechnol*. 18:555–558.

INDEX

Microbiologically Safe Foods, Edited by Norma Heredia, Irene Wesley, and Santos García